MANUAL OF CLINICAL PROBLEMS IN OBSTETRICS AND GYNECOLOGY

FOURTH EDITION

EDITED BY

MICHEL E. RIVLIN, M.D.
Associate Professor of Obstetrics and Gynecology and Director of Ambulatory Obstetrics and Gynecology, University of Mississippi Medical Center, Jackson, Mississippi

RICK W. MARTIN, M.D.
Associate Professor of Obstetrics and Gynecology, University of Mississippi Medical Center, Jackson, Mississippi

FOREWORD BY
WINFRED L. WISER, M.D.
Chairman and Professor of Obstetrics and Gynecology, University of Mississippi Medical Center, Jackson, Mississippi

LITTLE, BROWN AND COMPANY
BOSTON/NEW YORK/TORONTO/LONDON

Library of Congress Cataloging-in-Publication Data

Manual of clinical problems in obstetrics and gynecology / edited by
    Michel E. Rivlin,,Rick W. Martin ; foreword by Winfred L. Wiser. —
    4th ed.
        p.   cm.
    Includes bibliographical references and index.
    ISBN 0-316-74777-7
    1. Pregnancy—Complications.   2. Gynecology.   I. Rivlin, Michel
E.   II. Martin, Rick W.
    [DNLM: 1. Gynecology—handbooks.   2. Obstetrics—handbooks.   WQ
39 M294   1994]
RG571.M28   1994
618—dc20
DNLM/DLC
for Library of Congress   93-35803
                                                                         CIP

Printed in the United States of America

SEM

Editorial: Nancy E. Chorpenning
Production Editor: Anne Holm
Copyeditor: Betty Notzon
Indexer: Ann Blum
Production Supervisor: Michael A. Granger
Cover Designer: Hannus Design Associates

For Sarah, Katy, Janice, Joel, and David

CONTENTS

OBSTETRICS

MANUAL OF CLINICAL PROBLEMS IN OBSTETRICS AND GYNECOLOGY

DM : 13 ? 7 5 → sacral agenal.

CONTRIBUTING AUTHORS

GARLAND D. ANDERSON, M.D.
Jennie Sealy Smith Professor and Chairman of Obstetrics and Gynecology, University of Texas Medical School at Galveston; Chairman of Obstetrics and Gynecology, University of Texas Medical School at Galveston Hospitals, Galveston, Texas

FRANK H. BOEHM, M.D.
Professor of Obstetrics and Gynecology, Vanderbilt University School of Medicine; Director of Maternal-Fetal Medicine, Vanderbilt University Medical Center, Nashville, Tennessee

JOSEPH P. BRUNER, M.D.
Assistant Professor of Obstetrics and Gynecology, Vanderbilt University School of Medicine; Director of Obstetric Ultrasound, Vanderbilt University Medical Center, Nashville, Tennessee

LINDA C. BUCHHEIT, R.D.M.S., L.P.N.
Head Sonographer, Department of Obstetrics and Gynecology, University of Missouri—Columbia Hospital and Clinics, Columbia, Missouri

SISTER CLARICE CARROLL, M.S.N.
Assistant Professor of Obstetrics and Gynecology, University of Mississippi Medical Center, Jackson, Mississippi

BRYAN D. COWAN, M.D.
Professor and Director of Reproductive Endocrinology, University of Mississippi Medical Center, Jackson, Mississippi

RICHARD O. DAVIS, M.D.
Professor of Obstetrics and Gynecology, University of Alabama School of Medicine, Birmingham, Alabama

RUDOLPH P. FEDRIZZI, M.D.
Chief Resident, Department of Obstetrics and Gynecology, Vanderbilt University Medical Center, Nashville, Tennessee

MICHAEL D. FOX, M.D.
Fellow, Division of Reproductive Endocrinology, University of Kentucky Medical Center, Lexington, Kentucky

CORNELIA R. GRAVES, M.D.
Instructor in Maternal-Fetal Medicine, Vanderbilt University School of Medicine, Nashville, Tennessee

HARRIETTE L. HAMPTON, M.D.
Assistant Professor of Obstetrics and Gynecology, University of Mississippi Medical Center, Jackson, Mississippi

BRUCE A. HARRIS, JR., M.D.
Charles E. Flowers Professor Emeritus of Obstetrics and Gynecology, University of Alabama School of Medicine; Honorary Staff, Department of Obstetrics and Gynecology, University of Alabama Hospitals, Birmingham, Alabama

DARLA B. HESS, M.D.
Assistant Professor of Obstetrics and Gynecology, University of Missouri—Columbia School of Medicine; Head, Adult Echocardiography Laboratory, University of Missouri—Columbia Hospital and Clinics, Columbia, Missouri

L. WAYNE HESS, M.D.
Associate Professor of Obstetrics and Gynecology, University of Missouri—
Columbia School of Medicine; Head, Obstetrics and Maternal-Fetal Medicine,
University of Missouri—Columbia Hospital and Clinics, Columbia, Missouri

JOHN A. HUNT, M.B., B.CH., F.R.C.S.
Clinical Professor of Surgery, Marshall University School of Medicine; Attending
Surgeon, Cabell-Huntington Hospital, Huntington, West Virginia

JOHN D. ISAACS, M.D.
Fellow, Division of Reproductive Endocrinology, Washington University School of
Medicine, St. Louis

STEPHEN R. LINCOLN, M.D.
Assistant Professor of Obstetrics and Gynecology, University of Mississippi Medical
Center, Jackson, Mississippi

CECIL A. LONG, M.D.
Assistant Professor of Obstetrics and Gynecology, University of Mississippi Medical
Center, Jackson, Mississippi

JAMES F. MCCAUL IV, M.D.
Director of Maternal-Fetal Medicine, Phoebe Putney Memorial Hospital, Albany,
Georgia

STERLING W. MCCOLGIN, M.D.
Director of Maternal-Fetal Medicine, Saint Joseph Hospital, Denver

RICK W. MARTIN, M.D.
Associate Professor of Obstetrics and Gynecology, University of Mississippi Medical
Center, Jackson, Mississippi

G. RODNEY MEEKS, M.D.
Professor of Obstetrics and Gynecology and Director of Gynecology, University of
Mississippi Medical Center, Jackson, Mississippi

SUE M. PALMER, M.D.
Vice Chair of Obstetrics and Gynecology and Maternal-Fetal Medicine, MacGregor
Medical Association, Houston

KENNETH G. PERRY, JR., M.D.
Assistant Professor of Obstetrics and Gynecology, University of Mississippi Medical
Center, Jackson, Mississippi

JOSEPH A. PRYOR, M.D.
Assistant Professor of Obstetrics and Gynecology, University of Mississippi Medical
Center, Jackson, Mississippi

MICHEL E. RIVLIN, M.D.
Associate Professor of Obstetrics and Gynecology and Director of Ambulatory
Obstetrics and Gynecology, University of Mississippi Medical Center, Jackson,
Mississippi

WILLIAM E. ROBERTS, M.D.
Assistant Professor of Obstetrics and Gynecology, University of Mississippi Medical
Center, Jackson, Mississippi

RICHARD L. ROSEMOND, M.D.
Assistant Professor of Obstetrics and Gynecology, Vanderbilt University School of
Medicine; Director of Maternal-Fetal Division, Baptist Hospital, Nashville,
Tennessee

ABRAHAM RUBIN, M.D.
Visiting Associate Professor of Obstetrics and Gynecology, University of Illinois
College of Medicine; Senior Attending Obstetrician/Gynecologist, Humana Michael
Reese Hospital, Chicago

BAHA M. SIBAI, M.D.
Professor and Chief of Maternal-Fetal Medicine, University of Tennessee, Memphis, College of Medicine; Chief of Maternal-Fetal Medicine, E. H. Crump Women's Hospital, Memphis, Tennessee

JAMES J. SOWASH, M.D.
Clinical Assistant Professor of Obstetrics and Gynecology, University of Missouri—Columbia School of Medicine; Attending Physician, Department of Obstetrics and Gynecology, University of Missouri—Columbia Hospital and Clinics, Columbia, Missouri

ERIC R. STRASBURG, M.D.
Assistant Professor of Reproductive Biology, Case Western Reserve University School of Medicine; Divisional Director of Gynecology, MetroHealth Medical Center, Cleveland

MARC VATIN, M.D.
Clinical Assistant Professor of Obstetrics and Gynecology, George Washington University School of Medicine and Health Sciences; Attending Physician, Department of Obstetrics and Gynecology, Columbia Hospital for Women, Washington, D.C.

NEIL S. WHITWORTH, PH.D.
Professor of Obstetrics and Gynecology, University of Mississippi Medical Center, Jackson, Mississippi

MENDLEY A. WULFSOHN, M.D.
Clinical Assistant Professor of Urology, Mount Sinai School of Medicine of the City University of New York, New York; Attending Physician, Division of Urology, General Hospital Center, Passaic, New Jersey

FOREWORD

This outstanding teaching volume in obstetrics and gynecology is unique in its approach to providing in-depth information about major topics in the specialty in a simple, readable fashion. The list of authors demonstrates a variety of qualified teachers and practitioners with the ability to provide crucial information in a succinct but forceful manner. The annotated references following each topic are invaluable to medical students and residents as well as the busy practicing physician.

Michel E. Rivlin is a dedicated, highly competent teacher who constantly strives to uncover improved vehicles for learning. This volume demonstrates his interest in providing better patient care through an improved method of learning.

Winfred L. Wiser, M.D.

PREFACE

It is said that half of what is thought and taught is incorrect and the problem lies in identifying which half is which. It is also said that the questions remain the same but the answers keep changing. Looking back over a dozen years of this manual, now in its fourth edition, it is clear that some "advances" have turned out to be blind alleys, while other, unpromising beginnings have turned into broad highways. Obstetrics and gynecology is now at the cutting edge of scientific medicine. Vaginal ultrasonography is revolutionizing diagnostic gynecology, while endoscopic surgery is rapidly becoming the standard in operative gynecology. In the field of maternal-fetal medicine, access to fetal blood vessels and anatomy with sophisticated ultrasound has more than ever enabled the obstetrician to function as a fetal pediatrician, not only in terms of diagnosis but in terms of treatment. It has been a pleasure and a privilege to regularly review the field for students and physicians.

We would like to thank Dr. Winfred Wiser for placing the facilities of his department at our disposal, the Vicksburg Hospital Medical Foundation for its continuing support, and Little, Brown and Company for its publishing expertise. Donna White, our secretarial maven, has now typed the manual four times and would doubtless pass her boards in a breeze. Our heartfelt thanks to her, to her outstanding colleague Gail Head, and also to Robema Carter, Peggy Manning, and Martha Roan for their help with the manuscript.

M. E. R.
R. W. M.

MANUAL OF
CLINICAL PROBLEMS IN
OBSTETRICS AND
GYNECOLOGY

OBSTETRICS

I. HEMORRHAGE IN PREGNANCY

Coreg: CHF 3.125 mg Bid with food.
double dose q 2 weeks as tolerated up
to max of 25mg Bid

1. ABORTION

Eric R. Strasburg

Abortion is the termination of pregnancy before the fetus is capable of extrauterine life, generally considered to be that taking place before the twentieth week of gestation or the conceptus achieving a mass of less than 500 g or a crown-rump length of 18 cm. The incidence of spontaneous abortion (also called miscarriage) has been estimated to constitute 10 to 20 percent of all pregnancies.

The most common cause of fetal death is an abnormality of the conceptus, probably occurring in 50 to 80 percent of spontaneous abortions. Malformations of the conceptus can be caused by such conditions as the defective implantation of a normal trophoblast, an abnormal embryo, maternal viral infections, chromosomal aberrations, or the maternal ingestion of cytotoxic agents. Chromosomally abnormal fetuses account for approximately 35 percent of these abortions. Two situations exist among the parents of chromosomally abnormal abortuses. In most instances, the couple is chromosomally normal and the chromosomal abnormalities occur in a random and sporadic fashion. In a small percentage of cases, one member of the couple is a carrier of a balanced translocation; the offspring of these parents may be repeatedly aborted. Other factors implicated include acute maternal bacterial infections, chronic maternal cardiac and renovascular disease, and maternal endocrine disorders. Some investigators have noted a higher incidence of toxoplasmosis, herpes simplex, cytomegalovirus, and T-strain mycoplasma among these patients. Lupus anticoagulant, anticardiolipin antibodies, and embryotoxic factors have also been shown to be associated with a history of repeated abortion, but this is controversial. In addition, clinical and laboratory investigations have shown that heretofore unexplained pregnancy losses can be caused by immunogenetic factors. Uterine developmental abnormalities and cervical incompetence may also trigger midtrimester spontaneous abortions. These disorders are often amenable to surgical correction (e.g., metroplasty and cervical cerclage).

Abortion is considered "threatened" when a pregnant woman experiences uterine bleeding. In this setting, pain, if present at all, is minimal, and the cervix is closed and uneffaced. The differential diagnosis includes ectopic pregnancy and trophoblastic disease. Pregnancy tests and ultrasound are helpful for determining diagnosis and prognosis. Management is limited to explaining the pathologic process and the prognosis to the patient. She is advised that there is no increase in fetal congenital anomalies when such pregnancies continue. Bed rest has not been shown to be beneficial and need not be recommended.

A spontaneous abortion is inevitable when bleeding is accompanied by pain and dilatation of the internal os. The abortion is incomplete when the products of conception protrude through the cervix. In pregnancies of 14 weeks or less, suction, sharp curettage, or both, are performed to evacuate the uterus. In pregnancies of more than 14 weeks, abortion can be expedited by the administration of intravenous oxytocin or prostaglandin E_2 vaginal suppositories. The abortion is considered complete when the uterus is empty. The term *missed abortion* is applied when the conceptus dies but is not delivered, and the term *anembryonic pregnancy* is applied when a gestational sac is present but no developing embryo is present. Diagnosis is confirmed by real-time ultrasonography. If the conceptus is retained for more than 4 weeks, there is a risk of disseminated intravascular coagulation (DIC). The uterus should therefore be evacuated once appropriate clotting studies are obtained.

Although any abortion may become infected, septicemia usually attends nonmedical interference. The infecting organisms are commonly aerobic and anaerobic, occurring in mixed culture. Generally, these are gram-negative bacilli, most commonly *Escherichia coli* and *Bacteroides fragilis*, and gram-positive cocci, particularly enterococcus and beta-hemolytic streptococcus. Other important organisms are *Clostridium perfringens* and *C. tetani*. The infection may be localized to the products of conception, or one may find endometritis with parametritis, salpingo-oophoritis, peritonitis, septic thrombophlebitis, or septicemia. Other major complications include renal failure, septic shock, uterine perforation, and DIC. Rapid resuscitation, adequate antibiotic therapy (penicillin, gentamicin, and clindamycin in severe cases), and evacuation of the uterus, usually within 12 hours of admission (by dilatation and curettage or laparotomy and hysterotomy), can minimize morbidity and mortality. Hysterectomy is occasionally indicated in the event of persistent hemorrhage, uterine perforation, or a gangrenous uterus.

Women who have three or more consecutive losses are defined as habitual aborters. The causes of the abortions are similar to those mentioned previously for spontaneous miscarriage. A full diagnostic evaluation is mandated, although the risk of further abortion is only 25 to 30 percent.

An induced abortion is the elective termination of a pregnancy before viability. The indications may be therapeutic or at the patient's request. In 1990 in the United States, the Centers for Disease Control reported that there were 1.4 million legal abortions. The earliest intervention is "menstrual regulation," which consists of aspiration of the endometrium within 14 days of a missed menstrual period when pregnancy has been confirmed by serum radioimmunoassay. After 6 weeks of gestation, dilatation of the cervix is required for evacuation of the uterus. The procedure of dilatation and suction curettage for termination of first-trimester pregnancies is usually performed under paracervical block, intravenous sedation, and analgesia as an outpatient procedure. The uterine contents must always be sent for histologic examination to rule out the possibility of ectopic pregnancy or trophoblastic disease. Complications include cervical laceration, uterine perforation, hemorrhage, and bowel injury. The complications must be immediately and adequately treated. Postabortal infection is an additional complication that can be reduced by performing preoperative cervical cultures for *Neisseria gonorrhoeae*, beta-hemolytic streptococcus, and *Chlamydia trachomatis*, and appropriate treatment instituted if positive. The use of intraoperative prophylactic antibiotics also reduces the incidence of postoperative infection.

Two highly successful orally administered medications have been introduced in Europe for the safe and noninvasive termination of early pregnancy (less than 56 days). The first is RU 486 (mifepristone), a progesterone receptor antagonist used either alone or in combination with prostaglandin vaginal pessaries (e.g., Gemeprost, which is 16,16-dimethyl-trans-delta$_2$-prostaglandin E$_1$ methyl ester). The second is Epostane, an inhibitor of 3-beta-hydroxysteroid dehydrogenase, an enzyme necessary for the synthesis of progesterone, which is essential to sustain pregnancy in the first 8 weeks. The ban on the importation of RU 486 into the United States is expected to be removed in 1993.

Second-trimester pregnancy terminations are more difficult and usually require admission to the hospital. The intraamniotic instillation of prostaglandin F$_{2\alpha}$, hypertonic saline, or hyperosmolar urea augmented by the intraamniotic instillation of prostaglandin F$_{2\alpha}$ has been used to manage second-trimester procedures. More recently, 15 methyl prostaglandin F$_{2\alpha}$, given intramuscularly, and, more commonly, prostaglandin E$_2$ vaginal suppositories have been used, either alone or to augment other techniques. *Laminaria japonica* or lamicels (osmotic cervical dilators made from absorbent polyvinyl alcohol sponges impregnated with magnesium sulfate) should be used to assist in dilating the cervix and reducing the incidence of complications. Labor may be supplemented by the intravenous administration of oxytocin once the membranes have ruptured, but uterine rupture has been noted when oxytocin is combined with prostaglandin agents. Hypertonic saline infusion may precipitate hypernatremia or DIC in rare instances. Dilatation and evacuation may also be performed between the twelfth and twentieth week, provided it is performed by surgeons skilled in the procedure. In late second-trimester procedures, this operation is also facilitated by the use of multiple *Laminaria* or lamicels (placed in the cervical canal 10 to 12 hours before the procedure), large dilators, and the intraamniotic administration of urea to produce fetal demise and maceration. The patient is spared a prolonged induction-to-delivery interval.

Induced abortion is safest, however, when performed before 9 weeks' gestation. The death-to-case ratio increases by approximately 40 to 60 percent with each week of delay after the eighth week. Hysterotomies and hysterectomies carry a relatively high morbidity and mortality, and should be avoided in the absence of specific indications. Although the rates for immediate and delayed complications resulting from legal abortions are low, the potential long-term effects of abortion on subsequent fertility await final evaluation. The findings from most recent studies suggest that there is not a higher spontaneous abortion rate or an increase in perinatal morbidity and mortality for pregnancies that occur subsequent to elective vaginal terminations of pregnancy.

Multifetal pregnancy reduction for multiple pregnancies that occur after in vitro procedures or ovulation induction is the most recent technique of pregnancy termination and is causing many ethical and legal dilemmas.

General

1. Edmonds, D. K., et al. Early embryonic mortality in women. *Fertil. Steril.* 38:447, 1982.
   Before 12 weeks of pregnancy, 61.9 percent of conceptuses are lost. Most of these losses (91.7%) occur subclinically without the knowledge of the mother.
2. Rock, J. A., and Zacur, H. A. The clinical management of repeated early pregnancy wastage. *Fertil. Steril.* 39:12, 1983.
   A good review with an extensive bibliography.
3. Castadot, R. G. Pregnancy termination: techniques, risks, and complications and their management. *Fertil. Steril.* 45:1, 1986.
   Review of the standard techniques with an excellent list of references.
4. Houwert-DeJong, M. H., et al. Habitual abortion: a review. *Eur. J. Obstet. Gynecol. Reprod. Biol.* 30:39, 1989.
   This is an excellent review article on habitual abortion and discusses many of the classic as well as new studies in the literature.
5. Ryan, K. J. Abortion or motherhood, suicide and madness. *Am. J. Obstet. Gynecol.* 166:1029, 1992.
   The author discusses the legal history of abortion in the United States and different ethical views on the subject.

Etiology

6. Stray-Pedersen, B., and Stray-Pedersen, S. Etiologic factors and subsequent reproductive performance in 195 couples with a prior history of habitual abortion. *Am. J. Obstet. Gynecol.* 148:140, 1984.
   Blighted ovum, chromosomal abnormalities, and uterine malformation are the most common causes of habitual abortion.
7. Coulam, C. B. Unexplained recurrent pregnancy loss: epilogue. *Clin. Obstet. Gynecol.* 29:999, 1986.
   This summarizes the relative frequency of the established causes of this complex problem and suggests appropriate tests for its evaluation.
8. Mishell, D. R., Jr. Recurrent abortion. *J. Reprod. Med.* 38:250, 1993.
   Most fetal causes of recurrent abortion consist of genetic or chromosomal abnormalities; most maternal causes are congenital or acquired uterine abnormalities.
9. Christian, O. B., and Christian, B. S. Prospective study of anticardiolipin antibodies in immunized and untreated women with recurrent spontaneous abortions. *Fertil. Steril.* 53:328, 1992.
   Anticardiolipin levels did not increase after the active immunization of women with recurrent spontaneous abortions. Prospectively, anticardiolipin-positive patients did not miscarry more often than did patients without this antibody.
10. Ecker, J. L., Laufer, M. R., and Hill, J. A. Measurement of embryotoxic factors is predictive of pregnancy outcome in women with a history of recurrent abortion. *Obstet. Gynecol.* 81:84,1993.
    In early pregnancy, the production of embryotoxic factors predicts a subsequent spontaneous abortion; absence of these factors predicts a viable pregnancy.
11. McIntyre, J. A., et al. Clinical, immunologic, and genetic definitions of primary and secondary recurrent spontaneous abortions. *Fertil. Steril.* 42:849, 1984.
    This elegant paper proposes that maternal antipaternal immunity can be related to spontaneous abortion, and thus supports the use of immunotherapy to prevent pregnancy losses in certain abortion-prone women.

12. Sider, D., et al. Cytogenetic studies in couples with recurrent pregnancy loss. *South. Med. J.* 81:1521, 1988.
    The lymphocyte karyotype of 232 couples with habitual abortion was studied. There was no significant difference in the incidence of chromosomal abnormalities between those having two losses and those having three or more. Because abnormalities were present in 6 percent, the authors recommend that this test be considered after two losses.
13. Clark, S. L. Bleeding during early pregnancy. *Female Patient* 14:71, 1989.
    This offers an excellent clinical approach to bleeding during early pregnancy. Abortion was most common, but other important entities were included in the differential diagnosis.

Diagnosis
14. Castle, D., and Bernstein, P. Cytogenetic analysis of 688 couples experiencing multiple spontaneous abortions. *Am. J. Med. Genet.* 29:549, 1988.
    Discusses the significance of balanced translocations, inversions, sex chromosome aneuploidies, and mosaicisms in the cause of multiple abortions.
15. Scott, J. P., et al. Immunologic aspects of recurrent abortion and fetal death. *Obstet. Gynecol.* 70:645, 1987.
    Mechanisms that prevent rejection of the conceptus and maternal immunologic aberrations that may cause repeated abortions are reviewed.
16. MacKenzie, W. E., et al. Spontaneous abortion rate in ultrasonographically viable pregnancies. *Obstet. Gynecol.* 71:81, 1988.
    Spontaneous abortion at less than 10 weeks' gestation was up to three times higher than that at greater than 10 weeks' gestation; this may have implications when deciding on the timing of first-trimester diagnostic procedures.
17. Cervenak, F. A., et al. The need for routine sonography prior to late abortion. *NY State J. Med.* 31:4, 1985.
    The need for an ultrasound study to document fetal age before performing abortion is recommended.

Treatment
18. Dicker, D., et al. Spontaneous abortion in patients with insulin-dependent diabetes mellitus: the effect of preconceptional diabetic control. *Am. J. Obstet. Gynecol.* 158:1161, 1988.
    The authors confirm the evidence accumulated in the recent literature that metabolic control around the time of conception and in the early weeks of pregnancy may be the determining factor favoring abortion, above the rate in the normal population, in women with insulin-dependent diabetes mellitus.
19. Fuchs, A. R., et al. Prostaglandin $F_{2\alpha}$, oxytocin, and uterine activation in hypertonic saline–induced abortion. *Am. J. Obstet. Gynecol.* 150:27, 1984.
    Discusses the possible mechanism of action of hypertonic saline in the induction of abortion.
20. Romero, R., et al. Sonographic monitoring to guide the performance of postabortal uterine curettage. *Am. J. Obstet. Gynecol.* 151:51, 1985.
    The information in this article is of particular value in the management of postabortal endometritis with retained products of conception.
21. Methods of mid-trimester Abortion. *ACOG Tech. Bull.* No. 109, October 1987.
    Despite reductions in the percentage of midtrimester abortions, each year in the United States more than 100,000 women obtain legal abortions at 13 menstrual weeks or more. Techniques, morbidity and mortality, and recommendations are presented.
22. Cameron, I. T., and Baird, D. T. Early pregnancy termination: a comparison between vacuum aspiration and medical abortion using prostaglandin (16,16 dimethyl-trans-delta$_2$-PGE$_1$ methyl ester) or the antiprogestogen RU 486. *Br. J. Obstet. Gynaecol.* 95:271, 1988.
    Compares the efficacy of these medical techniques with vacuum aspiration.
23. Ulmann, A., et al. Medical termination of early pregnancy with mifepristone

(RU 486) followed by a prostaglandin analogue. *Acta Obstet. Gynecol.* 71:278, 1992.

This study conducted in 16,369 women is the largest to date and shows that the administration of RU 486 followed by a prostaglandin analogue provides an efficient and safe medical alternative to surgical intervention for early pregnancy termination, provided that the recommended protocol is adequately followed and the contraindications to prostaglandins are respected.

24. El-Refaey, H., et al. Medical management of missed abortion and anembryonic pregnancy. *Br. Med. J.* 305:1399, 1992.

The article shows that these conditions can be managed medically up to 13 weeks' gestation without the need to resort to surgery or anesthesia.

25. Henshaw, R. C., et al. Medical management of miscarriage: non-surgical uterine evacuation of incomplete and inevitable spontaneous abortion. *Br. Med. J.* 306;894, 1993.

The use of antigestagens and prostaglandins may replace operative evacuation in the treatment of miscarriage, thus freeing up surgical resources for other means.

26. Johnson, N. Intracervical tents: usage and mode of action. *Obstet. Gynecol. Surv.* 44:410, 1989.

A comprehensive review of the use of these adjuncts to cervical dilatation.

27. Jacot, F.R.M., et al. A five-year experience with second-trimester induced abortions: no increase in complication rate as compared to the first trimester. *Am. J. Obstet. Gynecol.* 168:633, 1993.

For suction curettage at less than 15 weeks, the complication rate was 5.1 percent versus 2.9 percent with dilatation and evacuation at 15 to 20 weeks.

Complications

28. Grimes, D. A., Cates, W., Jr., and Selik, R. M. Fetal septic abortion in the United States. *Obstet. Gynecol.* 57:739, 1981.

Fetal septic abortion remains an important national health problem. Reducing the patient's reliance on hazardous illegal abortions is an important means of eliminating septic abortion deaths.

29. Fackow, E. C., and Astiz, M. E. Pathophysiology and treatment of septic shock. *J.A.M.A.* 266:548, 1991.

Septic abortion persists as a cause of septic shock. Newer therapeutic modalities including immunologic interventions and pharmacologic therapies are described. Excellent review with extensive bibliography.

30. Berkowitz, R. L., et al. Selective reduction of multifetal pregnancies in the first trimester. *N. Engl. J. Med.* 318; 1043, 1988.

Discusses the practical techniques and ethical dilemmas involved in this procedure.

31. Boulot, P., et al. Multifetal pregnancy reduction: a consecutive series of 61 cases. *Br. J. Obstet. Gynaecol.* 100:63, 1993.

Selective termination reduces but does not prevent early preterm labor. The procedure is of value in pregnancies with more than three fetuses and should be considered carefully for triplet pregnancies.

32. Chervenak, F. A., et al. When is termination of pregnancy during the third trimester morally justifiable? *N. Engl. J. Med.* 310:501, 1984.

This landmark article addresses the very difficult question of when termination of pregnancy can be carried out in the third trimester.

2. ECTOPIC PREGNANCY
Michel E. Rivlin

A pregnancy in which the fertilized ovum implants on any tissue other than the endometrium is considered an ectopic pregnancy (EP). Approximately 95 percent of the cases of EP occur in the fallopian tube, then in the ampullary (81%), infundibular, isthmic, and cornual (interstitial) segments in descending frequency. Nonoviductal EP occurs in the abdominal cavity, ovaries, or cervix, between the layers of the broad ligament (intraligamentous), or in a congenital rudimentary uterine horn. The coexistence of both an intrauterine and extrauterine gestation (heterotopic pregnancy) is extremely rare, but does occur. The rate of occurrence of EP increased from 4.5 to 16.8 per 1000 pregnancies between 1970 and 1987. Paradoxically, the case-fatality rate decreased from 35.5 to 3.4 per 10,000 EPs over the same period.

The destruction of the normal tubal anatomy remains the major cause of EP and is the explanation in about 50 percent of the cases. The histologic changes associated with pelvic inflammatory disease (PID) are found in about half of the tubes removed for EP. Previous operation for an EP, previous tubal ligation, and conservative tubal procedures for the treatment of infertility are also important risk factors. Probably related to PID are other important risk indicators, such as age and ethnicity (i.e., a threefold increased incidence in women older than 35 years of age versus those younger than 35 and a 60 percent higher risk in black or Hispanic women than in white women). Although the use of oral contraceptives reduces the risk of EP by about 90 percent, the use of an intrauterine device (IUD) may increase the risk of EP, in that, when pregnancy does occur (<2%), about 4 to 17 percent will be an EP. The greatest risk occurs during the first year after removal of the IUD and when the device has been in place for more than 2 years. Similarly, although less than 3 percent of women become pregnant after tubal sterilization, 15 to 50 percent of these pregnancies are ectopic. Salpingitis isthmica nodosa, the microscopic presence of tubal epithelium in the oviductal wall generally in the proximal portion, also predisposes to EP.

The other occurrences of EP are probably a result of hormonal imbalance, aberrations in tubal motility, and abnormalities in the embryo, including transmigration to the opposite tube and genetic abnormalities. Hormonal factors that have been implicated include an increased incidence of EP with the use of the progesterone mini-pill, postcoital estrogens, and the progesterone-containing IUD. Congenital tubal anomalies secondary to intrauterine diethylstilbestrol exposure are associated with a fivefold increased risk of EP. Women undergoing in vitro fertilization and ovulation induction are also at increased risk, although this risk is probably related to associated tubal disease. Approximately 60 percent of the fetuses of EPs are malformed, and 30 percent have grossly abnormal chromosomal patterns. Previously induced abortion does not seem to be a risk factor for the occurrence of EP.

As with an intrauterine pregnancy, tubal gestation does not reside within the lumen but within the tubal wall. The trophoblast also invades vessel walls, so that the usual vasoconstrictive response to hemorrhage cannot occur. Embryonic death and tubal abortion are the most common outcomes of EP. Hemorrhage is frequently self-limiting, and, in some cases, a pelvic hematocele forms, composed of bowel, omentum, and dense adhesions. This is referred to as *chronic EP*.

Rarely, secondary implantation on another pelvic structure results in an abdominal pregnancy. Abdominal pregnancy resulting from primary implantation is even less common than that after secondary implantation. Cervical pregnancy occurs when the placenta attaches below the peritoneal reflection and the uterine vessels. Ovarian pregnancy is diagnosed when Spiegelberg's criteria are met: the tube is intact, ovarian tissue is present in the sac wall, and the sac is in the normal position of the ovary. Rudimentary horn pregnancy results from nidation in the atretic horn of a bicornuate uterus.

About 70 percent of those patients who are not diagnosed early present with the classic triad of symptoms, consisting of amenorrhea, abdominal pain, and abnormal vaginal bleeding. Symptoms of pregnancy are uncommon, whereas dizziness, shoulder pain, and syncope occur only when blood loss is heavy. Irregular bleeding stems from sloughing of the decidua, occasionally as a "decidual cast." Pain is most often experienced in the pelvis or abdomen, and usually occurs at approximately 4 to 6 weeks of gestation. Rupture with intraperitoneal bleeding generally occurs at 6 to 10 weeks. Abdominal and pelvic tenderness is the most consistent sign. In only half of the cases can an adnexal mass be palpated. The uterus is enlarged in about 30 percent of the cases, but rarely beyond 8 weeks' gestation size. Cul-de-sac fullness, orthostatic hypotension, and other evidence of intraperitoneal bleeding may be present. The most common misdiagnoses include PID, abortion, a ruptured corpus luteum cyst, appendicitis, adnexal torsion, endometriosis, dysfunctional uterine bleeding, and gastroenteritis. Leukocytosis is found in one third of the cases of EP, and temperature elevations above 38°C are found in approximately 20 percent.

Another group of patients present earlier in the natural course of the disease, and this group is growing more common, such that, in some centers, more than 80 percent of the patients are now diagnosed before tubal rupture. This diagnostic advance has primarily followed upon the availability of quantitative radioimmunoassays of the beta-subunit of human chorionic gonadotropin (hCG). During the first 40 days of pregnancy, the hCG titer doubles approximately every 2 days. Failure to do so is strong evidence of abnormal gestation. Another valuable diagnostic tool is the level of serum progesterone. Low levels are associated with EP or impending abortion, high levels with normal pregnancy. Unfortunately, there is considerable overlap in the ranges, such that the result is often not diagnostically helpful. The additional performance of vaginal ultrasonography greatly enhances the information supplied by the hCG reading, generally to exclude EP by demonstrating an intrauterine gestational sac (5–6 weeks), fetal pole, yolk sac, or fetal heartbeat (7–8 weeks). The level of hCG at which the sac becomes visible is referred to as the *discriminatory zone,* and many centers have reported this to range from 2000 to 3000 mIU/ml. (For abdominal ultrasound, this level is generally about 6500 mIU/ml.) The quantitation of hCG may be reported using one of two reference standards. It is vital that the standard used be stated. The levels just given are quoted from the International Reference Preparation (I.R.P.; 1 ng hCG = 10 mIU); the other standard is the Second International Reference Standard (Second IS; 1 ng hCG = 5 mIU). Sonography identifies a tubal gestational sac in less than one fourth of the EP cases; however, a solid adnexal mass or fluid in the cul-de-sac are highly important findings.

Uterine curettage may be helpful when the patient does not desire pregnancy and may reveal chorionic villi. The presence of decidual changes or the Arias-Stella reaction in the absence of villi is highly suggestive of EP. Culdocentesis is very helpful in symptomatic cases because 70 to 97 percent of these patients have enough intraperitoneal blood to permit aspiration via the cul-de-sac. A hematocrit of over 15 percent in the fluid indicates significant bleeding. A value of less than 15 percent is more frequently associated with a ruptured ovarian cyst or inflammatory and adhesional disease. False-positive rates vary from 5 to 10 percent, and false-negative rates vary from 11 to 14 percent. Because the procedure is painful, it should not be used unless the information obtained would alter the management plan. Laparoscopy is used in confusing cases, and false-positive and false-negative findings occur in 2 to 5 percent of the laparoscopies.

Treatment of the hemodynamically unstable patient includes volume resuscitation with the administration of crystalloid and type-specific blood as needed, together with early operation. Salpingectomy, the traditional treatment, is associated with a significant subsequent reduction in fertility (intrauterine pregnancy rate, approximately 40% after the procedure) and a 10 to 15 percent rate of recurrent EP in the contralateral tube. In recent years, the use of more conservative surgical procedures has been associated with higher pregnancy rates, without an increase in the rate of EP. These methods are used in women with isthmic or ampullary gestations who desire future pregnancies and are hemodynamically stable. The procedures include linear salpingostomy and segmental resection. Each may be performed via a laparoscope or by laparotomy. The laparoscopic approach is favored for small unruptured gestations. Recently, several nonsurgical methods have been used in the treatment of small unruptured tubal gestations. These methods include expectant management while awaiting spontaneous regression, and may have merit in those patients with persistent low hCG levels after a conservative tubal surgical procedure for EP. Another technique is the use of chemotherapy (methotrexate or actinomycin D), which is effective in the treatment of trophoblastic disease. These drugs have major side

effects and may or may not be safer than surgical techniques. Posttherapy pregnancy and recurrent ectopic rates also need to be compared with those after surgical intervention.
Traditionally, the prognosis with respect to fertility after EP was guarded. Approximately one third of the patients became infertile, one third had subsequent pregnancy loss (miscarriage or repeat ectopic), and one third had a full-term intrauterine pregnancy. However, with conservative surgical treatment, viable pregnancy rates of 50 to 85 percent have been reported. Results are better if the oviduct has not ruptured, emphasizing the importance of early diagnosis.

Reviews

1. Maymon, R., et al. Ectopic pregnancy, the new gynecological epidemic disease: review of the modern work-up and the nonsurgical treatment option. *Int. J. Fertil.* 37:146, 1992.
   Includes a review of 328 patients from the literature treated with various nonsurgical options; surgical interventions were avoided in 86 percent. This also includes an algorithm for the care of stable patients when ectopic pregnancy is suspected.
2. Ectopic Pregnancy. *ACOG Tech. Bull.* No. 150, December 1990. *Int. J. Gynecol. Obstet.* 37:213, 1992.
   Guidelines from the American College of Obstetricians and Gynecologists with regard to the management of EP.
3. Ory, S. J. New options for diagnosis and treatment of ectopic pregnancy. *J.A.M.A.* 267:534, 1992.
   Of the 88,000 women with EP in the United States annually, at least 30 percent are infertile afterwards.
4. Marchbanks, P. A., et al. Risk factors for ectopic pregnancy. A population-based study. *J.A.M.A.* 259:1823, 1988.
   Four variables remained as strong and independent factors: current IUD use, a history of infertility, a history of PID, and prior tubal surgery.

Etiology

5. Phillips, R. S., et al. The effect of cigarette smoking, *Chlamydia trachomatis* infection, and vaginal douching on ectopic pregnancy. *Obstet. Gynecol.* 79:85, 1992.
   Only current cigarette smoking was associated with EP. However, patients were more likely than controls to be nulliparous, nonwhite, and unmarried, and to have a high school education or less.
6. Tomaževič, T., and Ribič-Pucelj, M. Ectopic pregnancy following the treatment of tubal infertility. *J. Reprod. Med.* 37:611, 1992.
   There was a high risk for EP after tubal surgery. The risk after in vitro fertilization was much lower, but still higher than the risk in the general population.
7. Holt, V. L., et al. Tubal sterilization and subsequent ectopic pregnancy: a case-control study. *J.A.M.A.* 266:242, 1991.
   Tubal sterilization provides some protection against extrauterine as well as intrauterine pregnancy; however, 75 percent of the pregnancies that occur after tubal ligation are likely to be EP.
8. Homm, R. J., Holtz, G., and Garvin, A. J. Isthmic ectopic pregnancy and salpingitis isthmica nodosa. *Fertil. Steril.* 48:756, 1987.
   Salpingitis isthmica nodosa was noted in 46 percent of the patients with isthmic EPs in this study.

Diagnosis

9. Shepherd, R.W., et al. Serial beta hCG measurements in early detection of ectopic pregnancy. *Obstet. Gynecol.* 75:417, 1990.
   Serum hCG can be detected as early as 1 week before the expected menses. An abnormal hCG doubling time over the course of 48 to 72 hours, in a large percentage of cases, is predictive of an EP or an intrauterine pregnancy destined to abort.
10. Stovall, T. G., et al. Serum progesterone and uterine curettage in differential diagnosis of ectopic pregnancy. *Fertil. Steril.* 57:456, 1992.

These workers instituted curettage when the serum progesterone level was less than 5 ng/ml. When villi were not identified, hCG levels were measured to differentiate an EP from a complete abortion.

11. Penzias, A. S., and Huang, P. L. Imaging in ectopic pregnancy. *J. Reprod. Med.* 37:47, 1992.
Ultrasound and Doppler flow studies used in conjunction with beta-hCG levels exhibit high sensitivity and specificity for detecting EP.

12. Cacciatore, B., Stenman, U.-H., and Ylostalo, P. Diagnosis of ectopic pregnancy by vaginal ultrasonography in combination with a discriminatory serum hCG level of 1000 Iu/L (IRP). *Br. J. Obstet. Gynaecol.* 97:904, 1990.
In patients with an initial level exceeding 1000 IU/L, an intrauterine sac was detected by vaginal ultrasound in all the intrauterine pregnancies but in none of the EPs.

13. Vande Krol, L., and Abbott, J. T. The current role of culdocentesis. *Am. J. Emerg. Med.* 10:354, 1992.
These authors maintain that needle aspiration of the pouch of Douglas for non-clotting blood in the diagnosis of EP still has a role, albeit limited, despite the advances in noninvasive diagnostic testing.

14. Grosskinsky, C. M., et al. hCG, progesterone, alpha-fetoprotein, and estradiol in the identification of ectopic pregnancy. *Obstet. Gynecol.* 81:705, 1993.
A combination of biochemical markers can be superior to a single progesterone level or clinical evaluation in the diagnosis of ectopic pregnancy.

Treatment

15. Lundorff, P., Thorburn, J., and Lindblom, B. Fertility outcome after conservative surgical treatment of ectopic pregnancy evaluated in a randomized trial. *Fertil. Steril.* 57:998, 1992.
A randomized trial compared conservative surgical treatment for EP performed via laparoscopy and via laparotomy. The fertility outcome was the same. A laparoscopic procedure leads to a significantly short hospital stay, and thereby reduces cost.

16. Prevost, R. R., Stovall, T. G., and Ling, F. W. Methotrexate for treatment of unruptured ectopic pregnancy. *Clin. Pharm.* 11:529, 1992.
Selection criteria for methotrexate treatment consist of: (1) unruptured EP less than 3.5 cm in greatest dimension on ultrasound, (2) no active renal or hepatic disease, and (3) no evidence of leukopenia or thrombocytopenia.

17. Ylostalo, P., et al. Expectant management of ectopic pregnancy. *Obstet. Gynecol.* 80:345, 1992.
Expectant management in conjunction with serial hCG levels and sonography was successful in 69 percent of a selected group of patients with proven EP. Laparoscopy was performed when hCG levels rose or clinical symptoms appeared.

18. Pansky, M., et al. Nonsurgical management of tubal pregnancy: necessity in view of the changing clinical appearance. *Am. J. Obstet. Gynecol.* 164:888, 1992.
Salpingocentesis is a technique in which methotrexate, potassium chloride, prostaglandins, or hyperosmotic glucose is injected into the gestational sac at laparoscopy or under transvaginal ultrasound guidance.

19. Lundorff, P., et al. Persistent trophoblast after conservative treatment of tubal pregnancy: prediction and detection. *Obstet. Gynecol.* 77:129, 1991.
The risk of persistent EP after conservative surgical treatment is about 5 percent. Diagnosis is based on follow-up serial hCG levels and on the symptomatology. Treatment may be medical or the patient may require a second surgical procedure.

20. Silva, P. D., Schaper, A. M., and Rooney, B. Reproductive outcome after 143 laparoscopic procedures for ectopic pregnancy. *Obstet. Gynecol.* 81:710, 1993.
The results were similar to those observed for laparotomy. The major variable was prior tubal damage.

Complications

21. Martin, J. N., Jr., and McCaul, J. F., IV. Emergent management of abdominal pregnancy. *Clin. Obstet. Gynecol.* 33:438, 1990.

The management of the placenta forms the crux of the problem once the diagnosis is established. In general, the placenta is usually best left in situ.

22. Herbertsson, G., Magnusson, S. S., and Benediktsdottir, K. Ovarian pregnancy and IUCD use in a defined complete population. *Acta Obstet. Gynecol. Scand.* 66:607, 1987.
    Ovarian implantation occurred in 10.7 percent of EPs among IUD users compared to 0.9 percent among nonusers.

23. Roussis, P., et al. Cervical pregnancy. A case report. *J. Reprod. Med.* 37:479, 1992.
    Nidation below the internal os may be misdiagnosed as an "abortion." Bleeding is often heavy and hysterectomy is the usual therapy, although successful medical and conservative surgical management has been reported.

24. Goldman, G. A., et al. Heterotopic pregnancy after assisted reproductive technologies. *Obstet. Gynecol. Surv.* 47:217, 1992.
    Estimates of simultaneous intrauterine and extrauterine gestations (heterotopic) range from 1:100 in an in vitro pregnancy population to 1:4000 in the general population.

3. GESTATIONAL TROPHOBLASTIC DISEASE
Michel E. Rivlin

Gestational trophoblastic neoplasms arise from fetal tissue in the mother and are composed of both syncytiotrophoblast and cytotrophoblast. Trophoblastic tissue produces human chorionic gonadotropin (hCG), and the amount produced correlates with the amount of tissue present. Gestational trophoblastic disease (GTD) includes hydatidiform mole, invasive mole, choriocarcinoma, and placental-site trophoblastic tumor. The latter three are also referred to as *gestational trophoblastic tumors* (GTTs). Classification is further based on high-risk and low-risk factors, and whether the disease is metastatic or nonmetastatic. A complete hydatidiform mole occurs in 1 of 1500 pregnancies in the United States. The incidence may be higher elsewhere, especially in the Far East, although these differences may be due to reporting problems. Choriocarcinoma occurs in 2 to 5 percent of the patients with GTD, after a hydatidiform mole in half of these cases, term pregnancy in one fourth, and abortion or ectopic pregnancy in the remainder. The risk of molar pregnancy is greater in adolescents and in women over 40, but most patients are aged 25 to 29.

Molar pregnancy consists of two separate entities, partial and complete mole. They differ in chromosomal pattern, histopathologic characteristics, and clinical presentation. The complete mole has a 46XX karyotype in 90 percent of the cases. The molar chromosomes are of paternal origin. In general, a haploid (23X) sperm fertilizes an ovum and then duplicates its own chromosomes; the maternal chromosomes are absent or inactivated. The remainder are 46XY, apparently resulting from the fertilization of an empty ovum by two separate sperm. Partial moles have a triploid karyotype (69 XXY or 69XYY), after the fertilization of a normal ovum by two sperm, in two thirds of the instances; the remainder have a diploid karyotype (46XX or 46XY). Diffuse swelling, absent villus vasculature, and trophoblastic hyperplasia characterize the chorionic villi in the setting of complete moles with no identifiable embryonic or fetal tissues. Partial moles exhibit focal swelling of the villi with focal trophoblastic hyperplasia, marked scalloping of the villi, and identifiable embryonic or fetal tissue. The fetuses identified with partial moles generally have the stigmata of triploidy, such as hydrocephalus, syndactyly, and growth retardation. If the fetus is normal, a twin pregnancy with a complete mole should be considered. About 25 percent of the hydatidiform moles are partial, as shown by histologic review. Complete moles give rise to persistent GTT in about 15 to 25 percent of the cases. In contrast, a postmolar tumor develops in only 4 to 9 percent of the patients with partial moles. Completing the spectrum of GTD is the uncommon placental-site trophoblastic tumor. This tumor is composed almost entirely of intermediate trophoblast, and, unlike the usual GTD, there is little necrosis or hemorrhage. Human chorionic gonadotropin is produced as in all forms of GTD, but at much lower levels, and the major secretion is human placental lactogen. Furthermore, unlike the other forms of GTD, the response to chemotherapy is poor, so that, when this rare diagnosis is made, hysterectomy is usually indicated because there is a definite risk of malignancy.

Vaginal bleeding is the most frequent early sign of an abnormal gestation. Anemia, hyperemesis, abdominal pain, and, rarely, the passage of grapelike vesicles are less common signs. In the setting of complete moles, one half of the patients present with a uterus 4 weeks or more larger than their dates in terms of gestational weeks. Bilateral theca-lutein ovarian cysts are present in 15 to 25 percent of the patients. Less frequently, clinical pregnancy-induced hypertension (10–15%) or hyperthyroidism may be seen. Patients with partial moles do not usually exhibit these clinical features. The differential diagnosis includes ectopic pregnancy and abortion. The diagnosis is made on the basis of very high levels of hCG, the demonstration of multiple echoes that display a "honeycomb" pattern on ultrasound images, or, occasionally, histologic examination of the aborted products of conception.

Initial management consists of suction curettage performed under general anesthesia, along with uterine stimulation by oxytocin. Although usually a safe procedure, complications include hemorrhage, infection, perforation, and acute respiratory failure secondary to pulmonary trophoblastic embolization. In the setting of nonmetastatic tumors and in older women who have completed having their families, a hysterectomy decreases the risk of choriocarcinoma and the need for further therapy. With primary hysterectomy, there is only a 3 percent chance that further treatment will be needed, which is well under the usual 15 percent expected incidence rate of the need for subsequent therapy. As a result, up to one third of molar pregnancies are managed by primary hysterectomy. Routine prophylactic chemotherapy has not been shown to clearly reduce the overall risk and is not generally advocated. Follow-up consists of obtaining weekly beta-hCG titers until negative for three consecutive determinations; thereafter, this should be done every 3 months for 1 year. Because an elevation in the hCG level owing to a new pregnancy would complicate follow-up, oral contraceptives should be prescribed and careful counseling is essential. Generally, patients should not conceive for at least 1 year. The risk of persistent disease is less than 0.5 percent if the beta-hCG determination is negative for 3 months, and 1 in 500 if negative for 6 months after molar evacuation. The risk of another mole in a future pregnancy is 1 in 60, and, if two molar pregnancies have occurred, it is 1 in 6.

The probability of persistent GTD can be estimated by assessing the epidemiologic risk factors, including a second molar pregnancy, older age, large uterus (over 16-week size), the presence of theca-lutein cysts, or a combination of these. The diagnosis is usually made when the beta-hCG level plateaus or rises over a 2-week period, as indicated by three serial levels. Sometimes curettage may reveal the presence of a lesion consistent with choriocarcinoma or very high levels may persist after curettage, a finding associated with a high risk of uterine perforation. The workup for persistent GTD includes chest x-ray studies, abdominal and head computed tomographic (CT) scans to search for metastatic lesions, and a pelvic sonogram to rule out the existence of a normal pregnancy. In the event of bleeding or the suspicion that evacuation has been incomplete, a repeat suction curettage may be considered, although there is a real risk of perforation.

Nonmetastatic GTD (confined to the uterus) is usually treated on an outpatient basis using single-agent chemotherapy consisting of either methotrexate or dactinomycin. The methotrexate course may include folinic acid rescue. Moderate nausea or vomiting occurs in 80 percent of the patients, but severe toxicity is rare. Dactinomycin produces some alopecia, and pigmentation problems may occur. Although both are known mutagens and teratogens, there does not seem to be an increased frequency of malformations in the offspring of treated patients. Once the hCG level has returned to normal, two or three courses should then be given to obtain a relapse rate well under 5 percent. If first-line therapy is unsuccessful, another first-line drug may be used, although many would then use multiple-drug regimens of middle-risk toxicity such as vincristine, cyclophosphamide, or etoposide, in various combinations. Current remission rates for nonmetastatic GTD approach 100 percent, and fertility can be preserved in most cases. Nonmetastatic GTD is practically synonymous with the postmolar trophoblastic disease seen after molar evacuation.

Low-risk metastatic GTD is diagnosed based on the absence of high-risk criteria. Specifically, these criteria comprise liver or brain metastases, prior failed chemotherapy, an interval of more than 4 months from the antecedent pregnancy to treatment, pretreatment serum hCG level of more than 40,000 mIU/ml, an antecedent term pregnancy, or a histologic diagnosis of choriocarcinoma or placental-site trophoblastic tumor.

Most patients with high-risk GTD have choriocarcinoma. Up to one third of the patients have no gynecologic symptoms; the rest have uterine disease with vaginal bleeding or discharge. If vaginal lesions are present, biopsy is contraindicated because of the possibility of hemorrhage. Extrapelvic masses include pulmonary (75%), cerebral, and hepatic metastases, which cause dyspnea, hemoptysis, respiratory embarrassment, severe headaches, nausea, vomiting, and neurologic symptoms. Visceral metastases may cause hemorrhage intraperitoneally or into the bowel. Magnetic resonance imaging and ultrasound scans are important diagnostic aids. The keystone of management is the beta-hCG assay, with the vital proviso that, even when hCG is no longer detected, 10^4 to 10^5 viable cells may still be present. Various prognostic staging-scoring systems are available to aid in the identification of patients at risk for treatment failure, in the hope that prompt treatment with more effective regimens may improve survival.

The management of high-risk disease entails the aggressive use of multiagent chemotherapy. The emphasis is placed on alternating non–cross-resistant drug regimens given frequently to prevent the emergence of drug-resistant clones of cells. For instance, one regimen alternates etoposide, dactinomycin, and methotrexate/folinic acid with vincristine and cyclophosphamide. From the beginning of therapy, drugs must be administered according to their most effective schedules, with nothing held in reserve for future use. Drug effects are predictable and not idiosyncratic. During treatment courses, daily blood counts and chemistries are determined. Therapy is suspended for white cell counts under 3000, platelet counts under 100,000, or significant changes in renal or hepatic function. Generally, 5-day courses are given every 7 to 10 days for several cycles. Consideration is given to altering drug therapy if hCG levels plateau or rise, or if the metastases increase in size or number. A plateau is defined as no change in the titer in three separate assays performed over 15 days. Surgical treatment may consist of a hysterectomy, thoracotomy, or craniotomy to remove well-localized disease. Radiotherapy should be used only for the management of nonresectable disease because the responses are usually incomplete. The therapy for high-risk disease should be left to experts. Occasionally, a high-risk patient has been treated with single-agent therapy, making subsequent multiagent therapy much more toxic and chances for response poor.

Complete remission is defined as an hCG titer that remains in the normal range for 3 consecutive weeks. Cure is considered achieved if the patient is disease-free for 5 years. Shadows on chest x-ray studies representing nonviable pulmonary metastases may persist for 6 months or more. Cerebral abnormalities on CT scans also persist for long periods; thus, while the serial hCG titers remain normal, these changes can be disregarded. Drug resistance lies at the heart of therapeutic failure, and no active drug should remain in reserve. Early diagnosis and treatment carried out at major centers prevents low-risk patients from becoming high-risk patients.

General
1. Berkowitz, R. S., Goldstein, D. P., and Bernstein M. R. Evolving concepts of molar pregnancy. *J. Reprod. Med.* 36:40, 1991.
   Patients with persistent disease after a partial molar pregnancy usually have nonmetastatic tumors.
2. Bagshawe, K. D., et al. Gestational trophoblastic tumours following initial diagnosis of partial hydatidiform mole. *Lancet* 335:1074, 1990.
   Although the risk for GTT after a partial molar pregnancy is of the order of 1 in 200, compared with 1 in 12 after a complete molar pregnancy, these patients still require gonadotropin follow-up to ensure that complete remission has taken place.

Etiology

3. Parazzini, F., et al. Dietary factors and risk of trophoblastic disease. *Am. J. Obstet Gynecol.* 158:93, 1988.

   The role of dietary factors has been studied repeatedly in the context of GTD because of the differences in incidence related to race and socioeconomic status. The etiology, however, remains largely unknown.

4. Bracken, M. B. Incidence and aetiology of hydatidiform mole: an epidemiological review. *Br. J. Obstet. Gynaecol.* 94:1123, 1987.

   The author states that reports of a very high incidence of GTD in Asia, Africa, and South Central America may have been exaggerated due primarily to selection bias in the patients studied at university hospitals.

5. Buckley, J. D., et al. Case-control study of gestational choriocarcinoma. *Cancer Res.* 48:1004, 1988.

   Various kinds of abnormal fertilization cause different molar syndromes. Because all the chromosomes in complete moles are paternal, they are complete allografts (transplants). The expression of human leukocyte antigens by molar tissue is similar to that of the normal first-trimester placenta.

Diagnosis

6. Kohorn, E. I. Molar pregnancy: presentation and diagnosis. *Clin. Obstet. Gynecol.* 27:181, 1984.

   Serial sonography in conjunction with serial hCG evaluation may occasionally be indicated, either early in the first trimester or when there is a live fetus with a focus of molar tissue in the placenta.

7. Fine, C., et al. Sonographic diagnosis of partial hydatidiform mole. *Obstet. Gynecol.* 73:414, 1989.

   Ultrasound can be of value in predicting a high likelihood of a partial mole before curettage.

8. Yedema, K. A., et al. Identification of patients with persistent trophoblastic disease by means of a normal human chorionic gonadotropin regression curve. *Am. J. Obstet. Gynecol.* 168:787, 1993.

   Identifies patients with persistent disease and allows an expectant attitude within the limits of the curve.

9. Smith, E. T., et al. Renal metastases of malignant gestational trophoblastic disease: the use of intravenous urography in staging. *Gynecol. Oncol.* 20:317, 1985.

   Renal metastases are documented in up to 48 percent of fatal cases of choriocarcinoma. In this study, intravenous urography proved to be a poor technique for staging, and CT scanning is recommended in its place.

10. Lage, J. M. Flow cytometric analysis of nuclear DNA content in gestational trophoblastic disease. *J. Reprod. Med.* 36:31, 1991.

    Aneuploidy in complete moles was associated with a high risk of persistent GTD. However, no correlation between cell-cycle kinetics and outcome was noted.

Treatment

11. Lurain, J. R., and Brewer, J. I. Treatment of high-risk gestational trophoblastic disease with methotrexate, actinomycin D and cyclophosphamide chemotherapy. *Obstet. Gynecol.* 65:830, 1985.

    The GTDs are the prototype human tumors used in investigating the pharmacokinetics of chemotherapy because of their sensitivity to the drugs and the presence of an ideal tumor marker (hCG) that accurately reflects the tumor burden.

12. Soper, J. T., and Hammond, C. B. Role of surgical therapy and radiotherapy in gestational trophoblastic disease. *J. Reprod. Med.* 32:663, 1987.

    The coordination of chronic aggressive multiagent chemotherapy, irradiation, and surgical intervention may be necessary in patients with GTD. Up to 25 percent of the deaths are due to the toxic complications of therapy in patients with resistant disease.

13. Rotmensch, J., Rosenshein, N. B., and Block, B. S. Comparison of human chorionic gonadotropin regression in molar pregnancies and post-molar nonmetastatic gestational trophoblastic neoplasia. *Gynecol. Oncol.* 29:82, 1988.

Once chemotherapy is started for postmolar nonmetastatic GTD, the disappearance of hCG is the same as that seen for spontaneously regressing postevacuation moles. The regression curves can therefore identify those at high risk for failure of primary therapy.

14. Sutton, G. P., et al. Ifosfamide alone and in combination in the treatment of refractory malignant gestational trophoblastic disease. *Am. J. Obstet. Gynecol.* 167:489, 1992.
   Ifosfamide, a congener of cyclophosphamide, requires the concurrent administration of mercaptoethane sodium sulfonate (mesna) to prevent otherwise prohibitive urothelial toxicity.

15. Finkler, N. J. Placental site trophoblastic tumor. Diagnosis, clinical behavior and treatment. *J. Reprod. Med.* 36:27, 1991.
   Because of the poor response to chemotherapy and the inability to predict the biologic behavior of this tumor, prompt hysterectomy is recommended.

16. Newlands, E. S., et al. Results with the EMA/CO (etoposide, methotrexate, actinomycin D, cyclophosphamide, vincristine) regimen in high risk gestational trophoblastic tumours, 1979 to 1989. *Br. J. Obstet. Gynecol.* 98:550, 1991.
   EMA/CO appears superior to the combination of methotrexate, actinomycin, and cyclophosphamide in the treatment of patients with prognostic scores of 8 or higher. Cisplatin is also active and many oncologists include this agent in treating high-risk patients.

Complications

17. Kumar, J., Ilancheran, A., and Ratnam, S. S. Pulmonary metastases in gestational trophoblastic disease. A review of 97 cases. *Br. J. Obstet. Gynecol.* 95:70, 1988.
   Beta-hCG titers should always be obtained from women with unexplained urinary, gastrointestinal, or pulmonary bleeding, as well as from those with central nervous system tumors or atypical pelvic malignancies.

18. Newman, R. B., and Eddy, G. L. Association of eclampsia and hydatidiform mole: case report and review of the literature. *Obstet. Gynecol. Surv.* 43:185, 1988.
   These authors recommend the liberal use of prophylactic antiseizure medication when treating GTD in women with hypertension, neurologic complaints, or other evidence of pregnancy-induced hypertension.

19. Jones, W. B., Wagner-Reiss, K. M., and Lewis, J. L., Jr. Intracerebral choriocarcinoma. *Gynecol. Oncol.* 38:234, 1990.
   Multiagent chemotherapy (methotrexate, actinomycin, and cyclophosphamide) with whole-brain radiotherapy was relatively ineffective, with a 25 percent survival.

20. Bakri, Y. N., et al. Liver metastases of gestational trophoblastic tumor. *Gynecol. Oncol.* 48:110, 1993.
   The incidence of hepatic involvement ranges from 5 to 20 percent of the cases of high-risk metastatic GTT. The best chemotherapeutic regimen is still undetermined.

21. Kelly, M. P., et al. Respiratory failure due to choriocarcinoma: a study of 103 dyspneic patients. *Gynecol. Oncol.* 38:149, 1990.
   The cause of respiratory insufficiency in patients with GTD is probably multifactorial, and includes trophoblastic embolization, toxemia, hyperthyroidism, and vigorous transfusion therapy.

Prognosis

22. Ozturk, M. Human chorionic gonadotropin, its free subunits and gestational trophoblastic disease. *J. Reprod. Med.* 36:21, 1991.
   Mean levels of free beta-hCG were 3.5-fold higher in the presence of a benign partial mole versus that in normal pregnancy, 11-fold higher in the presence of benign complete mole, and 30-fold higher in patients with choriocarcinoma.

23. Dubuc-Lissoir, J., et al. Metastatic gestational trophoblastic disease: a comparison of prognostic classification systems. *Gynecol. Oncol.* 45:40, 1992.
   The three available classification systems are the FIGO staging system, the NIH prognosis classification, and the WHO scoring system.

24. Berkowitz, R. S., Goldstein, D. P., and Bernstein, M. R. Reproductive experience

after complete and partial molar pregnancy and gestational trophoblastic tumors. *J. Reprod. Med.* 36:3, 1991.
These patients can expect a normal reproductive outcome in the future if successfully treated with chemotherapy alone.
25. Wenzel, L., et al. The psychological, social, and sexual consequences of gestational trophoblastic disease. *Gynecol. Oncol.* 46:74, 1992.
Significant levels of anxiety, anger, fatigue, confusion, sexual problems, and pregnancy concerns persist for a protracted period.

4. PLACENTA PREVIA
Kenneth G. Perry, Jr.

Placenta previa is defined as the abnormal implantation of the placenta in the lower uterine segment over the internal cervical os, and accounts for approximately 20 percent of all cases of antepartum hemorrhage. Placenta previa may be classified according to the degree of placental encroachment on the cervical os. A total placenta previa completely covers the internal os, and may be central, anterior, or posterior. In the case of a partial placenta previa, the placenta covers part of the internal os, while a marginal placenta previa just reaches the edge of the internal os. In a low-lying placenta, the placental edge is within 5 cm of the cervix but does not reach the internal os. In the second trimester, a complete previa is found in approximately 5 percent of all pregnancies, with over 90 percent of them resolving by the time of delivery. The overall incidence of placenta previa is 1 in 200 deliveries at term. Because all forms of placenta previa have the potential for leading to severe antepartum hemorrhage and maternal and perinatal morbidity, management is based on the clinical presentation and not the classification.

Factors that have been associated with implantation in the lower uterine segment and placenta previa include advanced maternal age, increased parity, multiple gestations, prior uterine operation, and a previous placenta previa. The risk of recurrence for placenta previa may be as high as 10 to 15 percent.

The risk of abnormal placental attachment (accreta, increta, or percreta) increases when placentation occurs in the lower uterine segment. This is especially true when a placenta previa is diagnosed in a patient who has undergone a previous cesarean section. The risk of a placenta accreta is approximately 5 percent in cases of previa without prior uterine surgery. This risk increases to 25 percent after one cesarean delivery and further increases to approximately 50 percent after two cesarean births.

The most common clinical manifestation of placenta previa is substantial bright red vaginal bleeding occurring in the third trimester, particularly at 28 to 34 weeks' gestation. This is the time when the lower uterine segment thins before parturition, and this may disrupt a portion of the implantation site. As many as 20 percent of these patients present with uterine contractions, while approximately 10 percent present with uterine irritability suggestive of placental abruption. The mean gestational age at the time of the first bleeding episode is 30 weeks, with 25 percent of the patients presenting before 30 weeks. Physical examination reveals a soft, nontender uterus, and the fetus may be unengaged in an abnormal lie, either transverse or breech. The differential diagnosis includes abruption, vasa previa, genital tract trauma, excessive show, cervical lesions, cervicitis, nongenital bleeding (rectum or bladder), and blood dyscrasias. In addition, one third to one half of the cases of third-trimester bleeding remain unexplained.

Placenta previa is almost exclusively diagnosed on the basis of ultrasound findings, and a pelvic examination is contraindicated until the diagnosis of previa is excluded. Transabdominal ultrasound is very accurate in the detection of placental location. Even so, a false-positive rate of 10 percent has been reported, usually attributed to an overdistended bladder or an anterior placenta. On the other hand, a false-negative rate of 7 percent has also been noted and may result from a posterior or lateral placental location that is obscured by the fetal head. Use of transvaginal ultrasound can confirm the diagnosis of placenta previa in almost 100 percent of the patients.

Clinically, the diagnosis of placenta previa can be made by palpation of the placenta through the cervix during a procedure known as a "double setup." Though rarely indicated today, the use of the double setup assumes delivery is indicated, adequate blood replacement is available, and the patient is in the operating room prepared for cesarean delivery with a complete operating team in attendance. A speculum examination is performed initially, followed by a digital examination. If placental tissue is palpated, then cesarean section is performed immediately. The only indication for a double setup is when the ultrasound finding is inconclusive, the patient's condition is stable, the patient appears to be in active labor, and vaginal delivery is a consideration.

Management of the pregnancy complicated by placenta previa depends on (1) the gestational age of the fetus, (2) the maternal and fetal condition, and (3) the extent of vaginal bleeding. As with any cause of substantial antepartum hemorrhage, the mother's condition should be stabilized, external fetal monitoring begun, blood studies carried out, and blood products made available. If the vaginal bleeding persists or severe fetal distress is noted, then immediate cesarean section is indicated. If bleeding ceases and the fetus is immature (< 36 weeks), then expectant management is appropriate, with modified bed rest in the hospital until significant bleeding occurs or fetal lung maturity is documented by amniocentesis. The maternal hematocrit should be maintained at 30 percent or greater by the administration of supplemental iron or blood transfusions, or both. In those cases complicated by uterine contractions in which abruption has been excluded, tocolysis in the form of magnesium sulfate therapy may be utilized. In addition, some advocate the use of steroids to accelerate fetal lung maturity in the gravida remote from term. Rh-negative patients are at risk for isoimmunization resulting from a fetal-maternal transfusion, and should be given RhoGAM (Rh$_0$[D] immune globulin). Serial ultrasound examinations performed at 2-week to 3-week intervals and weekly fetal assessments in the form of a nonstress test or biophysical profile are useful. An ultrasound examination can document normal fetal growth and show placental migration, should it occur.

If delivery becomes necessary, cesarean section is the method of choice, with the type of uterine incision depending on placental location. In general, the placenta should be avoided during delivery, thus mandating a low-segment vertical or classic incision. In the setting of a posterior placenta and a well-developed lower uterine segment, a low-segment transverse cesarean incision may be chosen with minimal attendant risk of additional blood loss. Irrespective of the uterine incision, the administration of prophylactic antibiotics is indicated.

The outcome for both mother and fetus in the setting of placenta previa is generally favorable. The maternal mortality rate is less than 1 per 1000 and is most often a complication of infection or severe hemorrhage associated with placenta accreta, uterine atony, or the placenta previa itself. Preterm delivery poses the greatest risk to the fetus; however, other perinatal complications include growth retardation, anemia, asphyxia, and acute blood loss. Because of these various complications, the clinical management of placenta previa requires a team approach, with close cooperation among the obstetric, neonatal, and anesthesia personnel.

General
1. Musick, S. C., and Cotton, D. B. Placenta Previa. In J. J. Sciarra (ed.), *Gynecology and Obstetrics,* Vol. 2. Philadelphia: J. B. Lippincott, 1987.
   A well-done contemporary overview of the clinical management aspects of placenta previa.
2. Cunningham, F. G., et al. Obstetrical Hemorrhage. In *Williams Obstetrics* (19th ed.). Norwalk, CT: Appleton & Lange, 1993.
   A time-honored classic in the management of placenta previa.
3. Gallagher, P., et al. Potential placenta previa: definition, frequency, and significance. *Am. J. Radiol.* 149:1013, 1987.
   A 5 percent incidence of second-trimester placenta previa is reported. Complete

forms of previa usually persist until the end of gestation, versus the infrequent persistence of the marginal or partial forms of "potential placenta previa."

Etiology

4. Rose, G. L., and Chapman, M. G. Aetiological factors in placenta praevia—a case controlled study. *Br. J. Obstet. Gynaecol.* 93:586, 1986.
   Previous cesarean delivery, uterine curettage, and spontaneous abortion followed by uterine curettage are important etiologic factors in placenta previa.

5. Grimes, D. A., and Techman, T. Legal abortion and placenta previa. *Am. J. Obstet. Gynecol.* 149:501, 1984.
   Absence of evidence to corroborate suspicions that elective pregnancy interruption, or interruptions, are an etiologic factor for later placenta previa.

6. Gorodseki, I. G., et al. Recurrent placenta previa. *Eur. J. Obstet. Gynecol. Reprod. Biol.* 12:7, 1981.
   Women over 36 who experienced placenta previa in a previous gestation are at six times greater risk for recurrent placenta previa.

7. Clark, S. L., Koonings, P. P., and Phelan, J. P. Placenta previa/accreta and prior cesarean section. *Obstet. Gynecol.* 66:89, 1985.
   Strikingly high incidence rates (25%, 50%, and 67%) of placenta accreta are to be expected when prior low-segment transverse cesarean section (one, two, or three, respectively) is coupled with placenta previa in the present gestation.

8. Newton, E. R., Barss, V., and Cetrulo, C. L. The epidemiology and clinical history of asymptomatic midtrimester placenta previa. *Am. J. Obstet. Gynecol.* 148:743, 1984.
   An etiologic and epidemiologic analysis of asymptomatic placenta previa between 20 and 30 weeks' gestation as a high-risk pregnancy marker transcending considerations of bleeding alone.

9. Williams, M. A., et al. Cigarette smoking during pregnancy in relation to placenta previa. *Am. J. Obstet. Gynecol.* 165:28, 1991.
   The relationship of cigarette smoking to the occurrence of placental hypertrophy and placenta previa is examined.

Diagnosis

10. Farine, D., et al. Vaginal ultrasound for diagnosis of placenta previa. *Am. J. Obstet. Gynecol.* 159:566, 1988.
    A comparison of transvaginal ultrasound with transabdominal ultrasound demonstrates the safety and accuracy of transvaginal ultrasound for the diagnosis of placenta previa.

11. Leerentveld, R. A., et al. Accuracy and safety of transvaginal sonographic placental localization. *Obstet. Gynecol.* 76:759, 1990.
    Transvaginal sonographic localization of the placenta is proved to be safe and accurate, with a high sensitivity and specificity as well as positive and negative predictive values.

12. Oppenheimer, L. W., et al. What is a low-lying placenta? *Am. J. Obstet. Gynecol.* 165:1036, 1991.
    A suggestion is made for performing transvaginal ultrasound in the management of delivery mode with low-lying placentas.

13. Timor-Tritsch, I. E., and Yunis, R. A. Confirming the safety of transvaginal sonography in patients suspected of placenta previa. *Obstet. Gynecol.* 81:742, 1993.
    Confirms the safety of transvaginal ultrasound in the diagnosis and management of placenta previa.

14. de Mendonca, L. K. Sonographic diagnosis of placenta accreta. Presentation of six cases. *J. Ultrasound Med.* 7:211, 1988.
    Encourages clinicians and sonographers to pay special attention to the presence or absence of an anechoic retroplacental complex and textural myometrial changes at the site of prior uterine incisions when there is placenta previa.

Treatment

15. Sauer, M., Parsons, M., and Sampson, M. Placenta previa: an analysis of three years experience. *Am. J. Perinatol.* 2:39, 1985.

A thorough retrospective analysis of one referral center's recent clinical experience (1981—1984) with central placenta previa management utilizing modern diagnostic and therapeutic modalities.

16. Arias, F. Cervical cerclage for the temporary treatment of patients with placenta previa. *Obstet. Gynecol.* 71:545, 1988.

    Despite the small size of this patient series, an argument is made for the unconventional use of midgestational cervical cerclage in gravidas with symptomatic placenta previa; benefits include better perinatal outcome and less total hospital costs.

17. Silver, R. Placenta previa: aggressive expectant management. *Am. J. Obstet. Gynecol.* 150:15, 1984.

    Another excellent series, with a 4.2 percent perinatal mortality.

18. Dingily, L. J., and Irwin, L. F. Conservative management of placenta previa: a cost-benefit analysis. *Am. J. Obstet. Gynecol.* 149:320, 1984.

    Addresses the actual monetary costs of current perinatal management practices for placenta previa.

19. Gorodeski, I. G., and Bahari, C. M. The effect of placenta previa localization upon maternal and fetal-neonatal outcome. *J. Perinat. Med.* 15:169, 1984.

    A well-presented institutional series consisting of 165 gravidas from Israel, which found no association between the type of placenta previa and the character or timing of hemorrhage; a wealth of maternal and perinatal data highlight this article.

20. Chervenak, F. A., et al. Role of attempted vaginal delivery in the management of placenta previa. *Obstet. Gynecol.* 64:798, 1984.

    The authors suggest that the double-setup finding of partial placenta previa near term can be managed by attempted vaginal delivery if blood loss is minimal during the examination and ensuing trial of labor.

21. Tomich, P. G. Prolonged use of tocolytic agents in the expectant management of placenta previa. *J. Reprod. Med.* 30:745, 1985.

    The use of tocolytic therapy, even for prolonged periods, appears to have a place in the treatment of stable gravidas with placenta previa and in preterm labor.

Complications

22. McShane, P. M., Heyl, P. S., and Epstein, M. F. Maternal and perinatal morbidity resulting from placenta previa. *Obstet. Gynecol.* 65:176, 1985.

    In cases of placenta previa, there is a significant correlation with the need for neonatal transfusion, the occurrence of neonatal anemia, and the amount of intrapartum blood loss; respiratory distress syndrome in the neonate was the major cause of death.

23. Breen, J. L., et al. Placenta accreta, increta, and percreta. *Obstet. Gynecol.* 49:43, 1977.

    An excellent clinical series consisting of 40 patients with this related placental complication.

24. Druzin, M. L. Packing of lower uterine segment for control of postcesarean bleeding in instances of placenta previa. *Surg. Gynecol. Obstet.* 169:543, 1989.

    Packing the lower uterine segment in the event of hemorrhage after cesarean section is proposed.

5. ABRUPTIO PLACENTAE
Kenneth G. Perry, Jr.

Abruptio placentae (placental abruption) is the premature separation of a normally implanted placenta from its attachment to the uterus before the delivery of the fetus. It is characterized by the triad of (1) vaginal bleeding, (2) uterine hypertonus, and (3) fetal distress. Abruption occurs in approximately 1 in 120 deliveries and is responsible for 15 percent of the third-trimester stillbirths. Severe abruptions are associated with an overall perinatal mortality in the range of 25 to 35 percent.

The precise cause of placental abruption is unknown, though several associated factors have been noted. Maternal hypertension, whether chronic or pregnancy induced, is the most frequent condition found in the setting of abruptions and may be seen in as many as 50 percent of the cases. Rapid decompression of an overdistended uterus has also been implicated, as in cases of multiple gestations after the delivery of the first twin or in hydramnios after rupture of the membranes. Other factors associated with placental abruption include maternal trauma, cocaine abuse, smoking, and a short umbilical cord. A prior history of an abruption is a significant risk factor, with a reported risk of recurrence ranging from 5 to 17 percent. Unfortunately, there are no biochemical or biophysical tests that can predict the likelihood of abruption in subsequent pregnancies.

Hemorrhage into the decidua basalis with formation of a decidual hematoma is thought to initiate placental separation. Anomalies of the spiral arterioles as well as arteriolar weakness may be involved as the underlying pathologic mechanism. This separation of the decidua from the basal plate predisposes to further hemorrhage and dissection of the membranes from the uterine wall, resulting in placental destruction and the loss of placental function. If placental destruction is considerable, then fetal distress and ultimately fetal death will occur. If blood dissects toward the cervix, then escape of blood into the vagina results in external hemorrhage. On the other hand, if blood dissects away from the cervix, the hemorrhage is said to be concealed, and this occurs in 10 to 20 percent of the cases of abruption. This condition may only be discovered after delivery when examination of the placenta reveals a circumscribed depression on the maternal surface that is filled with a blood clot. In addition, blood may infiltrate the myometrium, resulting in a Couvelaire uterus.

Placental abruptions may be classified according to the clinical and laboratory findings. Grade I, or mild, abruptions occur in 40 percent of the cases and are characterized by slight vaginal bleeding associated with mild uterine activity in the absence of maternal hypotension or fetal distress. Forty-five percent of the abruptions are grade II, and there is moderate uterine bleeding and uterine contractions without evidence of maternal shock or fetal distress. Coagulopathy, if present, is only mild. In the presence of severe abruptions, grade III, found in 15 percent of the cases, there is severe uterine bleeding that results in maternal shock, coagulopathy, and fetal death.

Clinically the diagnosis of placental abruption should be suspected in any patient who presents with vaginal bleeding, uterine hyperactivity, and fetal distress. Even so, the signs and symptoms of placental abruption vary considerably. Approximately 80 percent of the patients present with vaginal bleeding and over 50 percent have uterine contractions. Two thirds of the patients with clinically significant abruptions complain of back pain, have uterine tenderness, or both. In the absence of vaginal bleeding, uterine tone and tenderness may be more pronounced, indicating a concealed abruption. Placenta previa as well as other causes of third-trimester hemorrhage should be ruled out. A degenerating leiomyomata, ovarian torsion, appendicitis, or any acute abdominal emergency must also be considered in the differential diagnosis.

Even though abruptio placentae is a clinical diagnosis, ultrasound may be useful, especially to rule out placenta previa as the cause of third-trimester hemorrhage. The ultrasound diagnosis of placental abruption can be made with certainty in only a minority of the cases because the characteristic retroplacental hematoma is identified less than 5 percent of the time. Because false-positive as well as false-negative results are a problem, negative ultrasound findings should not be used as a basis to rule out abruptio placenta.

Abruption is the most common cause of acute disseminated intravascular coagulopathy (DIC) in pregnancy. As many as 20 percent of gravidas with moderate to severe abruptions have clotting defects. Activation of the clotting cascade probably results from the release of thrombogenic material into the maternal circulation from the retroplacental clot. This results in an increase in fibrin split products, hypofibrinogenemia, and prolonged coagulation, with or without thrombocytopenia. Clinical manifestations of acute DIC include epistaxis, hematuria, oozing from puncture sites, purpura, and petechiae. Management of the patient with DIC includes delivery of the infant and supportive therapy in the form of volume replacement, transfusion of specific blood products, and the maintenance of cardiopulmonary integrity. Fortunately, postpartum hemorrhage is not usually a problem and the administration of oxytocin for uterine atony is usually effective.

Prompt and aggressive treatment of the patient with abruptio placentae is aimed at avoiding the complications of (1) hemorrhagic shock, (2) DIC, and (3) ischemia necrosis of vital organs (i.e., acute tubular necrosis resulting in renal failure). Vigorous blood and volume replacement with packed red blood cells and crystalloid is the initial therapy. Supplemental oxygen is indicated to decrease tissue hypoxia. A Foley catheter should be placed to monitor urine output and central monitoring implemented as needed. Continuous electronic fetal monitoring is useful in ruling out fetal distress. Initial laboratory studies include a complete blood count; measurement of creatinine, blood urea nitrogen, fibrin split product, and fibrinogen levels; prothrombin time; and a partial thromboplastin time. These tests need to be repeated every 4 to 6 hours until delivery, and thereafter as indicated. The patient should be typed and crossmatched for four units of packed red blood cells. If DIC is evident, then delivery of the infant is always appropriate, and blood, fluid volume, and clotting factors (fresh frozen plasma or cryoprecipitate) are replaced while proceeding toward delivery. The timing and mode of delivery depend on the fetal status and maternal condition, as well as the severity of the abruption. In general, a term pregnancy complicated by a mild abruption in the absence of fetal distress may be delivered vaginally. Amniotomy and the general use of oxytocin can facilitate delivery. If, however, the fetus is immature and the abruption is mild, expectant management and the use of tocolytics in the form of magnesium sulfate is advocated by some authorities. Such conservative management protocols mandate close maternal and fetal monitoring, as rapid deterioration can occur unexpectedly. On the other hand, fetal distress in a viable fetus mandates immediate delivery by cesarean section if vaginal delivery is not imminent. If fetal demise complicates the abruption and the maternal condition is stable, then vaginal delivery should be attempted.

General
1. Cunningham, F. G., et al. Obstetrical Hemorrhage. In *Williams Obstetrics* (19th ed.). Norwalk, CT: Appleton & Lange, 1993.
   A premier review strengthened by decades of firsthand study and clinical observation.
2. Karegard, M., and Gennser, G. Incidence and recurrence rate of abruptio placentae in Sweden. *Obstet. Gynecol.* 67:523, 1986.
   From the Swedish nationwide birth registry system comes this landmark review of pertinent maternal and perinatal data from almost 4000 pregnancies that were complicated by placental abruption; a wealth of clinically useful information is succinctly summarized.
3. Blumenfeld, M., and Gabbe, S. G. Placental Abruption. In J. J. Sciarra (ed.), *Gynecology and Obstetrics*, Vol. 2. Philadelphia: J. B. Lippincott, 1991.
   An excellent overview of placental abruption.
4. Pritchard, J. A., et al. On reducing the frequency of severe abruptio placentae. *Am. J. Obstet. Gynecol.* 165:1345, 1991.
   An overview of the experience at Parkland Memorial Hospital, with a reduced frequency of placental abruption in the past 20 years.
5. Abdella, T. N., et al. Relationship of hypertensive disease to abruptio placentae. *Obstet. Gynecol.* 63:635, 1984.
   A major review of the association between placental; abruption and specific types of hypertension; the highest incidence of abruption occurred in association with eclampsia (24%).
6. Voigt, L. F., et al. The relationship of abruptio placentae with maternal smoking and small for gestational age infants. *Obstet. Gynecol.* 75:771, 1990.
   Maternal smoking appears to be associated with abruptio placenta, and the birth

of small-for-gestational age infants in these mothers is probably the result of placental dysfunction.

7. Higgins, S. D., and Garite, T. J. Late abruptio placenta in trauma patients: implications for monitoring. *Obstet. Gynecol.* 63:10S, 1984.
   The importance of continuous fetal monitoring for 48 hours after severe maternal trauma is emphasized.

8. Kettel, L. M., Branch, D. W., and Scott, J. R. Occult placental abruption after maternal hemorrhage. *Obstet. Gynecol.* 71:449, 1988.
   Maternal trauma–induced occult placental abruption (no vaginal bleeding or uterine pain) can occur and be detectable only by continuous long-term fetal monitoring.

9. Landy, H. J., and Hinson, J. Placental abruption associated with cocaine use: case report. *Reprod. Toxicol.* 1:203, 1988.
   Substance abuse, particularly with cocaine, in the third trimester appears to be associated with a significant risk of placental abruption.

10. Gonen, R., Hannah, M. E., and Milligan, J. E. Does prolonged preterm premature rupture of the membranes predispose to abruptio placentae? *Obstet. Gynecol.* 74:347, 1989.
    The clinician should be aware of the association between the prolonged preterm rupture of membranes and abruption.

11. Darby, M. J., Caritis, S. N., and Shen-Schwarz, S. Placental abruption in the preterm gestation: an association with chorioamnionitis. *Obstet. Gynecol.* 74:88, 1989.
    There is a significant association between abruptio placentae and histologically confirmed chorioamnionitis.

Diagnosis

12. Nyberg, D. A., et al. Placental abruption and placental hemorrhage: correlation of sonographic findings with fetal outcome. *Radiology* 164:357, 1987.
    Excellent review of the various sonographic findings attendant to placental abruption and how these correlate with perinatal outcome.

13. Sauerbrei, E. E., and Pham, D. H. Placental abruption and subchorionic hemorrhage in the first half of pregnancy: U.S. appearance and clinical outcome. *Radiology* 160:109, 1986.
    Sonographic features of placental abruption and factors related to prognosis are discussed for gravidas suffering from vaginal bleeding between 10 and 20 weeks of gestation.

14. Mintz, M. C., et al. Abruptio placentae: apparent thickening of the placenta caused by hyperechoic retroplacental clot. *J. Ultrasound Med.* 5:411, 1986.
    Apparent thickening of the placenta may be the only sonographic sign of placental abruption.

Treatment

15. Hurd, W. W., et al. Selective management of abruptio placentae: a prospective study. *Obstet. Gynecol.* 61:467, 1983.
    Evaluates the place of individualized management of placental abruption and emphasizes that vaginal delivery for the less than 1500-g fetus can be achieved safely if safeguards are built in.

16. Sholl, J. S. Abruptio placentae: clinical management in nonacute cases. *Am. J. Obstet. Gynecol.* 156:40, 1987.
    Frequent inpatient fetal heart rate monitoring, tocolysis if indicated, and timely cesarean delivery are indicated in the event of nonacute preterm placental abruption.

17. Heinonen, P. K., Kajan, M., and Saarikoski, S. Cardiotocographic findings in abruptio placentae. *Eur. J. Obstet. Gynecol. Reprod. Biol.* 23:75, 1986.
    Tocographic monitor tracings associated with placental abruption are discussed as a diagnostic aid and management tool.

18. Grimes, D. A., Steele, A. O., and Hatcher, R. A. Rh immunoglobulin use with placenta previa and abruptio placentae. *South. Med. J.* 76:743, 1983.

Six of 25 Rh-negative gravidas with obstetric hemorrhage resulting from abruptio placentae or placenta previa required more than 300 μg of Rh immune globulin.

Complications
19. Weiner, C. P. Disseminated Intravascular Coagulopathy Associated with Pregnancy. In S. L. Clark, et al. (eds.), *Critical Care Obstetrics* (2nd ed.). Boston: Blackwell Scientific Publications, 1991.
    Placental abruption is the most common obstetric cause of acute DIC; the goals of therapy, a simple management protocol, critical laboratory tests, and important considerations are well detailed in this superbly done treatise.
20. Knab, D. R. Abruptio placentae: an assessment of the time and method of delivery. *Obstet. Gynecol.* 52:625, 1978.
    Analysis of 338 cases of abruptio placentae indicated that 75 percent of the fetal deaths occurred more than 90 minutes after admission to the hospital, and almost 70 percent of all perinatal mortality occurred in infants who were delivered more than 2 hours after the time of diagnosis.
21. Harris, B. A., Jr., Gore, H., and Flowers, C. E., Jr. Peripheral placental separation: a possible relationship to premature labor. *Obstet. Gynecol.* 66:774, 1985.
    A clinicopathologic investigation which suggests that peripheral placental separation ("marginal rupture") may play a role in some cases of preterm labor.
22. Neilson, E. C., Varner, M. W., and Scott, J. R. The outcome of pregnancies complicated by bleeding during the second trimester. *Surg. Gynecol. Obstet.* 173:371, 1991.
    Perinatal mortality is high among pregnancies complicated by second-trimester hemorrhage, and especially those attributed to placental abruption. The mortality rate decreased in those gestations maintained into the third trimester.

II. HYPERTENSION IN PREGNANCY

6. ESSENTIAL HYPERTENSION
Garland D. Anderson

Hypertension is one of the most common medical complications of pregnancy and its reported incidence rate ranges from 6 to 30 percent. One third to one half of these patients are women with essential hypertension. In women with a mean arterial pressure greater than 90 mm Hg during the second trimester, there is a significant increase in the rate of stillbirths, pregnancy-induced hypertension (PIH), and small-for-gestational age (SGA) infants. The overall perinatal mortality rate is reported to be 8 to 15 percent, but it is even higher in the setting of superimposed PIH. However, essentially all the increase in perinatal mortality occurs in those women who acquire superimposed PIH. Women with mild to moderate hypertension who do not suffer superimposed PIH do as well as the general obstetric population.

Differentiating chronic essential hypertension complicating pregnancy from PIH can be very difficult. All obstetric patients experience a decrease in blood pressure in the second trimester because the placenta is a low-resistance system parallel to the mother's circulation. Women with moderate chronic hypertension may therefore be considered to have normal blood pressure readings if first seen during midpregnancy. In late pregnancy, however, when the blood pressure rises to prepregnancy levels, the hypertension may then be erroneously attributed to PIH.

The diagnosis of preexisting hypertension is secure only if it is confirmed before pregnancy or if the patient exhibits elevated pressure before the twentieth week of gestation. Essential hypertension is also suspected, in retrospect, in the patient who receives the diagnosis of chronic preexisting hypertension postpartum. Clues that favor the diagnosis of chronic preexisting hypertension include (1) hypertension associated with chronic diseases such as diabetes mellitus, renal disease, or collagen vascular disease; (2) abnormal optic fundi (e.g., hemorrhages or exudates); and (3) abnormal renal function test results (e.g., blood urea nitrogen level > 20 mg/dl or plasma creatinine level > 1 g/dl).

Besides essential hypertension, other chronic causes of elevated blood pressure must be considered. Conditions such as vascular abnormalities (e.g., renal vascular disease and coarctation of the aorta), endocrinopathies (e.g., diabetes mellitus, pheochromocytoma, and hyperaldosteronism), and renal disease (e.g., glomerulonephritis, pyelonephritis, collagen vascular disease with renal involvement, and polycystic disease) should be included in the differential diagnosis. A flank bruit is suggestive of renovascular hypertension, whereas coarctation of the aorta can be detected by comparing arterial pressures in the upper and lower extremities and by palpating the femoral arteries.

The greatest threat of chronic essential hypertension to the obstetric patient is the increased prevalence of superimposed PIH. Although a diastolic pressure of 95 mm Hg or more has been shown to increase the risk of fetal death, it is the development of superimposed PIH that jeopardizes the mother's life. The three most common signs are accelerating hypertension, the onset of proteinuria, and worsening nondependent edema. The diagnosis can be based on one sign if it is severe, but the diagnosis is more secure if at least two signs are present. The sudden onset of headaches, visual disturbances, tremulousness, or epigastric pain often means impending convulsion. The incidence of abruptio placentae is increased in women with chronic hypertension, with a reported incidence rate that ranges between 2.5 and 17.9 percent. In a retrospective review of 265 cases of abruptio placentae, the incidence rate in the total obstetric population was 1.17 percent, compared with 10 percent in women with chronic hypertension.

Accurate documentation of gestational age is extremely important in the management of pregnant women with hypertension. Besides the risk of superimposed PIH, many of the fetuses in these women will be SGA. Any early correlation of uterine size with menstrual dates and documentation of first fetal heart tones heard by fetoscope are important data. Because of the increased incidence of SGA infants in the setting of maternal hypertension, serial ultrasonography should be performed in these women. Growth retardation in the fetus is more common in patients with chronic hypertension than in patients with PIH. Serial measurements that show increases in fundal height, progressive increases in estimated fetal weight, and appropriate increments in maternal weight are indications of fetal growth.

The plasma volume is reduced in pregnant women with chronic hypertension compared to that in normotensive gravidas. In addition, failure of the plasma volume to expand is associated with intrauterine growth retardation and intrauterine fetal demise.

Initial evaluation of the pregnant women with essential hypertension should include careful examination of the optic fundi as well as renal evaluation by assessment of a 24-hour urine specimen for protein and creatinine clearance. In addition, a chest x-ray study and electrocardiogram are appropriate if the hypertension has been long-standing or if there is any question of heart disease. Because of the high mortality rate in pregnant women with undiagnosed pheochromocytoma, a screening urine metanephrine test may be useful in the evaluation of women with severe hypertension.

Ideally, women of childbearing age who suffer from chronic hypertension should be counseled before they become pregnant, but this is not always possible. A patient with chronic hypertension and a history of severe PIH or eclampsia has at least a 50 percent chance of recurrent PIH, whereas the normotensive patient with a past history of severe PIH or eclampsia has a one-in-four chance of recurrence. Unfortunately, the next episode is often more severe than the prior one and occurs at an earlier stage of pregnancy.

The management of a pregnancy complicated by essential hypertension is controversial. The only point of universal agreement is restriction of physical activity. In addition to increased bed rest, the hypertensive gravida should limit household duties, shopping, and exercise. Dietary counseling is often neglected. Although sodium consumption may exacerbate hypertension, its restriction may decrease placental perfusion. In the appropriate diet, 2 g of sodium or 6 g of table salt per day is not exceeded, but this is not a "low-salt diet." Most patients with mild to moderate hypertension do not require medication during pregnancy.

One of the major unresolved questions in management is whether there is autoregulation of uterine blood flow in humans. If there is no autoregulation, placental perfusion will vary directly with maternal arterial pressure, in which case a reduction in blood pressure might be detrimental to the fetus. On the other hand, if there is autoregulation, a reduction in blood pressure to "normal" would pose no problem. European obstetricians have been more aggressive in their treatment of women with chronic hypertension by attempting to maintain diastolic blood pressure under 90 to 100 mm Hg, but obstetricians in the United States usually do not institute therapy until the diastolic blood pressure exceeds 100 mm Hg because of fetal perfusion considerations.

Two management questions frequently arise: What is the agent of choice, and what course is proper for the pregnant patient who is already on an established antihypertensive regimen? Methyldopa (Aldomet) is the preferred oral medication. The customary initial dose is 750 mg/day (250 mg 3 times a day). This may be increased to a total of 3 g daily, but occasionally it is necessary to add oral hydralazine. Pressures lower than 90 to 100 mm Hg are not desirable because of possible adverse effects on placental perfusion. Medications should not be prescribed for the patient with suspected PIH, but rather for the chronic hypertensive patient whose diastolic pressure exceeds 100 to 110 mm Hg.

Diuretics are contraindicated in pregnancy, except in the rare patient with pulmonary edema or congestive heart failure. Diuretics acutely reduce placental blood flow (as measured by the placental clearance of dehydroisoandrosterone sulfate). Women with chronic hypertension who receive diuretics during pregnancy have lower blood volumes than do hypertensive women who do not receive diuretics. When diuretic use is discontinued, there is then an increase in the plasma volume. Evidence also suggests that the long-term use of diuretics leads to reduced birth weight in the infants of such mothers, while making maternal pancreatitis more likely. Electrolyte disturbances, fetal thrombocytopenia, and neonatal jaundice are also well-established consequences of diuretic therapy. Most authorities discontinue diuretics in their patients once pregnancy is discovered, but oral methyldopa and oral hydralazine may be continued.

Fetal surveillance is important in women with chronic hypertension. In addition to serial ultrasonography, antepartum testing should be performed. Most commonly this consists of a weekly nonstress test, a weekly biophysical profile, or a weekly contraction stress test. In women with mild hypertension, antepartum fetal heart rate tests should be instituted at 34 weeks' gestation. In women with severe hypertension, a history of stillbirths, or a suspicion of an SGA fetus, these tests should be initiated at 28 to 32 weeks.

The timing of delivery is a crucial question in all high-risk pregnancies. This decision is easy when the fetus is mature and the cervix is favorable for induction. Even in the presence of mild hypertension, there is no benefit from procrastination, and a well-monitored induction of labor is indicated. When there is evidence of superimposed PIH or if severe intrauterine growth retardation is suspected, it is necessary to deliver the infant, even if preterm. In this situation, it is comforting to know that maternal hypertension is associated with accelerated maturation of the fetal lungs. After 32 to 34 weeks' gestation, the risk of severe respiratory distress syndrome in the neonate is therefore diminished compared to that in newborns who are products of normal pregnancies of the same duration. When superimposed PIH occurs, convulsions should be prevented by use of magnesium sulfate, and any severe hypertension (systolic pressure >160 mm Hg; diastolic pressure >110 mm Hg) should be controlled with the intravenous administration of hydralazine. Once superimposed PIH is established, delivery is the only cure. Induction of labor with oxytocin is recommended, unless an obstetric indication necessitates cesarean birth.

General

1. Gant, N. F., and Worley, F. J. *Hypertension and Pregnancy.* Norwalk, CT: Appleton-Century-Crofts, 1980.
   An excellent book-length review of both the basic science aspects and clinical management. Includes a critical analysis of major diagnostic and therapeutic questions on this subject.
2. Roberts, J. M., and Perloff, D. L. Hypertension and the obstetrician-gynecologist. *Am. J. Obstet. Gynecol.* 127:316, 1977.
   Concise review of hypertensive problems in the female patient.
3. Rubin, P.C. Hypertension in pregnancy. *J. Hypertension* 5:84, 1987.
   General article that summarizes current practice principles in the management of hypertension in pregnancy.

Etiology

4. Lindheimer, M. D., and Katz, A. I. Hypertension in pregnancy: advances and controversies. *Clin. Nephrol.* 36:4, 1991.
   The advances made and remaining controversies regarding hypertension in pregnancy are discussed.
5. Marx, J. L. Natriuretic hormone linked to hypertension. *Science* 212:1255, 1981.
   The author proposes that excess salt in the diet may produce hypertension by causing the release of a natriuretic hormone into the bloodstream. The effect of this mechanism is outlined.
6. Page, E. W., and Christianson, R. The impact of mean arterial pressure in the middle trimester upon the outcome of pregnancy. *Am. J. Obstet. Gynecol.* 125:740, 1976.
   Presents a simple formula for calculating the mean arterial pressure and demonstrates that perinatal mortality increases as the mean arterial pressure increases.
7. Hunyor, S. N. Vascular, volume, and cardiac response to normal and hypertensive pregnancy. *Hypertension* 6:196, 1984.
   Hypertension during pregnancy may blunt the normal increase in plasma volume.
8. de Boer, K., et al. Enhanced thrombin generation in normal and hypertensive pregnancy. *Am. J. Obstet. Gynecol.* 160:95, 1989.
   The authors studied 79 women who were normotensive compared to 24 who were

hypertensive. In the former, there was an increase in the plasma thrombin–antithrombin III levels and a decrease in the protein S levels, whereas, in the hypertensive patients, there was a reduction in the antithrombin III and protein C levels. The authors conclude that there is evidence for a prethrombotic state in normal pregnancy that is accentuated in those with hypertension.

9. White, W. B., et al. Average daily blood pressure, not office blood pressure, determines cardiac function in patients with hypertension. *J.A.M.A.* 261:873, 1989.
   In this study, 720 patients underwent ambulatory blood pressure monitoring, and, when their readings at home were compared to those in the office, it was found that a significant portion were hypertensive only while visiting the physician.

Diagnosis

10. Sibai, B. M., and Anderson, G. D. Clues from blood volume changes in hypertensive pregnancies. *Contemp. Ob/Gyn* 21:241, 1983.
    Plasma volume determinations are useful in identifying babies at risk for intrauterine growth retardation and intrauterine fetal demise.

11. Nicholas, W. C., et al. Does blood pressure cuff size make a difference in blood pressure readings? *J. Miss. State Med. Assoc.* 26:31, 1985.
    A large error in blood pressure measurement can result from using an inappropriate cuff size.

12. Moutquin, J. M., et al. A prospective study of blood pressure in pregnancy. *Am. J. Obstet. Gynecol.* 151:191, 1985.
    In 1000 patients, the sensitivity of simple but exact blood pressure assessment in predicting preeclampsia 9 to 12 weeks before clinical signs developed was evident.

13. Thompson, J. A., et al. Echocardiographic left ventricular mass to differentiate chronic hypertension from preeclampsia during pregnancy. *Am. J. Obstet. Gynecol.* 155:994, 1986.
    Describes results that indicate increased left ventricular size in chronic hypertensive women.

14. Villar, M. A., and Sibai, B. M. Clinical significance of elevated mean arterial blood pressure in second trimester and threshold increase in systolic or diastolic blood pressure during third trimester. *Am. J. Obstet. Gynecol.* 160:419, 1989.
    The authors studied (longitudinally) 700 normotensive gravidas in an effort to predict preeclampsia. Neither a mean arterial pressure in the second trimester greater than 90 mm Hg nor a threshold increase in the systolic/diastolic blood pressure during the third trimester was predictive.

15. Sibai, B. M. Diagnosis and management of chronic hypertension in pregnancy. *Obstet. Gynecol.* 78:451, 1991.
    The author reviews the diagnosis and management of hypertension in pregnancy and evaluates several treatment trials.

Treatment

16. Lieb, S. M., et al. Nitroprusside-induced hemodynamic alterations in normotensive and hypertensive pregnant sheep. *Am. J. Obstet. Gynecol.* 139:925, 1981.
    The treatment of severe hypertension with sodium nitroprusside was studied in pregnant ewes. This agent was shown to reduce hypertension; the reduction in blood pressure was shown to increase uterine blood flow.

17. Berkowitz, R. L. Anti-hypertensive drugs in the pregnant patient. *Obstet. Gynecol. Surv.* 35:191, 1980.
    A comprehensive and up-to-date review of all ramifications of antihypertensive therapy during pregnancy.

18. Redman, C. W. G., et al. Fetal outcome in trial of antihypertensive treatment in pregnancy. *Lancet* 2:753, 1976.
    Often-quoted paper defending use of methyldopa during pregnancy.

19. Dudley, D. K. L. Minibolus diazoxide in the management of severe hypertension in pregnancy. *Am. J. Obstet. Gynecol.* 151:196, 1985.
    Small dosages of intravenous diazoxide used in 34 patients with severe hypertension produced excellent results compared to those observed for conventional hydralazine therapy.

20. Mirro, R., Miley, J. F., and Holzman, I. R. The effects of sodium nitroprusside on blood flow and oxygen delivery to the organs of the hypoxemic newborn lamb. *Pediatr. Res.* 19:15, 1985.
    The use of nitroprusside, which is normally a vasodilator, can decrease oxygen delivery to vital organs in the fetus and neonate during hypoxia.
21. Black, H. R. Fixed-dose combination therapy for hypertension. *Drug Ther.* 19:80, 1989.
    The authors detail multiple combinations of antihypertensives formulated by a joint committee on the detection, evaluation, and treatment of high blood pressure. This is a must reading for those who treat such patients.
22. Knott, C. The treatment of hypertension in pregnancy—clinical pharmacokinetic considerations. *Clin. Pharmacokinet.* 21:233, 1991.
    The author discusses the pharmacokinetic considerations with regard to different drugs used to treat hypertension in pregnancy.

Complications
23. Sibai, B. M., Abdella, T. N., and Anderson, G. D. Pregnancy outcome in 211 patients with mild chronic hypertension. *Obstet. Gynecol.* 61:571, 1983.
    Presents data on pregnancy outcome in women with mild hypertension.
24. Abdella, T. N., et al. Relationship of hypertensive disease to abruptio placentae. *Obstet. Gynecol.* 63:365, 1984.
    A retrospective review of abruptio placentae in women with hypertension.
25. Mabie, W. C., Pernoll, M. S., and Biswas, M. K. Chronic hypertension in pregnancy. *Obstet. Gynecol.* 67:197, 1986.
    This report describes the outcome of 69 pregnancies in women with chronic hypertension.

7. PREGNANCY-INDUCED HYPERTENSION
Garland D. Anderson

Hypertension unique to pregnancy is best termed *pregnancy-induced hypertension (PIH)*. PIH is synonymous with preeclampsia-eclampsia (eclampsia being an extension of the preeclamptic process) and replaced the older term *toxemia*. Although the cause is unknown, there are many theories; none of these hypotheses, however, fully explain the disease entity. It is likely that the cause of PIH will be found to be multifactorial. Socioeconomic factors, nutritional deficiencies, and slow disseminated intravascular coagulation (DIC) have been postulated as etiologic agents, but may actually be only associated factors. Recent immunologic explanations are intriguing but not proved. There is a familial tendency observed for preeclampsia. In one large follow-up study of eclamptic women, preeclampsia occurred in 27 percent of the first pregnancies of sisters of eclamptic women. In 14 percent of the women who have severe PIH, severe preeclampsia develops in the second pregnancy. Any theory of PIH must explain the following observations: (1) PIH is principally a disease of primigravid women; (2) it is unique to humans; (3) it is associated with a large amount of trophoblast; (4) there is coordination with chronic vascular disease; (5) there is a genetic predisposition; and (6) a viable fetus is not always present.

In terms of the basic physiology involved, hypertension is a consequence of either cardiac output or peripheral vascular resistance. Because the cardiac output remains normal during pregnancy, this shows that PIH is the result of increased peripheral vascular resistance. This vascular resistance is caused by the generalized vasospasm so characteristic of hypertension. Early in normal pregnancy, the mother's arteries become more refractory to the effects of pressor agents such as angiotensin II (the most potent pressor substance). The cause of this normal increase in vascular refractoriness is not known, but prostaglandins do play a role. Many weeks before the onset of clinically detectable PIH, there is a loss of refractoriness to infused angiotensin.

The results of angiotensin infusions can actually predict which normotensive patients are destined to acquire PIH. After the loss of vascular refractoriness to angiotensin, but, before the onset of clinical hypertension, there is a decrease in placental perfusion (as measured by the clearance of dehydroisoandrosterone sulfate). It is now understood that PIH is a chronic disease process and that hypertension occurs relatively late in its course. By the time elevated blood pressure is detected, the disease is well established.

The diagnosis of PIH is determined by the presence of hypertension in conjunction with proteinuria, edema, or both, after the twentieth week of pregnancy. It is primarily a disease of the first pregnancy, and it occurs with higher frequency in younger (adolescent) and older (older than 35) primigravidas. The diagnosis of PIH in the multigravid woman is often incorrect and should be made only after ruling out cardiovascular and renal disease. *Hypertension* is defined as a blood pressure reading of greater than 140/90 mm Hg, or a reading that represents an increase of 30 mm Hg systolic or 15 mm Hg diastolic over the baseline measurements. Two blood pressure readings taken at least 6 hours apart are required for determining this. For example, a blood pressure of 130/80 mm Hg may constitute hypertension in the young primigravida with a previous baseline pressure of 90/50 mm Hg. Proteinuria is a more important diagnostic criterion than is nondependent edema, but both normally occur later than does hypertension. Significant proteinuria is defined as a protein level of 500 mg/dl or more per 24 hours, which approximates a 2+ urinary protein level. Edema is such a common occurrence that it is often not helpful for diagnosis. Nondependent edema is significant, but as many as 8 in 10 normotensive women exhibit dependent edema.

Many authorities differentiate between mild and severe PIH. Mild disease consists of minimal to moderate elevations in blood pressure (systolic, <160 mm Hg; diastolic, <100 mm Hg), nondependent edema, and a proteinuria of less than 2 g in 24 hours. When one or more of the following occur, PIH is classified as severe: blood pressure greater than 160/110 mm Hg, proteinuria greater than 5 g in 24 hours, oliguria (<400 ml in 24 hours), visual blurring or scotomata, and pulmonary edema or cyanosis.

The diagnosis of PIH usually mandates hospitalization, but ambulatory treatment in questionable or mild cases with frequent follow-up also has a place in treating PIH. Management must then be individualized according to the maturity of the fetus and the severity of PIH. If PIH arises at 37 or more weeks' gestation, little can be gained from procrastination. Even in the presence of mild PIH, oxytocin induction is indicated, particularly if the cervix is favorable. Severe PIH, even if associated with a premature fetus, demands intervention. There are also distinct warnings that eclampsia is imminent; these consist of accelerating hypertension, headache, visual blurring or scotomata, epigastric or upper quadrant abdominal pain, and tremulousness. The prompt administration of magnesium sulfate to prevent convulsions is needed when these signs are present.

Conservative management is appropriate only when the fetus is premature and the hypertension is not severe. The patient is allowed a regular hospital diet and light ambulation. Vital signs should be checked four times daily while she is awake. Weight is checked daily, and the urine protein level is checked frequently. Creatinine clearance is determined weekly, and serial sonography is performed every 3 weeks. The mother may be asked to record fetal movements, although nonstress tests, contraction stress tests, biophysical profiles, Coppler blood flow studies, or a combination of these assessment tests is usually conducted weekly or twice weekly in those who are managed conservatively. Biochemical monitoring consisting of the measurement of estriol, human placental lactogen, and pregnancy-specific protein levels is not usually helpful.

Once the patient is hospitalized, a spontaneous diuresis can be expected within the first 24 hours. This diuresis is reflected by a decrease in weight and an improvement in blood pressure, in addition to a large urinary output. If the patient becomes normotensive, it must be decided whether to continue hospitalization until delivery. However, it should be borne in mind that maternal hospital care is often less expensive than the great cost of neonatal intensive care resulting from exacerbation of disease and subsequent premature delivery. For the woman who is unwilling or unable to accept hospitalization, home bed rest with daily blood pressure monitoring is the next best therapy. Whenever severe preeclampsia occurs, management is straightforward and consists of the prevention of convulsions with magnesium sulfate, control of hypertension with intermittent hydralazine therapy, and delivery.

Magnesium sulfate ($MgSO_4 \cdot 7H_2O$ USP) is a safe and efficient agent to prevent convulsions and can be given by the intramuscular or intravenous route. The standard intravenous dose used for many years was a 4-g loading dose (20%) delivered over 5 to 10 minutes followed by 1 g/hr (10 g of $MgSO_4 \cdot 7H_2O$ USP added to 1000 ml of 5% dextrose in lactated Ringer's solution given at 100 ml/hr). Because of the low serum magnesium levels achieved at these dosages, the recommended regimen is now a 4-g to 6-g loading dose delivered over 15 to 20 minutes followed by a maintenance dose of 2 g/hr. The intravenous method requires the use of continuous-infusion pumps, available personnel for infusion monitoring, the documentation of adequate renal function, and preferably the ability to determine serum magnesium levels on a rapid basis. The initial intramuscular dose is 10 g (50%), given after the intravenous loading dose and followed by 5 g given intramuscularly every 4 hours. Each 5 g of $MgSO_4$ consists of 10 ml of a 50% solution that is given in the upper, outer quadrant of the buttock through a 3-inch (7.5-cm), 20-gauge needle. One milliliter of 2% xylocaine can be added to each dose for analgesia.

Maintenance of $MgSO_4$ may be continued without serial measurements of the serum magnesium level if the following criteria are met: (1) patellar reflex is present, (2) respirations are normal, and (3) urine output is at least 100 ml every 4 hours. Before any treatment, the normal serum magnesium level is 1.5 to 2 mEq/liter, whereas the therapeutic maintenance range is 4 to 7 mEq/liter. The earliest sign of magnesium toxicity is loss of the patellar reflex; this occurs at 7 to 10 mEq/liter. Respiratory depression begins at 10 to 15 mEq/liter and cardiac arrest at 30 mEq/liter. Calcium gluconate is the antidote to $MgSO_4$ toxicity and the dose is 1 g (10 ml of a 10% solution) given slowly over 3 minutes. Mechanical respiratory support may be necessary in these cases. An interesting subgroup of women with preeclampsia may present with the HELLP syndrome (hemolysis, elevated liver enzyme levels, and a low platelet count). Other coagulation tests such as the prothrombin time, the fibrinogen level, and partial thromboplastic time are normal. In some women who present with the HELLP syndrome, the diagnosis of PIH is delayed, or they may be diagnosed as having hypertension and begun on antihypertensive therapy. Women who have the HELLP syndrome should be stabilized with $MgSO_4$ treatment and undergo prompt delivery.

Antihypertensive medication is reserved for patients with a diastolic pressure greater than 110 mm Hg, and hydralazine is the drug of choice in this setting. It can be given by intermittent intravenous bolus infusion (5–10 mg); the preferred method is in 5-mg increments. It can also be given by continuous infusion (180 mg in 500 ml of 5% dextrose in water). To prevent hypotension, the continuous infusion should be discontinued when diastolic blood pressures enter the 90 to 100 mm Hg range. Because of vasospasm, the patient with PIH has a contracted blood volume. This knowledge is important in management because volume contraction prohibits either volume expansion or depletion. Injudicious fluid therapy may then precipitate overload and pulmonary edema. In contrast, salt restriction or the use of diuretics may cause decreased placental perfusion. As a consequence of the diminished blood volume, the patient with PIH cannot withstand the same degree of blood loss at delivery that a normal woman can. A sudden reduction in blood pressure at delivery is usually the result of a profound blood loss.

Invasive hemodynamic monitoring has proved helpful in the management of a subset of patients with severe PIH and additional complications such as pulmonary edema, oliguria unresponsive to fluid challenge, sepsis, and the clinical need for blood transfusion or massive volume replacement. The pulmonary artery catheter is the technology of choice, owing to the limited and erroneous information that a central venous pressure may reveal in a patient with PIH.

Severe PIH and its sequela, eclampsia, are largely preventable. The key to prevention is astute management. Patient education, close monitoring, and attention to subtle detail can reduce the morbidity, mortality, and expense associated with this disease.

General

1. Cunningham, F. G. et al. Hypertensive Disorders in Pregnancy. In *Williams Obstetrics* (19th ed.). Norwalk, CT: Appleton & Lange, 1993.
   A most complete review of PIH.
2. Soutte, W. P. The haemodynamic pathophysiology of preeclampsia. *S. Afr. Med. J.* 58:351, 1980.
   Reviews the hemodynamic characteristics of PIH. The overall role of therapeutic management is discussed.

Etiology

3. Yamaguchi, M., and Mori, N. 6-Keto prostaglandin F_{1a}, thromboxane B_2, and 13,14-dihydro-15-keto prostaglandin F concentrations of normotensive and preeclamptic patients during pregnancy, delivery, and the postpartum period. *Am. J. Obstet. Gynecol.* 151:121, 1985.
   This elegant article giving details on the metabolites of prostaglandins demonstrates that prostacyclin plays an important role in the etiology of preeclampsia.
4. Page, E. W. On the pathogenesis of pre-eclampsia and eclampsia. *Br. J. Obstet. Gynaecol.* 79:883, 1972.
   A most complete work regarding the pathogenesis of preeclampsia and eclampsia. This work promotes McKay's theory regarding DIC.
5. Jouppila, P., et al. Failure of exogenous prostacyclin to change placental and fetal blood flow in preeclampsia. *Am. J. Obstet. Gynecol.* 151:661, 1985.
   Prostaglandins, specifically a deficiency in prostacyclin, are thought to be intimately involved with the development of preeclampsia. In this study, prostacyclin was given to 13 women with the disease, but no change in placental or umbilical blood flow occurred.
6. Zlutnik, F. K., et al. Dietary protein and preeclampsia. *Am. J. Obstet. Gynecol.* 90:837, 1983.
   The relationship of protein intake to the incidence of preeclampsia is examined.
7. Alderman, B. W. An epidemiological study of the immunogenetic aetiology of preeclampsia. *Br. Med. J.* 292:372, 1986.
   Presents a population-based study evaluating the incidence of PIH compared to race dissimilarities of the father and mother.
8. Benedetto, C., et al. Reduced serum inhibition of platelet-activating factor activity in preeclampsia. *Am. J. Obstet. Gynecol.* 160:100, 1989.
   The authors carefully studied women with preeclampsia, looking specifically at the inhibition of platelet-activating factor activity. They found this in most of the preeclamptics and consider that it might contribute toward the hemostatic defect noted in these patients.
9. Arngrimsson, R., et al. Genetic and familial predisposition to eclampsia and preeclampsia in a defined population. *Br. J. Obstet. Gynaecol.* 97:762, 1990.
   The authors discuss the role of genetic and familial predisposition in the development of eclampsia and preeclampsia.
10. Zuspan, F. P. New concepts in the understanding of hypertensive disorders of pregnancy: an overview. *Clin. Perinatol.* 18:643, 1991.
    The authors present the new concept regarding the pathophysiology of preeclampsia.

Diagnosis

11. Phelan, J. P., et al. Severe preeclampsia. I. Peripartum hemodynamic monitoring. *Am. J. Obstet. Gynecol.* 144:17, 1982.
    The cardiovascular changes that occur in the setting of severe preeclampsia are described for women who underwent Swan-Ganz monitoring during labor.
12. Chesley, L. C. Diagnosis of preeclampsia. *Obstet. Gynecol.* 65:423, 1985.
    The diagnosis of mild preeclampsia may be wrong in more than half of the cases,

although the clinical management appears to be correct for those women suspected of having the disorder.

13. Hays, P. M., Cruikshank, D. P., and Dunn, L. J. Plasma volume determination in normal and preeclamptic pregnancies. *Am. J. Obstet. Gynaecol.* 151:958, 1985.
    Plasma volume determination using the Evans blue technique was performed in normal and preeclamptic patients. Those who were preeclamptic had a smaller plasma volume expansion and their offspring were more likely to be growth retarded.

14. Sibai, B. M., et al. Effect of magnesium sulfate on electroencephalographic findings in preeclampsia-eclampsia. *Obstet. Gynecol.* 64:261, 1984.
    Abnormal electroencephalographic recordings are common in patients with severe preeclampsia and are not altered by $MgSO_4$ treatment.

15. Romero, R., et al. Clinical significance, prevalence, and natural history of thrombocytopenia in pregnancy-induced hypertension. *Am. J. Perinatol.* 6:32, 1989.
    The authors of this study found that thrombocytopenia was encountered in 11.6 percent of the patients with PIH and, when present, was correlated with a higher incidence of preterm delivery and intrauterine growth retardation. The lowest platelet count usually appeared 48 hours after delivery and recovery likewise took 2 additional days.

Treatment

16. Berkowitz, R. Anti-hypertensive drugs in the pregnant patient. *Obstet. Gynecol. Surv.* 35:81, 1980.
    Comprehensive, recent review of all the ramifications of antihypertensive therapy during pregnancy.

17. Sibai, B. M., et al. Reassessment of intravenous $MgSO_4$ therapy in preeclampsia-eclampsia. *Obstet. Gynecol.* 57:199, 1981.
    The authors indicate that the standard dosage of $MgSO_4$ may be insufficient for many patients; they recommend adjusting the intravenous dosage of $MgSO_4$ for each patient.

18. Sibai, B. M., Graham, J. M., and McCubbin, J. H. A comparison of intravenous and intramuscular magnesium sulfate regimens in preeclampsia. *Am. J. Obstet. Gynecol.* 150;728, 1984.
    Intravenously and intramuscularly administered $MgSO_4$ was used in patients with severe preeclampsia. At 1 g/hr given, intravenously, the circulating level was significantly lower than that associated with the intramuscular regimen.

19. Mabie, W. C., et al. A comparative trial of labetalol and hydralazine in the acute management of severe hypertension complicating pregnancy. *Obstet. Gynecol.* 70:134, 1987.
    Study describes the use of labetalol in the treatment of a hypertensive crisis, compared to hydralazine treatment. Supports the contention that labetalol may be a safe and effective alternative.

20. Schwartz, M. L., and Brenner, W. Severe preeclampsia with persistent postpartum hemolysis and thrombocytopenia treated by plasmapheresis. *Obstet. Gynecol.* 65:53S, 1985.
    Plasmapheresis was used to treat a patient with severe PIH, with good results.

21. Clark, S. L., et al. Severe preeclampsia with persistent oliguria. Management of hemodynamic subsets. *Am. J. Obstet. Gynecol.* 154:3, 1986.
    Based on results of the study, the authors advise treatment based on hemodynamic variables evaluated by means of pulmonary artery catheterization.

22. Clark, S. L., and Cotton, D. B. Clinical indications for pulmonary artery catheterization in the patient with severe preeclampsia. *Am. J. Obstet. Gynecol.* 158:3, 1988.
    The authors review their own past experience with invasive hemodynamic monitoring in PIH patients, and recommend its use in those women who are unresponsive to antihypertensives, develop pulmonary edema, or have persistent oliguria, and in some patients requiring conduction anesthesia.

23. Ramanathon, J. Anesthetic considerations in pre-eclampsia. *Clin. Perinatol.* 18:876, 1991.
    The author discusses the special factors that should be considered before giving anesthesia to the woman with preeclampsia.

8. ECLAMPSIA   *(0% mortality)*
Garland D. Anderson

Eclampsia is the extension of pregnancy-induced hypertension (PIH) to the point of convulsion, coma, or both. Eclampsia can cause significant morbidity and mortality in both the mother and baby. The maternal mortality rate may be as high as 10 percent, and the perinatal mortality rate ranges from 8.6 to 27.8 percent. Fortunately, eclampsia is a largely preventable illness. The following are considered warnings that convulsion is imminent: acceleration of hypertension, epigastric right upper quadrant abdominal pain, visual blurring or scotomata, headache, and tremulousness. The presence of any of these signs demands the prompt administration of magnesium sulfate ($MgSO_4$). However, approximately 20 percent of the women in whom eclampsia develops have only mildly elevated blood pressure (80–90 mm Hg diastolic), often without proteinuria or edema. For this reason, all patients in labor who meet the blood pressure criterion of PIH should receive $MgSO_4$ therapy.

The cause of eclamptic convulsions is unknown. Both cerebral vasospasm and cerebral edema are incriminated but unproved as etiologic agents. One half of the cases of convulsions occur before labor, one fourth during labor, and most of the remainder within 48 hours postpartum. Occasionally, eclampsia arises before 20 weeks' gestation and often 48 hours postpartum. Eclampsia appearing more than 48 hours postpartum is relatively common, and now represents 10 percent of the total cases of eclampsia. The most striking feature of eclampsia that arises later than 48 hours postpartum is an immediate diuresis after the convulsion. Urine outputs greater than 500 ml in the first hour after the seizure are common. The seizures are grand mal in character, and typically there is no antecedent aura. Tongue biting, urinary and fecal incontinence, injury from falls, and occasionally fractures are observed, as are transient apnea and cyanosis.

Care during the actual convulsion consists of gentle constraint and maintenance of an airway, then the administration of oxygen as soon as the convulsion ceases. A chest x-ray study is obtained to rule out aspiration. Blood is drawn for a complete blood count, liver profile, and serum electrolyte measurements, and an indwelling catheter is placed in the bladder for the measurement of hourly urine output. A stage of agitation is common after the postictal patient regains partial consciousness. A quiet room with subdued light and the presence of a family member are helpful. The management of eclampsia is straightforward. The convulsions are treated, blood pressure is controlled, and delivery is accomplished as soon as possible after stabilization of the mother's condition. Timing of delivery does not depend on the maturity of the fetus.

The agent of choice for the treatment of convulsions is $MgSO_4$. The following regimen has proved efficacious: 4 to 6 g of $MgSO_4$ in 20% solution given intravenously over 5 to 10 minutes, followed by a continuous maintenance infusion of 2 g/hr if there is no sign of maternal respiratory depression. If the patient has a recurrent seizure, another bolus of 2 to 4 g of $MgSO_4$ can be given over 3 to 5 minutes. We no longer use the maintenance dose of 1 g/hr of $MgSO_4$, because this does not achieve therapeutic levels. Occasionally the maintenance dose has to be increased to greater than 2 g/hr if the urinary output is high. Another regimen frequently used is 4 g of $MgSO_4$ given intravenously over 4 minutes, followed immediately by 5 g (50%) given intramuscularly in each buttock and an intramuscular injection of 5 g every 4 hours. This 14-g loading dose can be given safely to any patient who has not already received $MgSO_4$. Another convulsion within 20 minutes or more after the initial dose is treated with additional intravenously administered (10%) MgSO₄ (with 2 g delivered slowly intravenously if the patient weighs less than 55 kg, or 4 g if the patient weighs more than 55 kg). The routine use of intravenous diazepam (Valium) or phenytoin sodium (Dilantin) in addition to the MgSO₄ should be avoided if possible. These combinations may lead to aspiration, respiratory distress, or cardiac arrest. Only rarely does the patient continue to convulse after the second intravenous bolus of MgSO₄. In these rare instances, intravenous sodium amobarbital (Amytal), titrated as needed, may be helpful.

MgSO₄ causes a peripheral neuromuscular blockage through interference with acetylcholine release and action. This is clinically important if succinylcholine is used, because less of the muscle relaxant is then required for cesarean delivery or other surgical procedures. The synergism between MgSO₄ and succinylcholine explains the cases of prolonged muscle paralysis that arise postoperatively. Vasodilatation and a central cerebral sedative effect are also noted as actions of MgSO₄. Before any therapy, the normal serum magnesium level is 1.5 to 2.0 mEq/liter. After a loading dose of 4 g, given intravenously, and the maintenance infusion of 1 g of MgSO₄ per hour, serum magnesium levels range from 2.2 to 4.1 mEq/liter within 2 hours. The levels return to normal within 6 hours if no further magnesium is given. A maintenance dose of 5 g, given intramuscularly every 4 hours, results in a therapeutic range of between 4 and 7 mEq/liter. Even with a 4-g loading dose of MgSO₄ and 1 g of MgSO₄ per hour, it may take 6 to 8 hours to achieve therapeutic levels. We now recommend a 6-g intravenous loading dose of MgSO₄, followed by a maintenance dose of 2 g/hr, to more rapidly arrive at a reasonable level.

Because magnesium is excreted by the kidneys, renal disease or oliguria requires a reduction in the dose or cessation of MgSO₄ treatment. The earliest sign of magnesium toxicity is loss of the patellar reflex, occurring at 7 to 10 mEq/liter. Respirations are depressed at 10 to 15 mEq/liter and cardiac arrest occurs at about 30 mEq/liter. A maintenance regimen of MgSO₄ (either delivered by the intramuscular or intravenous route) should not be administered without obtaining serial serum magnesium levels, unless the following criteria are confirmed: (1) the patellar reflex is present, (2) respirations are normal, and (3) urine output is at least 100 ml every 4 hours. The intramuscular regimen consists of 5 g given every 4 hours up to 24 hours postpartum, whereas the intravenous maintenance is 2 g/hr up to 24 hours postpartum. Calcium gluconate is the antidote to MgSO₄. The dose in the event of respiratory depression is 1 g (10 ml of a 10% calcium gluconate solution) administered intravenously over 3 minutes. Mechanical respiratory support may be necessary if respiratory depression develops.

The blood pressure may be normal immediately after a convulsion, although the hypertension usually resumes. If the patient remains normotensive or if the convulsion occurs more than 48 hours postpartum, causes of convulsions other than eclampsia should be considered, although eclampsia can occur more than 48 hours postpartum. Other causes include epilepsy, a cerebrovascular accident, central nervous system tumor, electrolyte disturbances, and hypoglycemia.

Intravenously administered hydralazine is the drug of choice to control the hypertension associated with eclampsia. Its use is reserved for a blood pressure of 170/110 mm Hg or greater. Hydralazine is given by intravenous bolus in 5-mg to 10-mg increments every 15 to 20 minutes. Blood pressure is measured every 5 minutes initially and every 15 minutes after becoming stable. The goal of therapy is to maintain the diastolic blood pressure between 90 and 100 mm Hg. If the diastolic blood pressure drops below 90 mm Hg, the injections should be discontinued. One may begin with 5 mg and increase (if necessary) in 5-mg increments until the diastolic pressure is 90 to 100 mm Hg. Rarely, hypotensive episodes may occur. Because hydralazine has a relatively long half-life, care must be taken to avoid hypotension.

The definitive cure of eclampsia is delivery, although it is best to wait until the mother's condition is stable on MgSO₄ therapy before proceeding to effect delivery. This is usually accomplished 4 to 8 hours after the last convulsion. Even if the cervix is unfavorable for induction, oxytocin stimulation may be successful. The fetus should be carefully monitored during labor. Many fetuses of eclamptic women have intrauterine growth retardation. They may have little placental reserve and may not tolerate labor. The incidence of placental abruption is also greatly increased in the setting of eclampsia, and this may lead to sudden fetal distress. The exception is the woman at less than 32 weeks' gestation, particularly if she has a long uneffaced cervix. In this type of woman, one usually opts for cesarean delivery.

The eclamptic patient, like the one with severe PIH, has a contracted blood volume. Hemoconcentration is a consistent finding. Puerperal hemorrhage, even of a magnitude tolerated by the normal pregnant patient, can lead to the dangerous underperfusion of vital organs in the eclamptic women. A sudden reduction in blood pressure at the time of delivery or immediately postpartum is usually the consequence of excessive blood loss. Because of their contracted blood volume, women with eclampsia should be typed and crossmatched for blood.

The patient may frequently inquire about the risk of recurrent severe PIH or eclampsia. The young primigravida who has experienced this disease has a much more favorable prognosis than the older multigravida with chronic hypertension and superimposed preeclampsia-eclampsia. There is a one-in-four chance of recurrent PIH if the patient is normotensive. In the setting of chronic hypertension, the recurrence risk is even higher. Women who suffer eclampsia do not appear to exhibit an increased incidence of hypertension later in life.

General
1. Villar, M. A., and Sibai, B. M. Eclampsia. *Obstet. Gynecol. North Am.* 15:355, 1968.
   An excellent and thorough review of the diagnosis, treatment, and management of eclampsia.
2. Zuspan, F. P. Toxemia of Pregnancy. In J. J. Sciarra and T. W. McElin (eds.), *Gynecology and Obstetrics,* Vol. 2. Hagerstown, MD: Harper & Row, 1985.
   A 20-page review of all aspects of PIH, with excellent references.
3. Mendlowitz, M. Toxemia of pregnancy and eclampsia. *Obstet. Gynecol. Surv.* 35:327, 1980.
   An in-depth review regarding the basic science aspects of the preeclampsia-eclampsia syndrome, with 70 references.
4. Wright, J. P. Anesthetic consideration in preeclampsia/eclampsia. *Anesth. Analg.* 62:590, 1983.
   A review of the anesthetic considerations in women with eclampsia, with 116 references.
5. Bergsjo, P. Familiar and remote clinical problems: remedies in 1922. *Acta Obstet. Gynecol. Scand.* 71:166, 1992.
   Historical account of the management and outcome of eclampsia in 1922.
6. Sibai, B. M., et al. Eclampsia VII, Pregnancy outcome after eclampsia and long-term prognosis. *Am. J. Obstet. Gynecol.* 166:1757, 1992.
   This article describes the long-term follow-up and prognosis in a large number of women who had eclampsia.

Etiology
7. Porapakkham, S. An epidemiologic study of eclampsia. *Obstet. Gynecol.* 54:26, 1979.
   The epidemiologic characteristics in 298 cases of eclampsia were studied. Inadequate antenatal care was a major factor in maternal and perinatal mortality.
8. Hankins, G. D. V., et al. Longitudinal evaluation of hemodynamic changes in eclampsia. *Am. J. Obstet. Gynecol.* 150:506, 1984.
   Extracellular and extravascular fluid mobilization occurs long after delivery in patients with eclampsia. Fluid management is particularly important in these patients.
9. Pitkin, R. M. Calcium metabolism in pregnancy and the perinatal period: a review. *Am. J. Obstet. Gynecol.* 151:99, 1985.
   Calcium homeostasis may be related to toxemia. This fine review containing 135 references dealing with calcium metabolism may help demonstrate this relationship.

10. Romero, R., et al. Toxemia: new concepts in an old disease. *Semin. Perinatol.* 12:302, 1988.
    Offers a very good diagrammatic depiction of what we know about the cause of toxemia, or PIH, with particular reference to eclampsia. It also contains 291 references.

Diagnosis

11. Sibai, B. M., et al. The late postpartum eclampsia controversy. *Obstet. Gynecol.* 55:74, 1980.
    Purportedly, eclampsia does not occur before the twentieth week and after a few days postpartum. This study deals with women who were diagnosed as eclamptic by exclusion, although the seizures occurred much later than is commonly acceptable for such a diagnosis.
12. Dahmus, M. A., et al. Cerebral imaging in eclampsia: Magnetic resonance imaging versus computed tomography. *Am. J. Obstet. Gynecol.* 167:935, 1992.
    This article focuses on the value of magnetic resonance imaging versus computed tomography in the evaluation of the eclamptic patient.
13. Watson, D. L., et al. Late postpartum eclampsia: an update. *South. Med. J.* 76:1487, 1983.
    The incidence of eclampsia and differential diagnosis in women who develop eclampsia more than 40 hours postpartum are discussed.

Treatment

14. Pritchard, J., and Pritchard, S. A. Standardized treatment of 154 consecutive cases of eclampsia. *Am. J. Obstet. Gynecol.* 123:543, 1975.
    A classic presentation of a successful management protocol prepared by authors with extensive experience.
15. Sibai, B. M., et al. Reassessment of intravenous MgSO₄ therapy in preeclampsia-eclampsia. *Obstet. Gynecol.* 57:199, 1981.
    This reference offers evidence that the current methods of MgSO₄ management in the treatment of eclampsia may not be adequate.
16. Zuspan, F. P., and Zuspan, K. J. Strategies for controlling eclampsia. *Contemp. Ob/Gyn* 18:135, 1981.
    An in-depth review of the therapeutic choices for treating eclampsia, with a detailed section on the delivery of the eclamptic patient.
17. Little, B. C., et al. Treatment of hypertension in pregnancy by relaxation and biofeedback. *Lancet* 1:865,1984.
    Biofeedback is used during pregnancy to lower blood pressure. Postpartum, this may prove helpful in eclamptic patients with high blood pressure.
18. Tondriaux, A., et al. Hemodynamic effects of magnesium sulfate in eclampsia. *Clin. Exp. Hypertens.* [E] 2:405, 1983.
    The hemodynamic effects of MgSO₄ are decreased venous compliance, decreased preload, and reduced cardiac output.
19. Sibai, B. M., et al. Eclampsia treatment and referral. *South. Med. J.* 75:267, 1982.
    Guidelines for the treatment and stabilization of patients for subsequent referral to a tertiary care center are offered.
20. Koontz, W. L., and Reid, K. H. The effect of pretreatment with magnesium sulfate on the initiation of seizure foci in anesthetized cats. *Am. J. Obstet. Gynecol.* 160:508, 1989.
    The effects of parenteral magnesium sulfate before the initiation of seizure foci in anesthetized cats were studied, and no significant difference in terms of benefit was found between the experimental group and the control groups not so treated. The mechanism of magnesium's therapeutic effect remains unknown.

Complications

21. Sibai, B. M., et al. Eclampsia. II. Clinical significance of laboratory findings. *Obstet. Gynecol.* 59:153, 1982.

Describes the significance of the laboratory findings in women with eclampsia.

22. Sibai, B. M., et al. Eclampsia. III. Neonatal outcome, growth and development. *Am. J. Obstet. Gynecol.* 146:307, 1983.
    The short-term follow-up in children whose mothers had eclampsia is detailed.

23. Mansa, K. J., et al. Hepatic hemorrhage without rupture in preeclampsia. *N. Engl. J. Med.* 312:424, 1985.
    Hepatic swelling with subsequent rupture is a dreadful complication of pre-eclampsia-eclampsia. This case report graphically describes such a case.

24. Hill, W. C., Gill, P. J., and Katz, M. Maternal paralytic ileus as a complication of magnesium sulfate tocolysis. *Am. J. Perinatol.* 2:47, 1985.
    The use of MgSO₄ for tocolysis or for the treatment of toxemia can result in paralytic ileus if too much of the medication is used, as demonstrated by this case report.

25. Montan, S., and Ingemarsson, I. Intrapartum fetal heart rate patterns in pregnancies complicated by hypertension. *Am. J. Obstet. Gynecol.* 160:283, 1989.
    Hypertensive pregnancies, particularly eclampsia, accounted for more than one fifth of all ominous intrapartum fetal heart rate tracings. A high index of suspicion for fetal distress should be kept in mind when eclampsia is diagnosed.

III. INFECTIONS IN PREGNANCY

9. VIRAL INFECTIONS DURING PREGNANCY
G. Rodney Meeks

Approximately 5 percent of pregnancies are complicated by maternal viral infections. Nonspecific infections such as the common cold are common, and fortunately mild. However, some infections are of considerable consequence. The proportion of congenital anomalies (3–6% of all infants) and spontaneous abortion (15–30% of all conceptions) directly attributable to viral infections is unknown. Viruses may cause localized or generalized infection of the fetus, inflammation of the placenta, chromosomal aberrations, or direct viral disease in the infant. The ultimate consequence of intrauterine infection may be any of the following: no significant problem, asymptomatic chronic infection, spontaneous abortion or intrauterine death, fetal malformation, or neonatal infection.

Approximately 6 to 11 percent of adult women are susceptible to rubella, an RNA virus. Susceptible individuals have no detectable serum antibodies. Infected individuals develop a typical mild exanthematous rash that is associated with postauricular lymphadenopathy and transient small joint arthralgia. The virus can be isolated from the nasopharynx, but infection is best documented by seroconversion. Hemagglutination inhibition, enzyme-linked immunosorbent assay, and indirect immunoassay are all methods that can detect rubella immunoglobulin M (IgM) and G (IgG) antibodies. Determinations of total rubella antibodies and complement fixation antibodies are now used infrequently. Rubella IgM can be detected with the onset of the rash; the level then peaks at 7 to 10 days and persists for 4 to 6 weeks. It is very specific for the presence of acute infection. If rubella IgM is not detected, this does not definitely exclude rubella infection, because there may be early waning of the antibody. Additional testing that utilizes acute and convalescent serum for the detection of rubella IgG is necessary. A substantial rise in the level of IgG antibodies confirms the diagnosis.

Primary rubella infection is associated with congenital infection in 80 percent of the conceptuses, and fetal anomalies, including cataracts, congenital heart defects, and neurosensory deafness, afflict approximately one fourth of the infected infants. The risk of anomalies is dependent on the gestational age. The risk of congenital defects is 90 percent when maternal infection occurs before 11 weeks' gestation, and this falls to 25 percent at 16 weeks' gestation. When infection occurs between 16 and 20 weeks, congenital defects are rare and seem to be confined to deafness, although the deafness may be severe. No congenital defects have been documented in infants when maternal infection occurs after 20 weeks' gestation. The spontaneous abortion rate in women who have rubella in the first trimester is approximately 50 percent. Because the risk of major congenital defects is great when maternal rubella occurs in the first trimester, termination of pregnancy should be considered. In addition, congenitally infected infants shed the virus and pose a threat to susceptible women.

Rubella vaccination is recommended for children at 12 to 15 months of age and for nonimmune women of childbearing age. The currently available live attenuated vaccines induce antibody formation 95 percent of the time, and more than 90 percent of vaccinated individuals have detectable antibody after 18 years. Although there is no evidence that rubella vaccine causes birth defects, on theoretic grounds alone, vaccination should be avoided during pregnancy. Susceptible puerperal women should be vaccinated. The virus may be shed in breast milk, but this seems to pose no threat to the fetus.

Acute viral hepatitis is manifested by malaise, fatigue, anorexia, nausea, right upper quadrant pain, jaundice, and cytomegaly. With the onset of symptoms, the serum concentrations of alanine aminotransferase (ALT; previously SGPT), aspartate aminotransferase (AST; previously SGOT), and bilirubin increase. With severe infection, coagulation abnormalities and hyperammonemia may also be present. Liver biopsy is rarely indicated, but may be performed for the purpose of excluding other liver diseases, even during pregnancy.

Hepatitis B, which is caused by a small DNA virus, is the most common of the five types of viral hepatitis that have been identified. Acute hepatitis B occurs in 2 per 1000 pregnancies and chronic hepatitis B occurs in 15 per 1000 pregnancies. Acute infection is documented by the presence of surface antigens (HBsAg) and the IgM core antibody (HBcAb). The presence of HBeAg indicates active viral replication. Chronic infection is associated with the persistence of HBsAg. Hepatitis B can be transmitted by either parental or sexual contact. Of great importance is the risk of vertical transmission. Approximately 20 percent of HBsAg-positive women who do not undergo immunoprophylaxis transmit the virus to their neonates. If HBeAg is present, the rate of transmission is 90 percent. Transmission is also dependent on gestational age. When acute maternal infection occurs in the first trimester, 10 percent of the neonates are seropositive for HBsAg, and this rises to 90 percent if infection occurs in the third trimester. Exposure to maternal blood and genital tract secretions is responsible for 90 percent of the transmissions, and transplacental dissemination of virus, breast-feeding, and personal contact account for the remaining 10 percent.

Prevention of infection is of paramount importance, because antiviral agents are not effective. Recombinant DNA vaccines produce seroconversion in 95 percent of the recipients and confer protection for up to 9 years. The Centers for Disease Control (CDC) now recommends the universal immunization of all infants. Infants of seronegative mothers should be vaccinated before discharge from the hospital and infants of seropositive mothers, within 12 hours of birth. In addition, infants of seropositive mothers should receive hepatitis B immune globulin. Combined active and passive immunization is 95 percent effective in preventing perinatal infection. All women should be routinely screened for HBsAg. If the screen yields positive results, further testing is necessary to delineate whether the infection is acute or chronic. Chronic carriers are at risk for suffering subsequent sclerosis and hepatocellular carcinoma.

The most common congenital infection in the United States and England is cytomegalovirus (CMV), which occurs in 0.5 to 1.5 percent of live births. This herpes-type virus can be spread from person to person by multiple routes, including venereal contacts. Most cases are asymptomatic. The virus may be cultured from the urine, nasopharynx, or cervix in 3 to 5 percent of pregnant women. Viral culture is the best way to document infection. Detection of the specific CMV IgM antibody is the most sensitive indication of primary infection, but it may persist for 9 months. Measurement of acute and convalescent IgG levels can help in the diagnosis of secondary infection. Congenital infections may arise after either primary or recurrent maternal infection. An additional 3 to 5 percent of neonates may become infected by exposure to infected cervical secretions, by the ingestion of infected breast milk, or by close oral contact. As many as 10 percent of these children may exhibit symptoms.

Therapeutic abortion is warranted in the rare situation of diagnosed primary maternal infection occurring early in pregnancy because of the teratogenic potential of CMV. The prognosis for those infants with obvious disease at birth is poor. Central nervous system abnormalities and perceptual disabilities are common. CMV represents an immense public health problem because of the potential for infection in large numbers of mothers and their offspring.

Venereal transmission of herpes simplex virus (HSV), a DNA virus, is common. The appearance of vesicles associated with pruritus, burning, or hyperesthesia of the skin is diagnostic. The vesicles form flat, nonindurated ulcers 2 to 5 mm in diameter that have a grayish white base, are extremely tender and painful, and resolve in 2 to 4 weeks, unless they become secondarily infected. Recurrent disease is less debilitating and has a shorter course. After infections, IgM antibodies are identifiable. Viral cultures, however, remain the most accurate way to confirm diagnosis. Transplacental herpes infection may result in spontaneous abortion or congenital infection, but this is much less likely than that that can occur with CMV or rubella infection. The incidence of neonatal HSV infection is 1 per 2000 live births. Ascending infection via the cervix is also rare in the absence of rupture of the membranes. Passage through an infected birth canal is the most significant cause of infection. The risk of systemic infection in an infant born vaginally to a mother with active primary infection is 40 to 80 percent, whereas the risk for an infant born to a mother with active recurrent infection is 5 percent. Systemic neonatal herpes carries a 60 to 90 percent mortality rate, and virtually no neonate is left unscathed. Unfortunately, 70 percent of the infants who acquire neonatal HSV are born to women with no clinical evidence of infection; therefore, the infection in these infants is not always preventable.

Viral cultures should be performed in women with symptoms of or exposure to HSV infection. Subsequent cultures in late pregnancy should be performed only if suspicious lesions or symptoms occur. If careful examination reveals the presence of no suspicious lesions when the woman is in labor, the fetus may be delivered vaginally. In women with recently positive culture results or with active lesions who present in labor, delivery should be accomplished by cesarean section. If the membranes have ruptured, cesarean section is still indicated, regardless of duration. Adenosine arabinoside has been effective in treating neonatal herpetic encephalitis, and acyclovir is capable of modifying the mucocutaneous lesions in the mother and baby, but has not yet been approved for use in pregnancy.

Approximately 15 percent of the women of childbearing age are susceptible to varicella, a herpes-type virus that is spread by direct contact. The macular rash involved progresses to become crops of pruritic lesions that may be seen at various stages (vesicular to crusting), and are more likely to be seen on the trunk. Approximately 5 percent of susceptible women who become infected with varicella during the first 16 weeks of gestation will bear children with congenital defects. Neonates of mothers infected during pregnancy usually escape severe infection because antibody of maternal origin is present and this alters the course of their disease. However, 30 percent of the infants whose mothers are infected within 4 days of delivery suffer severe disseminated infection, presumably because they have no maternal antibody protection. Infants born to these mothers should receive high-titer varicella-zoster immune globulin, which provides protection through passive immunity, and also alters the course of the disease in the event of severe neonatal infection.

The human immunodeficiency virus (HIV) is responsible for producing the acquired immunodeficiency syndrome (AIDS). This retrovirus may be transmitted by sexual contact, exposure to infected blood or blood products, or perinatal transmission from the mother to the fetus or neonate. The thymic-derived T-helper lymphocyte (T4) fully supports viral replication, and is clearly a major target of the virus. Women at high risk for getting AIDS include (1) those who have used illegal intravenous drugs, (2) those native to countries where heterosexual transmission is significant, (3) those who engage in prostitution, and (4) those who are or have been sexual partners of men who abuse drugs, are bisexual, have hemophilia, are native to countries where heterosexual transmission is significant, or have evidence of HIV infection.

The CDC has proposed a hierarchical classification system for HIV infection. Currently, the stage of infection is designated by Roman numerals. Group I represents initial infection, proved by seroconversion for the HIV antibody; most patients in this group are asymptomatic. Group II is asymptomatic infection but there are laboratory-detected abnormalities, such as anemia, leukopenia, and a decreased T-helper lymphocyte count (less than $400/mm^3$). The T4/T8 ratio (helper lymphocyte to suppressor lymphocyte ratio) is less than 1 in 75 percent of these patients. Group III constitutes persistent generalized lymphadenopathy, and patients in group IV have other constitutional diseases such as diarrhea, myelopathy, and opportunistic infections (*Pneumocystis carinii* pneumonia, toxoplasmosis, tuberculosis, and cervical cancer). For the most part, patients in group IV are designated as having AIDS, and those in groups II and III are designated as having the AIDS-related complex (ARC). Infection with HIV is documented by enzyme immunoassay (EIA) and a confirmatory Western blot assay. These tests should be repeated for confirmation, when results are positive. The sensitivity of EIA is 99 percent when performed under optimal conditions. Therefore, the probability of a false-negative result is remote, except in those weeks just following initial infection. The specificity is also 99 percent when repeatedly reactive tests are considered.

Perinatal transmission is principally responsible for the cases of AIDS among infants and children. The presence of AIDS in an infant indicates a substantial risk in the mother and an increased risk in subsequent siblings for the development of AIDS. This is true, even if the mother exhibited no evidence of ARC or AIDS during the index pregnancy. For infants infected in utero, the median interval from birth to the appearance of symptoms is 8 months. A dysmorphic syndrome, consisting of microcephaly, prominent boxlike forehead, flattened nasal bridge, wide palpebral fissures, hypertelorism, blue sclerae, and short philtrum, has been described in association with in utero infection. Women who are pregnant or contemplating pregnancy should be tested for HIV. Women who are at high risk for HIV infection or women who have been repeatedly exposed to the virus should be tested repeatedly, because seroconversion may not take place for up to 4 months after exposure (although a frequency has not been determined). Seropositive pregnant women should be counseled regarding their own risk as well as the fetal and neonatal risk. Women with T4 (CD4) counts less than 500/mm^3 should receive zidovudine prophylaxis. Because the risk of developing opportunistic infections is great in infected women, those with T4 counts less than 200/mm^3 should be treated with trimethoprim, sulfamethoxazole, and pentamidine. The effects of these medications on the fetus have not been fully evaluated. Neonatal jaundice may occur when any sulfa medication is taken during late pregnancy. Seropositive women should not breast-feed. The isolation practices in these patients are not different from those adopted in patients with other infectious diseases, such as hepatitis.

Rubeola, mumps, influenza, smallpox, and vaccinia have all been proved to cause perinatal infection and congenital malformations. However, a consistent pattern of congenital deformities, newborn infections, or increased early abortion has not been documented in the setting of these infections.

Rubella

1. Herrman, K. L. Rubella in the United States: toward a strategy for disease control and elimination. *Epidemiol. Infect.* 107:43, 1991.
   A mechanism by which susceptible women are identified and then immunized is outlined.
2. Rubella and Pregnancy. *ACOG Tech. Bull.* No. 171, August 1992.
   Management recommendations are outlined for the identification of seronegative individuals and for the immunization of children, adolescents, and adults. An outline for the documentation of suspected rubella infection is also provided.
3. Freij, B. J., South, M. A., and Sever, J. L. Maternal rubella and the congenital rubella syndrome. *Clin. Perinatol.* 15:247, 1988.
   The most common abnormalities in the congenital rubella syndrome are hearing loss, mental retardation, cardiac malformation, and eye defects. Diabetes mellitus, thyroid disease, and glaucoma are delayed manifestations.
4. Munro, N. D., et al. Temporal relations between maternal rubella and congenital defects. *Lancet* 2:201, 1987.
   Approximately 80 percent of the infants whose mothers had rubella at less than 12 weeks' gestation became infected, and all had congenital defects. Only 25 percent of the infants whose mothers had rubella beyond 17 weeks' gestation became infected, and the risk of congenital rubella is small after the seventeenth week. At least 40 percent of all infected infants were ultimately able to attend regular school.
5. Preblud, S. R., and Williams, N. M. Fetal risk associated with rubella vaccine: implications for vaccination of susceptible women. *Obstet. Gynecol.* 66:1121, 1985.
   In a registry of pregnant women who received rubella vaccine, the CDC found that the virus could cross the placenta, but no congenital infections occurred. These data support the vaccination of puerperal women.
6. Markowitz, L. E., et al. Patterns of transmission in measles outbreaks in the United States, 1985–1986. *N. Engl. J. Med.* 320:75, 1989.
   Rubella outbreaks during 1985 and 1986 were analyzed by these epidemiologists. Their data suggest that there are deficiencies in the national measles elimination strategy, and that other approaches, such as selective or mass revaccination, may be necessary to prevent continued outbreaks of rubella.

Cytomegalovirus

7. Yow, M. A., et al. Epidemiologic characteristics of cytomegalovirus infection in mothers and their infants. *Am. J. Obstet. Gynecol.* 158:1189, 1988.
   Half of the pregnant women screened for CMV are susceptible. Only 2 percent become infected, but 25 percent of those with primary infection transmit the infection to their fetus. Infected infants are likely to suffer hearing loss, hepatitis, and developmental delay.

8. Doerr, H. W. Cytomegalovirus infection in pregnancy. *J. Virol.* 17:127, 1987.
   Sources of vertical transmission are semen, maternal viremia, ascending genital infection, cervical secretions, breast milk, and saliva. Vertical transmission is more common in the presence of primary maternal infection and may result in deafness, mental retardation, and infection in the infant.

9. Pass, R. F., et al. Young children as a probable source of maternal and congenital cytomegalovirus infection. *N. Engl. J. Med.* 316:1366, 1987.
   The children of women who have an infant with congenital infection are often the source of such infection.

10. Stagno, S., et al. Primary infection in pregnancy. Incidence, transmission and clinical outcome. *J.A.M.A.* 256:1904, 1986.
    Primary CMV infection varies from 1 to 3 percent, and vertical transmission occurs in one third of these cases. An adverse outcome is most likely if infection occurs during the first trimester.

Herpes

11. Hirsch, M. S. Treatment of herpes virus infections (Part 2). *N. Engl. J. Med.* 309:1034, 1984.
    The current therapy for neonates infected with one of the herpes family of viruses is outlined. Although not ideal, these new drugs, specifically acyclovir, offer great promise.

12. Prover, C. G., et al. Use of routine viral cultures at delivery to identify neonates exposed to herpes simplex virus. *N. Engl. J. Med.* 318:887, 1988.
    In a general population, 0.2 percent of asymptomatic women were noted to shed HSV. It seems that most neonatal exposure cannot be predicted.

13. Perinatal herpes simplex infections. *ACOG Tech. Bull.* No. 122, November 1988.
    The most recent American College of Obstetricians and Gynecologists recommendations on the management of patients with HSV infection are outlined. Cultures are not recommended for asymptomatic women with a history of past infection. Women who have no identifiable lesions are candidates for vaginal delivery.

14. Toltzis, P. Current issues in neonatal herpes simplex virus infection. *Clin. Perinatol.* 2:193, 1991.
    The methods for establishing an accurate diagnosis, prevention strategies, pitfalls, and fetal and neonatal risks are discussed.

15. Brown, A. Z., et al. Effects on infants of a first episode of genital herpes during pregnancy. *N. Engl. J. Med.* 317:1246, 1987.
    Primary maternal infection with HSV is associated with serious perinatal morbidity in 40 percent of the infants of such pregnancies. Primary infection is also associated with premature birth, intrauterine growth retardation, and neonatal infection.

Varicella

16. Weibel, R. E., et al. Live attenuated varicella virus vaccine. Efficacy trial in healthy children. *N. Engl. J. Med.* 310:1409, 1984.
    A vaccine for varicella was 100 percent effective in preventing the disease in 468 children. No spread to sibling controls or pregnant women was noted.

17. Peryani, S. G., and Arvin, A. M. Intrauterine infection with varicella-zoster virus after maternal varicella. *N. Engl. J. Med.* 314:1542, 1987.
    The occurrence of maternal morbidity and mortality is increased during pregnancy, and morbidity includes pneumonia and premature labor. The varicella syndrome seems to occur in 10 percent of the infants delivered to women with varicella. No associated risks were noted for herpes zoster.

18. Higa, K., Dan, K., and Manabe, H. Varicella-zoster virus infection during pregnancy: hypothesis concerning the mechanism of congenital malformations. *Obstet. Gynecol.* 69:214, 1987.
Congenital infection seems to be limited to those infants who contracted varicella in the first 20 weeks of gestation. Clinical features include abnormalities of the skin, peripheral nervous system, and autonomic nervous system, or those attributed to encephalitis.

Human Immunodeficiency Virus
19. MacGregor, S. N. Human immunodeficiency virus in pregnancy. *Clin. Perinatol.* 1:33, 1991.
All aspects of AIDS are discussed. What practicing physicians can do to educate the public, to identify women at risk, and to manage women who are seropositive for HIV is emphasized. The medical, social, and ethical dilemmas faced by obstetricians as HIV infection becomes more common are discussed.
20. Weiss, S. H. HIV infection and the health care worker. *Med. Clin. North Am.* 1:269, 1992.
Precautions to prevent the transmission of HIV and other pathogens to health-care workers and the risks to patients posed by seropositive health-care workers are detailed. Emphasis is placed on the CDC recommendations regarding the performance of invasive procedures.
21. Minkoff, H. L., et al. Serious infections during pregnancy among women with advanced immunodeficiency virus infection. *Am. J. Obstet. Gynecol.* 162:30, 1990.
Serious infections occur in seropositive pregnant women who had CD4 counts less than 300/mm³, while the rate of infections in seropositive women with counts greater than 300/mm³ was similar to that in seronegative women.
22. Minkoff, H. L., et al. Pregnancies resulting in infants with acquired immunodeficiency syndrome or AIDS-related complex. *Obstet. Gynecol.* 69:285, 1987.
Few of the mothers in this series were symptomatic. Low birth weight, preterm birth, and premature rupture of membranes were common. The age at which infected children became symptomatic did not correlate with the birth weight, gestational age, status of membranes, or mode of delivery.
23. Falloon, J., et al. Human immunodeficiency virus infection in children. *J. Pediatr.* 114:1, 1989.
This is the most complete article on children with HIV infection yet to be published. It has 244 references and offers a wealth of information helpful in counseling women who are pregnant or just given birth.

10. URINARY TRACT INFECTION IN PREGNANCY
Mendley A. Wulfsohn

Urinary tract infection (UTI) in pregnancy may be asymptomatic or symptomatic. To detect asymptomatic bacteriuria (ASB), which occurs in 4 to 7 percent of pregnant women, a routine urine assessment, most often a urinalysis and urine culture, should be performed at the first prenatal visit. A higher incidence of ASB is associated with multiparity as well as the sickle cell trait, and it is found more commonly in the lower socioeconomic group.

Symptomatic UTI most often reflects an exacerbation of preexisting ASB, facilitated by the changes that take place in the urinary tract during pregnancy. Patients who have an antenatal history of UTI and are found to have ASB in early pregnancy have a considerable chance of acquiring active UTI during pregnancy. In addition, women with a previous history of UTI have a 35 to 50 percent chance of having ASB and may develop active UTI in late pregnancy. Therefore, despite initially negative urine culture results at the first visit, further culture should be done in this group of women at the beginning of the third trimester. Patients who have an initially positive culture result usually remain positive throughout pregnancy, unless they receive treatment, and acute pyelonephritis may develop in 28 to 65 percent of them, compared to only 1 percent of the women with negative culture findings. It has been conclusively shown that progression to pyelonephritis can be effectively prevented in 97 percent of the cases by adequate antibiotic treatment of ASB.

Persistence or recurrence of infection despite adequate treatment suggests the presence of an underlying urologic disease, such as vesicoureteral reflux, obstructive uropathy, or urinary tract calculi. This is an indication for a urologic workup once the pregnancy has been terminated.

Symptomatic UTI may be confined to the bladder, and cause cystitis, or may be manifested as acute pyelonephritis. The initial symptoms of cystitis consist of frequent urination, nocturia, urgency, and suprapubic discomfort. Hemorrhagic cystitis occasionally occurs. Cystitis must be distinguished from urethral syndrome (frequency-urgency syndrome), interstitial cystitis, and the physiologic frequency occurring during pregnancy. Patients with simple cystitis are usually afebrile, and the diagnosis rests on positive culture findings.

Acute pyelonephritis is more serious and is most commonly caused by *Escherichia coli*. Less commonly offending organisms are the *Klebsiella, Enterobacter, Proteus,* and *Pseudomonas* species. Rarely, gram-positive cocci (e.g., coagulase-negative staphylococci and enterococci) are found. Ascending infection from the bladder is more likely to occur during gestation, accounting for the increased incidence of acute pyelonephritis during pregnancy. The usual presentation consists of acute flank pain and tenderness, more commonly on the right side. Irritative bladder symptoms as well as fever and chills are usually present because bacteremia is common. Pyelonephritis may be a dangerous illness in pregnancy, with a 3 percent incidence of septic shock, and the attendant potential for maternal death. Pyelonephritis may also precipitate premature labor.

Urinary stasis is an important component of the pathophysiologic mechanism responsible for UTI in pregnancy. Hydronephrosis is found on the right side in 90 percent of pregnant women, compared to 60 percent on the left side. Ureteral dilatation begins during the seventh week and progresses until term. The dilated collecting system may hold up to 200 ml of urine, making it an ideal reservoir for UTI. The cause of hydronephrosis and right-sided predominance has never been satisfactorily explained. Obstruction occurs at the level of the pelvic brim because hydronephrosis extends only to this level. The enlarged uterus may compress the ureter against the pelvic brim, and the ovarian veins, which dilate tremendously during late pregnancy, are also implicated. In addition, high progesterone levels may cause ureteral atonicity, as well as hypertrophy of the longitudinal muscle below the pelvic brim (Waldeyer's sheath). The right-sided predominance may stem from the fact that the right ureter crosses the pelvic brim at a sharper angle. In addition, the uterus more commonly lies toward the right, and a right-sided placenta is more common. After delivery, hydronephrosis gradually resolves and is usually completely resolved in all patients by the eighth week postpartum. Other factors that may be important in promoting UTI are the high position of the bladder as well as hypotonicity of the detrusor muscle. A decreased concentrating ability of the kidneys may cause the antibacterial activity of the urine to be diminished. The glycosuria of pregnancy may also lower the patient's resistance to microorganisms.

When UTI does not respond to appropriate therapy, the presence of urinary calculi should be considered. The presence of a urea-splitting organism, particularly one of the *Proteus* species, and a persistently alkaline urine suggests calculus disease. The usual symptoms of severe renal colic may be absent during pregnancy, owing to the poor tone of the ureters. Although most calculi can be treated expectantly, an infected kidney that is obstructed by a ureteral calculus may require emergency decompression by the passage of a ureteral catheter or indwelling ureteral stent via a cystoscope or through a percutaneous nephrostomy. Rarely, endoscopic or operative removal of a ureteral calculus becomes necessary. The use of lithotripsy is contraindicated in pregnancy. Diagnosis of calculi during pregnancy may be difficult in view of the reluctance to perform x-ray studies. An excretory urogram (intravenous pyelogram), however, can be limited to a plain film and a 20-minute film, which is usually sufficient to arrive at a diagnosis. Ultrasonography is useful in detecting hydronephrosis. It can detect a stone in the kidney but usually not a ureteral calculus.

Acute pyelonephritis is associated with premature labor and delivery. Mild UTIs appear to have little effect on perinatal morbidity and mortality. There is evidence to suggest that labor may be triggered by phospholipase A, which can be produced by *E. coli* and other gram-negative organisms. This in turn stimulates the production of prostaglandins E_2 and F_2, which initiates labor.

The diagnosis of UTI is based on the findings yielded by urine culture. A midstream clean-catch urine specimen should be obtained, and culture should be performed within 1 hour. A dip culture medium is best used as an inexpensive screen for bacteriuria. Routine catheterization to obtain specimens should be avoided during pregnancy and labor, because there is a significant danger of this introducing infection. During pregnancy, catheterization carries a 4 to 6 percent risk of producing symptomatic UTI, and some of these patients could eventually suffer chronic UTI and pyelonephritis. The suprapubic aspiration of urine is a safe and accurate method of collection, but is poorly accepted by both patients and physicians. Bacteriuria is considered significant if greater than 10^5 colonies of a single organism are present on culture. A colony count of 10^2 to 10^4 in an acutely symptomatic patient also signifies infection. On routine culture, a count of 10^4 to 10^5 colonies is equivocal, and the culture should be repeated; less than 10^4 is not significant. The presence of any bacteria after suprapubic aspiration or catheterization is an important finding.

Pyuria alone is a poor indicator of UTI and indicates inflammation (infective or noninfective) in the urinary tract. Abacterial pyuria is commonly due to vaginal contamination or the use of antibiotics before culture is taken. The possibility of anaerobic or other fastidious organisms should not be overlooked. These include *Gardnerella vaginalis, Lactobacilli,* microaerophilic *Streptococci,* and *Ureaplasma urealyticum.* Persistent abacterial pyuria may also be caused by tumors, ureteral calculi, analgesic abuse, and renal tuberculosis.

ASB in early pregnancy or simple cystitis should be treated with antibiotics for 7 to 10 days. Preferred agents are ampicillin, nitrofurantoin, and cephalexin. Sulfa drugs are usually avoided in late pregnancy because they may produce jaundice in the infant. Tetracycline should not be used during pregnancy. Careful follow-up is essential after treatment. Reculture of the urine should be done 1 week after cessation of the treatment and monthly thereafter. Recurrent infection may require repeated courses or continuous low-dose antibiotic therapy throughout pregnancy (e.g., nitrofurantoin at bedtime). Failure to respond to the initial course of treatment necessitates a second course of appropriate antibiotic, based on sensitivity results. Further relapse of infection is highly suggestive of an underlying urologic abnormality, which requires evaluation postpartum.

Patients with acute pyelonephritis are usually toxic and dehydrated and may be in premature labor. They should be hospitalized, and treatment should consist of the administration of intravenous fluids and correction of electrolyte imbalances. The intravenous administration of antibiotics is advisable. Ampicillin or a first-generation cephalosporin is the initial antibiotic of choice. Aztreonam or a second- or third-generation cephalosporin may be needed, as indicated by the sensitivity results. If the infection does not respond to the appropriate antibiotics, obstructive uropathy and renal or perirenal abscess must be suspected. Occasionally, abscesses may form in a localized area of pyelonephritis, and these may require percutaneous or operative drainage. Termination of pregnancy to control UTI is rarely indicated.

In summary, UTI during pregnancy can usually be prevented by intense prenatal assessment and treatment. If it does occur, however, it should be treated promptly; otherwise, maternal and fetal compromise can occur. Comprehensive follow-up of patients with this problem is strongly indicated.

General
1. Patterson, T. F., and Andriole, V. T. Bacteriuria in pregnancy. *Infect. Dis. Clin. North Am.* 1:807, 1987.
   A general review of 76 references is offered on the etiology, pathogenesis, diagnosis, and management of UTI in pregnancy.
2. Farrar, W. E., Jr. Infections of the urinary tract. *Med. Clin. North Am.* 67:187, 1983.
   An updated review of UTI. Emphasizes the importance of screening for UTIs in early pregnancy and reviews subsequent management.
3. Wait, R. B. Urinary tract infection during pregnancy. *Postgrad. Med.* 75:153, 1984.
   This article answers three important questions. Why is it important to treat ASB in pregnancy? What is the predominant organism in the vast majority of cases of acute cystitis and acute pyelonephritis? When should urologic evaluation be done in the pregnant patient with pyelonephritis?
4. Dempsey, C., et al. Characteristics of bacteriuria in a homogeneous maternal hospital population. *Eur. J. Obstet. Gynecol. Reprod. Biol.* 44:89, 1992.
   A prospective study of over 3000 antenatal women revealed a 4.74 percent incidence of bacteriuria. Sixty-seven percent of these patients were asymptomatic or had a previous history of UTI. The mainstay of treatment was nitrofurantoin. There were no fetal or maternal complications.

Etiology
5. Andriole, V. T., and Patterson, T. F. Epidemiology, natural history, and management of urinary tract infections in pregnancy. *Med. Clin. North Am.* 75:359, 1991.
   ASB is the major risk factor for symptomatic UTI developing in pregnancy. Short-course therapy should be followed by repeat culture to document resolution of the bacteriuria.
6. Martinell, J., Jodal, U., and Linin-Janson, G. Pregnancies in women with and without renal scarring after urinary infections in childhood. *Br. Med. J.* 300:840, 1990.
   Preexisting renal scarring and vesicoureteral reflux predispose to the occurrence of acute pyelonephritis in pregnancy.
7. Jones, W. A., Correa, R. J., and Ansell, J. S. Urolithiasis associated with pregnancy. *J. Urol.* 122:335, 1979.
   There were 20 cases of calculi in 34,081 deliveries observed over a 12-year period.
8. Gilbert, G. L., et al. Bacteriuria due to *Ureaplasma* and other fastidious organisms during pregnancy: prevalence and significance. *Pediatr. Infect. Dis.* 5:293, 1986.
   Ureaplasma urealyticum and Gardnerella vaginalis can be detected quite commonly in apparently healthy pregnant women. Women with Ureaplasma bacteriuria detected at the first antenatal visit are three times more likely to suffer preeclampsia.

Diagnosis
9. Chang, P. K., and Hall, M. H. Antenatal prediction of urinary tract infection in pregnancy. *Br. J. Obstet. Gynaecol.* 89:8, 1982.
   A combination of ASB and a history of UTIs signifies a considerable risk; such a woman is ten times more likely to suffer active infection during pregnancy than a normal woman.
10. Kincaid-Smith, P. Bacteriuria in Pregnancy. In E. H. Kass (ed.), *Progress in Pyelonephritis*. Philadelphia: Davis, 1965.
    Screening for bacteriuria in early pregnancy allows for the prevention of acute pyelonephritis and diagnosis of underlying urinary tract abnormalities. A classic original chapter on this subject.

11. Pollock, H. M. Laboratory techniques for detection of urinary tract infection and assessment of value. *Am. J. Med.* 75:79, 1983.
    Review of laboratory methods for detecting bacteriuria and their importance. The finding of bacteria on uncentrifuged gram-stained smears correlates with the presence of significant bacteriuria. The possible presence of anaerobic organisms and Mycoplasma should not be overlooked.
12. Platt, R. Quantitative definition of bacteriuria. *Am. J. Med.* 75:44, 1983.
    Existing data strongly support the threshold of 10^5 colonies per milliliter as the criterion for diagnosis of pyelonephritis and ASB.
13. Peake, S. L., Roxburgh, H. B., and Langlois, S. LeP. Ultrasonic assessment of hydronephrosis of pregnancy. *Radiology* 146:167, 1983.
    Ultrasonography performed during the routine examination of pregnant women confirmed the high incidence of hydronephrosis.
14. North, D. H., et al. Correlation of urinary tract infection with urinary screening at the first antepartum visit. *J. Miss. State Med. Assoc.* 31:331, 1990.
    A cost-effective outpatient assessment of ASB is presented. Single-dose antibiotic therapy was effective.
15. Stenqvist, K., et al. Bacteriuria in pregnancy. Frequency and risk of acquisition. *Am. J. Epidemiol.* 129:372, 1989.
    The sixteenth gestational week is the optimal time for a single screening for bacteriuria in pregnancy.

Treatment
16. Hankins, G. D. V., and Whalley, P. J. Acute urinary tract infections in pregnancy. *Clin. Obstet. Gynecol.* 28:266, 1985.
    Routine screening for ASB in pregnancy, followed by adequate therapy and urine culture surveillance, are important preventive measures. The considerable maternal morbidity associated with the development of acute pyelonephritis more than justifies the effort and expense necessary to implement screening methods. This article also gives an excellent general review of the subject.
17. Adelson, M. D., Graves, W. L., and Osborne, N. G. Treatment of urinary infections in pregnancy using single versus 10-day dosing. *J. Natl. Med. Assoc.* 84:73, 1992.
    Single-dose therapy did not provide adequate cure or prevent reinfection.
18. Tan, J. S., and File, T. M., Jr. Urinary tract infections in obstetrics and gynecology. *J. Reprod. Med.* 35:339, 1990.
    Antimicrobial therapy using an agent that contains a beta-lactamase inhibitor is preferred.
19. Cunha, B. A. Nitrofurantoin: an update. *Obstet. Gynecol. Surv.* 44:399, 1989.
    Nitrofurantoin has a solid safety record in the treatment of ASB in pregnancy.

Complications
20. Rosenfield, J. A. Renal disease and pregnancy. *Am. Fam. Physician* 39:209, 1989.
    Women with preexisting renal disease usually do well during pregnancy if renal function is normal and hypertension is not present.
21. Davison, J. M., Sprott, M. S., and Selkon, J. B. The effect of covert bacteriuria on renal function in schoolgirls at 18 years and during pregnancy. *Lancet* 2:651, 1984.
    ASB treated by antibiotic coverage prevents clinical renal damage that is more evident in the pregnant than in the nonpregnant state.
22. Hill, J. A., Devoe, L. D., and Bryans, C. I. Frequency of asymptomatic bacteriuria in preeclampsia. *Obstet. Gynecol.* 67:52, 1986.
    A significant difference in the rate of ASB was found in patients with preeclampsia versus that in control subjects. In addition, preeclamptic patients with bacteriuria had substantially lower total serum protein and albumin levels.
23. Yasin, S. Y., and Doun, S. N. B. Hemodialysis in pregnancy. *Obstet. Gynecol. Surv.* 43:655, 1988.
    Chronic UTIs during pregnancy may lead to renal disease severe enough to re-

quire hemodialysis. The authors have reviewed the literature in this exhaustive search and find that hemodialysis can be accomplished safely, if done properly.

11. VENEREAL DISEASES IN PREGNANCY
Bryan D. Cowan

Venereal diseases are usually asymptomatic; few of the women who have signs seek medical advice because their symptoms are mild and transient. Furthermore, the clinical course of venereal disease may be even milder in pregnancy. The common venereal diseases that may be contracted in pregnancy include trichomoniasis, gonorrhea, condyloma acuminatum, herpes, and syphilis.

Trichomonas vaginalis is transmitted by sexual intercourse, and women usually have more symptoms than men. The subjective symptoms include a profuse, frothy, foul-smelling vaginal discharge, accompanied by vulvar itching, dyspareunia, and dysuria. The wet smear, or occasionally the more sensitive *T. vaginalis* culture medium, is used to establish diagnosis. The most effective therapeutic agent is metronidazole (Flagyl), which may be administered orally in doses of either 250 mg three times a day for 7 days or 2 g orally in one dose. Metronidazole may be safely administered in the second and third trimester of pregnancy but its use is contraindicated during the first trimester. Local measures, such as povidone-iodine (Betadine) sitz baths and sulfur creams, are advocated for relief in the first trimester but have low cure rates. Clotrimazole, in a 100-mg vaginal suppository inserted at bedtime for 7 days, may also provide symptomatic relief. Treatment of the sexual partner is strongly recommended, especially in the setting of recurrent cases. Lactating women may be treated with metronidazole, 2.0 g orally in a single dose, but should stop breast-feeding for 24 hours after taking it.

Gonorrhea is the most commonly reported venereal disease in the United States, with more than one million cases reported annually. The incidence rate of gonorrhea in the pregnant population is 2 to 5 percent; 90 percent of these cases are asymptomatic. *Neisseria gonorrhoeae* is almost always spread by genital or oral contact. The gonococcus is most commonly found in the endocervix. From the cervix the gonococcus may move into the endometrium, oviducts, and pelvic peritoneum. During pregnancy, the infection rarely ascends to the upper genital tract, although it can disseminate to other organs, such as the joints and skin, by hematogenous pathways. Patients with disseminated gonococcal infection usually initially exhibit a pyogenic arthritis accompanied by chills and fever. In uncomplicated cases, the gonorrhea usually involves a transient dysuria, mild vaginal discharge, pharyngeal infection, or any combination of these symptoms.

The definitive diagnosis of gonorrhea is based on the results of culture on modified Thayer-Martin medium in an enriched (5–10%) carbon dioxide atmosphere. Gram's staining, even if the results are positive, may be an inaccurate method. Endocervical cultures yield the best results, although anorectal and pharyngeal sources for cultures should be considered. Both sexual partners should be examined and treated. Finally, a diagnostic serologic test for concomitant syphilis is strongly recommended.

The recommended treatment for uncomplicated asymptomatic pregnant patients with gonorrhea consists of the single intramuscular administration of 250 mg of ceftriaxone. If chlamydial diagnostic testing is not available, empirical treatment for chlamydia should also be given. Because tetracyclines are contraindicated in pregnancy, this treatment should consist of erythromycin base 500 mg (or equivalent) taken orally four times a day for 7 days. Pregnant women who are allergic to beta-lactams should be treated with spectinomycin, 2 g intramuscularly, plus erythromycin. In pregnant patients hospitalized with severe infections, ceftriaxone, ceftizoxime, or cefotaxime may be given intravenously, or, if the infecting organism proves to be penicillin sensitive, parenteral penicillin may be used. Details of this therapy and of the treatment of neonates, infants, and children are beyond the scope of this chapter. Appropriate cultures should be performed 4 to 7 days after treatment is completed. Women with known recent exposure to gonorrhea should be treated as just described.

Condyloma acuminatum (venereal warts) represent a viral venereal disease spread by sexual contact. The warts are most commonly found in the genital area during the years of maximal sexual activity. The Papanicolaou (Pap) smear is not useful for diagnostic purposes because there are no specific cytologic findings involved. The initial lesion is usually a rough, cauliflower-like warty papilloma that appears in the perineal area. During pregnancy, the condyloma acuminatum may grow more rapidly and hinder vaginal delivery. The pregnant patient with condyloma acuminatum poses special problems because the usual treatment, topically administered podophyllin, should be avoided throughout pregnancy owing to its toxic properties. Thus, during pregnancy, destructive methods of therapy (e.g., electrocautery, cryosurgery, or laser), combined with povidone-iodine douches and sitz baths, are helpful. In the event of recurrent and persistent condyloma acuminatum, an autogenous vaccine has been used successfully.

Syphilis is primarily a sexually transmitted disease, and approximately 30 percent of the 25,000 annual cases occur in women. Additionally, there are 350 cases of congenital syphilis reported every year. During pregnancy, transplacental infection of the fetus may occur, resulting either in an asymptomatic newborn who later shows the stigmata of congenital syphilis or in fetal death. Syphilis is a chronic infectious process caused by the spirochete *Treponema pallidum*. Owing to its small size, it can be identified only by dark-field microscopy. After a 10- to 90-day incubation period, an indurated, nontender ulcer develops, known as a *chancre*. This primary lesion, accompanied by painless regional lymphadenopathy, usually appears on the external genitalia, in the vagina, or on the cervix. The chancre is followed by a bacteremic, or secondary, stage if the disease is not treated. The clinical manifestations of secondary syphilis include skin rash, lesions on the palms and soles, mucous patches on mucosal surfaces, and wartlike growths in the genital area (condyloma latum). In the absence of therapy, the clinical manifestations of tertiary syphilis ensue some years after the initial infection, and include gummatous involvement of various organs as well as abnormalities in the cardiovascular and central nervous systems.

The effect of syphilis on the fetus depends on when the disease was contracted in relation to the time of gestation, and on the effectiveness of treatment. It has been shown that the placenta is permeable to the *Treponema* organism throughout pregnancy. Clinical observation, however, has shown that, if a pregnant patient contracts syphilis during the first 16 to 18 weeks of gestation, it is less likely that the fetus will be affected. Nevertheless, untreated syphilis in pregnancy may result in early spontaneous abortion, premature labor, stillbirth, neonatal death, or congenital syphilis.

The diagnosis of syphilis is best established by serologic testing, or, if primary or secondary lesions are present, by dark-field examination, as serologic tests may still be nonreactive. Nonspecific (Venereal Disease Research Laboratory [VDRL]) and reagin (rapid plasma reagin [RPR]) tests are nontreponemal screening serologic tests that should be performed on the first prenatal visit. These tests are insensitive in the setting of very early or latent disease. Results may also be positive in patients without syphilis. Therefore, confirmation of the diagnosis requires a *Treponema*-specific test that can detect specific antibodies to *T. pallidum* (the fluorescent treponemal antibody absorption test [FTA-ABS] and *T. pallidum* immobilization test). Congenital syphilis can be confirmed by either a dark-field examination, if lesions are present, or by determining the immunoglobulin M (IgM)–FTA-ABS titer, which represents infant IgM antibodies produced as a result of active syphilic infection.

The treatment of incubating syphilis and syphilis of less than 1 year's duration includes benzathine penicillin G (2.4 million units total), half given intramuscularly in each buttock. For gravidas with syphilis of more than 1 year's duration or of unknown duration, the treatment of choice is also benzathine penicillin G (2.4 million units given intramuscularly weekly for 3 successive weeks, for a total of 7.2

million units). Patients allergic to penicillin should undergo skin testing and desensitization, if necessary, done in collaboration with an expert. Finally, the treatment of syphilis with long-acting penicillin is not always effective in pregnant patients owing to the lower serum levels of antibiotics attained during pregnancy, versus those in the nonpregnant patient. Thus, the course of the pregnant patient should be monitored by the performance of monthly quantitative nontreponemal serologic tests, and the patient should be retreated if the titer rises.

Chancroid, caused by *Haemophilus ducreyi,* is an acute, autoinoculable, and painful infection of the external genitalia and regional lymph nodes (bubo). It can be transmitted sexually. The diagnosis is made on the basis of findings yielded either by culturing material from the ulcers or bubo in a blood-containing medium or by biopsy of these lesions. Treatment with erythromycin or ceftriaxone is recommended, and sulfonamide therapy may be effective.

Granuloma inguinale, caused by *Calymmatobacterium granulomatis* (also called *Donovania granulomatis*), is a disease with a low incidence, and infection is spread by sexual intercourse. The initial lesion consists of a raised, painless papule that develops into central ulcerations accompanied by local, deep destruction of tissues and the formation of rectovaginal fistulas and pseudobuboes. The diagnosis is made by the finding of characteristic Donovan bodies in material aspirated from lymph nodes. Culture of *C. granulomatis* is also helpful. Tetracycline and erythromycin are effective agents in the treatment of early lesions, although only the latter can be used in pregnancy. Surgical intervention may be required for correction of advanced tissue destruction.

Lymphogranuloma venereum, caused by *Chlamydia trachomatis,* is a disease that is usually transmitted through sexual intercourse, and primarily affects the lymphatics and the lymph nodes (inguinal buboes). Common complications of the disease include rectovaginal fistulas, perirectal abscesses, and polypoid growths of the colon, with occasional malignant degeneration. The definitive diagnosis of lymphogranuloma venereum is made by a complement fixation test. Biopsy of the lesions, biochemical tests, and the Frei intradermal test (nonspecific) can also be used diagnostically. The recommended treatment in pregnancy consists of sulfonamides or erythromycin given for at least 2 weeks.

Molluscum contagiosum is a sexually transmitted viral (poxvirus group) cutaneous disease that involves the genital area. The diagnosis is based on the findings from microscopic examination of the lesion. Cryosurgery and electrocautery are utilized as methods of treatment.

Chlamydia trachomatis is the most prevalent sexually transmitted bacterial pathogen in the United States today. Because laboratory screening for this pathogen is becoming widely available, pregnant women who are at high risk for sexually transmitted disease should be routinely cultured in the third trimester. Treatment should be instituted in women with proven *C. trachomatis* infection or women whose sexual partners have nongonococcal urethritis or epididymitis. During pregnancy, the suggested treatment is erythromycin. When treatment fails, patients should be retreated, and male sexual partners should be treated with tetracycline or doxycycline.

Genital herpes infection is a viral disease that may appear acutely or chronically during pregnancy. No antiviral therapy for herpes simplex virus infection has been shown to be effective during pregnancy, and the safety of systemic acyclovir treatment in pregnant women has not been established. Treatment is generally topical, and consists of sitz baths and locally applied agents to reduce pain. Because of the risk of neonatal transfer, frequent perineal inspection during pregnancy is important, as is notification of the pediatric personnel.

The growing threat that the human immunodeficiency virus (HIV) poses to reproduction is of increasing concern. It is estimated that one million people are infected with the virus in the United States, and that 10 percent of these are women. The acquired immunodeficiency syndrome (AIDS) has been diagnosed in nearly 17,000 women in the United States by early 1991, and this syndrome is expected to be a leading cause of death in women of reproductive age in the United States.

It is estimated that there are almost 6000 HIV-infected infants born annually in the United States. Most prospective studies indicate that vertical HIV transmission (mother to infant) occurs uniformly in approximately 25 to 35 percent of such pregnancies. Additionally, the rate of transmission in women with low CD4 cell counts ($<400/mm^3$) seems to be higher.

The first task in caring for a pregnant woman with HIV is to provide counseling that will allow an informed reproductive choice. HIV-positive women should be screened for other sexually transmitted infections, including syphilis, gonorrhea, chlamydia, and hepatitis B. Tuberculosis should also be excluded. Antibody titers of cytomegalovirus (CMV) and *Toxoplasma* should be measured. Counseling concerning the risk of vertical transmission should be provided and the reproductive options outlined.

The CD4 cell counts in patients with HIV infection should be monitored. If the counts fall below $500/mm^3$, consultation concerning the institution of antiviral therapy should be initiated. Patients with low CD4 counts are at risk for suffering opportunistic infections. If counts fall below $200/mm^3$, prophylaxis against *Pneumocystis carinii* should be instituted.

Pneumocystis carinii is the most common opportunistic infection seen in patients with AIDS. Standard treatment consists of orally or intravenously administered trimethoprim and sulfamethoxazole (Bactrim). Additionally, prophylaxis with Bactrim should be considered when the CD4 counts fall below $200/mm^3$. Antiviral therapy with zidovudine has not been commonly carried out in pregnant women. Although no fetal malformations have been shown to be attributable to the use of zidovudine, in general, the duration of pregnancy is short compared with the course of HIV infection, and the risk of exposing the fetus to this agent may not be justifiable.

There is no evidence that the mode of delivery alters the rate of HIV transmission. However, commonsense measures, such as the avoidance of direct contact of the infected mother's vaginal secretions with the fetal blood (such as might occur during fetal scalp sampling or electronic scalp electrode application), should be taken. Finally, there is little information regarding the postpartum management of HIV-infected women. Recent evidence suggests that HIV vertical transmission can occur during breast-feeding, and, therefore, HIV-infected patients should be advised not to breast-feed their infants.

General
1. Ross, S. M. Sexually transmitted diseases in pregnancy. *Clin. Obstet. Gynecol.* 9:565, 1982.
   A discussion of 12 venereal diseases and their impact on pregnancy.
2. Charles, D. Syphilis. *Clin. Obstet. Gynecol.* 26:125, 1983.
   This comprehensive article details the diagnosis and treatment of syphilis during pregnancy.
3. Human immunodeficiency virus infections. *ACOG Tech. Bull.* No. 169, June 1992.
   A concise review of the etiology, diagnosis, and vertical transmission of HIV in pregnancy. Worth reading.

Etiology
4. Blanchard, A. C., Pastonek, J. G., and Weeks, T. Pelvic inflammatory disease including pregnancy. *South. Med. J.* 80:136, 1987.
   The authors report on three cases of acute gonococcal salpingitis that coexisted with pregnancy.
5. Holmes, K. K. The chlamydia epidemic. *J.A.M.A.* 245:1718, 1981.
   This article considers chlamydia and how it affects pregnant and nonpregnant women. This is must reading for those interested in the chlamydia epidemic in the country.
6. Hardy, P. H., et al. Prevalence of six sexually transmitted disease agents among pregnant inner-city adolescents and pregnancy outcome. *Lancet* 2:333, 1984.
   This study demonstrated that Trichomonas vaginalis *infection, either alone or in conjunction with* Chlamydia trachomatis *or* Candida *infection, was associated with small-for-gestational-age and low-birth-weight infants.*

Diagnosis
7. Wendel, G. D. Gestational and congenital syphilis. *Clin. Perinatol.* 15:287, 1988.
   In this review, the author outlines the current status, epidemiology, and complications of syphilis. The presentation on maternal and neonatal syphilis is nicely organized.
8. Brown, S. T., et al. Serological response to syphilis treatment. A new analysis of old data. *J.A.M.A.* 253:1296, 1985.
   This article describes a curve for following the VDRL titer, which allows the clinician to identify early treatment failures and reinfections.
9. Stamm, W. E., et al. Diagnosis of *Chlamydia trachomatis* infections by direct immunofluorescence staining of genital secretions. *Ann. Intern. Med.* 101:638, 1984.
   Direct immunofluorescence staining of genital secretions for Chlamydia trachomatis *in men, women, and pregnant women demonstrated high sensitivity and specificity and offers an alternative diagnostic approach to cell culture.*
10. Zbella, E. A., Deppe, G., and Elrad, H. Gonococcal arthritis in pregnancy. *Obstet. Gynecol. Surv.* 39:81, 1984.
    A review of the clinical presentation, diagnostic criteria, and recommended treatment for women with gonococcal arthritis in pregnancy.

Treatment
11. Ryan, G. M., Jr. Ambulatory Management of Venereal Disease. In G. M. Ryan, Jr. (ed.), *Ambulatory Care in Obstetrics and Gynecology.* New York: Grune & Stratton, 1980.
    The author describes the ambulatory management of gonorrhea and syphilis in both pregnant and nonpregnant patients.
12. Centers for Disease Control. 1989 STD treatment guidelines. *M.M.W.R.* 38:8S, 1989.
    Treatment guidelines for sexually transmitted diseases established by the CDC.
13. U.S. Department of Health and Human Services. Guidelines for the prevention and control of congenital syphilis. *M.M.W.R.* 37:1S, 1988.
    Recommendations of the CDC for the prevention and treatment of neonatally acquired syphilis.

Complications
14. Nguyen, D. Gonorrhea in pregnancy and in the newborn. *Am. Fam. Physician* 29:185, 1984.
    The prevalence of gonorrhea in pregnancy ranges from 0.2 to 15 percent. Maternal gonococcal infection is associated with ectopic pregnancy, premature birth, and ophthalmia neonatorum.
15. Solola, A. S., Ryan, G. M., Jr., and Ling, F. W. Gonorrhea during the intrapartum period. *Am. J. Obstet. Gynecol.* 144:351, 1982.
    A 1-month surveillance of 148 randomly selected women in labor detected 9.5 percent with a positive gonococcal culture. The authors recommend initial prenatal screening and repeat screening until term in high-risk populations.
16. Mascola, L., et al. Congenital syphilis. Why is it still occurring? *J.A.M.A.* 252:1719, 1984.
    A CDC epidemiologic review of 50 cases of congenital syphilis. Improved prenatal care in high-risk populations and refined care efforts to control infectious syphilis would reduce this complication.
17. Public Health Service Guidelines for Counseling and Antibody Testing to Prevent HIV Infection and AIDS. *M.M.W.R.* 36:509, 1987.
    In this document, the CDC outlines recommendations for counseling and testing with regard to HIV infection.
18. Henrion, R. Pregnancy and AIDS. *Hum. Reprod.* 3:257, 1988.
    A review of the maternal and neonatal impact of an ever-increasing number of pregnancies complicated by HIV infection. Recommends abortion in the first trimester, open decision in the second trimester, and natural delivery for the third trimester.

19. Minkoff, H., et al. Pregnancies resulting in infants with acquired immunodeficiency syndrome or AIDS-related complex: follow-up of mother, children and subsequently born siblings. *Obstet. Gynecol.* 69:288, 1987.
    Follow-up in 34 children with AIDS or the AIDS-related complex indicates that the development of disease in a child indicates a high risk for the development of illness in the mother and subsequently born children.

IV. PREEXISTING DISEASES AND PREGNANCY

12. PULMONARY DISEASE IN PREGNANCY
Sterling W. McColgin

The maternal respiratory tract alterations that take place during pregnancy facilitate increased oxygen transfer to the fetus. In normal pregnancy, there are appreciable increases in the tidal volume, minute ventilation, and minute oxygen uptake, with a decrease in the residual volume, total pulmonary resistance, and functional residual capacity. These events account for a significant increase in oxygen transfer to the fetus. At the same time, major compensatory mechanisms exist in the fetus that facilitate increased oxygen transport. Most respiratory diseases are not adversely affected by pregnancy and do not interfere with gestation, unless oxygenation is significantly reduced.

Asthma is defined by the American Thoracic Society as reversible airway obstruction. It is characterized by paroxysmal episodes of wheezing, dyspnea, and cough. The variable airway obstruction seen during an asthmatic attack is produced by mucous plugging and bronchial constriction, inflammation, and edema. An exacerbation of bronchial asthma that does not respond to standard therapy is called *status asthmaticus*. Asthma affects approximately 1 percent of women of reproductive age, and appears to be more severe in blacks than whites and most severe among adolescent pregnant girls (6.6%). Increased perinatal mortality and morbidity appear to be particularly heightened among those women with more severe forms of asthma.

Although most asthmatics do well during pregnancy, it may be helpful to consult with a specialist in pulmonary disease to assist with management, perform pulmonary function testing, be available in the event of an acute asthmatic attack, and carry out long-term care after pregnancy has ended. Routine pregnancy care should include (1) frequent individualized prenatal visits, (2) serial pulmonary function tests (PFTs), (3) auscultation of the lungs at every visit, (4) the identification and elimination of potential allergens, (5) measurement of theophylline levels, if indicated, (6) reduction of stress and heavy exercise, and (7) avoidance of iodine-containing compounds. PFTs should be performed in all asthmatics, even if they are asymptomatic, to obtain a baseline for future comparison. The forced expiratory volume at 1 second (FEV_1) and midexpiratory flow rates ($FEF_{25\%-75\%}$) are most influential in oxygen transport to the fetus. These values should remain at the 80 to 85 percent (of normal) or greater range. Although a less sensitive method of assessing airway disease than formal PFTs, peak flowmeters that measure peak expiratory flow rates (PEFRs) are enjoying increased use. These tests can be easily performed by the patient at home on a daily basis, or if any respiratory difficulty develops. Predicted values range between 400 to 550 liters/min, but a baseline must be established for each patient. A decline of 10 percent generally indicates a need for an increase in medication, while a decline of 20 percent frequently dictates a need for acute intervention.

Beta$_2$-adrenergic agonist inhalers are the principal therapeutic medications utilized in pregnancy. These agents facilitate smooth muscle relaxation, mucociliary clearance, and a decreased release of cell mediators. The primary beta$_2$-adrenergic agonists used are albuterol, metaproterenol, and terbutaline. Two sprays administered in a metered dose inhaler every 4 to 6 hours, as needed, provides adequate control in most patients. In the event of worsening symptoms or decreased PFT values, this medication should be administered on a regular basis. A cromolyn sodium inhaler, two puffs every 6 hours preceded by two puffs of the beta$_2$-adrenergic agonist, may be indicated in atopic patients and patients with more persistent asthmatic symptoms. Cromolyn takes 4 to 6 weeks to achieve appropriate efficacy, but a corticosteroid burst frequently promotes a more rapid onset of effects. This can be given in the form of 40 mg of prednisone daily, followed by use of the corticosteroid inhaler on the fifth day, two to four sprays 4 times a day. Once the patient's condition is stable, a maintenance dose of two to four sprays 4 times a day can be given. The methylxanthines are not utilized as frequently as they once were due to concerns about maternal toxicity.

Asthmatic attacks do not occur as frequently with our modern agents as they did in the past, but should still be viewed as a medical emergency. They should be "broken" as rapidly as possible, because of the serious fetal hypoxia that may occur during an attack. Beta$_2$-adrenergic agonists are now considered the therapy of choice for acute asthma. These can be administered sequentially by a handheld nebulizer every 30 minutes for up to three doses, and this achieves at least as much bronchodilatation as does subcutaneously administered epinephrine or terbutaline, with the same rapidity of onset but less toxicity. Other measures include the supplemental administration of oxygen, serial blood gas measurements, intravenously performed hydration, and the involvement of a pulmonary specialist. Epinephrine, aminophylline, and steroids are other agents that can be considered for use in resistant cases.

Pneumonia in pregnancy is the second leading cause of nonobstetric maternal death. Although maternal mortality has declined significantly in recent years, preterm labor has been reported to be as high as 44 percent, with a 36 percent rate of preterm delivery in such patients. The most prevalent bacterial organisms are *Streptococcus pneumoniae* and *Diplococcus pneumoniae,* with *Haemophilus influenzae, Staphylococcus aureus, Klebsiella pneumoniae,* and *Legionella pneumophila* also possible organisms. A patient with bacterial pneumonia first exhibits an acute illness characterized by the abrupt onset of shaking chills, followed rapidly by high fever, headache, malaise, dyspnea, and cough, which is frequently purulent, blood tinged, or both. A chest x-ray film reveals consolidation, with air bronchograms and occasionally pleural effusion. Leukocytosis is common, with bacteremia occurring in 25 to 30 percent of such patients. Mortality still ranges between 17 and 30 percent and is highest in patients contracting pneumonia in the third trimester of pregnancy, as well as in immunocompromised patients. An attempt should be made to identify organisms in induced sputum specimens and blood cultures. Prompt hospitalization, antibiotic therapy directed against the suspected organism, serial measurement of the arterial oxygen tension (PaO$_2$), oxygen therapy, and vigorous pulmonary toilet are all indicated. *Mycoplasma* pneumonia is the most common atypical pneumonia and has a more insidious presentation. These patients are more likely to have a low-grade fever, nonproductive cough, and often only mildly elevated leukocytosis. Infiltrates in these patients are more likely to be patchy. Diagnosis is often suggested by the presence of cold agglutinins (found in 70% of the patients) and by characteristic x-ray findings. The treatment of choice is erythromycin.

Influenza pneumonia can be deadly, particularly during pregnancy. This entity should be suspected in a patient with respiratory symptoms who is otherwise recovering from a flulike illness. Amantadine hydrochloride is effective for prophylaxis in the treatment of influenza A infections. Just as important, influenza immunization is indicated for those pregnant women with heart disease, chronic anemia, diabetes mellitus, any chronic lung disease, or an altered immune response, and should be carried out after the first trimester to minimize fetal risk. Although antibiotics are not effective against these viruses, they are valuable for the treatment of secondary bacterial pneumonia (most often pneumococci and staphylococci), which is most often the cause of death in these women.

Although varicella pneumonia is rare in childhood, it appears frequently in adults with chickenpox, and pregnant women appear to be particularly susceptible. Presentation usually consists of pleuritic chest pain, cough, dyspnea, and tachypnea arising 2 to 6 days after the onset of the cutaneous eruptions from varicella. Because of increased virulence in adulthood, patients should be cautioned to report any pulmonary complaints or presumed upper respiratory infections. These patients are at significant risk for contracting varicella pneumonia. The maternal mortality rate has been reported to be as high as 40 percent. Contracting varicella just before delivery also poses a serious threat to the newborn. In some instances, the infant will acquire disseminated visceral and central nervous system disease, which is often fatal (65% mortality before the advent of acyclovir treatment). This is most frequently associated with maternal evidence of a varicella rash occurring between 4 days before delivery and 2 days postpartum. Varicella zoster immune globulin should be administered to the neonate whenever the onset of maternal disease occurs during this time. Acyclovir is now the drug of choice in treating pregnant patients and their neonates with varicella pneumonia. Delivery should be delayed in patients with active disease unless the patient's condition is terminal.

The most significant of the fungal and parasitic infections arise in severely immunocompromised patients, particularly those with acquired immunodeficiency syndrome (AIDS). These patients are most susceptible to *Pneumocystis carinii* pneumonia (PCP), which is the most common opportunistic infection in AIDS patients. It is frequently the presenting infection that leads to the diagnosis of AIDS. The mortality rate for one episode of PCP is greater than 25 percent. Reports on its occurrence in pregnancy reveal that the outcome most often is fatal. Therapy consists of the intravenous administration of trimethoprim-sulfamethoxazole, pentamidine, or diaminodiphenylsulfone. There is concern about the fetal effects of all these medications, but the mother must be treated to have any hope of survival. Treatment usually lasts about 3 weeks, but recurrence is common. Maintenance therapy is being investigated for the prevention of recurrences.

Aspiration pneumonia continues to be the leading cause of maternal mortality secondary to anesthetic use, and is responsible for over a hundred maternal deaths per year in the United States. The focus of the treatment of aspiration pneumonia is on prevention. Neutralization of gastric acid with an antacid, coupled with continuous cricoid pressure at the time of intubation and then careful extubation only after the patient is fully awake, can minimize the risk of aspiration at the time of general anesthesia. Measures for treating aspiration include immediate clearance of the airway and adequate oxygenation, use of bronchodilators, and suctioning. Mechanical ventilation with positive end-expiratory pressure is often required, with the goal of therapy keeping the oxygen saturation at least at 90%. If superimposed infection is strongly suspected, it is very important to obtain adequate culture specimens so that proper antibiotic therapy can be planned. Bacterial superinfections generally develop 2 to 3 days after the initial injury. Many of the patients require intubation and assisted ventilation because of the exhaustion resulting from the effort needed for adequate oxygenation.

There has been a resurgence of tuberculosis worldwide arising from the migration of members of certain high-risk ethnic groups and the increased number of individuals who are immunosuppressed. The members of certain high-risk groups need to undergo testing, and these groups include (1) Haitian and Southeast Asian immigrants, (2) prison inmates, (3) individuals who have had contact with known tuberculosis patients, (4) immunocompromised patients, and (5) those with symptoms compatible with tuberculosis. If the purified protein derivative (PPD) test result is positive, a chest radiograph should be obtained, with the abdomen shielded. If no active disease is discovered, prophylaxis should probably be withheld until after pregnancy, unless the patient is a known recent converter. In this situation, isoniazid (INH) therapy should be started after the first trimester. If active disease is revealed, pulmonary consultation should be obtained and chemotherapy instituted during pregnancy. The compounds most commonly utilized for this purpose are INH, rifampin, and ethambutol. The serum glutamic-oxaloacetic transaminase (SGOT) level should be measured every 3 months in patients taking INH because of the risk of INH hepatitis developing. Should the SGOT level become significantly elevated during pregnancy, INH treatment should be discontinued. Supplemental pyridoxine (15 mg/day) should be given in conjunction with the INH. INH and ethambutol, given in combination, are probably the first two drugs of choice for pregnant women with active disease and need to be given for 18 months. The combination of INH and rifampin need only be taken for 9 months, but the risk of fetal malformations caused by rifampin makes it a less desirable medication. Pyrazinamide may well allow for shorter courses of therapy in the future, but remains an investigational agent at the present time. Streptomycin should not be utilized because of its ototoxic properties and ethionamide should not be given because it is generally considered a teratogen. The three-drug regimen, consisting of INH, ethambutol, and rifampin, should be used in patients in whom INH resistance is strongly suspected. Because of the significant risk to neonates, the newborns of mothers with active tuberculosis should receive chemoprophylaxis with INH after delivery. This should be given for 3 months, or until the sputum cultures from the mother yield negative findings. If, after 3 months, the neonate is tuberculin negative and has a normal chest radiograph, treatment can be terminated. If active disease is discovered in the neonate, a two-drug regimen, consisting of INH plus rifampin, is indicated and should be maintained for 6 months. Separation of the mother and infant should be considered if the mother is highly infectious, untreated, or noncompliant with therapy.

Adult respiratory distress syndrome (ARDS) results from damage to the cells of the pulmonary alveolar lining or pulmonary capillary endothelium, or both. The most common preexisting factors that predispose to the development of ARDS include sepsis, aspiration, and disseminated intravascular coagulation. Other causes include diabetic ketoacidosis, sickle cell crisis, substance abuse, burns, and severe pregnancy-induced hypertension. Acute lung injury follows the inciting event by 12 to 72 hours before the symptom complex becomes apparent. The mechanism responsible for ARDS is as follows. Increased alveolar-capillary permeability with leakage of protein causes interstitial edema, resulting in collapse of the alveoli. As compliance decreases, right-to-left shunting ensues. Inadequate blood supply to the pulmonary tree causes the formation of type II pneumocytes to be inhibited, and this results in alteration and depletion of surfactant. This further contributes to decreased compliance. A ventilation-perfusion mismatch then leads to severe hypoxemia.

The first clinical evidence of ARDS is generally what appears to be pulmonary edema. Tachypnea, tachycardia, dyspnea, and cyanosis rapidly follow. A chest x-ray study reveals bilateral diffuse infiltrates along with pleural effusions that rapidly progress until there is evidence of massive pulmonary involvement. Severe hypoxemia ensues with PaO_2 levels less than 50 mm Hg when the fraction of inspired oxygen (FIO_2) is greater than 0.6. A normal or near-normal Swan-Ganz pulmonary capillary wedge pressure helps exclude the presence of left ventricular heart failure. Management of the ARDS patient involves elimination of the underlying cause and aggressive cardiorespiratory supportive care. The combination of mechanical ventilation, hemodynamic monitoring, and adequate nutrition is the cornerstone of treatment. The care of an intensivist or pulmonologist is absolutely essential in giving the patient an optimal chance for survival. Steroid, diuretic, inotropic, and antibiotic agents are administered as indicated. Anemia, alkalosis, and hyperphosphatemia should be monitored and corrected on an ongoing basis. Fluids need to be meticulously managed, as these patients are particularly susceptible to fluid overload. Hyperalimentation should be started early in the recuperative course, along with the prophylactic administration of antacids to prevent stress ulcers from forming. These patients are particularly prone to nosocomial infections and must be constantly monitored for evidence of pneumonia, cystitis, and sinusitis. Delivery should be undertaken if a pregnancy-related event is the cause of the ARDS or if there are obstetric indications. Other therapeutic pitfalls, besides fluid overload, include oxygen toxicity, barotrauma, and iatrogenic lung injury.

Maternal cigarette smoking during pregnancy and during the early life of a child is associated with substantial risks of fetal death, prematurity, low birth weight, abnormal breast feeding, and respiratory disease in the child. The degree of risk to the fetus is clearly dose related, and, if a woman stops smoking by her fourth month of gestation, the risk to the fetus is substantially reduced. Nicorette gum (containing nicotine polacrilex) and the nicotine patch are class X drugs that are contraindicated for use in pregnancy, but hold some hope, pending investigation, for use in those mothers who are heavy smokers. Pregnancy represents an excellent opportunity and impetus to educate both parents to the hazards of smoking to themselves and to their fetus. This should offer a time for both parents to embark on a joint effort to stop smoking. The medical and economic benefits accruing to them and their family far outweigh any inconvenience or distress involved with the cessation of smoking.

General
1. McColgin, S. W., Glee, L., and Brian, B. A. Pulmonary disorders complicating pregnancy. *Obstet. Gynecol. Clin. North Am.* 19:697, 1992.
   A more detailed review of the pulmonary physiology and pathology in pregnancy.

Physiology
2. Rosman, J. Pulmonary Physiology. In N. Gleicher (ed.), *Principles and Practice of Medical Therapy in Pregnancy*. Norwalk, CT: Appleton-Lange, 1992.
   An in-depth review of pulmonary physiologic alterations that take place in pregnancy.

Asthma
3. Hankins, G. D. V., and Cunningham, F. G. Asthma Complicating Pregnancy. In *Williams Obstetrics* Suppl. 15, Norwalk, CT: Appleton-Lange, 1992.
   An excellent review of the evaluation and treatment of asthma in pregnancy.
4. Wollner, A., and Duncan, S. R. Update: management of asthma. *Compr. Ther.* 16:24, 1990.
   An overview of asthma with particular emphasis on medications.
5. Schriver, L. Asthma. In N. Gleicher (ed.), *Principles and Practice of Medical Therapy in Pregnancy*. Norwalk, CT: Appleton-Lange, 1992.
   Review of asthma management in pregnancy.

Pneumonia
6. Maccato, M. L. Pneumonia and pulmonary tuberculosis in pregnancy. *Obstet. Gynecol. Clin. North Am.* 16:417, 1989.
   An overview of pneumonia and tuberculosis in pregnancy.
7. Duff, P. Pneumococcal Infections. In N. Gleicher (ed.), *Principles and Practice of Medical Therapy in Pregnancy*. Norwalk, CT: Appleton-Lange, 1992.
   A review of the most common type of pneumonia encountered in pregnancy.
8. Madinger, N. E., Greenspoon, J. S., and Ellrodt, A. G. Pneumonia during pregnancy: has modern technology improved maternal and fetal outcome? *Am. J. Obstet. Gynecol.* 161:657, 1989.
   A review of the maternal and perinatal morbidity and mortality associated with pneumonia.
9. Harstad, T. W., and Gilstrap, L. C., III. Respiratory infections with *Mycoplasma pneumoniae*. *Obstet. Gynecol. Clin. North Am.* 15:615, 1988.
   Current treatment modalities for Mycoplasma *pneumonia.*
10. Cox, S. M., Cunningham, F. G., and Luby, J. Management of varicella pneumonia complicating pregnancy. *Am. J. Perinatol.* 7:300, 1990.
    Guidelines for the treatment of varicella pneumonia and for the evaluation and treatment of the neonate after delivery.
11. Minkoff, H., et al. *Pneumocystis carinii* pneumonia associated with adult immunodeficiency syndrome in pregnancy: a report of three maternal deaths. *Obstet. Gynecol.* 67:284, 1986.
    A review of the deadly nature of Pneumocystis carinii *pneumonia associated with AIDS in pregnancy.*
12. Gibbs, C. P., Rolbin, S. H., and Norman, P. Cause and prevention of maternal aspiration. *Anesthesiology* 61:111, 1984.
    A review of the most commonly encountered anesthetic risks associated with maternal aspiration and measures for their prevention.
13. McKay, S., and Mahan, C. How can aspiration of vomitus in obstetrics best be prevented? *Birth* 15:222, 1988.
    Techniques for decreasing the risk of aspiration pneumonia, particularly in patients with a full stomach, are discussed.

Tuberculosis
14. Collop, N. A., and Harman, E. M. Pulmonary problems in pregnancy. *Compr. Ther.* 4:17, 1990.
    An excellent review of the chemotherapeutic agents used in the treatment of tuberculosis in pregnancy.
15. Benson, C. A. Mycobacterial Infections. In N. Gleicher (ed.), *Principles and Practice of Medical Therapy in Pregnancy*. Norwalk, CT: Appleton-Lange, 1992.
    Current medical practices associated with the evaluation and treatment of tuberculosis.

Adult Respiratory Distress Syndrome
16. Hankins, G. D. V. Acute Pulmonary Injury and Respiratory Failure During Pregnancy. In S. L. Clark, D. B. Cotton, and G. D. V. Hankins (eds.), *Critical Care Obstetrics* (2nd ed.). Boston: Blackwell Scientific, 1991.
    An in-depth dissertation concerning the etiology, evaluation, treatment, and pitfalls in the treatment of patients with ARDS.
17. Erickson, V. L., and Parisi, V. M. Adult respiratory distress syndrome and pregnancy. *Semin. Perinatol.* 14:68, 1990.
    A synopsis of the evaluation and treatment of ARDS in the setting of pregnancy.

Smoking
18. U.S. Department of Health and Human Services. The health benefits of smoking cessation: a report of the Surgeon General. Washington, DC: DHHS Publication No. (CDG) 90–3416, 1990.
    The most current Surgeon General's report concerning smoking and the associated pregnancy risk.
19. Floyd, R. L., et al. Smoking during pregnancy: prevalence, effects, and intervention strategies. *Birth* 18:48, 1991.
    An outline of a smoking cessation program that is enjoying success in the author's private practice.

13. CARDIOVASCULAR DISEASE IN PREGNANCY
Sterling W. McColgin

In the past thirty years, a dramatic shift has occurred in the etiology of cardiovascular lesions. Previously, acquired disease (usually rheumatic fever) was twenty times more common than congenital heart disease. Today, that ratio has shifted dramatically due to the decline in rheumatic heart disease and also to increased longevity in women with congenital heart disease. Infectious cardiac disease does still occur, and recently has been on the rise because of the increased number of women who are intravenous drug abusers and who are immunocompromised. Regardless of the cause, cardiovascular disease continues to be a leading nonobstetric cause of maternal death.

The physiologic cardiac changes that take place in pregnancy result in marked increases in oxygen and nutrient transport to the developing fetus. The normal heart readily adapts to this increased workload, whereas pregnant patients with underlying cardiac disease may be profoundly affected. The physiologic changes of the cardiovascular system during pregnancy include significant increases in cardiac output, stroke volume, and heart rate, combined with decreased peripheral vascular resistance. Two other considerations particularly pertinent to patients with heart disease include the hypercoagulable state associated with pregnancy and the marked fluctuations in cardiac output seen in the intrapartum and postpartum periods. Early cardiovascular alterations appear to primarily stem from the increased blood volume (40–50%) and the decreased peripheral vascular resistance. The increase in stroke volume is initiated early in pregnancy, peaks in the late second trimester, and then falls to almost normal by term. There is a gradual increase in heart rate that peaks at term at approximately 15 beats per minute greater than nonpregnant levels. The cardiac output fluctuates depending on the body position. The greatest effect (25% decrease) is seen in the supine position, owing to uterine compression of the vena cava. The reverse is true (25% increase) when the patient changes from the supine to the left lateral decubitus position. During labor, cardiac output increases by 25 percent over prelabor values during uterine contractions, with a further rise (20–60%) at delivery. The postpartum cardiac output abates, owing to blood loss, the rapid involution of the uterus with resultant increased venous return, a decreased intravascular space, and the administration of oxytocics.

The New York Heart Association classifies patients with heart disease according to their functional capacity. Patients in classes I and II have little or no limitation to activity, and these patients generally do well in pregnancy. Patients in classes III and IV are markedly limited in their ability to engage in physical activity and represent that group of patients at highest risk for maternal and perinatal morbidity and mortality. These patients generally should be advised not to become pregnant until their functional capacity can be improved to class I or II through medical or surgical means. Usually cardiac disease has already been diagnosed in these patients, but, occasionally, it is initially suspected only during pregnancy. Such patients must then undergo thorough cardiac evaluation that includes appropriate consultation, chest x-ray studies, electrocardiography, and echocardiography. Holter monitoring can be performed for those patients with arrhythmias. Other more invasive procedures can be performed if indicated. In those patients found to be in class III or IV, efforts should be made to improve their cardiac status to class I or II.

Several cardiac lesions are usually well tolerated in pregnancy, as many patients are in class I or II. These lesions include mild mitral, aortic, or pulmonary valvular disease, idiopathic hypertrophic subaortic stenosis (IHSS), mitral valve prolapse, and small shunts such as an atrial septal defect, ventricular septal defect, and patent ductus arteriosus. Patients with class III or IV cardiac disease of any nature, including primary pulmonary hypertension, Eisenmenger's syndrome, complicated coarctation of the aorta, Marfan's syndrome with aortic involvement, and peripartal myocardiopathy, are considered to have severe cardiac disease that is a contraindication to pregnancy. These patients carry a 25 to 50 percent risk of mortality during pregnancy. There is an intermediate classification of disease severity, with a maternal mortality rate of between 5 and 15 percent, in those patients with significant mitral or aortic stenosis, coarctation of the aorta without valvular involvement, uncorrected tetralogy of Fallot, previous myocardial infarction, Marfan's syndrome with a normal aortic root, and mitral stenosis with atrial fibrillation, and this classification also includes patients with prosthetic heart valves. In this subset of patients it is prudent to have a conference involving a high-risk obstetric specialist and a cardiologist or cardiovascular surgeon, together with the patient and her family, before she attempts pregnancy to discuss the risk-benefit ratio of pregnancy or of continuing a pregnancy should it already be present.

Mitral stenosis is still the most common lesion resulting from rheumatic heart disease. This condition involves decreased ventricular diastolic filling, which results in a relatively fixed cardiac output. If the mitral stenosis is severe and deemed class III or IV disease, pregnancy should not be undertaken. Such patients who do become pregnant must be monitored carefully during pregnancy for the development of tachycardia, atrial fibrillation, and pulmonary edema. Patients with chronic or paroxysmal atrial fibrillation, left atrial clot, or a prior embolic history must be treated with anticoagulants. Heparin remains the drug of choice. These patients are best managed with bed rest, careful diuresis, and aggressive intervention in the event of any evidence of tachycardia, pulmonary edema, or atrial fibrillation. Closed mitral commissurotomy or valvular replacement has been accomplished safely during pregnancy, but operation should be avoided if possible. These patients need to receive appropriate subacute bacterial endocarditis (SBE) prophylaxis during labor and delivery, with prophylaxis given throughout pregnancy should the lesion be rheumatic in origin. Should atrial fibrillation develop, digoxin treatment should be considered to control the ventricular rate. The most dangerous time for patients with serious disease is the intrapartum and postpartum eras, because of the attendant marked fluctuations in blood volume. Some advocate beta-blocker therapy for those patients whose pulse rate exceeds 90 beats per minute. Obtaining pulmonary capillary wedge pressure readings intrapartum should be considered in patients with more significant disease, with close attention to the patient's volume status. Maintaining the wedge pressure at or below 14 to 16 mm Hg should minimize volume shifts.

Aortic stenosis is most commonly a result of a rheumatic heart disease and often occurs in conjunction with other lesions. Patients with this entity also require careful monitoring throughout pregnancy, and it has been associated with high fetal and maternal mortality, particularly in those patients with more severe disease. Patients with class III or IV disease should be advised against pregnancy before surgical correction. If pregnancy does occur, bed rest in the left lateral decubitus position and avoidance of medication that might decrease cardiac output are recommended. Physical activity must be limited in such patients. Preload is necessary to maintain the already fixed stroke volume, and thus diuretics should be avoided. These patients may also have ischemic heart disease, placing them at significant risk for myocardial infarction. Pulmonary artery catheterization should also be considered intrapartum, with the capillary wedge pressures maintained at the high normal range to prevent hypovolemia. If the lesion is rheumatic in origin, SBE prophylaxis is recommended.

Coarctation of the aorta should be managed individually according to the patient's functional classification, associated defects, and severity. There is an increased risk of maternal death in those patients with an anomalous or bicuspid aortic valve in association with the aortic coarctation. Associated anomalies include ventricular septal defects, patent ductus arteriosus, and intracranial aneurysms of the circle of Willis. If these risk factors exist, the risk of death approaches 15 percent and such patients should be counseled accordingly. Maternal risk is substantially increased in these patients if pregnancy-induced hypertension develops.

Patients with corrected tetralogy of Fallot generally do well during pregnancy if they are in functional class I or II. Patients with uncorrected tetralogy of Fallot with class III or IV disease should be strongly counseled concerning the advisability of pregnancy. Women with Marfan's syndrome, even without aortic involvement, must be monitored closely for the onset of aortic dissection during pregnancy. The pregnancy-associated mortality rate in women with an aortic root diameter greater than 40 mm may be as high as 50 percent. It may be prudent to serially assess the aortic root diameters in these women throughout pregnancy. In counseling patients with Marfan's syndrome and IHSS, patients need to understand that these are autosomal dominant conditions, with a theoretical 50 percent chance of transmitting the disease to their offspring. In general, pregnant patients who have other congenital heart disease transfer a risk to their offspring of between 2 and 10 percent. However, the transmission rate for congenital aortic stenosis or coarctation may be as high as 18 percent. The risk of congenital transmission, if the father of the child is affected, ranges between 1 and 3 percent.

Pregnant women with prosthetic heart valves pose a particular dilemma. Certainly those patients with class III or IV disease should be advised against pregnancy. Porcine prosthetic valves are generally preferable in women of reproductive age because these patients may not have to undergo anticoagulation. However, there is a potential risk of accelerated deterioration of the valve during pregnancy. All patients with mechanical heart valves need to undergo anticoagulation. Patients with porcine valves likewise need to undergo anticoagulation should they have a history of atrial fibrillation, atrial hypertrophy, or thromboembolism. It is the prevalent opinion in the United States to treat patients needing anticoagulation with subcutaneous heparin two or three times a day, maintaining a partial thromboplastin time of 1½ to 2 times control or appropriate heparin levels.

For patients with significant cardiovascular lesions, early and prolonged hospitalization is frequently necessary. These patients must be seen more frequently by both the obstetrician and the cardiologist throughout pregnancy, and must be monitored for worsening signs and symptoms, such as diminished exercise tolerance, increased dyspnea, the development of cyanosis, or sudden weight gain. Signs of atrial fibrillation and venous congestion (hallmarks of pulmonary edema) should be looked for at each visit. Activity should generally be restricted, and frequent rest should be encouraged. Diuretic treatment, a limited salt diet, and early hospital admission if any evidence of pulmonary congestion appears are basic measures in preventing congestive heart failure. Alcohol ingestion and smoking should be avoided because of their negative impact on cardiac output.

Many cardiac patients are maintained on cardiac medications throughout pregnancy, as indicated. Digoxin, beta-blockers, diuretics, and antiarrhythmic medications (such as quinidine, procainamide, lidocaine, and verapamil) have been shown to be relatively safe during pregnancy. All of these should be used judiciously and with appropriate monitoring. Dilantin (phenytoin) should particularly be avoided in the first trimester, if possible, because of the risk of precipitating fetal hydantoin syndrome.

Fetal surveillance is important in patients with cardiac disease, owing to the increased incidence of intrauterine growth retardation and stillbirth. Kick counts can be started in the third trimester and supplemented with additional fetal surveillance as indicated. The obstetrician, cardiologist, and anesthesiologist should work together as a team during the intrapartum and postpartum periods. It is generally best to plan for delivery once fetal lung maturity is ascertained, or if fetal distress is noted or maternal disease worsens. Intense hemodynamic monitoring may be beneficial during labor and delivery in patients at risk for the development of pulmonary edema. Epidural anesthesia remains the treatment of choice for pain relief in most patients with cardiac disease, but must be avoided in patients with conditions in which decreased systemic vascular resistance is contraindicated, including aortic stenosis, IHSS, and pulmonary hypertension. As an alternative, small doses of systemic narcotics may be given in these cases. A semisitting position appears to be optimal for the laboring cardiac patient in labor. The lithotomy position is discouraged for delivery, owing to the increased volume load in the immediate peripartum period. Antibiotics for SBE prophylaxis should be administered in appropriate patients starting early in the course of labor or immediately after cesarean section, with at least two doses given 8 hours apart after delivery and a total of at least three doses.

Peripartal cardiomyopathy is a syndrome of cardiac failure that occurs late in pregnancy or postpartum without an obvious cause in a woman with a previously normal heart. The mortality rate associated with this condition is quite high, with most deaths occurring within the first 3 months postpartum. Medical management of this condition parallels the conventional treatment for heart failure, including digoxin, diuretics, and sodium restriction. The risk associated with future pregnancies depends on the residual cardiomegaly. These patients must be appropriately counseled.

Sterilization should be offered to cardiac patients with significant disease. A viable option for those patients undergoing vaginal delivery for whom operation is contraindicated is a vasectomy in the spouse. In patients desiring sterilization who have undergone vaginal delivery, the nonpregnant cardiovascular condition should be regained before performing sterilization procedures in most cases. Contraception for the postpartum cardiac patient is particularly complex because of the relative contraindications to both oral contraceptives and intrauterine devices in these patients. Norplant certainly offers a viable option for intermediate-term contraception. Likewise, barrier contraceptives are safe, but carry a higher risk of contraceptive failure.

General
1. Cardiac Disease in Pregnancy. *ACOG Tech. Bull.* No. 168, 1992.
   The American College of Obstetrics and Gynecology guidelines for the evaluation and treatment of patients with cardiac disease in pregnancy.
2. Hess, D. B., and Hess, L. W. Management of cardiovascular disease in pregnancy. *Obstet. Gynecol. Clin. North Am.* 19:679, 1992.
   A current review of the evaluation, treatment, and counseling of patients with heart disease who are contemplating pregnancy.
3. Clark, S. L. Cardiac disease in pregnancy. *Crit. Care Clin.* 7:777, 1991.
   Current management guidelines for cardiac disease in pregnancy, with particular emphasis on specific lesions.

Physiology
4. Yeomans, E. R., and Hankins, G. D. V. Cardiovascular physiology and invasive cardiac monitoring. *Clin. Obstet. Gynecol.* 32:2, 1989.
   An overview of the physiologic changes that take place in the heart patient who is pregnant, and the cardiac monitoring involved.
5. Clark S. L., et al. Central hemodynamic assessment of normal term pregnancy. *Am. J. Obstet. Gynecol.* 161:1439, 1989.
   The article focuses on the hemodynamics measured in normal pregnancies antepartum and postpartum using pulmonary capillary wedge pressure monitoring.

Specific Lesions
6. Easterling, T. R., et al. Aortic stenosis in pregnancy. *Obstet. Gynecol.* 72:113, 1988.
   Discussion of aortic stenosis in pregnancy, with management guidelines.
7. Clark, S. L. How labor and delivery influence mitral stenosis. *Contemp. Ob/Gyn* 27:127, 1986.
   An overview of mitral stenosis with particular emphasis on management during labor and delivery.
8. McColgin, S. W., Martin, J. N., and Morrison, J. C. Pregnant women with prosthetic heart valves. *Clin. Obstet. Gynecol.* 32:76, 1989.
   Extensive review of pregnancy in patients with prosthetic heart valves.
9. Rotmensch, H., Rotmensch, C., and Elkayam, U. Management of cardiac arrhythmias during pregnancy. *Drugs* 33:623, 1987.
   A review of cardiac arrhythmias and the antiarrhythmic drugs that can be used during pregnancy.
10. Nolan, T. E., and Hankins, G. D. V. Myocardial infarction in pregnancy. *Clin. Obstet. Gynecol.* 32:68, 1989.
    Management guidelines for the pregnant patient with a myocardial infarction.

Treatment
11. Little, B. B., and Gilstrap, L. C., III. Cardiovascular drugs during pregnancy. *Clin. Obstet. Gynecol.* 32:13, 1989.
    Current recommendations concerning cardiovascular drug use and management during pregnancy.
12. Roberts, S. L., and Chestnut, D. H. Anesthesia for the obstetric patient with cardiac disease. *Clin. Obstet. Gynecol.* 30:601, 1987.
    The anesthesia management of labor and delivery in patients with cardiac disease is outlined.
13. Frishman, W. H., and Chesner, M. Beta-adrenergic blockers in pregnancy. *Am. Heart J.* 115:147, 1988.
    The role of beta-adrenergic blockers in pregnancy is discussed.
14. Clark, S. L. Labor and delivery in the patient with structural cardiac disease. *Clin. Perinatol.* 13:695, 1986.
    Guidelines for the management of cardiac patients in labor are presented.
15. Dajani, A. D., et al. Prevention of bacterial endocarditis. Recommendations by the American Heart Association. *J.A.M.A.* 264:2919, 1990.
    Current guidelines for the prophylaxis and treatment of subacute bacterial endocarditis.

Counseling
16. Whittemore, R., Hobbins, J. C., and Engle, M. A. Pregnancy and its outcome in women with and without surgical treatment of congenital heart disease. *Am. J. Cardiol.* 50:641, 1982.
    Counseling a patient with congenital heart disease prior to pregnancy and for subsequent pregnancy.
17. Nora, J. J., and Nora, A. H. Maternal transmission of congenital heart diseases: new recurrence risk figures and the questions of cytoplasmic inheritance and vulnerability to teratogens. *Am. J. Cardiol.* 59:459, 1987.
    The recurrence risk in the offspring if either parent has congenital heart disease. Particularly valuable is Table IV in this article.
18. Filkins, K. Recurrence risks for congenital heart defects. *Contemp. Ob/Gyn* 32:19, 1988.
    The recurrence risk if a previous child has had a congenital heart defect averages 3 to 4 percent for the next gestation.
19. Mabie, W. C., Hackman, B. B., and Sibai, B. M. Pulmonary edema associated with pregnancy: echocardiographic insights and implications for treatment. *Obstet. Gynecol.* 81:227, 1993.
    Forty-seven percent of pregnant women with pulmonary edema proved to have unsuspected findings on an echocardiogram, which altered long-term management.

28 - 30 weeks   weekly clinic.

14. DIABETES MELLITUS ASSOCIATED WITH PREGNANCY
Rick W. Martin

Diabetes mellitus is a metabolic disorder associated with hyperglycemia, which results in an increased rate of congenital malformations and perinatal morbidity and mortality. Gestational diabetes can arise in 3 to 12 percent of all pregnancies, and this represents approximately 90 percent of all cases of diabetes occurring during pregnancy. Fortunately, with control of the hyperglycemia, the complications of diabetes can be reduced.

Outside of pregnancy, diabetic patients are typically classified as having either type I disease, insulin-dependent diabetes, or type II disease, non–insulin-dependent diabetes mellitus. Although type II patients may require insulin therapy, they are not usually prone to suffering ketoacidosis. In pregnancy, White's classification is generally used. This classification categorizes patients according to gestational versus preexisting diabetes, and also classifies patients according to the age at onset and duration of diabetes as well as any systemic involvement.

Women known to have diabetes should undergo evaluation before pregnancy. The risk of a congenital anomaly has been shown to be increased in women with poor glucose control, as reflected by the hemoglobin A_1C level. The most common malformations include cardiac and neural tube defects. Ideal metabolic control during pregnancy is generally accepted to be a plasma glucose fasting level of 60 to 90 mg/dl, and a before-meal glucose level of 60 to 105 mg/dl. Two-hour postprandial glucose levels should be less than 120 mg/dl. Most pregnant women require approximately 2200 calories a day, divided among three meals and a bedtime snack. A mid-morning and mid-afternoon snack may also be prescribed. Insulin therapy is usually given twice daily and, as a rule, two thirds of the insulin is given in the morning and one third is given in the evening. Combinations of intermediate-acting insulins, such as NPH, and a shorter-acting insulin, such as regular insulin, are prescribed. Usually human insulin generated by recombinant techniques is preferable to animal-derived insulin.

Laboratory evaluation of the insulin-dependent diabetic includes an assessment for systemic involvement, consisting of a 24-hour urine specimen for determination of the creatinine clearance of protein, an electrocardiogram, and urine culture. An ophthalmologic evaluation is performed in each trimester, and the patient is seen every 1 to 2 weeks throughout her pregnancy.

At each clinical visit, the maternal weight gain is assessed, and blood glucose levels, determined by a reflectance meter, are measured by the patient at home four times a day on a daily basis, and these records are reviewed. Most would agree that serial sonographic examinations are indicated to evaluate fetal growth. An alphafetoprotein level is determined and a targeted sonogram performed in the second trimester to evaluate for any possible fetal anomalies. Antepartum fetal surveillance is usually begun at 32 weeks' gestation, but may be instituted sooner in individual cases. If the nonstress test is to be used, it should be performed on a twice-weekly basis. Others prefer a combination of nonstress and contraction stress testing. When results of these tests are positive, they are evaluated in the context of the biophysical profile, or the physician may decide to induce delivery, especially when the fetus is mature. Delivery is usually planned before the fortieth week of gestation, and some advise amniocentesis to document fetal lung maturity, especially in cases in which glycemic control has been poor. Fetal lung maturation may not proceed as predicted in diabetic pregnancies, and often a phosphatidylglycerol evaluation is performed, in addition to determination of the L:S (lecithin-to-sphingomyelin) ratio.

At the onset of labor, or should induction be chosen, glucose control remains important. To maintain a maternal glucose level at approximately 100 mg/dl, a continuous infusion of regular insulin is administered in a 5% dextrose solution. The mother is evaluated regularly throughout labor. Using this protocol will decrease the risk of neonatal hypoglycemia resulting from the appearance of hyperinsulinemia, which is a response to elevated glucose levels in utero.

Glyburide safe for DM pregnancy.

maintains glucose level 110 mg/dl during labor

In the postpartum period, glucose control is relaxed somewhat, with the aim to prevent ketoacidosis, and glucose values of 150 to 200 mg/dl are then considered acceptable. The insulin regimen is decreased significantly from prepregnancy values, and hypoglycemia frequently occurs at this time.

The detection of those women who will suffer diabetes during pregnancy involves screening those at risk. The presence of typical risk factors, a family history of diabetes, obesity, maternal age greater than 25, or the previous birth of a macrosomic infant, will only reveal half of these patients. Some practitioners prefer to test all women during pregnancy. The most commonly employed technique involves the use of a 50-g glucose drink administered orally, with the plasma glucose level determined 1 hour later. If values exceed 140 mg/dl, then a formal 3-hour glucose tolerance test is carried out. For this procedure, at least 3 days of an unrestricted diet, with more than 150 g of carbohydrates consumed daily, is recommended. With the patient at rest, fasting 1-, 2-, and 3-hour plasma glucose levels are determined, with normal levels being less than 105, 190, 165, and 145 mg/dl, respectively. If the patient exhibits two or more values that exceed these levels, she is considered to have gestational diabetes.

The gestational diabetic may be managed by dietary measures alone, but she should be evaluated at 1- to 2-week intervals and, if fasting levels exceed 105 mg/dl or the 2-hour postprandial glucose level is 120 mg/dl, the patient is placed on an insulin regimen similar to that used in the patient with preexisting diabetes. Fetal surveillance in the setting of gestational diabetes is begun at 30 to 32 weeks in the insulin-dependent gestational diabetic, and at 40 weeks in the non–insulin dependent diabetic. The patient with diabetes should be monitored frequently for the presence of hypertension, as this may coexist with the diabetes, or she should be monitored for the development of pregnancy-induced hypertension. Although vaginal delivery may usually be accomplished, particular attention should be given to an estimation of fetal weight, as fetal macrosomia and subsequent shoulder dystocia may occur.

Contraception for the diabetic patient is a difficult problem. The barrier methods are less effective, but would not exert systemic effects, as would be expected with oral contraceptives. The possibility of undergoing permanent sterilization at the completion of childbearing should also be discussed.

General
1. Management of Diabetes Mellitus in Pregnancy. *ACOG Tech. Bull.* No. 92, May 1986.
   Overview of the accepted classification of diabetes in pregnancy and recommended screening techniques. General guidelines for pregnancy management are also given.
2. Landon, M. B. Diabetes Mellitus and Other Endocrine Diseases. In S. G. Gabbe, J. R. Niebyl, and J. L. Simpson (eds.), *Obstetrics: Normal and Problem Pregnancies* (2nd ed.). New York: Churchill Livingstone, 1991.
   An excellent summary of the problem of diabetes in pregnancy and a detailed algorithm for clinical management are presented.

Diabetes Screening
3. Cousins, S. L., et al. Screening recommendations for gestational diabetes mellitus. *Am. J. Obstet. Gynecol.* 165:493, 1991.
   A screening threshold no higher than 140 mg/dl is recommended after the 50-g oral glucose challenge test.
4. Lindsay, M. K., Graves, W., and Klein L. The relationship of one abnormal glucose tolerance test value and pregnancy complications. *Obstet. Gynecol.* 73:103, 1989.
   Pregnant women with one abnormal value during the oral glucose tolerance test were at risk for fetal macrosomia and preeclampsia.
5. Reece, E. A., et al. Assessment of carbohydrate tolerance in pregnancy. *Obstet. Gynecol. Surv.* 46:1, 1990.
   A comprehensive discussion of all aspects of diabetes screening during preg-

metformin: may ("B" catagory) used in pregnancy

Basal need +300 kcal for singleton.

nancy is presented, including the method of glucose loading and laboratory test
procedures. *Carbohydrate counting·*

Management

6. Jovanovic-Peterson, L., Kitzmiller, J. L., and Peterson, C. M. Randomized trial of human versus animal species insulin in diabetic pregnant women: improved glycemic control, not fewer antibodies to insulin, influences birth weight. *Am. J. Obstet. Gynecol.* 167:1325, 1992.
   The use of human insulin was associated with less maternal hyperglycemia or hypoglycemia, fewer macrosomic infants, fewer large-for-gestational-age infants, and less neonatal hyperinsulinemia.

7. Landon, M. B., et al. Fetal surveillance in pregnancies complicated by insulin-dependent diabetes mellitus. *Am. J. Obstet. Gynecol.* 167:617, 1992.
   Pregnancies complicated by vascular disease were at greatest risk for abnormal findings during fetal testing, requiring early delivery.

8. Coustan, D. R., et al. A randomized clinical trial of insulin pump versus intensive conventional therapy in diabetic pregnancies. *J.A.M.A.* 255:631, 1986.
   Excellent glucose control was obtained with either the insulin pump or conventional therapy.

9. Barrett, J. M., Salyer, S. L., and Boehm, F. H. The nonstress test: an evaluation of 1000 patients. *Am. J. Obstet. Gynecol.* 141:153, 1981.
   Weekly nonstress testing was not adequate for evaluation in patients with diabetes mellitus.

10. Landon, M. B., Gabbe, S. G., and Sachs, L. Management of diabetes mellitus in pregnancy: a survey of obstetricians and maternal-fetal specialists. *Obstet. Gynecol.* 75:635, 1990.
    Intensive fetal surveillance, elective delivery, and high cesarean delivery rates are common in pregnancies complicated by insulin-dependent diabetes. Most clinicians practice universal screening for diabetes.

11. Coustan, D. R., and Imarah, J. Prophylactic insulin treatment of gestational diabetes reduced the incidence of macrosomia, operative delivery, and birth trauma. *Am. J. Obstet. Gynecol.* 150:836, 1984.
    The incidence of fetal macrosomia was 7 percent in the insulin-treated group, 17.8 percent in the untreated group, and 18.5 percent in a diet-only–treated group of women with gestational diabetes.

Complications

12. Miller, E., et al. Elevated maternal hemoglobin A_1C in early pregnancy and major congenital anomalies in infants of diabetic mothers. *N. Engl. J. Med.* 304:1331, 1981.
    There was a 3.4 percent risk of major congenital anomalies when the hemoglobin A_1C value was below 8.5 percent, and the risk was 22.4 percent when the value was greater than 8.5 percent.

13. Elman, K. D., et al. Diabetic retinopathy in pregnancy: a review. *Obstet. Gynecol.* 75:119, 1990.
    The authors discuss the impact of diabetic retinopathy in pregnancy and evaluate current treatment methods.

14. Mills, J. L., et al. Incidence of spontaneous abortion among normal women and insulin-dependent diabetic women whose pregnancies were identified within 21 days of conception. *N. Engl. J. Med.* 319:1617, 1988.
    Women with poorly controlled diabetes had a significantly increased risk of spontaneous abortion.

15. Ojomo, E. O., and Coustan, D. R. Absence of evidence of pulmonary maturity at amniocentesis in term infants of diabetic mothers. *Am. J. Obstet. Gynecol.* 163:954, 1990.
    In 21 percent of women with gestational diabetes, no phosphatidylglycerol was detected in the amniotic fluid as late as 38 weeks' gestation.

16. Ballard, J. L., et al. Diabetic fetal macrosomia: significance of disproportionate growth. *J. Pediatr.* 122:115, 1993.

insulin: 1st trimester: 0.7-0.8 units/kg/day
2nd   0.8 - 1.0,
0.9 - 1.2

food log,

Infants with dysproportional macrosomia, as reflected by a high weight-to-length ratio, were most likely to exhibit hypoglycemia, acidosis, and hyperbilirubinemia.

17. Kjaer, K., et al. Infertility and pregnancy outcome in an unselected group of women with insulin-dependent diabetes mellitus. *Am. J. Obstet. Gynecol.* 166:1412, 1992.

   Insulin-dependent diabetic women had a normal ability to conceive, but had fewer pregnancies and fewer births per pregnancy than did controls.

18. Reece, A., et al. Diabetic nephropathy: pregnancy performance and fetomaternal outcome. *Am. J. Obstet. Gynecol.* 159:56, 1988.

   With the current methods of managing insulin-dependent diabetes, the risk of adverse outcome in women with diabetic nephropathy was not excessive.

15. THYROID DISEASE IN PREGNANCY
Sue M. Palmer

The functioning of the thyroid gland is altered by the metabolic and hormonal changes that take place during pregnancy. Likewise, the reproductive outcome may be affected by diseases of this organ. Because all forms of thyroid disease are three to four times more common in women than in men, disorders of this gland are not uncommon during pregnancy.

The hormonal milieu of pregnancy complicates interpretation of the results of thyroid function studies. The triiodothyronine (T_3) resin uptake (T_3RU) decreases secondary to the increase in carrier proteins (thyroid-binding globulin, albumin, and prealbumin). By creating a fraction of the normal for T_3RU (measured T_3RU over the mean of normal) and multiplying that times the thyroxine (T_4) level, the functional (free) T_4 level can be estimated. An example of this is as follows. If the normal mean for T_3RU is 30 percent and the patient's T_3RU level is 15 percent, then 15 divided by 30 times a T_4 of 16 μg/dl equals 8 μg/dl, a level that is within normal limits for free T_4. This can also be done for T_3. For the T_3RIA (normal, 80–200 ng/dl), a nonpregnant value of 250 ng/dl is reduced to 125 ng/dl during pregnancy. These calculations are necessary to evaluate any patient in an increased estrogenic state, whether owing to pregnancy or exogenous estrogen therapy.

Tests that are the most important in diagnosing the various thyroid disease states are the T_3RU, T_4, T_7, or free thyroid index (which is a multiple of T_3RU and T_4 and eliminates hormonal influence), and determining the level of the thyroid-stimulating hormone (TSH), a pituitary hormone that is not altered either by changes in pregnancy hormone levels or by carrier protein levels. Measuring the TSH level is most important in diagnosing hypothyroidism and monitoring such patients, whereas the T_3RIA is most important in diagnosing hyperthyroidism.

The placenta is essentially impermeable to T_4, T_3, and TSH, but not to iodine, so that the fetal thyroid develops independently of the maternal system. During pregnancy, therefore, radioiodine uptake assessment of thyroid function is contraindicated because of resultant fetal hypothyroidism. Neonatal and fetal thyroid function laboratory values are slightly higher than maternal values, with increased fetal free T_4, T_3, and TSH levels that decrease by the fifth day after delivery to normal nonpregnant adult values.

Maternal hypothyroidism is relatively uncommon in the pregnant patient because menstrual irregularities, oligoovulation, and spontaneous abortion are hallmarks of this disorder. Hypothyroidism is generally thought to be an immunologic disease with a multifactorial inheritance found predominantly in females. One of the more common causes is iatrogenic, that is, patients are told to stop taking thyroid replacement medications to observe for possible resolution of the condition. The primary condition is usually associated with a goiter (owing to the gland's inability to produce T_4 and T_3, which results in hypertrophy of the organ). The goiter is generally multinodular and can enlarge to cause potential airway management problems. Primary hypothyroidism is usually secondary to chronic thyroiditis, prior radioactive iodine therapy, thyroidectomy (surgical or iodine 131), or the ingestion of goitrogens (e.g., thiocyanate, lithium carbonate, or amiodarone). Secondary hypothyroidism, resulting from a chromophobe adenoma of the pituitary gland, Sheehan's syndrome, and so on, is rare. Idiopathic hypothyroidism has a much more protracted onset and is usually related to the presence of Hashimoto's disease.

Complaints of fatigue, obesity, coarse skin, thinning of the hair (particularly the eyebrows), myxedematous changes (facial or tibial), macroglossia, and a subnormal body temperature are typical signs of hypothyroidism. Paresthesias and delayed deep tendon reflexes are early symptoms in about 75 percent of the patients. Postpartum amenorrhea and galactorrhea may be presenting complaints of hypothyroidism after pregnancy has ended. Thyroid antibodies are frequently detected in these cases. This scenario occurs more commonly after parturition than in nonpregnant patients.

The laboratory diagnosis of hypothyroidism rests on a reduction in the T_4 level and in the T_3RU, the presence of anemia, and an elevated TSH level. Once the diagnosis of hypothyroidism is established, therapy should be instituted, but care must be taken in the older patient to gradually increase the dose of thyroid replacement medication, because cardiovascular insults can occur if the thyroid deficiency is corrected too rapidly. Most patients with early hypothyroidism may be started on 50 to 100 μg per day of levothyroxine, increasing the dosage by 25 μg per day every week until the patient is euthyroid. Most patients require 100 to 200 μg of thyroxine per day for maintenance therapy. Optimal maintenance therapy can be determined by the patient's clinical status, TSH levels, and free thyroxine index. The prognosis for both the mother and fetus is excellent when hypothyroidism is corrected, although antepartum fetal assessment in the third trimester is indicated, owing to a small increase in the stillbirth rate.

Maternal hyperthyroidism is not uncommon, ranging from 0.05 to 0.2 percent during pregnancy. Hyperthyroidism during pregnancy is associated with an increase in neonatal wastage and low-birth-weight infants. There is no evidence that the pregnancy per se makes the disease process more difficult to control, although there is a propensity for relapse during the postpartum period. The most common causes, in descending order of frequency, are toxic diffuse goiter (Graves' disease), acute thyroiditis, toxic nodular goiter (Plummer's disease), and toxic adenoma. Graves' disease occurs frequently during pregnancy, and is usually diagnosed based on the presence of the classic symptoms of weight loss, ocular signs, pretibial myxedema, a resting pulse rate above 100 beats per minute (bpm) that fails to slow during a Valsalva maneuver, muscular wasting, and nervousness. The serum T_4 level exceeds normal pregnancy values (>12 μg/dl). Similarly, a T_3RU in the normal nonpregnant range is indicative of thyrotoxicosis during pregnancy.

Treatment is basically medical, with surgical removal infrequently advocated and radioactive iodine therapy contraindicated. All therapies of hyperthyroidism initially center around slowing the release or stopping conversion of T_4 to T_3. In pregnancy, propylthiouracil (PTU) is the drug of choice. In the setting of severe hyperthyroidism, a dosage of 100 to 200 mg 4 times daily may be required. Mild hyperthyroidism usually responds to a dosage of 100 mg 3 times daily. Symptoms of hyperthyroidism usually decrease 2 to 3 weeks after institution of the least-effective dose to maintain the T_4 at about 14 μg/dl (usually, <200 mg per day). In the face of impending thyroid storm, therapy to avoid decompensation is important. Treatment of the hyperthermia with acetaminophen suppositories (aspirin should be avoided because it can cause displacement of T_4 from T_4-binding globulin) and the application of cooling blankets can be effective. General therapy should also include the use of intravenous multivitamin preparations, glucose as well as fluids, and electrolytes. The administration of 100 mg of hydrocortisone intravenously every 6 to 8 hours may also be indicated. Corticosteroid use also confers the additional benefit of blocking of the conversion of T_4 to T_3.

Propranolol has been the standard beta-blocking agent used in the treatment of thyroid storm because of its physiologic role in controlling heart rate as well as blocking peripheral conversion of T_4 to T_3. The dosage of propranolol for the patient in thyroid storm is 60 to 120 mg given orally every 6 hours until a pulse rate of less than 90 bpm is reached, at which time the dosage can be halved. In the patient who will need emergent cesarean section, use of the intravenous formulation for rapid control is preferred. It is of utmost importance to remember that the intravenous preparation is extremely potent. The starting dosage of propranolol is 0.5 to 1.0 mg followed by 2.0 to 3.0 mg every 10 to 15 minutes. Again, a heart rate of less than 90 bpm is the desired end-point. If the patient has a history of bronchospasm, the use of propranolol is contraindicated. In this situation, metoprolol tartrate (Lopressor), a $beta_1$-blocking agent, should be used instead. The dosage for metoprolol is 5 mg every 2 minutes to a maximum dosage of 15 mg.

Graves' disease is a cyclic disease and may subside spontaneously. With adequate treatment and follow-up, the long-term maternal prognosis is excellent. Fetal prognosis in the setting of well-controlled hyperthyroidism is also excellent. However, two fetal precautions are necessary. First, a few studies have revealed an increased stillbirth rate in the presence of maternal hyperthyroidism, and antepartum fetal assessment is therefore indicated in the third trimester. Second, a fetal goiter may rarely be responsible for a face presentation at delivery, thus necessitating operative delivery. Skilled resuscitation of the newborn after delivery may be needed if the airway is obstructed by a goiter.

Neonatal hypothyroidism is a remediable condition that occurs in 1 in 4000 deliveries. Early diagnosis and treatment are extremely important because the age at which treatment is initiated has a bearing on the prognosis; thus, all neonates should be screened for it. Endemic cretinism occurs in areas of the world where iodine deficiency is relatively common, but parents usually have evidence of a goiter. Thyroid hormone replacement in the infant will return thyroid hormone levels to normal, but does not reverse the associated neurologic deficits (e.g., deaf-mutism and spasticity) acquired in utero, which appear to be due to the lack of iodine in the developing brain.

Patients who have taken PTU may give birth to infants with a small goiter, although there is no evidence that PTU or other drugs have a detrimental long-term effect in terms of growth and development. In contrast, iodine ingestion by the mother has been associated with large neonatal goiters at birth. One of the most important problems caused by these large goiters is respiratory distress owing to laryngeal pressure. In most infants with goiters, a low serum T_4 level (<9.5 $\mu g/dl$) and a normal T_3RU are diagnostic of hypothyroidism.

Thyrotoxicosis is even more common in the newborn than in the mother. Although some infants will receive the 7S immunoglobulin, long-acting thyroid stimulator (LATS), from the mother by means of placental transfer, diagnosis is usually made on the basis of the total clinical picture, which includes maternal symptoms of the disease in conjunction with goiter, tachycardia, increased T_4 levels, and hyperirritability in the infant. Occasionally, the serum T_4 level may not be raised and the goiter may be absent; thus, the positive assay for LATS is helpful in some infants. Cardiac decompensation, hepatosplenomegaly, and jaundice have also been seen in these infants. If the hyperthyroidism is mild, usually no treatment is needed. If treatment is necessary, Lugol's solution (1 drop 3 times a day) or PTU (10 mg every 8 hours) is utilized. Propranolol is reserved for thyrotoxic infants with severe cardiac decompensation. The infants are usually treated for 3 to 6 weeks; after that time, they require no further treatment.

General
1. Kaplan, M. Thyroid Diseases. In N. Gleicher (ed.), *Principles and Practice of Medical Therapy in Pregnancy*. Norwalk, CT: Appleton-Lange, 1992.
   A comprehensive review of the basic and clinical considerations regarding thyroid gland function during pregnancy. The effects of hypothyroid and hyperthyroid states on the neonate and fetus are discussed.
2. Endocrine Disorders in Pregnancy. In A. B. Galway and G. N. Burrow (eds.), *Medicine of the Fetus and Mother*. Philadelphia: Lippincott, 1992.
   A detailed review of the thyroid gland, including the clinical assessment and treatment in the abnormal state in the nonpregnant and pregnant patient.

Etiology

3. Kennedy, R. L., et al. Thyrotoxicosis and hyperemesis gravidarum associated with a serum activity which stimulates human thyroid cells in vitro. *Clin. Endocrinol.* 36:83, 1992.
   This represents a detailed evaluation of the sera response in five patients with biochemical hyperthyroidism and hyperemesis. The stimulatory activity could not be neutralized by depleting the sera of human chorionic gonadotropin.

4. Hayskip, C. C., et al. The value of serum antimicrosomal testing in screening for symptomatic thyroid dysfunction. *Am. J. Obstet. Gynecol.* 159:203, 1988.
   Samples were drawn from 1034 consecutive women on their second postpartum day for the detection of antimicrosomal (AMA) and antithyroglobulin antibodies. Biochemical thyroid dysfunction developed in 34 (67%) of 51 of the AMA-positive women.

5. Learoyd, D. L., et al. Postpartum thyroid dysfunction. *Thyroid* 2:73, 1992.
   This is a review article which shows that in approximately 5 to 9 percent of women thyroid dysfunction develops in the postpartum period, which appears to be related to a rebound from the relative immune tolerance of pregnancy.

6. Othman, S. Iodine metabolism in postpartum thyroiditis. *Thyroid* 2:107, 1992.
   This is the report on a prospective study of 1996 women during the second trimester of pregnancy. It was noted that, in the immediate postpartum period, the iodine excretion of 152 women matched with 235 antibody-positive women did not differ, and neither did the iodine excretion in the 73 women who developed postpartum thyroiditis, compared to controls. Iodine intake is thus unlikely to affect the prevalence of postpartum thyroiditis.

Diagnosis

7. Zimmerman, P., et al. Ultrasonography of the thyroid gland in pregnancies complicated by autoimmune thyroid disease. *J. Clin. Ultrasound* 21:109, 1993.
   A detailed review of the ultrasound findings in both pregnancy and disease states.

8. Gerstein, H. Incidence of postpartum thyroid dysfunction in patients with type I diabetes mellitus. *Ann. Intern. Med.* 118:419, 1993.
   This was a prospective study to examine postpartum thyroid dysfunction in women with type I diabetes. It was noted that this dysfunction occurred in 10 of 40 patients, for a 25 percent incidence. This strongly supports routine thyroid function screening at postpartum visits in type I diabetics.

9. Gerhard, I., et al. Thyroid and ovarian function in infertile women. *Hum. Reprod.* 6:338, 1991.
   This prospective study examined the impact of thyroid function and the pituitary-ovarian axis in infertile women. One hundred eighty-five infertile women without clinical signs of thyroid dysfunction were given a TRH test. Seventy-four were found to be euthyroid, 31 had latent hyperthyroidism, and 80 had preclinical hypothyroidism.

10. Klein, R. Z., et al. Prevalence of thyroid deficiency in pregnant women. *Clin. Endocrinol.* 35:41, 1991.
    This study was carried out to determine the extent of gestational hypothyroidism and was made up of 2000 consecutive women in Maine who were tested for alpha-fetoprotein concentrations. Hypothyroidism was noted in 0.3 percent and hyperthyroidism in 0.3 percent.

11. Goodwin, T. M., et al. Transient hyperthyroidism and hyperemesis gravidarum: clinical aspects. *Am. J. Obstet. Gynecol.* 167:648, 1992.
    Sixty-seven patients with hyperemesis gravidarum were studied prospectively, and 66 percent were found to have biochemical hyperthyroidism. Clinically, this was a self-limited disorder, resolving by 18 weeks' gestation, but the incidence of abnormal electrolyte levels was found to be higher in these patients, and the liver enzyme levels were also increased.

12. Perelman, A. H., et al. Intrauterine diagnosis and treatment of fetal goitrous hyperthyroidism. *J. Clin. Endocrinol. Metab.* 71:618, 1990.
    This is the report of a case study that examined the utilization of percutaneous umbilical blood sampling to diagnose fetal hypothyroidism and the treatment of

the fetus in vitro with intraamniotic injections of T_4. This treatment led to normal thyroid functions at birth with subsequently normal neonatal development.

13. Fort, P., et al. Neonatal thyroid disease: differential expression in three successive offspring. *J. Clin. Endocrinol. Metab.* 66:645, 1988.
   This is an interesting description of a mother with hyperthyroidism and its impact on three children who had different forms of thyroid dysfunction at birth. The first child was clinically normal, the second child had transient neonatal hyperthyroidism, and the third child had neonatal hypothyroidism. This spectrum of neonatal thyroid disease differs depending on whether stimulating or blocking antibodies predominate in the mother.

Treatment

14. Cooper, D. Antithyroid drugs: to breast-feed or not to breast-feed. *Am. J. Obstet. Gynecol.* 157:234, 1987.
   A review article with 14 references that summarize the known data on the effect of antithyroid medicine in infants exposed through breast milk. PTU is the drug of choice in this situation, because it does not cross membranes readily and the milk concentrations are low.

15. Messer, P. M., et al. Antithyroid treatment of Graves' disease in pregnancy: long-term effects on somatic growth, intellectual development and thyroid function of the offspring. *Acta Endocrinol.* 123:311, 1990.
   Comparison was made between 17 children of 13 hyperthyroid mothers receiving antithyroid drug treatment with 25 children of 15 mothers who were euthyroid. There were no adverse effects noted as the result of antithyroid drug treatment during pregnancy.

16. Hashizume, K., et al. Effect of administration of thyroxine on the risk of postpartum recurrence of hyperthyroid Graves' disease. *J. Clin. Endocrinol. Metab.* 75:6, 1992.
   It was found that T_4 administration during pregnancy and after delivery was effective in decreasing the level of antibodies to TSH receptors and in preventing postpartum recurrence of hyperthyroidism.

17. Leung, A. S., et al. Perinatal outcome in hypothyroid pregnancies. *Obstet. Gynecol.* 81:349, 1993.
   Sixty-eight hypothyroid patients were divided into two groups, 23 with overt and 45 with subclinical hypothyroidism. It was noted that gestational hypertension and pregnancy-induced hypertension were significantly more common in the patients with overt and subclinical hypothyroidism, with rates of 22 and 15 percent compared to 7.5 percent in the general population. Low birth weight was higher in the offspring of these pregancies due to delivery for pregnancy-induced hypertension or eclampsia.

18. Matsura, N., et al. Transient hypothyroidism in infants born to mothers with chronic thyroiditis—a nationwide study of 23 cases. *Endocrinol. Jpn.* 37:369, 1990.
   It was found that the children of mothers whose maternal thyroid function during pregnancy was mild or corrected exhibited normal development, in contrast with clinical impairment in the offspring of mothers with abnormal thyroid function. This suggests that maternal thyroid function during pregnancy is an important factor in the prognosis of infants born to mothers with chronic thyroiditis.

Complications

19. Davis, L. E., et al. Thyrotoxicosis complicating pregnancy. *Am. J. Obstet. Gynecol.* 160:63, 1989.
   This 12-year study involved 120,000 women, of which 60 had overt thyrotoxicosis (1:2000). This was diagnosed in 32 women during pregnancy. Because of the preponderance of morbidity in such mothers, the authors advise the institution of aggressive medical therapy, particularly when pregnancy is advanced.

20. Tamaki, H., et al. Evaluation of TSH receptor antibody by "natural in vivo human assay" in neonates born to mothers with Graves' disease. *Clin. Endocrinol.* 30:493, 1989.

Maternal serum thyroid antibody indices showed highly significant correlations with the serum T_4 index and free T_3 index in neonates 5 to 10 days after birth. Further evaluation of the relationship between antibodies and the stimulation index showed that in vitro assays using animal thyroid cells as an index of response are suitable for detecting circulating thyroid stimulating activity in vivo.

21. Page, D. V., et al. The pathology of intrauterine thyrotoxicosis: two case reports. *Obstet. Gynecol.* 72:479, 1988.

    This article reviews in detail the autopsy findings in two infants of mothers with hyperthyroidism. The autopsy findings suggest the presence of intrauterine thyrotoxicosis secondary to transplacental thyroid-stimulating immunoglobulin.

V. MORE HIGH-RISK PREGNANCIES

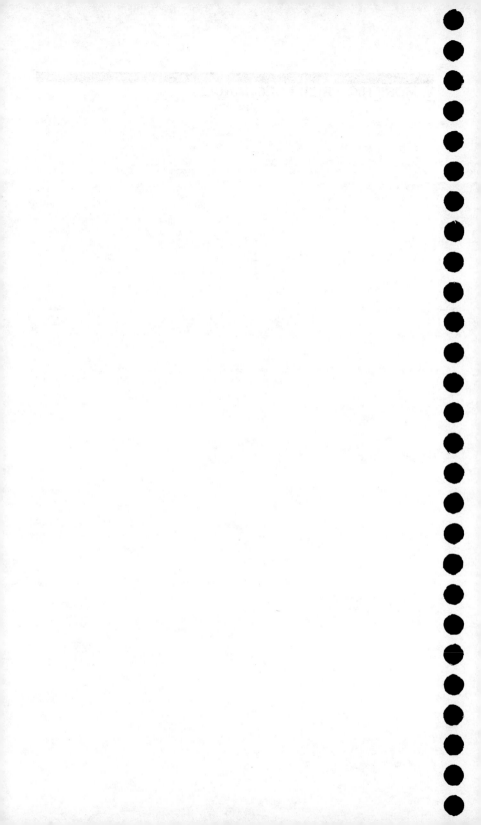

16. PREGNANCY IN THE ADOLESCENT

Sister Clarice Carroll

Of all the developed and industrialized nations in the world, the United States continues to rank as one of the highest in terms of pregnancy and childbearing. Each year more than 1.1 million adolescents (10% of female adolescents) become pregnant. The births resulting from these pregnancies account for 20 percent of the total births in the United States. Two fifths of all American adolescent girls will have conceived by the age of 19, and 400,000 will have an abortion. Despite the availability of contraceptive information and methods and the legalization of abortion, pregnancy prevention in adolescent females has not been successful.

The incidence of adolescent pregnancy is not bound by social class or race; however, the most vulnerable adolescents are those who are disadvantaged socially, economically, and ethnically. Black adolescent girls from low-income families continue to rank the highest among all pregnancies in the United States. It is a known and proven fact that adolescents living in poverty are more likely than their middle-class peers to become sexually active earlier.

All too frequently, adolescent pregnancy is not only unplanned but unwanted. Adolescent pregnancy has a negative impact on the physical, social, emotional, educational, and economic conditions of the teenaged woman. Too early she becomes a child-mother with a vulnerable, and perhaps neglected and abused, newborn.

The change in the age of menarche from just over 14 years to 12.5 years, with fertility occurring by age 14, has influenced the high rate of adolescent pregnancy. Increased sexual activity at younger ages, with one fifth of adolescents having had intercourse by age 16 and two thirds by age 19, has also contributed to the rising pregnancy rate. Many of these teenagers have misinformation on human anatomy and reproduction. They may be biologically immature, yet one half of premarital first pregnancies occur in adolescent girls within 6 months of beginning sexual intercourse, and one fifth occur in the first month.

The psychologic factors associated with the motivation for pregnancy in the adolescent are complex. These may include a desire to establish her identity as an "adult," escape from responsibility, rebellion against authority figures, and a desire for or the need to give love. Pregnancy may also temporarily bolster her self-esteem through peer acceptance, or serve as a mechanism through which a relationship with a significant male can be established or maintained. In addition, adolescents who become pregnant have a poor self-image and self-esteem. Their own identity is incomplete, and they do not have the necessary skills to form their baby's identity. Repeat pregnancy among adolescent mothers is a major problem. Immature child-mothers are poorly equipped to face the demands of caring for the newborn, much less several newborns. Burdened grandmothers are frequently unskilled and ill-educated themselves. There is evidence that the younger sisters of childbearing adolescents are at risk for adolescent childbearing as well. Explanations might include social modeling and shared parenting. Attention seeking may also be a factor.

Adolescent pregnancy has been associated with an increased incidence of both obstetric and social complications—twice that of women in their twenties. There is an increased risk of anemia, pregnancy-induced hypertension (PIH), perinatal death, sexually transmitted diseases, human immunodeficiency virus infection, and premature delivery. The increased risk of PIH is significant, especially if the pregnancy occurs within 24 months of menarche. There is an increased incidence of cephalopelvic disproportion in women younger than 15 years of age, which is related to the relative skeletal immaturity of the pelvis, leading to a higher incidence of cesarean delivery, a surgical procedure associated with greater maternal morbidity. Pregnant adolescents are also more likely to experience abnormal labor patterns such as prolonged or precipitous labors, and both may be associated with neonatal sequelae. These teenagers may also experience an increased incidence of postpartum infection and hemorrhage. Adolescent mothers may also have unhealthy habits. Smoking, alcohol consumption, and the use of drugs are common among pregnant teenagers and may lead to sudden infant death syndrome, growth retardation, and neurologic dysfunction.

Adolescence is normally a period of high nutritional needs, owing to the rapid growth and development of the body. Pregnancy imposes additional nutritional demands on the growing body and may rapidly deplete already limited reserves. The increased incidence of poor nutrition among adolescents owing to limitations in economic resources, poor eating habits, and lack of knowledge regarding nutrition has been directly related to the increased incidence of low-birth-weight infants, who are themselves susceptible to increased mortality as well as developmental and neurologic handicaps. Pregnant adolescents may be deficient in calcium, iron, and vitamins A and C, although they usually have adequate calories, protein, and other vitamins. Because a high proportion of pregnant adolescents are nutritionally at risk and require nutritional intervention throughout their pregnancy and postpartum period, a nutrition consultant who can skillfully establish rapport with them is essential. The pregnant adolescent needs professional help in identifying food sources to supplement or improve her nutrient intake, not only during her pregnancy but well into the postpartum period.

The psychologic ramifications of adolescent pregnancy are enormous. Adolescence is a period of maturational crisis in which the role of child must evolve into the role of adult. The familiar prepubescent body image must be revised to that of a woman accommodating the changes of normal hormonal development. Psychologic inconsistence with unpredictable reactions is characteristic of adolescents, and this produces confusion and frustration both in themselves and in those around them. Experimentation is essential for the adolescent and may play a major role in pregnancy. Likewise, pregnancy may also be viewed as a maturational crisis in which the familiar role of a single individual is exchanged for the role of mother and provider. When pregnancy occurs during adolescence, the young person must deal with two maturational crises at the same time, and satisfactory resolution is seldom possible. A "syndrome of failure" associated with adolescent pregnancy has been described. It includes failure to (1) fulfill developmental tasks of adolescence, (2) remain in school, (3) limit family size, (4) establish stable families, (5) be self-supporting, and (6) have healthy children.

The long-term consequences to adolescent parents can be extremely costly to both society and the individuals involved. Extensive study has revealed that both adolescent mothers and fathers have substantially less education than their peers, and the degree of educational deprivation is related to the age of the parent at the time of the infant's birth. Teenagers who become pregnant before completing the twelfth grade usually drop out of school and never return. The earlier she drops out of school, the less chance that she will complete her education.

Adolescent mothers account for 17 percent of the parturients with 8 years of education or less. Adolescent parents are also much more likely to hold low-prestige jobs, owing to their relatively low educational attainment. Reduced occupational attainment also means lower income and greater job dissatisfaction. A young pregnant teenager is not likely to support herself; she bears an unwanted child who is born into poverty and exposed to inadequate parenting. She is dependent on family and governmental agencies for monetary assistance and child-care support. The majority of adolescent pregnancies do not result in marriage, and those that do are frequently dissolved.

Factors that influence the reproductive behavior of adolescents are peers, sexual partners, family, religion, schools, media, and the health-care system. A poorly planned pregnancy occurring during the adolescent years also adversely affects intrapersonal relationships. Social skills as well as intrapersonal relationship skills may not develop adequately; both have long-term social ramifications. Relationships with family members as well as with men may be jeopardized, leading to the development of further social or psychologic complications.

Delivery of health care to the adolescent presents a complex challenge. No single health-care provider can meet the many needs of the adolescent, but a team of health-care providers can be invaluable. Her primary medical care will not differ significantly from the prenatal care of other women, although she may need more privacy and confidentiality. She is more likely to keep prenatal appointments and comply with medical regimens if a trusting, nonjudgmental relationship has been established. The pregnant adolescent will often delay obtaining prenatal care because of the many fears that she has developed: fear of being pregnant, fear of her family being informed, and fear of being examined. She sometimes delays because she hopes that a more meaningful relationship between her and the father will develop. Professionals who work with adolescents on health-care issues need to know about adolescent development, sexuality, and counseling. As part of the health-care team, a nutritionist is necessary to discuss the adolescent's body needs and food requirements peculiar to pregnancy, thereby helping to provide the nutritional requirements for both the mother's growth as well as the growth of her unborn baby. A social worker can provide referral information and counseling regarding pregnancy alternatives. Above all, the pregnant adolescent needs the cooperation and understanding of her parents and school authorities, so that it may be possible for her to receive early and comprehensive prenatal care.

Consideration and support must also be given to the adolescent father, so that he may be included in health-care decisions, labor and delivery, and care of the infant, if he so chooses. Contrary to popular belief, most infants born to teenagers are not fathered by teenagers; however, the exact number of adolescent fathers cannot be determined because many adolescent mothers refuse to give identifying information about the father.

Adolescent pregnancy is not solely a medical problem, and all solutions cannot be found within the scope of medical practice. Prevention of this problem is an important goal and ultimately may be reached through comprehensive educational programs. Such educational programs need to be directed toward the formation of healthy, mature attitudes about sexuality and childbearing. Courses should be integrated into the elementary curriculum before the teenage years and continued throughout childhood and adolescence. Basic information about human reproduction and conception, contraception, fetal growth, antenatal developments, and intrapartum experiences as well as infant care should be included. Discussions between adolescents and parents within the structure of religious institutions and schools may prove beneficial in reducing misconceptions regarding sexuality and pregnancy.

The consequences of childbearing for adolescent parents, their children, and society are severe. Much stress has been placed on the consequences of adolescent sexual activity, namely pregnancy. An even more serious consequence is the acquiring of sexually transmitted diseases, particularly the acquired immunodeficiency syndrome. Information alone will not prevent adolescent pregnancy, nor will increased communication between parents and teenagers and teachers and teenagers. Only abstinence from sexual activity alone can prevent adolescent pregnancy.

General
1. East, P. L., and Felice, M. E. Pregnancy risk among the younger sisters of pregnant and childbearing adolescents. *J. Dev. Behav. Pediatr.* 13:128, 1992.
   There is increasing evidence that the younger sisters of childbearing teenagers are at risk for adolescent childbearing.
2. Brooks-Gunn, J., and Paikoff, R. L. Promoting healthy behavior in adolescence: the case of sexuality and pregnancy. *Bull. N.Y. Acad. Med.* 67:527, 1991.
   Multiple pathways of sexual well-being are possible.
3. Fielding, J. E., and Williams, C. A. Adolescent pregnancy in the United States: a review and recommendations for clinicians and research needs. *Am. J. Prev. Med.* 7:47, 1991.
   Clinicians have an important role in providing guidance for teenagers and their parents, as well as in influencing schools and community leadership in providing sex education.
4. Stevens-Simon, C., and White, M. M. Adolescent pregnancy. *Pediatr. Ann.* 20: 322, 1991.
   The United States must improve its efforts to reduce teenage pregnancy.
5. O'Sullivan, A. L. Tertiary prevention with adolescent mothers: rehabilitation after the first pregnancy. *Birth Defects* 27:57, 1991.

A large number of diverse local programs and specific projects exist across the nation.

6. Nelson, P. B. Repeat pregnancy among adolescent mothers: a review of the literature. *J. Natl. Black Nurses Assoc.* 4:28, 1990.
   Repeat pregnancy among adolescent mothers is a major problem facing health-care providers today.
7. Davis, S. Pregnancy in adolescents. *Pediatr. Clin. North Am.* 36:665, 1989.
   The United States must improve its effort to reduce teenage pregnancy.
8. McAnarney, E. R., and Hendee, W. R. The prevention of adolescent pregnancy. *J.A.M.A.* 7:262, 1989.
   Prevention of adolescent pregnancy is problematic because adolescents become biologically mature at an earlier age.

Etiology
9. Sowers, J. G. Preventive strategies in education: history, current practices, and future trends regarding substance abuse and pregnancy prevention. *Bull. N.Y. Acad. Med.* 67:256, 1991.
   The most effective prevention of adolescent pregnancies consists of positive life and health promotion strategies.
10. Smith, L. A critique of family-focused tertiary prevention with the adolescent mother and her child. *Birth Defects* 27:155, 1991.
    The complexity of problems related to pregnant adolescents requires a coordinated multidisciplinary approach.
11. Gordon, D. E. Formal operational thinking: the role of cognitive-developmental processes in adolescent decision-making about pregnancy and contraception. *Am. J. Orthopsychiatry* 60:346, 1990.
    Adolescents who become pregnant have difficulty in envisioning alternatives.

Diagnosis
12. Perkins, J. L. Primary prevention of adolescent pregnancy. *Birth Defects* 27:29, 1991.
    Programs that contribute to the prevention of adolescent pregnancy and an understanding of life options in adolescents are counterbalanced by cost.
13. Raines, T. G. Family-founded primary prevention of adolescent pregnancy. *Birth Defects* 29:87, 1991.
    There is a need for expertise and influence in the area of primary prevention of adolescent pregnancy.
14. Flick, L. H. A critique of community-based tertiary prevention with the adolescent parent and child. *Birth Defects* 27:250, 1991.
    The characteristics and circumstances that increase the likelihood of early child-bearing also increase the chances of harmful consequences to the young mother, child, and perhaps the father.
15. Kokotailo, P. K., and Adger, H., Jr. Substance use by pregnant adolescents. *Clin. Perinatol.* 18:125, 1991.
    Research is needed to determine the prevalence of substance abuse among pregnant adolescents.
16. Nash, E. S. Teenage pregnancy—need a child bear a child? *S. Afr. Med. J.* 77:147, 1990.
    International and local evidence suggests that the incidence of unplanned pregnancy in teenage girls is unacceptably high.

Treatment
17. Zabin, L. S. Adolescent pregnancy: the clinician's role in intervention. *J. Gen. Intern. Med.* 5:S81, 1990.
    This report reviews research on adolescent development and sexual behavior.
18. Stahler, G. J., DuCette, J., and McBride, D. The evaluation component in adolescent pregnancy care projects: is it adequate? *Fam. Plann. Perspect.* 21:123, 1989.
    A review of the activities promoted by the adolescent Family Life Act—projects designed to care for pregnant teenagers.

19. Stephenson, J. N. Pregnancy testing and counseling. *Pediatr. Clin. North Am.* 36:681, 1989.
    Pregnancy testing and counseling are increasingly accepted as necessary services for adolescents.
20. Nutrition management of adolescent pregnancy: technical support paper. *J. Am. Diet Assoc.* 89:105, 1989.
    A high proportion of pregnant teenagers are nutritionally at risk and require nutrition intervention.

Complications
21. Stevens-Simon, C., Roghmann, K. J., and McAnarney, E. R. Repeat adolescent pregnancy and low birth weight: methods issues. *J. Adolesc. Health Care* 11:114, 1990.
    The results of birth order and birth weight studies conducted among adolescent mothers are conflicting.
22. Hechtman, L. Teenage mothers and their children: risks and problems: a review (abstract). *Can. J. Psychiatry* 34:569, 1989.
    To identify positive instrumentation, factors that influence the physical and psychologic health of adolescents must be recognized.
23. Slap, G. B., and Schwartz, J. S. Risk factors for low birth weight to adolescent mothers. *J. Adolesc. Health Care* 10:267, 1989.
    A study of mothers under 20 years of age who delivered babies weighing 2500 g or less.
24. Furstenberg, F. F., Jr., Brooks-Gunn, J., and Chase-Lansdale, L. Teenaged pregnancy and childbearing. *Am. Psychol.* 44:313, 1989.
    This study supports evidence that there is a need for more integration and availability of services to the adolescent needy.
25. Silva, M. O., Cabral, H., and Zuckerman, B. Adolescent pregnancy in Portugal: effectiveness of continuity of care by an obstetrician. *Obstet. Gynecol.* 81:142, 1993.
    Pregnant adolescents in this study received care from the same obstetrician and were followed in a special clinic. Maternal weight gain and infant weights were greater than those noted for controls, and the number of prenatal visits in the study group were twice those in the control group.

17. ADVANCED MATERNAL AGE AND MANAGEMENT OF THE GRAND MULTIPARA
Rick W. Martin

Deliveries of women older than 35 years of age have increased in number over the past decade and represent almost 7 percent of all births. Postponed childbearing in women born between 1945 and 1965 probably accounts for most of the phenomenon.

The wide availability of safe and effective contraceptives has allowed these women to delay childbearing. Other factors accounting for advanced maternal age include pursuit of a career, the lack of a suitable partner, the beginning of a second marriage, and a desire for greater financial security. Many physicians find that these women ask more questions and have higher expectations than their younger counterparts. These patients may also be better prepared for childbirth than younger women, and most obstetricians find it enjoyable to care for such parturients.

The nature of counseling in women older than 35 years differs from that in younger women. Fertility decreases with age, and many of these women have less time for the evaluation of problems that may arise. The incidence of chromosomal anomalies, including Down syndrome, in live born infants rises to about 1 in 20 in mothers 45 years of age or older. Genetic counseling is discussed in Chapter 44. The incidence of spontaneous abortion also rises with increased maternal age. Many of these women have concerns about the effect of age on their pregnancy and the impact of an abnormal pregnancy on their careers and personal lives.

Various medical diseases, such as diabetes and hypertension, are more common as age increases. In general, the risk of diabetes in this older age group of women is 6 percent, compared to 3 percent in younger age groups. Hypertension affects approximately 6 percent of women older than 35 years of age, whereas, in general, chronic vascular disease complicates less than 2 percent of gestations. In most patient series, no difference in perinatal outcome with advancing maternal age has been noted, unless there is associated diabetes, hypertension, or obesity. However, the parity of the more mature woman does seem to have a bearing on the obstetric outcome. One epidemiologic study revealed that there was more intrauterine growth retardation and lower developmental scores in this group, but only in primiparas. Several authors have noted prolonged labor to be associated with increasing maternal age. In particular, there is a greater incidence of secondary arrest and a longer second stage. Primary cesarean delivery rates are consistently higher in this age group, even when the data are controlled for such factors as fetal distress. One factor that may be responsible for this is increased physician attentiveness to problems in this age group and more aggressive management of these problems.

Maternal mortality appears to be increased in pregnant women older than 35 years, compared to their nonpregnant counterparts. In one large study, the leading cause of maternal death was obstetric hemorrhage and embolism. Other studies have shown an increase in maternal mortality owing to pregnancy-induced hypertension, placenta previa, and postpartum hemorrhage. In particular, the mortality at age 45 years may be as high as 200 times that of younger pregnant patients. The figures also show that race is an important factor; the mortality in black women 35 years or older is higher than that in whites in the same age group. Additionally, underlying maternal conditions such as hypertension and diabetes greatly increase the chances for maternal death.

Fetal risks seem to be more related to maternal disease states than to maternal age alone, although vascular changes such as sclerotic lesions in the myometrial arteries are found more frequently in older patients. Intrapartum deaths do not seem to be increased in association with advanced maternal age; however, the observations from some studies suggest that antepartum fetal loss may be more common. There is a slight increase in birth weight with advanced maternal age, and the childhood IQ scores in the offspring of parturients in this group are higher.

Although probably the best approach to contraception in this age group of women is permanent sterilization, many (especially those of lower parity) may not have completed their families. The older patient is more likely to be in a stable relationship and presumably has a better understanding of barrier devices; therefore, this method is also most suitable. Although many of the intrauterine devices have been removed from distribution, they may also constitute an alternative method. Oral contraceptive agents with less than 50 μg of estrogen may also be suitable, as long as the patient has no risk factors (e.g., smoking or obesity).

The definition of the grand multipara is a woman who has given birth seven times or more to an infant or infants weighing at least 500 g. Many early reports warned of increases in hypertension, abruptio placentae, malpresentation, cesarean delivery, and postpartum hemorrhage in these women. Thus, because of the increased maternal mortality in this group, sterilization was advocated. The findings from more recent surveys have contradicted these findings, however, with no maternal deaths encountered in one series consisting of more than 5000 grand multiparas. One would expect conditions such as diabetes and hypertension that primarily affect the older population to be more prevalent in grand multiparas, but there appears to be no significant difference in their incidence versus that in younger patients.

Many physicians anticipate obstetric problems in the grand multipara. Because the uterus contains less muscle and more connective tissue with increased parity, uterine inertia and abnormal presentations would be expected to be more likely, but this is not the case. Instead, multiple gestation is increased 2.5 times in these grand multiparas, compared to that in mothers of lower parity.

According to the findings from older studies, the risk of uterine rupture in the grand multipara appeared to be increased 20 times that of the woman of lower parity, but the findings from recent studies do not confirm this. Nevertheless, the use of oxytocin in these patients is controversial. Although there are case reports of rupture with oxytocin use in the grand multipara, the results of most series do not substantiate this. The judicious administration of dilute oxytocin by means of a controlled infusion device in conjunction with internal uterine pressure monitoring provides an adequate defense against uterine rupture.

In summary, the aging of the obstetric population brings new problems for the obstetricians involved. Most pregnancies in older parturients are safely negotiated. Although, in general, the average parity is decreasing, the grand multipara occasionally requires the attention of practitioners who are less experienced with the obstetric management required. However, the individual patient can be reassured by the modern advances in obstetrics care. The outcome in such women now appears to be no different from that in women of lower parity.

Maternal Age
1. Buehler, J. W., et al. Maternal mortality in women aged 35 years or older: United States. *J.A.M.A.* 255:53, 1986.
   During a 5-year period beginning in 1974, the leading causes of maternal death in women aged 35 and older were found to be obstetric hemorrhage and embolism.
2. Cnattingius, S., et al. Delayed childbearing and risk of adverse perinatal outcome. *J.A.M.A.* 268:886, 1992.
   The rates of low-birth-weight infants and preterm delivery were higher in nulliparous women over 35 years compared to controls.
3. Davies, B. L., and Doran, T. A. Factors in a woman's decision to undergo genetic amniocentesis for advanced maternal age. *Nurs. Res.* 31:56, 1982.
   The major concern of women undergoing amniocentesis was concern about the effect of maternal age on the developing child.
4. Schwartz, D., and Mayaux, M. J. Female fecundity as a function of age. *N. Engl. J. Med.* 306:404, 1982.
   The fertility in women undergoing artificial insemination with no diagnosis other than oligospermia in their partners was found to be decreased with greater maternal age.
5. Fonteyn, V. J., and Isada, N. B. Nongenetic implications of childbearing after age thirty-five. *Obstet. Gynecol. Surv.* 43:709, 1988.
   In women older than 35 years, the prenatal diagnosis, recognition, and management of high-risk pregnancies have led to dramatic reductions in the problems associated with age. A management plan for these patients is introduced.
6. Friede, A., et al. Older age and infant mortality in the United States. *Obstet. Gynecol.* 72:152, 1988.
   The perinatal risks were not greatly elevated until women were aged 40 to 49 years, suggesting that it is relatively safe for women to postpone childbearing until the middle or late thirties.
7. Friedman, E. A., and Sachtleben, M. R. Relation of maternal age to the course of labor. *Am. J. Obstet. Gynecol.* 91:915, 1965.
   Secondary arrest of labor and a prolonged second stage of labor were observed with increasing maternal age.
8. Hansen, J. P. Older maternal age and pregnancy outcome: a review of the literature. *Obstet. Gynecol. Surv.* 41:726, 1986.
   A comprehensive review of the effect of maternal age on pregnancy.
9. Hershey, D. W., Crandall, B. F., and Perdue, S. Combining maternal age and serum alpha fetoprotein to predict the risk of Down's syndrome. *Obstet. Gynecol.* 68:177, 1986.
   Guidelines for counseling women with a low serum alpha fetoprotein level are provided.
10. Hook, E. B. Rates of chromosomal abnormalities at different maternal ages. *Obstet. Gynecol.* 58:282, 1981.
    The estimated rates of chromosomal abnormalities for a range of maternal ages are the standards used for counseling most women before amniocentesis.

11. Kirz, D. S., Dorchester, W., and Freeman, R. K. Advanced maternal age: the mature gravida. *Am. J. Obstet. Gynecol.* 152:7, 1985.
The pregnancies of older women delivered in the 1980s may have been at no greater risk for adverse outcomes than those of younger patients.
12. Mishell, D. R. Use of oral contraceptives in women of older reproductive age. *Am. J. Obstet. Gynecol.* 158:1652, 1988.
There is no increased risk of cardiovascular disease in patients taking low-dose oral contraceptives, except in those women with other risk factors and those who smoke.
13. Naeye, R. L. Maternal age, obstetric complications, and the outcome of pregnancy. *Obstet. Gynecol.* 61:210, 1983.
An increase in sclerosis of the myometrial arteries found in autopsy specimens from nonpregnant women is associated with increasing maternal age, and this factor may explain the rise in conditions reflecting underperfusion of the uterus that occur with advanced maternal age.
14. Sauer, M. V., Paulson, R. J., and Lobo, R. A. Reversing the natural decline in human fertility. An extended clinical trial of oocyte donation to women of advanced reproductive age. *J.A.M.A.* 268:1275, 1992.
The age-related decline in fertility was not demonstrated with respect to oocyte donation. The perinatal outcomes were generally good.
15. Peipert, J. F., and Bracken, M. B. Maternal age: an independent risk factor for cesarean delivery. *Obstet. Gynecol.* 81:200, 1993.
Advanced maternal age was found to be an independent risk factor for cesarean delivery.
16. Sauer, M. V., Paulson, R. J., and Rogerio, A. L. Pregnancy after age 50: application of oocyte donation to women after natural menopause. *Lancet* 341:321, 1993.
This reports on eight pregnancies resulting from oocyte donation in menopausal women ages 50 to 59 years. Two of three women who delivered had preeclampsia.
17. Spellacy, W. N., Miller, S. J., and Winegar, A. Pregnancy after 40 years of age. *Obstet. Gynecol.* 68:452, 1986.
The major factors in determining an adverse outcome in women of advanced maternal age were maternal weight and parity rather than age itself.
18. Witter, F. R., Repke, J. T., and Niebyl, J. R. The effect of maternal age on primary cesarean section rate. *Int. J. Gynecol. Obstet.* 27:51, 1988.
The likelihood of cesarean section increases with maternal age, and fetal distress may be partially responsible for this rise.
19. Tuck, S. M., Yudkin, P. L., and Turnbull, A. C. Pregnancy outcome in elderly primigravidae with and without a history of infertility. *Obstet. Gynecol. Surv.* 44:35, 1988.
This excellent article reveals the risk for adverse pregnancy outcome is higher for women who deliver when they are older than 35 years of age. Principally, there was a high rate of preterm delivery, cesarean section, forceps deliveries, chronic hypertension, and uterine myomas.

Grand Multiparity
20. Eastman, N. J. The hazards of pregnancy and labor in the grand multipara. *NY State Med. J.* 40:1708, 1940.
Because of the high maternal and fetal mortality associated with parity of nine or more, permanent sterilization is recommended after the eighth child.
21. Eidelman, A. I., et al. The grand multipara: is she still at risk? *Am. J. Obstet. Gynecol.* 158:389, 1988.
In the absence of coincidental medical conditions, grand multiparity is not a risk factor for adverse perinatal outcome.
22. Evaldson, G. R. The grand multipara in modern obstetrics. *Gynecol. Obstet. Invest.* 30:217, 1990.
The frequency of diabetes, transverse lie, uterine inertia, fetal heart rate abnormalities, and postpartum hemorrhage was higher in grand multiparous women compared to that in other multiparas.

23. Fuchs, K., et al. The "grand multipara"—is it a problem? A review of 5785 cases. *Int. J. Gynecol. Obstet.* 23:321, 1985.
   Rupture of the uterus was found to be about 20 times more frequent in grand multiparas than that in the general population.
24. King, P. A., Duthie, S. J., and Ma, H. K. Grand multiparity: a reappraisal of the risks. *Int. J. Gynecol. Obstet.* 36:13, 1991.
   The outcome in 168 women of low socioeconomic status with parity greater than five was similar to that in women of lower parity.

18. MULTIFETAL GESTATIONS
William E. Roberts

The disproportionately high perinatal morbidity and mortality associated with multifetal gestations underscores this issue as a significant contemporary challenge. The incidence of twins in the United States is about 1 in 90 live births (11–12 per 1000) and the incidence of triplets is about 1 per 8000 live births. The use of routine sonography early in gestation has revealed that the incidence of twin conceptions is much higher than was suspected (3–5%), with the occasional unrecognized loss of one twin. Multiple births occur most frequently in blacks and least frequently in Asians. Increasing maternal age and parity are also generally associated with higher rates of twinning. A higher incidence of multifetal gestation occurs under the following circumstances: women who are themselves a dizygotic twin, women who conceive within 1 month of the cessation of oral contraceptives, women who have undergone ovulation induction with gonadotropin (20–40%) or clomiphene (13%) therapy, and women whose pregnancy results from in vitro fertilization. In terms of triplet or higher gestations, less than one third now occur naturally; the remainder result from the use of potent ovulating drugs or other assisted reproductive technologies.

Multiple gestations can arise from one or more ova. The division of a single ovum into two embryos is termed *monozygotic*, or *identical twinning*. If the fertilized ovum divides within the first 72 hours after fertilization, a diamniotic, dichorionic, monozygotic twin pregnancy will ensue, involving either two distinct or a single-fused placenta. Ovum division between the fourth and eighth day of development produces a diamniotic, monochorionic, monozygotic twin pregnancy. After the eighth day, the amniotic cavity is established and division results in a monoamniotic, monochorionic, monozygotic twin pregnancy. Varieties of conjoined twins result if division of the already formed embryonic disk is initiated after 13 days.

Placental examination at delivery can help determine the nature of zygosity. The existence of either one sac (one chorion, one amnion) or a monochorionic placenta with only amnions forming the intervening membrane is evidence of monozygosity. If neonates are of the same sex, blood group testing or human leukocyte antigen typing is useful for establishing zygosity. The frequency of monozygotic twins remains relatively constant worldwide at 1 in 250 births, whereas the frequency of dizygotic twins is influenced by parental age, race, parity, or fertility therapy.

Although not strictly twins, *dizygotic* twins result from the maturation and fertilization of two ova from either the same or different ovaries. The two placentas, whether proximate or separated, have separate amniotic and chorionic membranes (diamniotic, dichorionic). A *superfecundation* is the fertilization of two ova from more than one act of coitus in the same menstrual cycle. *Superfetation* is the fertilization of two ova from different menstrual cycles and is rare in humans. A third type of twinning has been postulated in which a single ovum is fertilized by two sperm with subsequent zygote division.

The enlarged multifetal uterine mass is frequently associated with maternal discomfort, aortocaval compression, peripheral dependent edema, varicosities, anemia, and fatigue. Uterine overdistention may contribute to the high frequency of premature labor, abnormal labor with hypotonic uterine dysfunction, and uterine atony with postpartum hemorrhage seen in multiple gestations. Hydramnios is also more likely to occur in a multifetal gestation. The acute form is more common in monozygotic than dizygotic twin pregnancies, often occurring secondary to extensive twin-to-twin transfusion remote from term with a high rate of fetal loss. The finding of late gestational hydramnios usually suggests the existence of a congenital anomaly affecting one fetus, especially if it is confined to a single sac. Pregnancy-induced hypertension (PIH) is about three times more common in twin pregnancies without regard to zygosity. Glucose intolerance is also more frequently observed.

In the United States, the perinatal death rate in the setting of twin gestations averages 15 percent, over 10 times that of singleton gestations. Spontaneous abortion is also more common, and preterm birth occurs in one half of all multifetal gestations. The normal duration of gestation for twins is 261 days, versus 280 for singletons; the mean birth weight is 2395 g, versus 3377 g for singletons. Because of an estimated 50 percent mortality in monoamniotic twins, secondary to intertwining umbilical cords, the overall perinatal death rate is 2.5 times greater in monozygotic twins than in dizygotic twins. As the number of fetuses in a pregnancy increases, the duration of gestation and the birth weight decrease, while the degree of growth retardation increases. The frequency of malformations is generally twice that seen for singletons, with that in monozygotics exceeding that in dizygotic twins. A reduction in the high perinatal mortality associated with multifetal gestations is best accomplished by decreasing the incidence of preterm birth.

The most important step in the antenatal care of patients with a multifetal gestation is early diagnosis. Clues to a multiple gestation include family history; the recent administration of clomiphene, gonadotropins, or oral contraceptives; and larger-than-expected uterine size. Clinical signs of a multifetal gestation include an increased transverse abdominal girth, multiple small palpable fetal parts, distinctly different fetal heart rates, a small fetal head in a large uterus, maternal anemia unresponsive to customary oral iron therapy, PIH, or preterm labor.

The increasingly routine use of early gestational ultrasound for pregnancy evaluation and fetal age determination has led to a declining incidence in undiagnosed multifetal gestations. By the end of the first trimester of pregnancy, abdominal real-time ultrasound can regularly identify fetal skulls. Two gestational sacs can be identified by 5 to 6 weeks, and a fetal body and heart motion can be detected by 7 to 8 weeks, especially with vaginal ultrasound scanning. As the number of fetuses increases, it becomes more difficult to determine the number of fetuses and to perform mensuration techniques. An inability to distinguish the fetal bodies, the identification of more than three vessels in a single umbilical cord, the lack of a separating membrane, or the presence of fetal anomalies should suggest the possibility of conjoined twins. If real-time ultrasound is not available, a confirmatory x-ray study of the maternal abdomen after 18 weeks of gestation may be obtained to determine fetal number. There is no biochemical test that can accurately discriminate multiple from singleton gestations. In multifetal pregnancies, each amniotic sac can be sampled for genetic studies with minimal complications. The injection of dilute indigo carmine into the first sample sac usually permits confirmation that the other sac has not been entered.

In the presence of triplet and higher multifetal gestations, some advocate consideration of first-trimester pregnancy reduction, as it is well established that the risk of perinatal morbidity and mortality as well as maternal morbidity are directly related to an increase in fetal number. Although multifetal pregnancy reduction represents a complex ethical issue, available data indicate that transvaginal embryo aspiration at 7 to 8 weeks' gestation or transabdominal fetal reduction at 9 to 14 weeks leads to an improved overall perinatal performance in the setting of quadruplet pregnancies, with a low procedure-related loss rate.

The management goals for multifetal gestation include (1) early diagnosis; (2) an optimal intrauterine environment; (3) prevention of preterm labor or delivery, or both; (4) close fetal surveillance to detect disorders, decreased growth, and distress; (5) atraumatic delivery; and (6) immediate expert neonatal care. The mother is encouraged to take frequent periods of lateral recumbent rest and to stop full-time employment to promote fetal growth. Dietary requirements are increased by increments of approximately 300 calories per day for each fetus, together with folate and iron supplementation. Frequent prenatal visits are scheduled to detect premature cervical dilatation and to assess uterine activity, and the patient is educated regarding the signs and symptoms of preterm labor—all in an attempt to reduce the incidence of preterm birth. Prophylactic cervical cerclage (unless otherwise indicated), prophylactic tocolytic (beta-mimetic) drug treatment, and progestin administration do not appear to be efficacious. The preterm rupture of membranes is usually managed conservatively, as in a singleton gestation.

Serial sonography is performed at the beginning of the second and third trimesters of pregnancy to verify the gestational age, and later to ascertain whether there is discordant fetal growth in the last trimester of pregnancy (17- to 28-day intervals after 28 weeks' gestation). When discordancy is suggested by a biparietal diameter (BPD) difference of 5 mm or more, or by an abdominal circumference difference of 30 mm or more, the fetal weight between or among fetuses should be estimated, with discordance generally defined as a 20 percent or greater difference.

Weekly nonstress testing (NST), beginning at 30 to 32 weeks, is usually performed. Because of its high rate of false-positive results and the fear of initiating preterm labor, contraction stress testing (CST) should be avoided in multifetal gestations except to evaluate a nonreactive NST or other worrisome clinical or ultrasound finding. Biophysical profiles and assessments of umbilical systolic-diastolic ratios are additional methods of fetal surveillance to alert the clinician to incipient fetal problems. Assessment of fetal lung maturation in the absence of labor is performed from a single sac if the BPDs of both fetuses are commensurate or if a second site is unavailable. A lecithin-sphingomyelin ratio of 2 or more is expected by 32 to 33 weeks' gestation in a twin pregnancy.

The intrapartum management of a multiple gestation remains controversial. If preterm labor is detected, the cervix is less than 4 cm dilated (80% effaced), and clinical evidence of compromising maternal or fetal disease is lacking, tocolytic agents in conjunction with lateral recumbent bed rest and appropriate hydration can be instituted to delay delivery. Corticosteroid therapy can be considered to accelerate fetal lung maturity. Magnesium sulfate is the tocolytic agent of choice in multifetal gestations, as beta-mimetic agents carry a greater risk of causing maternal pulmonary edema.

Optimally, the gravida in a laboring multiple gestation is referred to a tertiary perinatal care center for maternal, fetal, and neonatal care. Monitoring of both fetal heart rates is performed. Blood for transfusion should be available, and a well-functioning intravenous line with large-bore catheter should be in place. The gestational age, as well as fetal position and presentation, will strongly influence the mode of delivery. Safe vaginal delivery is usually possible for vertex-vertex presentations, whereas other combinations most often necessitate abdominal birth. The presenting twin's birth weight often bears no relationship to the weight of the second twin. Liberal use of low vertical cesarean section, often through a low vertical abdominal incision, is recommended in the settings of gross discordance in fetal sizes, fetal distress, umbilical cord prolapse, hypertonic uterine dysfunction, severe preterm preeclampsia, a contracted cervix after delivery of the first twin, a gestation of three or more fetuses, or a first-twin breech presentation. Either skillfully executed conduction anesthesia by an epidural catheter or general anesthesia is used for multifetal delivery. In all cases, sound medical judgment of the individual patient is essential to ensure optimal results.

General
1. O'Grady, J. P. Twins and beyond: management guide. *Contemp. Ob/Gyn* 36:45, 1991.
   Covering every important aspect of twinning, this concise article considers the full range of pertinent considerations, from physiology to diagnosis and delivery.
2. Herruzo, A. J., et al. Perinatal morbidity and mortality in twin pregnancies. *Int. J. Gynecol. Obstet.* 36:17, 1991.

A thorough discussion of the antenatal, intrapartum, and postpartum complications in the multifetal gestation, along with a review of early neonatal morbidity and mortality.

3. Fleming, A. D., et al. Perinatal outcomes of twin pregnancies at term. *J. Reprod. Med.* 35:881, 1990.
   A review of the antepartum and postpartum complications encountered in twin gestations after 36 weeks' gestation.

4. Weissman, A., et al. Management of triplet pregnancies in the 1980s—are we doing better? *Am. J. Perinatol.* 8:333, 1990.
   The authors review their experience with 29 triplet gestations encountered over a 10-year period. They conclude that there has been no significant decrease in perinatal mortality in spite of early sonographic diagnosis, the increased use of tocolytic agents, and the placement of prophylactic cervical sutures.

5. Walker, E. M., and Patel, N. B. Maternal serum alpha-fetoprotein, birthweight and perinatal death in twin pregnancy. *Br. J. Obstet. Gynaecol.* 93:1191, 1986.
   Although a high maternal serum alpha-fetoprotein level alerts the clinician to a possible multifetal pregnancy, it does not appear to identify the twin gestation at increased risk for preterm delivery, growth retardation, or neonatal or infant mortality.

Etiology

6. Benirschke, K. Multiple Gestation: Incidence, Etiology, and Inheritance. In R. Creasy and R. Resnik (eds.), *Maternal-Fetal Medicine: Principles and Practice.* Philadelphia: Saunders, 1989.
   A thorough, inclusive review of the physiologic principles and clinical practices pertaining to multifetal gestations.

7. Levene, M. I., et al. Higher multiple births and the modern management of infertility in Britain. *Br. J. Obstet. Gynaecol.* 99:607, 1992.
   This review of 156 triplet and higher pregnancies revealed that only 47 (31%) were conceived naturally. Assisted reproductive techniques were responsible for all quadruplet and quintuplet pregnancies.

Diagnosis

8. Yarkoni, S., et al. Estimated fetal weight in the evaluation of growth in twin gestations: a prospective longitudinal study. *Obstet. Gynecol.* 69:636, 1987.
   Nomograms of fetal weight gain, measurements, and growth patterns have been formulated based on a careful prospective longitudinal study of 35 normal twin gestations.

9. Landy, H. J., et al. The "vanishing twin": ultrasonographic assessment of fetal disappearance in the first trimester. *Am. J. Obstet. Gynecol.* 78:739, 1991.
   The true incidence of multiple gestations in the first trimester ranges from 3.3 to 5.4 percent; in one of five such pregnancies, one twin will subsequently "vanish" in association with vaginal bleeding, with a good prognosis for the remaining twin.

10. Michaels, W. H., et al. Ultrasound surveillance of the cervix in twin gestations: management of cervical incompetency. *Obstet. Gynecol.* 78:739, 1991.
    The authors describe a study utilizing ultrasound and clinical assessment to diagnose cervical incompetency in twin gestations. Use of this protocol led to a lower preterm delivery rate and perinatal mortality in comparison to the findings in the control group.

11. Allen, S. R., et al. Ultrasonographic diagnosis of congenital anomalies in twins. *Am. J. Obstet. Gynecol.* 165:1056, 1991.
    The authors present data to substantiate their contention that targeted ultrasound scanning in twin gestations is useful for detecting noncardiac anomalies.

12. Watson, W. J. Sonographic evaluation of growth discordance in twin gestations. *Am. J. Perinatol.* 8:342, 1991.
    Study data demonstrate that the accuracy of ultrasound in the detection of weight discordance in twin gestations is acceptable.

13. Shah, Y. G., et al. Doppler velocimetry in concordant and discordant twin gestations. *Obstet. Gynecol.* 80:272, 1992.
    These authors conclude from the results of their study of 63 pairs of concordant and 17 pairs of discordant twins that the systolic-diastolic ratio is useful in identifying the small discordant twin.
14. Giles, W. B., et al. Doppler umbilical artery studies in the twin-twin transfusion syndrome. *Obstet. Gynecol.* 76:1097, 1990.
    In this study of 11 cases of twin-twin transfusion syndrome that were followed serially, no intertwin difference was detected in the umbilical artery systolic-diastolic ratio.
15. Pruggmayer, M. R. K., et al. Genetic amniocentesis in twin pregnancies: results of a multicenter study of 529 cases. *Ultrasound Obstet. Gynecol.* 2:6, 1992.
    In this multicenter study, the spontaneous abortion rate after genetic amniocentesis was found to be 3.7 percent. Although this rate is higher than the 1.7 percent reported for singleton gestations, the authors did not believe it was substantially higher than the normal biologic loss rate in twin pregnancies.

Treatment
16. Dewan, D. M. Anesthesia for preterm delivery, breech presentation, and multifetal gestation. *Clin. Obstet. Gynecol.* 30:566, 1987.
    A well-summarized review of current recommendations for anesthesia in the delivery of gravidas with multifetal gestations.
17. Davison, L., et al. Breech extraction of low-birthweight second twins: Can cesarean section be justified? *Am. J. Obstet. Gynecol.* 166:497, 1992.
    The authors conclude from a review of their data that routine cesarean section is not justified for the delivery of nonvertex second twins expected to weigh less than 2000 g.
18. Laros, R. K., Jr., and Dattel, B. J. Management of twin pregnancy: the vaginal route is still safe. *Am. J. Obstet. Gynecol.* 158:1330, 1988.
    The case for vaginal delivery of twin pregnancy is made and debated in this paper, which includes commentaries from its discussants.
19. Ahn, M. O., and Phelan, J. P. Multiple pregnancy: antepartum management. *Clin. Perinatol.* 15:55, 1988.
    The authors offer a comprehensive management plan for the antepartum treatment of multiple pregnancy. There are 97 references.
20. Younis, J. S., et al. Twin gestations and prophylactic hospitalization. *Int. J. Gynecol. Obstet.* 32:325, 1990.
    Despite a slight increase in the birth weights of infants of twin gestations whose mothers were hospitalized as a prophylactic measure, there was no significant reduction in perinatal morbidity or mortality.
21. Itskovitz, E. J., et al. Transvaginal embryo aspiration—a safe method for selective reduction in multiple pregnancies. *Fertil. Steril.* 58:351, 1992.
    Nineteen cases of reduction by transvaginal embryo aspiration are described, with a pregnancy loss rate of 5.2 percent.
22. Melgar, C. A., et al. Perinatal outcome after multifetal reduction to twins compared with nonreduced multiple pregnancies. *Obstet. Gynecol.* 78:763, 1991.
    The data from this study demonstrate a clinical advantage associated with multifetal reduction for quadruplet pregnancies but not for triplet gestations.
23. Committee on Ethics. Multifetal pregnancy reduction and selective termination. *ACOG Committee Opinion,* No. 94, April 1991.
    Excellent discussion of the ethical issues surrounding multifetal pregnancy reduction and selective termination.

Complications
24. Hagay, Z. J., et al. Management and outcome of multiple pregnancies complicated by the antenatal death of one fetus. *J. Reprod. Med.* 31:717, 1986.
    The management protocol for this complication of multiple gestation should be based on the type of placentation as well as gestational age.

25. Sakala, E. P. Obstetric management of conjoined twins. *Obstet. Gynecol.* 67:21S, 1986.
   An obstetric plan for the management of this unusual problem is proposed and illustrated with three case studies.
26. Lee, C. Y. Management of monoamniotic twins diagnosed by ultrasound. *Am. J. Gynecol. Health* 6:25, 1992.
   Criteria for the antenatal diagnosis, details of prenatal care, and recommendations for operative delivery highlight this presentation on the topic of multifetal gestation's most dangerous circumstance.
27. Weiner, C. P. Challenge of twin-twin transfusion syndrome. *Contemp. Ob/Gyn* 37:83, 1992.
   A plea is made for the performance of invasive procedures to establish an accurate diagnosis. An algorithm for the antenatal evaluation of a monochorionic twin gestation complicated by acute hydramnios and a stuck twin is presented.
28. Long, P. A., and Oats, J. N. Preeclampsia in twin pregnancy—severity and pathogenesis. *Aust. N.Z. J. Obstet. Gynaecol.* 27:1, 1987.
   From Australia comes this excellent review of 166 twin pregnancies complicated by preeclampsia in the mother, 75 of whom had severe disease. The more common occurrence, earlier onset, and greater severity of preeclampsia in the setting of twin versus singleton gestation are emphasized.
29. Belfort, M. A., et al. The use of color flow Doppler ultrasonography to diagnose umbilical cord entanglement in monoamniotic twin gestations. *Am. J. Obstet. Gynecol.* 168:601, 1993.
   Color flow Doppler proved to be a useful method of monitoring for evidence of cord compression.

19. Rh ISOIMMUNIZATION
G. Rodney Meeks

More than a hundred blood group antigens have been identified. Maternal isoimmunization to approximately one third of these antigens can stimulate the formation of sufficient maternal antibody to precipitate hemolytic disease of the fetus or newborn (HDN). For hemolysis to occur, the fetus must possess an antigen lacking in the mother, and the parturient must be sensitized to that antigen. The maternal antibody produced must be immunoglobulin G (IgG), which is the only immunoglobulin capable of placental transfer. ABO incompatibility is responsible for two thirds of all cases of HDN. Affected infants tend to exhibit jaundice in the first 24 hours of neonatal life, but rarely require exchange transfusion for the treatment of anemia or hyperbilirubinemia. Most cases occur in the setting of a type O mother and a type A, or occasionally type B, fetus. Type O mothers make IgG isoantibodies, whereas type A and B mothers make immunoglobulin M (IgM) isoantibodies.

Rh incompatibility is the second most common cause of HDN but is more significant because of its severity. The Rh antigens are found only on red blood cells; therefore, isoimmunization occurs only by exposure to Rh-positive erythrocytes. Since Rh typing became widely available and the transfusion of incompatible blood largely avoidable, the most common cause of Rh isoimmunization is pregnancy. Approximately 10 percent of pregnancies in Caucasian Rh-negative women result in an Rh-positive conceptus. The incidence for blacks and Asians is approximately 17 percent. When the mother and fetus are ABO incompatible, a protective effect is noted as fetal cells that enter into the maternal circulation are immediately destroyed by maternal AB isoantibodies.

The degree of fetal hemolysis depends on the amount of antibody transferred by the mother to the fetus and the affinity of the antibody for the fetal red blood cells. If the rate of red blood cell destruction exceeds the compensatory capacity of the fetus, anemia results and extramedullary hematopoiesis becomes intense. Portal vein hypertension develops, followed by ascites, hypoproteinemia, and hepatic failure. Ultimately, generalized anasarca (hydrops fetalis) occurs. The fetus is not commonly jaundiced at birth because the bilirubin is transferred to the mother. Hyperbilirubinemia may rapidly develop in the neonate, after delivery, however. Bilirubin uptake by the heavily myelinated cells of the basal ganglia, hippocampus, and cerebellum results in kernicterus. Surviving infants with kernicterus are afflicted with cerebral palsy, deafness, and some degree of mental retardation.

The management of isoimmunization begins at the first prenatal visit when the Rh factor and ABO group are determined. An indirect Coombs' test, regardless of Rh type, should be performed to identify those women who may have isoimmunization to one of the irregular antigens, the Rh factor, or ABO groups. Rh antibody determinations in Rh-negative women may be repeated monthly, even if no antibody was identified at the first visit. If antibody is detected at any stage, more frequent determinations are indicated. A positive indirect Coombs' test result alerts the physician to the presence of isoimmunization. Antigen identification lets the physician know whether the antigen is causing erythroblastosis. In a previously unsensitized woman, the indirect Coombs' titer provides an estimate of the degree of fetal hemolysis that can be expected. Serial antibody titers usually reflect the condition of the fetus, because the onset, duration, and strength of immunization are known. A titer of $1:16$ is believed to be safe because no intrauterine deaths have occurred at this level. In subsequent immunized pregnancies, however, the titers do not accurately reflect the condition of the fetus. If antibodies are present at the beginning of pregnancy, the fetus may be more severely affected than if this same level of antibody developed later in pregnancy. Thus, serial amniotic fluid analysis should be performed if the Rh antibody titer is greater than $1:16$ in a first immunized pregnancy and in all subsequent immunized pregnancies.

In the immunized parturient, the clinician must weigh two potentially hazardous conditions: intrauterine death and prematurity. Intrauterine death may be avoided by performing spectrophotometric analysis of the amniotic fluid for determination of the indirect bilirubin content. Liley defined a nomogram that compared the optical density of amniotic fluid at 450 nm with the gestational age. Unfortunately, nomogram curves have not been constructed for the second trimester, and evaluation of the fetal status must rely on serial amniotic fluid assessments. This method can be used to identify those infants at risk and to predict fetal outcome. Prematurity can be prevented by determining the lecithin-sphingomyelin (L/S) ratio, which assesses functional lung maturity. In severe cases of HDN, early delivery may be mandatory and is also carried out once functional lung maturity is adequate. The timing of delivery depends on the degree of fetal hemolysis (determined through analysis of the amniotic fluid), fetal lung maturity (the L/S ratio), and clinical acumen. Other methods to assess fetal status include Doppler wave-form studies, evaluation of fetal movement, fetal cardiotocography, and the biophysical profile.

Hemolysis may be so severe that the fetus's condition begins to deteriorate too early in gestation for it to survive if delivered. At less than 32 weeks, intrauterine transfusion is indicated to supply the fetus with sufficient Rh-negative blood to survive until it is mature enough to be delivered. Initially this involved the transfusion of red cells into the fetal peritoneal cavity, but now they are administered directly into the fetal circulation through the use of percutaneous umbilical vessel blood sampling (PUBS). In utero transfusion continues to be associated with a 10 percent risk of fetal death. For those infants at 32 weeks' gestation or greater, delivery can be effective. The gestational age when delivery is preferred to intrauterine transfusion needs to be constantly reevaluated as the survival of infants delivered preterm increases.

Sensitized women should be sent to high-risk centers to receive intensive clinical management when antibodies are first detected. Perinatal mortality secondary to Rh isoimmunization has decreased from 45 to 8 percent in the past 15 years owing, at least in part, to the efforts of these intense management programs. The neonatologist should be present in the delivery room so that appropriate care can be initiated immediately, if necessary. Because the newborn may be so anemic as to need immediate transfusion, O-negative maternal-compatible blood should be available. Crossmatching against maternal blood ensures that any antibody that may have crossed transplacentally to the fetus will not cause a transfusion reaction. Treatment of the affected neonate is aimed at preventing death from anemia and brain damage from kernicterus. By monitoring the hematocrit and bilirubin concentrations, one can know when to perform an exchange transfusion.

Rh immunoglobulin harvested from previously isoimmunized patients is usually successful in preventing sensitization to the Rh antigen in subsequent pregnancies. When high-titer anti-Rh immunoglobulin (RhoGAM) is given within 72 hours of delivery, less than 1 percent of treated individuals acquire subsequent Rh isoimmunization. Unusually excessive fetal-maternal hemorrhage may occur in the setting of abruptio placentae, cesarean section, manual removal of the placenta, or traumatic vaginal delivery. In these situations, more than the standard dosage of immunoglobulin may be required. The dosage needed may be determined by the Kleihauer-Betke assay for fetal erythrocytes. The incidence of Rh isoimmunization after abortion or ectopic pregnancy is 4 to 5 percent, and Rh immunoglobulin is indicated for protection. Rh immunoglobulin is also indicated after amniocentesis, antenatal obstetric hemorrhage, and routinely at 28 to 32 weeks' gestation in Rh-negative unsensitized women.

When an Rh_o(D)-negative woman delivers an Rh_o(D)-positive infant, she becomes a candidate for Rh_o(D)-immunoglobulin therapy. The following conditions, however, must be met: (1) she must be both D negative and Du negative with no anti-D antibodies in her serum; (2) her infant must be D positive or Du positive; and (3) the result of the direct Coombs' test performed on the infant's cord blood must be negative. If the result of the maternal indirect Coombs' test or fetal direct Coombs' test is positive, but due to antibody other than D, Rh_o(D) immunoglobulin should be administered.

Rh isoimmunization is uncommon now because Rh disease has been controlled by the administration of Rh immunoglobulin. Unfortunately, isoimmunization will continue to be a problem because of treatment failures, lack of therapy, and disease associated with the rare antigens.

General
1. Frigoletto, F. D., Jewett, J. F., and Konugres, A. A. *Rh Hemolytic Disease—New Strategy for Eradication.* Boston: G. K. Hall, 1982.
   An excellent reference that reviews the history, pathophysiology, maternal management, and prevention of Rh disease, as well as the neonatal management of hemolytic disease of the newborn.
2. Tannirandorn, Y., and Rodeck, C. H. New approaches in the treatment of hemolytic disease of the fetus. *Ballieres Clin. Haematol.* 3:289, 1990.
   The articles included in this series review all aspects of isoimmunization.
3. Stangenberg, M., et al. Rhesus immunization: new perspectives in maternal fetal medicine. *Obstet. Gynecol. Surv.* 16:189, 1991.
   An excellent review article detailing the approach to antenatal screening for isoimmunization, diagnostic assessment for fetal hemolytic disease, treatment of hemolytic disease of the newborn, and prophylaxis.
4. Management of Isoimmunization in Pregnancy. *ACOG Tech. Bull.* No. 90, January 1986.
   Provides up-to-date diagnostic and management advice regarding Rh isoimmunization.

Etiology
5. Tovey, L. A. Haemolytic disease of the newborn—the changing scene. *Br. J. Obstet. Gynaecol.* 93:960, 1986.
   With the advent of Rh immunoglobulin, the number of sensitized pregnant women has decreased by 70 percent and fetal death has decreased by 96 percent. The frequency of isoimmunization resulting from antigens other than Rh(D) now exceeds that for Rh(D).

6. Bowman, J. M. Treatment options for the fetus with alloimmune hemolytic disease. *Transfus. Med. Rev.* 4:191, 1990.
   The Rh blood group system is actually made up of at least five antigens capable of causing isoimmunization. The most common and significant antigen is D, and currently it is the only one that can be prevented. Other antibodies to antigens within the Kell, Kidd, Duffey, and MNS blood group systems have been associated with severe hemolysis. Currently prophylaxis is unavailable for these antigens.

Diagnosis

7. Wang, X. H., and Zipursky, A. Maternal erythrocytes in the fetal circulation. *Am. J. Clin. Pathol.* 88:346, 1987.
   Maternal-fetal hemorrhage can be documented in 14 percent of Rh-negative infants born to Rh-positive mothers. This may explain some cases of sensitization in primigravid women.
8. Polesky, H. F., and Sebring, E. S. Evaluation of methods for detection and quantitation of fetal cells and their effects on Rh IgG usage. *Am. J. Clin. Pathol.* 76:525, 1981.
   An accurate index of the amount of fetomaternal hemorrhage is necessary to know how much Rh immunoglobulin to administer. If the amount of hemorrhage is not quantitated, a single injection may be inadequate and result in treatment failures.
9. Frigoletto, F. D., et al. Fetal surveillance in the management of isoimmunized pregnancy. *N. Engl. J. Med.* 315:430, 1986.
   Utilizing modern surveillance techniques, fetuses who by former standards would be candidates for delivery or intrauterine transfusion can be managed expectantly for longer periods.
10. Reece, E. A., et al. Diagnostic fetal umbilical blood sampling in the management of isoimmunization. *Am. J. Obstet. Gynecol.* 159:1057, 1988.
    The authors managed Rh isoimmunization in five patients by PUBS. Their diagnostic accuracy was increased, and their complication rate did not rise with continued experience.
11. Voutilainen, P. E. J., et al. Amniotic fluid erythropoietin predicts fetal distress in Rh-immunized pregnancies. *Am. J. Obstet. Gynecol.* 160:429, 1989.
    Amniotic fluid erythropoietin measurements in 23 Rh-isoimmunized pregnancies were evaluated as an indication of fetal distress. Increasing levels of this substance reliably predicted fetal distress during labor.

Treatment

12. Parer, J. T. Severe Rh isoimmunization—current methods of in utero diagnosis and treatment. *Am. J. Obstet. Gynecol.* 158:1323, 1988.
    Severely isoimmunized patients now have greater than a 90 percent chance of a successful pregnancy outcome when management consists of high-resolution ultrasonography, cordocentesis, intravascular fetal transfusion, and meticulous fetal surveillance.
13. Berkowitz, R. L., et al. Intravascular monitoring and management of erythroblastosis fetalis. *Am. J. Obstet. Gynecol.* 158:783, 1988.
    Percutaneous transfusions or exchange transfusions performed under ultrasonic guidance were successful in 87 percent of the patients.
14. Whittle, M. J. Rhesus haemolytic disease. *Arch. Dis. Child.* 67:65, 1992.
    A protocol to evaluate and treat the newborn with hemolysis associated with isoimmunization is outlined.
15. Watson, W. J., Katz, V. L., and Bowes, W. A., Jr. Plasmapheresis during pregnancy. *Obstet. Gynecol.* 76:451, 1990.
    Maternal plasmapheresis performed twice weekly may protect the fetus during the first trimester before the time when intrauterine transfusion becomes an option.
16. Ronkin, S., et al. Intravascular exchange and bolus transfusion in the severely isoimmunized fetus. *Am. J. Obstet. Gynecol.* 160:407, 1989.
    Rh-sensitized fetuses were treated with 31 intravascular transfusions (PUBS). Bleeding from the puncture site was found in one third, but this was without apparent maternal or fetal consequence.

Complications
17. Frigoletto, F. D., Jr., et al. Intrauterine fetal transfusion in 365 fetuses during fifteen years. *Am. J. Obstet. Gynecol.* 139:781, 1981.
    This article reviewed 365 consecutive cases of fetuses who received intrauterine fetal transfusions from 22 to 32 weeks of gestation; 45 percent survived. Direct ultrasound guidance confers increased success in this procedure.
18. Grannun, P. A. T., and Copel, J. A prevention of Rh isoimmunization and treatment of the compromised fetus. *Semin. Perinatol.* 12:324, 1988.
    This article is replete with details on the use of Rh immunoglobulin and has a nice table on the various doses of the drug to use for each condition. It likewise provides a very well-organized treatment approach to the severely affected fetus.

Prophylaxis
19. Tovey, L. A., and Taverner, J. M. A case for the antenatal administration of anti-D immunoglobulin. *Lancet* 1:878, 1981.
    The authors believe that RhoGAM given antepartum is cost effective and recommend its routine use.
20. Bowman, J. M. Controversies in Rh prophylaxis. Who needs immune globulin and when should it be given? *Am. J. Obstet. Gynecol.* 151:289, 1985.
    To suppress Rh isoimmunization to its lowest possible level (2–4 per 10,000 pregnancies), Rh immunoglobulin must be given to all Rh-negative nonimmunized women who (1) deliver Rh-positive babies, (2) abort, (3) have ectopic pregnancies, or (4) undergo amniocentesis, except when the husband is Rh negative. The dose should be at least 300 μg per 30 ml of fetal blood.
21. Prevention of D Isoimmunization. *ACOG Tech. Bull.* No. 147, October 1990.
    The most current recommendations of the American College of Obstetricians and Gynecologists concerning the administration of Rh immunoglobulin are detailed.
22. Bowman, J. M. Antenatal suppression of Rh alloimmunization. *Clin. Obstet. Gynecol.* 34:296, 1991.
    Routine use of antenatal Rh immunoglobulin at 28 to 30 weeks' gestation and again 12 weeks later if the patient is undelivered resulted in the incidence of Rh(D) isoimmunization declining from 1.8 to 0.1 percent. This method of administration is cost effective and apparently safe for both the mother and fetus.

20. POSTTERM PREGNANCY
Rick W. Martin

Postterm pregnancy is a gestation lasting 42 weeks or more, and occurs in 3 to 12 percent of pregnancies. Although only 20 percent of postterm infants exhibit the postmaturity syndrome, other problems are frequent. Without intervention, the perinatal mortality doubles from 10.5 to 20.0 deaths per 1000 births during 39 to 41 weeks. It doubles again by 44 weeks. There are also 50 percent more congenital anomalies associated with postterm pregnancies than with term pregnancies. In addition, placental insufficiency or oligohydramnios may be responsible for causing an abnormal fetal heart rate or even fetal death. Fetal macrosomia, and associated birth trauma, is three to seven times more common than they are in a term birth. In about 24 to 30 percent of postterm pregnancies, meconium aspiration syndrome may occur.

The correct diagnosis of postterm pregnancy depends on accurate determination of the gestational age. Although ultrasound performed before the twentieth week of gestation is accurate to within 1 week, it can vary by 3 weeks in the third trimester. Calculation of the gestational age from the last menstrual period is very helpful when a reliable patient can provide such information. Using Nägele's rule, the expected date of confinement may be calculated by subtracting 3 months from the first day of the last menstrual period and adding 7 days. This must be correlated with the clinical findings, however, especially when the patient's history is unreliable. The time of the patient's first perception of fetal movement (16–20 weeks) or of the initial auscultation of the fetal heartbeat with a nonelectronic stethoscope (18–20 weeks) may also provide acceptable documentation of the gestational age. An experienced practitioner can determine uterine size during the first trimester, and the fundal height reaches 20 cm above the symphysis pubis (same level as the maternal umbilicus) at 20 weeks' gestation.

Many physicians prefer to induce labor at 42 completed weeks of gestation, but the cesarean section rate would likely be increased in patients with an unfavorable Bishop score. Others prefer to maintain continued surveillance. The time to initiate antepartum testing varies in the opinion of obstetricians. All would begin assessment at 42 weeks, but some would begin at 41 weeks. The nonstress test (NST) is a noninvasive test that is relatively easy to perform. Traditionally, this test is done on a weekly basis; however, there is some evidence that twice weekly testing may be indicated for the postterm pregnancy. Despite a reactive test result, intervention is often recommended if spontaneous fetal heart rate decelerations are noted. The contraction stress test (CST) is an excellent method of fetal monitoring in the postdates pregnancy. In one series, more than 679 postdates infants were delivered without a single perinatal death. Although originally the contractions were induced through the administration of oxytocin, this is now done by nipple stimulation. This approach has also greatly reduced the expense and time involved in performing the CST.

The fetal biophysical profile is another test of fetal well-being that assesses such factors as fetal tone, gross body movements, amniotic fluid volume, and fetal breathing; this profile also includes the NST. One important component of the biophysical profile is the amniotic fluid volume, and some recommend assessing this on a weekly basis in postterm pregnancies. In fact, the combination of the NST and amniotic fluid volume determinations yields results equally as good as those yielded by the CST. The amniotic fluid volume may be assessed using the rule that a vertical diameter of 1 cm or less is abnormal. The amniotic fluid index, as calculated by assessment of the vertical pockets in four quadrants centered about the umbilicus, can also be utilized. An amniotic fluid index less than 5 cm is considered low. Doppler ultrasound is used less frequently to evaluate the postterm fetus, but it appears that umbilical artery systolic-diastolic ratios above 2.40 should be considered abnormal, whereas a higher value is satisfactory in other high-risk pregnancy situations.

Induction of labor at 42 weeks' gestation is an acceptable method of managing the postterm pregnancy. Concerns about the difficulty of inducing labor with oxytocin have led to a search for other means to "ripen" the cervix. Prostaglandin E_2 gel has been administered, either intravaginally or into the cervical os, with good results. Fetal monitoring is recommended during this procedure, as cases of hyperstimulation and fetal distress have been reported. Mechanical ripening of the cervix has been accomplished with *Laminaria* tents. Newer synthetic forms of *Laminaria* would seem to pose less risk of infection than the natural *Laminaria*. Others propose "sweeping" or "stripping" the fetal membranes away from the cervix by a vigorous digital examination. One study revealed that such stripping of the membranes beginning at 40 weeks' gestation significantly reduces the number of postterm pregnancies.

Labor is usually induced by the administration of a dilute oxytocin infusion. As already mentioned, cervical ripening may or may not be chosen by the obstetrician. Electronic surveillance is definitely recommended, as the incidence of fetal distress is increased in the setting of postterm pregnancy. In addition, an early amniotomy should be performed to assess for meconium-stained fluid and to allow placement of the fetal scalp electrode if needed. An ultrasound estimation of fetal weight may be helpful, although this is known to be highly inaccurate when the estimated fetal weight exceeds 4500 g. A cesarean section is often performed to prevent shoulder dystocia. Because of the risk of fetal macrosomia, the obstetrician should be prepared to initiate maneuvers to relieve a shoulder dystocia at the time of vaginal delivery. During labor, decelerations may occur, especially variable decelerations, which are often noted with oligohydramnios. Some authors have noted rather bizarre fetal heart rates in postdates pregnancies, which may indicate fetal distress. In about 25 to 30 percent of pregnancies at 42 weeks, there may be meconium-stained amniotic fluid. In the presence of oligohydramnios, there is little dilution and the meconium is likely to be thicker. DeLee suction of the fetal nose and pharynx after delivery of the head is performed, and trained personnel should be available to carry out endotracheal suctioning once the infant is delivered. Because of in utero aspiration, the neonatal meconium aspiration syndrome may be unavoidable in some cases.

In summary, the postterm pregnancy presents special problems for the attending physicians. Not only must they deal with an anxious mother who is anticipating delivery, but they must be prepared to handle the many medical situations that can arise. At this time, both continued surveillance and induction of labor are acceptable methods of management. Surveillance may be appropriate, especially in patients with poor gestational dating. The presence of oligohydramnios or an abnormal fetal heart rate indicates a need for intervention.

General
1. Diagnosis and Management of Postterm Pregnancy. *ACOG Tech. Bull.* No. 130. July 1989.
   The current management opproach to postterm pregnancy is provided.
2. Postterm Pregnancy. *ACOG Committee Opinion.* No. 57. October 1987.
   Obstetricians are alerted to six important aspects of the management of postterm fetuses.
3. Lagrew, D. C., and Freeman, R. K. Management of postdate pregnancy. *Am. J. Obstet. Gynecol.* 154:8, 1986.
   Excellent review of postdate pregnancies.
4. Dyson, D. C., Miller, P. D., and Armstrong, M. A. Management of prolonged pregnancy: induction of labor versus antepartum fetal testing. *Am. J. Obstet. Gynecol.* 156:928, 1987.
   In a prospective study, the rates of meconium, fetal distress, and cesarean section were higher in the antepartum surveillance group compared to those undergoing PGE_2 gel ripening and induction.
5. Hannah, M. E., et al. Induction of labor as compared with serial antenatal monitoring in postterm pregnancy. *N. Engl. J. Med.* 326:1587, 1992.
   Induction of labor resulted in a lower rate of cesarean section compared to serial monitoring. The rates of perinatal mortality and morbidity were similar.
6. Freeman, R. K., et al. Postdate pregnancy: utilization of contraction stress testing for primary fetal surveillance. *Am. J. Obstet. Gynecol.* 140:128, 1981.
   The CST was used to evaluate 679 patients for postterm pregnancies, without a single related perinatal death.
7. Small, M. L., et al. An active management approach to the postdate fetus with a reactive nonstress test and fetal heart rate decelerations. *Obstet. Gynecol.* 70: 636, 1987.
   The authors recommend induction of labor when fetal heart rate decelerations occur in conjunction with a reactive NST.
8. Phelan, J. P. The postdate pregnancy: an overview. *Clin. Obstet. Gynecol.* 32:221, 1989.
   Excellent summary of the subject of postdate pregnancy.

Cervical Ripening
9. McColgin, S. W., et al. Stripping membranes at term: can it safely reduce the incidence of postterm pregnancies? *Obstet. Gynecol.* 76:678, 1990.
   Women who had undergone membrane stripping beginning at 38 weeks had earlier deliveries and fewer postterm deliveries than did those in a controlled group. The effect was most notable in nulliparous women.
10. Kadar, N., Tapp, A., and Wong, A. The influence of nipple stimulation at term on the duration of pregnancy. *J. Perinatol.* 10:164, 1990.
    Nipple stimulation did not influence either the duration of pregnancy or the cesarean section rate. Patient compliance was poor.
11. Rayburn, W., and Husslein, P. Use of prostaglandins for induction of labor. *Semin. Perinatol.* 15:173, 1991.
    Overview of prostaglandin use for cervical ripening.

12. Rayburn, W. F. Prostaglandin E_2 gel for cervical ripening and induction of labor: a critical analysis. *Am. J. Obstet. Gynecol.* 160:529, 1989.
    This report summarizes the observations from 3313 pregnancies in 59 clinical trials evaluating the use of prostaglandin E_2 gel for cervical ripening.
13. Nicholas, J. Intracervical tents: usage and mode of action. *Obstet. Gynecol. Surv.* 44:410, 1989.
    Overview of the use of Laminaria.

Miscellaneous
14. Pollack, R. N., Hauer-Pollack, G., and Divon, M. Y. Macrosomia postdate pregnancies: the accuracy of routine ultrasonic screening. *Am. J. Obstet. Gynecol.* 167:7, 1992.
    Routine ultrasound for the detection of macrosomia in postterm pregnancies predicted only 56 percent of such infants.
15. Macri, C. J., et al. Prophylactic amnioinfusion improves outcome of pregnancy complicated by thick meconium and oligohydramnios. *Am. J. Obstet. Gynecol.* 167:117, 1992.
    A lower frequency of fetal distress, cesarean section, and meconium aspiration was observed for term and postterm patients in the presence of thick meconium and oligohydramnios who underwent amnioinfusion.
16. Roberts, L. J., and Young, K. R. The management of prolonged pregnancy—an analysis of women's attitudes before and after term. *Br. J. Obstet. Gynaecol.* 98:1102, 1991.
    Most pregnant women were unwilling to accept conservative management of a prolonged pregnancy.
17. Fischer, R. L., et al. Doppler evaluation of the umbilical and uterine arcuate arteries in the postdate pregnancy. *Obstet. Gynecol.* 78:363, 1991.
    An umbilical artery systolic-diastolic ratio of 2.4 was recommended rather than 3.0 as a threshold to identify high-risk postdates pregnancies.
18. Phelan, J. P. Medical-legal considerations in the post date pregnancy. *Clin. Obstet. Gynecol.* 32:294, 1989.
    Because of the increased risk of perinatal morbidity, it is important for the physician to maintain his or her knowledge and skills in the management of postterm pregnancy.
19. Niswander, K. R. EFM and brain damage in term and postterm infants. *Contemp. Ob/Gyn* 36:39, 1991.
    An abnormal electronic fetal monitoring tracing is a poor predictor of cerebral palsy in the newborn. Several fetal heart rate patterns may be suggestive of an infant with existing fetal brain damage.

21. ANEMIAS AND HEMOGLOBINOPATHIES IN PREGNANCY

Joseph A. Pryor

Anemia is one of the most frequently encountered complications of pregnancy. In the second trimester, a relative anemia is noted in most pregnancies secondary to a proportionately larger increase in the plasma volume relative to the red blood cell (RBC) mass. Absolute anemias occur because of decreased erythrocyte production, increased RBC destruction, or accentuated erythrocyte loss. The most common cause of anemia other than obvious blood loss is decreased erythrocyte production (95%). These anemias are collectively called *hypoproliferative anemias*. These processes usually stem from deficiency of an essential subcellular component, such as iron, folic acid, or vitamin B_{12}. Most of these anemias are acquired. In contrast, anemia may be congenital, as in the hemoglobinopathies, which are biochemical disorders that function at a molecular level and affect either the production rate (thalassemia) or the structural integrity (sickle hemoglobin [Hb]) of the normal Hb molecule. Homozygous sickle cell anemia, Hb SC disease, and Hb S–thalassemia are the most clinically significant, and constitute what is known as *sickle cell disease* (SCD). The incidence of SCD ranges from 1 in 400 to 1 in 600 patients.

The effect of anemia on gestation is variable. Deterioration in the maternal condition is not usually noted unless the Hb level is less than 4 to 6 g/dl and the packed cell volume (PCV) is less than 12 to 18 percent. In patients with isovolemic anemia, hemodynamic stability at rest was noted with PCVs of 5 to 10 percent. Increased bleeding time, longer recuperation, and a prolonged hospital stay may be the outcome in the moderately anemic parturient (Hb ≤8 g/dl; PCV <25%). Mild anemia (Hb <10–11 g/dl; PCV <30%) may result in intrauterine growth retardation (IUGR).

The nature of the laboratory assessment is changed by the pregnancy itself, but most of the necessary tests can be performed on an ambulatory basis. When the anemia is severe or serious hematologic disease is suspected, hospitalization may be indicated. Classically, the pregnant patient with an Hb less than 10 g/dl, a PCV less than 30 percent, or both, is considered anemic. Blood smears and indices may be helpful. If the mean corpuscular Hb concentration (MCHC) is less than 30 μg/dl/RBC, an absolute anemia is almost always present. In pregnancy, the reticulocyte count should be 1 to 3 percent; however, when this is not the case, a hypoproliferative disorder usually exists. This situation usually indicates a primary toxic effect, a hereditary disorder (thalassemia), or a lack of essential nutrients such as iron and folic acid. On the other hand, the parturient with an anemia and a reticulocyte count of greater than 3 percent usually has accelerated RBC production in response to excessive blood loss.

Iron deficiency anemia (IDA) can be implicated in up to 75 percent of all anemias during pregnancy. The iron requirement during a normal gestation is more than 1000 mg, exceeding by 300 to 400 mg the amount of iron available even with the best diets. Therefore, there is a rationale for prescribing supplemental iron in all pregnant women. The diagnosis of IDA can be made by the findings of a hypochromic, microcytic RBC smear together with an MCHC of less than 30 μg/dl/RBC, an unsaturated iron-binding capacity of greater than 300 μg/dl, a serum iron level of less than 60 μg/ml, and a low serum ferritin level. The treatment of IDA should involve the administration of 60 mg of elemental iron (300 mg of ferrous sulfate) taken 3 times a day with meals.

Folic acid deficiency constitutes 20 to 22 percent of the cases of anemia during pregnancy. Therefore, together folic acid deficiency and IDA account for approximately 97 percent of all anemias that occur during the reproductive years. The use of recombinant human erythropoietin has been shown to be effective in the treatment of postpartum anemia; however, its use in pregnant women has been very limited and is not recommended at this time. Most vitamin preparations have enough folic acid (1 mg) and suffice if the diet is adequate. Laboratory findings indicating folate deficiency include hypersegmented neutrophils, macrocytic and hyperchromatic changes in the RBC, and a low serum folate level. Neural tube defects (NTDs) are associated with reduced folic acid intake. Folic acid (4 mg daily before and during early pregnancy) reduced the recurrence of NTDs by 71 percent in women who had already had a child with NTD. The American College of Obstetricians and Gynecologists recommend the use of folic acid (4 mg daily for 1 month before and continuing through the first 3 months of pregnancy) in high-risk patients.

Anemias associated with the defective production of erythrocytes are numerous, but they are rarely seen clinically. Various toxins may give rise to an aplastic anemia, whereas antiinflammatory agents or severe acute infections may also be toxic to the bone marrow. A mortality rate of up to 75 percent has been reported in patients with aplastic anemia; however, pregnancy itself usually does not affect the disorder adversely. Chronic inflammation, as seen in the autoimmune diseases and neoplasia, may also result in an anemia.

Hemolytic anemias of pregnancy include those in which RBCs are destroyed prematurely. Diseases such as the HELLP (hemolysis, elevated liver enzymes, low platelets) syndrome, spherocytosis, and porphyria exhibit blood smear abnormalities that feature very bizarrely shaped cells. The social, family, and individual history may be informative in these cases. Mild hemoglobinopathies such as heterozygous thalassemia or sickle cell trait are common, and pregnancies usually proceed routinely. In contrast, patients with SCD face a significant risk for maternal difficulties and increased perinatal morbidity and mortality. There is an increased incidence of vasoocclusive crises caused by hydrophobic bonding of the sickle Hb in patients with SCD. This condition is aggravated by infections, pregnancy, high altitudes, hypoxia, and acidosis.

Since 1970, intensive medical therapy, as well as the use of prophylactic transfusions, has been more successful in yielding good maternal-fetal outcomes in patients with SCD. There has also been a dramatic decrease in the number of premature or low-birth-weight babies born to mothers with SCD when these intensive measures are instituted. If transfusions are used, one must counsel patients about their risks, including hepatitis, transfusion reaction, isosensitization, and potential exposure to human immunodeficiency virus infection. There are those who favor the use of prophylactic transfusions on a regular basis to prevent complications, whereas others prefer to use blood component therapy only when symptoms are severe. Both methods appear to yield good results for the mother and the neonate. It should be noted, however, that, when the reactive approach is adopted, as many as 50 percent of the patients will receive transfusions for complications, versus a less than 5 to 15 percent complication rate in those who receive prophylactic transfusions. Buffy-coat poor, washed RBCs are usually administered on an ambulatory basis by erythrocytopheresis in transfusions. A reduction in the Hb S level to less than 50 percent and an increase in the Hb A concentration to at least 40 percent is desirable. In most of these instances, the PCV will be between 30 and 35 percent after transfusion.

The method of follow-up after transfusion is fairly standardized. In most centers, an Hb electrophoresis is carried out at least every 2 weeks to assess for a possible change in the Hb A and S levels. Most authors agree that retransfusion should be performed if the Hb A level falls below 20 percent. Antisickling agents, such as urea and thiocyanate, are not recommended during pregnancy, because their effect on the fetus is unknown. Regardless of whether transfusions are given, there should be frequent fetal health assessment and careful management in such patients during the intrapartum period. Electronic monitoring of the fetal heart rate and assessment of maternal blood gases is advised. Fetal scalp pH determinations, when abnormal fetal heart rate tracings are noted, may also be used. Oxygen, delivered at 4 to 6 liters/min, should be administered, and labor should be managed with the patient in the lateral semirecumbent position. Anesthesia for delivery can be regional, pudendal, or local. Balanced general anesthesia for cesarean birth is most acceptable, although care must be taken postoperatively to prevent atelectasis. Obviously, conduction anesthesia for abdominal delivery is also acceptable, if approved by the anesthesiologist. Postpartum care should include intensive assessment for infections. The hospital stay in most patients managed with transfusion therapy is not prolonged unless infections are evident.

Genetic counseling and education are of paramount importance in patients with SCD. The father should also be tested so that some prediction of the risk to the infant can be made. Cord blood is screened so that the genetic condition of the fetus is known and genetic counseling can take place. Therapeutic abortion for maternal reasons is usually not recommended unless severe maternal disease is already present. It is possible to diagnose various states of SCD using chorionic villus sampling, percutaneous umbilical blood sampling, or amniocentesis utilizing restriction endonuclease assessment. These tests should be offered to the patients, while the education of the patient and interpregnancy care should be coordinated with a hematologist.

General

1. Morrison, J. C., and Gookin, K. S. Anemia Associated With Pregnancy. In J. J. Sciarra (ed.), *Gynecology and Obstetrics*, Vol. 3. Philadelphia: Lippincott, 1988. *An in-depth review of the various causes of anemia and how they relate to pregnancy. A nice section is also included on laboratory determinations.*

2. Samson, D. The anemia of chronic disorders. *Postgrad. Med.* 59:543, 1983. *Chronic disease such as infection, inflammatory disease, or malignancy is the*

most common known cause of normochromic, normocytic anemia. This article classifies the methods of diagnosis as well as the clinical manifestations and contains more than 50 references.

3. Sergeant, G. R. Sickle haemoglobin and pregnancy. *Br. Med. J.* 287:628, 1983.
   This timely overall review of the subject by a noted authority with 25 years of experience is concise, to the point, and good basic reading for the person interested in sickle cell hemoglobinopathies.

4. Savitt, T. L., and Goldberg, M. F. Herrick's 1910 case report of sickle cell anemia. The rest of the story. *J.A.M.A.* 261:266, 1989.
   This special communications article is a very lucid report on the first publication involving sickle cell anemia. Eighty-two references of very early medical works make it must reading for those interested in this subject.

5. Institute of Medicine (U.S.). Subcommittee on Nutritional Status and Weight Gain During Pregnancy. *Nutrition During Pregnancy.* Washington, D.C.: National Academy Press, 1990.
   An in-depth text with practical guidelines on nutrition in pregnancy.

Etiology

6. Pryor, J. A., and Morrison, J. C. Nutritional Anemia. In M. Bern and F. Frigoletto (ed.), *Hematologic Contribution to Fetal Health.* New York: Liss, 1989.
   A review of the etiology, diagnosis, complications, and treatment of nutritional anemia, with 37 references.

7. Steinberg, M. H., and Hebbel, R. P. Clinical diversity of sickle cell anemia: genetic and cellular modulation of disease severity. *Am. J. Hematol.* 14:405, 1983.
   Various cellular and genetic factors may play a role in modulating the clinical effects of the sickle Hb gene, which may explain why the clinical spectrum ranges from incapacitating problems to an absence of clinical symptomatology.

Diagnosis

8. Roberts, W. E., Morrison, J. C., and Blake, P. G. Evaluation of Anemia in Pregnancy. In D. Z. Kitay (ed.), *Hematologic Problems in Pregnancy.* New York: Grune & Stratton, 1985.
   Describes the essentials in the diagnosis of anemia during pregnancy in the setting of all acquired disorders. Thirty-three references are included.

9. McClure, S., Custer, E., and Bessman, J. D. Improved detection of early iron deficiency in nonanemic subjects. *J.A.M.A.* 253:1021, 1985.
   The RBC distribution width was 100 percent sensitive in correlating with decreased serum iron saturation in nonanemic subjects.

10. Butler, E. The common anemias. *J.A.M.A.* 259:2433, 1988.
    A concise review of the common anemias, including an especially applicable discussion of the diagnosis of iron-deficiency anemia and many recent references.

11. Alter, B. P. Prenatal diagnosis of hemoglobinopathies: development of methods for study of fetal red cells and fibroblasts. *Am. J. Pediatr. Hematol. Oncol.* 5:378, 1983.
    Since 1974, prenatal testing for hemoglobinopathies has been performed, with 2000 cases studied by fetal globin synthesis and approximately 100 by restriction enzyme techniques.

12. Hogge, W. A. Prenatal diagnosis of sickle cell anemia. *Contemp. Ob/Gyn* 33:21, 1989.
    This is a short but well-defined article with good diagrams illustrating how the prenatal diagnosis of sickle cell anemia is undertaken.

13. Osborne, P. T., et al. An evaluation of red blood cell heterogeneity (increased red blood cell distribution width) in iron deficiency of pregnancy. *Am. J. Obstet. Gynecol.* 160:336, 1989.
    Early iron deficiency without anemia is infrequently identified by classic means. A new classification, making use of the mean corpuscular volume, was evaluated in 331 patients in this study and did not improve the diagnostic accuracy among those without frank anemia.

Treatment

14. Morrison, J. C., Martin, J. N., Jr., and McKay, M. L. DIC, ITP and Hemoglobinopathies. In R. A. Knuppel (ed.), *High Risk Obstetrics: A Team Approach.* Philadelphia: Saunders, 1986.
    Causes of anemia that are related to various pathologic disorders in obstetrics are detailed and their treatment is elucidated.

15. Food and Nutrition Board, National Research Council. *Recommended Dietary Allowances.* Washington, D.C.: National Academy of Sciences, 1980.
    A detailed listing of nutritional requirements.

16. IV iron dextrose therapy. *Drug Information Bull.* Vol. 18, No. 3, March–April 1984.
    Review of the indications, techniques, and complications of parenteral iron therapy.

17. Morrison, J. C., et al. Prophylactic transfusions in pregnant patients with sickle hemoglobinopathies: benefit versus risk. *Obstet. Gynecol.* 56:274, 1980.
    Analyses of 75 patients with severe sickle cell hemoglobinopathies who received prophylactic exchange transfusions are outlined.

18. Perry, K. G., Jr., and Morrison, J. C. The diagnosis and management of hemoglobinopathies during pregnancy. *Semin. Perinatol.* 14:90, 1990.
    A review of the physiology, diagnosis, and appropriate therapeutic interventions in pregnant patients with a hemoglobinopathy.

19. Embury, S. H. Effects of oxygen inhalation on endogenous erythropoietin kinetics, erythropoiesis, and properties of blood cells in sickle-cell anemia. *N. Engl. J. Med.* 311:291, 1984.
    The effect of continuous oxygen inhalation during SCD crises was tested. The number of irreversibly sickled cells increased after the cessation of oxygen therapy (rebound effect). Oxygen should be administered intermittently rather than continuously.

20. James, J., Oakhill, A., and Evans, J. Preventing iron deficiency in at-risk communities. *Lancet* 1:40, 1989.
    The authors offer tips on how to appropriately counsel patients about dietary indiscretions that may lead to IDA. They were able to reduce the frequency of IDA in those patients who participated in nutritional counseling.

21. Huch, A., et al. Recombinant human erythropoietin in the treatment of postpartum anemia. *Obstet. Gynecol.* 80:127, 1992.
    A comparative study of women with postpartum anemia. This article contains succinct review and discussion of erythropoietin and its effectiveness in the postpartum anemic patient.

Complications

22. Agarwal, R. M. D., Tripathi, A. M., and Agarwal, K. N. Neonatal hematological values in maternal anemia. *Indian J. Pediatr.* 20:369, 1983.
    Details on and the neonatal hematologic profile in the offspring of anemic and nonanemic parturients. The hematologic values were significantly higher in the newborns of anemic mothers through the first 7 postnatal days based on the presence of mild chronic hypoxia.

23. Reid, C. D. The national sickle cell disease program. *Am. J. Hematol.* 14:265, 1983.
    Data on specific symptomatology in those with SCD are offered. Particularly interesting are the data on infection in the context of SCD.

24. Pastorek, J. G., II, and Seiler, B. Maternal death associated with sickle cell trait. *Am. J. Obstet. Gynecol.* 151:295, 1985.
    A patient with sickle cell trait can be at risk for severe morbidity and death if faced with a condition that aggravates intravascular sickling.

25. MRC Vitamin Study Research Group. Prevention of neural tube defects: results of the medical research council vitamin study. *Lancet* 338:131, 1991.
    The results and discussion of a randomized double-blind prevention trial of folic acid therapy in patients at high risk for having children with NTDs.

26. Committee on Obstetrics: Maternal and Fetal Medicine. Folic acid for the pre-

vention of recurrent neural tube defects. *ACOG Committee Opinion* No. 120, March 1993.
Recommendations concerning the use of folic acid in patients at high risk for bearing children with an NTD.

22. PRETERM LABOR
Rick W. Martin

Preterm delivery occurs in 8 to 10 percent of all births and is responsible for over 50 percent of the cases of perinatal morbidity and mortality. There are many causes of preterm delivery, including preterm labor, premature rupture of the membranes, maternal medical or obstetric complications, and fetal distress. Obviously, not all cases of preterm birth are preventable. There are several known risk factors for preterm labor, most important of which is its occurrence in a previous pregnancy. In the mother who has had one previous preterm delivery, the risk is approximately 30 percent and this may increase to 50 percent if there have been two previous preterm births. Other factors, such as multiple gestation, cervical incompetence, uterine or cervical abnormalities, placental abnormalities, second-trimester bleeding, and serious maternal infection, are also known to increase the likelihood of preterm delivery. Several investigators have developed scoring systems to identify those women at risk of preterm birth. Once such women are identified, they are placed in the care of special clinics, where they receive enhanced education, make frequent clinic visits, and undergo periodic cervical examination. These programs have been particularly successful in France, and have been shown to bring about a decline in the number of preterm births in the years since the programs have been implemented. Typically, approximately 10 percent of pregnant women who are at risk are identified, though only 30 percent of these women actually go on to develop preterm labor.

Preterm labor is diagnosed when a woman experiences regular uterine contractions accompanied by a change in effacement or dilatation of the cervix. If there has been no cervical change, then the patient is not in preterm labor and should not receive tocolytic therapy. Hydration is sometimes effective for the patient in false labor, but sedation is usually avoided during preterm gestations. Documentation of the gestational age is very important in these cases, and early examination and reliable information about the dates of the last menstrual period are helpful in this regard. Ultrasound performed in the third trimester is less accurate in determining gestational age than it is in earlier trimesters. Amniocentesis is sometimes indicated to document fetal pulmonary maturity.

In the setting of certain maternal conditions, such as severe preeclampsia, or fetal conditions, such as a severe intrauterine growth retarded fetus, or in the event of fetal distress, medical therapy for preterm labor may be contraindicated. The beta-agonist drugs and magnesium sulfate are the most commonly used medications for tocolysis. Ritodrine is the only drug approved by the Food and Drug Administration (FDA) for tocolysis. The initial dosage consists of 50 to 100 μg/min, given intravenously, and this is increased by 50 μg/min every 10 minutes until contractions cease or until a maximum dosage of 350 μg/min is reached. Ritodrine is noted for its cardiovascular effects, and the maternal pulse and blood pressure should therefore be checked frequently. Fetal tachycardia may also occur with its use. Intravenous ritodrine therapy is usually followed by oral ritodrine, in a dosage of 10 mg every 2 hours for the first 24 hours followed by 10 to 20 mg every 4 to 6 hours. The physician should be particularly cautious about using ritodrine in the presence of multifetal gestation or pyelonephritis, as pulmonary edema can develop. Another beta-agonist, terbutaline, remains to be approved by the FDA for use in preterm labor. Many protocols use a dosage of 2.5 μg/min, given intravenously, and increase this to a maximum of 20 μg/min. Orally administered terbutaline, 5 mg every 4 to 6 hours, may follow the intravenous regimen. Although magnesium sulfate is not approved by the FDA for use as a tocolytic drug, it is also an effective tocolytic agent and seems to have fewer cardiovascular side effects than the beta-agonists. Magnesium sulfate has been available for the treatment of preeclampsia for many years, and obstetricians are therefore very familiar with its use. The usual dosage consists of a 4- to 6-g loading dose, followed by an infusion of 2 to 4 g/hr until the situation resolves. Because magnesium is excreted by the kidneys, normal renal function should be documented and urine output recorded regularly. After the intravenous magnesium sulfate therapy, oral maintenance is usually provided with a beta-agonist drug or magnesium. Magnesium gluconate may be given in a dosage of 2 g taken orally every 4 hours, though there may be gastrointestinal side effects. Tocolytic drugs are most effective when given before marked cervical dilatation takes place.

Newer agents are usually considered as second-line therapy for preterm labor. Indomethacin has shown good results, and an oral dose of 25 mg every 4 to 6 hours may be given. The medication may also be given as a rectal suppository. The prolonged use of indomethacin is discouraged, as oligohydramnios can occur. The drug is not recommended beyond 32 weeks' gestation because of concerns about it causing premature closure of the fetal ductus arteriosus. Calcium channel–blocking drugs, such as nifedipine, have also been used as a second choice. When preterm delivery is anticipated, the administration of glucocorticoids may enhance fetal lung maturity. There is wide experience with betamethasone, given in a dosage of two doses of 12 mg, 24 hours apart, or dexamethasone, four doses of 6 mg given every 12 hours.

Should efforts to delay delivery fail, intrapartum management becomes very important. Electronic heart rate monitoring of the fragile preterm fetus is desirable. Vaginal birth seems appropriate for the preterm infant in the vertex presentation, as long as there are no signs of fetal distress. Most would perform cesarean section for the preterm infant in the breech position. Should a cesarean section be required, special attention should be paid to making an adequate incision for delivery, as the lower uterine segment is often thick and may cause trauma to the infant. At the time of delivery, medical staff should be available for resuscitation of the preterm infant.

General
1. Smith, C. V. Antepartum fetal surveillance in the preterm fetus. *Clin. Perinatol.* 19:437, 1992.
   An outline of the indications for antepartum fetal surveillance in the preterm fetus is given.
2. Preterm Labor. *ACOG Tech. Bull.* No. 133, October 1989.
   Infant survival as it relates to gestational age is discussed and common tocolytic drug therapy is described.
3. Graber, E. A. Prematurity—1992. *Obstet. Gynecol. Surv.* 47:521, 1992.
   Brief review of the topic of prematurity. The ethical and financial issues are also discussed.
4. Gibbs, R. S., et al. A review of premature birth and subclinical infection. *Am. J. Obstet. Gynecol.* 166:1515, 1992.
   The authors conclude that preterm birth results in part from infection caused by genital tract bacteria.
5. Amon, E., Nshyken, J. M., and Sibai, B. M. How small is too small and how early is too early? A survey of American obstetricians specializing in high-risk pregnancies. *Am. J. Perinatol.* 9:17, 1992.
   Four hundred five maternal-fetal medicine specialists were surveyed to determine their clinical opinions regarding intrapartum management of the severely preterm fetus.
6. Korenbrot, C. C., Aalto, L. H., and Laros, R. K. The cost effectiveness of stopping preterm labor with beta-adrenergic treatment. *N. Engl. J. Med.* 310:691, 1984.
   The increased cost of medical care for treating preterm labor was offset by decreased costs of neonatal medical care before 34 weeks' gestation.
7. Romero, R., Mazor, M., and Oyarzun, E. Role of intraamniotic infection in preterm labor. *Contemp. Ob/Gyn* 32:94, 1988.
   The authors discuss the association between intraamniotic infection and preterm labor.

8. Romero, R., et al. Meta-analysis of the relationship between asymptomatic bacteriuria and preterm delivery/low birth weight. *Obstet. Gynecol.* 73:576, 1989.
   A strong association exists between untreated asymptomatic bacteriuria and preterm delivery.
9. Gibbs, R. S., et al. A review of premature birth and subclinical infection. *Am. J. Obstet. Gynecol.* 166:1515, 1992.
   Comprehensive analysis of the role of infection and preterm birth.

Risk Assessment
10. Creasy, R. K. Preterm birth prevention: where are we? *Am. J. Obstet. Gynecol.* 168:1223, 1993.
    Overview of preterm birth and the problems associated with diagnosis and management.
11. Creasy, R. K., Gummer, B. A., and Liggins, G. C. System for predicting spontaneous preterm birth. *Obstet. Gynecol.* 55:692, 1980.
    A risk scoring system is presented that can identify approximately 10 percent of the patients. Only one third of the patients identified actually went on to experience preterm labor.
12. Morrison, J. C., et al. Oncofetal fibronectin in patients with false labor as a predictor of preterm delivery. *Am. J. Obstet. Gynecol.* 168:538, 1993.
    A positive fetal fibronectin level in women who have false labor indicated a significant risk for preterm labor and early delivery.
13. Morrison, J. C., et al. Prevention of preterm birth by ambulatory assessment of uterine activity: a randomized study. *Am. J. Obstet. Gynecol.* 156:536, 1987.
    Use of a device that could be used at home for monitoring uterine activity led to a greater number of patients reaching term than was seen for a control group.
14. Papiernik, E., et al. Prevention of preterm births: A perinatal study in Haguenau grants. *Pediatrics* 76:154, 1985.
    A reduction in preterm births was accomplished through the implementation of a comprehensive program for the management of patients at risk.
15. Grimes, D. A., and Schulz, K. F. Randomized control trials of home uterine activity monitoring: a review and critique. *Obstet. Gynecol.* 79:137, 1992.
    The authors questioned the efficacy of home uterine monitoring.
16. Leveno, K. J., Cox, K., and Roark, M. L. Cervical dilatation and prematurity revisited. *Obstet. Gynecol.* 68:434, 1986.
    Findings from early third-trimester cervical examination predicted preterm delivery.

Treatment
17. Kirshbaum, T. Antibiotics in the treatment of preterm labor. *Am. J. Obstet. Gynecol.* 168:239, 1993.
    The author reviews only the data from randomized, prospective studies examining the management of preterm labor with antibiotic therapy.
18. Petrie, R. H. Tocolysis using magnesium sulfate. *Semin. Perinatol.* 5:266, 1981.
    A thorough review of magnesium sulfate as a tocolytic drug.
19. Martin, R. W., and Morrison, J. C. Oral magnesium for tocolysis. *Contemp. Ob/Gyn* 30:111, 1987.
    Various oral magnesium preparations are reviewed, as well as their use for management after parenteral magnesium sulfate treatment.
20. Murray, C., et al. Nifedipine for treatment of preterm labor: a historic prospective study. *Am. J. Obstet. Gynecol.* 167:52, 1992.
    Nifedipine proved to be a well-tolerated and safe tocolytic agent.
21. King, J. F., et al. Beta-mimetics in preterm labor: an overview of the randomized controlled trials. *Br. J. Obstet Gynaecol.* 95:211, 1988.
    The administration of beta-agonists for tocolysis delays delivery, and this is reflected by a reduction in preterm births.
22. Allbert, J. R., et al. Subcutaneous tocolytic infusion therapy for patients at very high risk for preterm birth. *J. Perinatol.* 12:28, 1992.

The use of a subcutaneous infusion pump is described for the management of preterm labor.

Neonatal Problems

23. Horbor, J. D., et al. A multicenter randomized, placebo-controlled trial of surfactant therapy for respiratory distress syndrome. *N. Engl. J. Med.* 320:959, 1989.
Treatment with single-dose surfactant reduces the severity of respiratory distress during the first 3 days after treatment, but did not lead to a significantly improved clinical status later in the neonatal period.

24. Saigai, S., et al. Intellectual and functional status at the school entry of children who weighed 1000 grams or less at birth. A regional perspective of births in the 1980's. *J. Pediatr.* 116:409, 1990.
Two thirds of the children were performing in the adequate range and the remainder in the moderately low to low range. Of the children with no impairments, 49 percent were identified to be at risk for future learning disabilities.

25. DePalma, R. T., et al. Birth weight threshold for postponing preterm birth. *Am. J. Obstet. Gynecol.* 167:1145, 1992.
Aggressive attempts to prevent preterm birth in infants whose weight exceeded 1900 g conferred few benefits.

26. Martin, G. I., and Sindel, B. D. Neonatal management of the very low birth weight infant: the use of surfactant. *Clin. Perinatol.* 19:461, 1992.
A review of the results from the administration of surfactant for the prevention of respiratory distress syndrome.

27. Robertson, P. A., et al. Neonatal morbidity according to gestational age and birth weight from five tertiary care centers in the United States, 1983 through 1986. *Am. J. Obstet. Gynecol.* 166:1629, 1992.
The incidence of respiratory distress syndrome and patent ductus arteriosus is decreased in association with increasing gestational age and birth weight. The incidence of severe intraventricular hemorrhage, necrotizing enterocolitis, and sepsis diminishes markedly after 34 weeks.

28. Escobar, G. J., Littenberg, B., and Petitti, D. B. Outcome among surviving very low birthweight infants: a meta-analysis. *Arch. Dis. Child.* 66:204, 1991.
A worldwide analysis of over 26,000 births of infants weighing less than 1500 g was performed. Forty-one percent of the infants died and 25 percent of the survivors were noted to have a disability.

23. PREMATURE RUPTURED MEMBRANES
James F. McCaul IV

Premature rupture of the membranes (PROM) can be a major obstetric complication, and constitutes the rupture of membranes before the onset of true labor, but is often difficult to document. It occurs in 6 to 20 percent of all parturients. When PROM occurs before 37 weeks (about 33%), it is associated with increased perinatal mortality directly related to prematurity. The incidence of placental abruption may be as high as 7 percent in the setting of PROM, and the prevalence of infection is estimated to be 20 percent. If PROM occurs at or near term (60–80%), the potential fetal sequelae are somewhat diminished, but the mother still faces the risk of infectious morbidity and those risks associated with abdominal delivery. Although the neonatal sepsis rate is increased in the presence of PROM, it does not correlate with the duration of ruptured membranes; rather, it is related to the extent of prematurity. When possible, fetal gestational age and lung maturity should be determined, as they are important elements for establishing a rational management plan. The ultimate goal is to formulate a plan that will yield a healthy neonate while also producing the fewest maternal complications. Thus, the decision whether to manage a given patient with induced labor, operative delivery, or expectant observation may be difficult at times.

The presumed causes of PROM are many. Trauma, an incompetent cervix, and uterine anomalies have all been implicated. Multiple sexual partners and sexually transmitted diseases are also risk factors. The vaginal infections most frequently encountered in association with PROM include bacterial vaginosis, as well as *Neisseria gonorrhoeae*, group B streptococcus, *Chlamydia, Mycoplasma, Ureaplasma,* and *Trichomonas* infections. The role of bacterial metabolic byproducts, such as collagenase and elastase (proteases), which may weaken the chorioamnionic membranes, has been a focus of research efforts. Maternal leukocytes recruited to combat infection may release elastases, which cause further weakening of the membranes and cervical changes. Some bacteria also produce phospholipases that release arachidonic acid from the fetal membranes and the decidua, thereby initiating prostaglandin production. Prostaglandins stimulate proteolytic activity, in addition to causing contractions.

The first step in the management of PROM is documentation. The time of rupture, presence of meconium, and appearance of symptoms that might herald infection should be noted. Next, the cervix should be inspected using a sterile speculum to note the presence of free-flowing amniotic fluid from the cervical os. Fluid from the posterior fornix may be tested for an alkaline pH (amniotic fluid) using nitrazine paper. A sample of the fluid should be allowed to dry on a slide; arborization or ferning will be observed microscopically if amniotic fluid is present. The presence of fetal fibronectin in the posterior fornix is diagnostic when there is a high index of suspicion for PROM, but the findings yielded by traditional diagnostic methods are inconclusive. Cervical specimens for culture for group B streptococcus and *N. gonorrhoeae* can be obtained during the speculum examination, and the degree of dilatation and effacement of the cervix should be estimated, as this may have predictive value in determining which patients can be managed expectantly. Internal digital examination of the cervix should not be performed unless induction of labor is anticipated. If acute cervicitis or vaginal lesions are present, the likelihood of successful expectant management is diminished. Cord prolapse may occasionally be noted and necessitates delivery.

Maternal hyperpyrexia and maternal or fetal tachycardia are excellent predictors (but relatively late signs) in the course of amnionitis. Abdominal tenderness or uterine irritability may also herald chorioamnionitis. Abdominal examination may be performed to help in determining fetal presentation (e.g., breech, vertex, or transverse), and occasionally a multifetal gestation will be identified.

Ultrasound examination can be performed to determine fetal head circumference, biparietal diameter (BPD), and femur or humerus length, and this information can be used to estimate gestational age. Additionally, fetal viability (cardiac activity), some fetal anomalies, fetal presentation, and multigestation can be documented. Ultrasound is also useful for placental localization and assessment of amniotic fluid volume. If possible, amniotic fluid should be obtained for fetal lung maturity studies when the estimated gestational age is greater than 32 weeks, as the sonographically obtained measurements are only approximate at this time. Amniocentesis performed under sonographic guidance will permit fluid recovery in over 50 percent of patients. Culture and Gram's staining of fluid collected transabdominally may be helpful in diagnosing amniotic bacterial colonization, but whether an immature fetus should be delivered in this setting (in the absence of apparent clinical chorioamnionitis) remains unclear. Cultures may be of benefit in guiding antimicrobial therapy if amnionitis develops. If free-flowing amniotic fluid can be obtained during the sterile speculum examination, the lecithin-sphingomyelin (L/S) ratio can be determined. The results are usually not significantly different from those yielded by the transabdominal samples; but, in the presence of blood or meconium, the L/S ratio may be artificially lowered. With a contaminated specimen, the presence of phosphatidylglycerol in amniotic fluid may be useful in confirming lung maturity if the fetus is beyond 36 weeks.

The laboratory assessment of amnionitis can be confusing because the infection is subclinical in many cases. The presence of leukocytes or organisms on Gram's stained amniotic fluid specimens obtained by amniocentesis (or an intrauterine catheter) has been correlated with an increased risk of amnionitis. Initially, cultures are not clinically useful but may be advantageous later if amnionitis develops. The maternal leukocyte count (>20,000 with a shift toward segmented neutrophils) may also be indicative of imminent amnionitis.

In those pregnancies with probable fetal lung maturity (>36 weeks), the management of PROM usually leans toward delivery. Because more than 80 percent of the patients at or near term will go into spontaneous labor within 12 hours of PROM, many practitioners advocate 4 to 24 hours of observation before inducing delivery. Others begin induction immediately, although this course of management may lead to more cesarean births (as high as 50% because of an unfavorable cervix), and may also lead to an increased maternal infectious morbidity, even in those delivered vaginally. Infectious sequelae occur in less than 3.5 percent of the patients treated conservatively, according to the findings from contemporary investigations. Maternal morbidity may be higher in those patients immediately receiving oxytocin because of the increased surgical and infectious morbidity associated with cesarean delivery. If the patient has latent genital herpes or the culture for cervical group B streptococcus is positive, induction is generally initiated as soon as is practical.

In preterm pregnancies in which pulmonary immaturity is documented, conservative management with observation is indicated. Intervention is undertaken only when signs of infection or fetal compromise are noted. Nonstress tests and the biophysical profile may be helpful in this regard. Tocolytic therapy can be considered if chorioamnionitis is not present. In practice, this is done infrequently, as spontaneous labor with PROM may be due to subclinical amnionitis. The use of maternal corticosteroids to enhance fetal lung maturation in the setting of PROM is controversial; most reports do not describe a clear benefit from this.

PROM occurring before 24 weeks' gestation may be further complicated by the theoretic increased risk of fetal compression deformities and pulmonary hypoplasia (unless fluid reaccumulates) while awaiting pulmonary maturity or spontaneous labor. A perinatal survival of only 13 to 17 percent is observed for such patients, and, of the infants involved, only between 33 and 66 percent will be developmentally normal. After having been presented with all the facts, the patient should ultimately decide between expectant management or pregnancy termination.

When hospital facilities permit and potential fetal viability has been reached (24–26 weeks), many advocate hospitalization until delivery, unless leakage stops and there is a reaccumulation of fluid. Others send the mother home after 72 hours of observation for the development of amnionitis and labor, if the fetus is vertex, or frank breech, and the cervix is less than 2 cm. In either case, external fetal and uterine monitors are usually utilized in the labor area for 4 to 24 hours to detect fetal compromise, amnionitis, or labor before sending a patient to an antepartum room. It is important to determine serial white blood cell counts and monitor vital signs in any inpatient or outpatient PROM management protocol.

If delivery is indicated, the infant is in the vertex position, and there are no signs of fetal compromise, oxytocin induction is begun. If the premature infant is in a breech or a transverse lie, cesarean delivery is indicated. Prophylactic antibiotics are frequently used in the management of preterm PROM without amnionitis, pending the results of cervical culture for group B streptococcus. At term, prophylaxis may also be considered if a long induction is anticipated. Patients with clinical amnionitis should be treated with broad-spectrum antibiotics (frequently ampicillin and gentamicin), unless delivery is imminent. In this case, therapy can be instituted after clamping the cord, so that neonatal cultures will then accurately reflect the status of neonatal bacteremia.

The effect of PROM on the incidence of respiratory distress syndrome (RDS) is unclear. Most physicians believe that 24 hours after rupture of the membranes, neonates are somewhat "protected" from the development of hyaline membrane disease. Unfortunately, the findings from several studies have not confirmed this apparent advantage, after weight and other variables are adjusted for. The documentation of fetal pulmonary maturity, or immaturity, is the most sensitive predictor of neonatal respiratory distress if delivery occurs.

General
1. Hertz, R. H., and Rosen, M. G. Clinical Management of Premature Rupture of the Membranes. In J. J. Sciarra (ed.), *Gynecology and Obstetrics,* Vol. 2. Hagerstown, MD: Harper & Row, 1985.
   A very practical approach to addressing the problems in the diagnosis and management of PROM is presented.
2. Schutte, M. F., et al. Management of premature rupture of membranes: the risk of vaginal examination to the infant. *Am. J. Obstet. Gynecol.* 146:395, 1983.
   The authors report on the outcome associated with conservative management in 6160 infants born after PROM. The risk of infection was related to gestational age and vaginal examination, but not to the duration of membrane rupture.
3. Cox, S. M., et al. The natural history of preterm ruptured membranes: what to expect of expectant management. *Obstet. Gynecol.* 71:558, 1988.
   The outcome of expectant management in the setting of PROM before 34 weeks' gestation was reviewed in an indigent population. Only 7 percent of the patients in this group were not in labor within 48 hours. The incidence of PROM in this population before 34 weeks' gestation was 1.7 percent, but accounted for 20 percent of the perinatal deaths.

Etiology
4. Lenihan, J. P., Jr. Relationship of antepartum pelvic examinations to premature rupture of the membranes. *Obstet. Gynecol.* 63:33, 1984.
   The incidence of PROM in 349 patients near term was greater if weekly pelvic examinations were performed.
5. Shubert, P. J., et al. Etiology of preterm premature rupture of membranes. *Obstet. Gynecol. Clin. North Am.* 19:251, 1992.
   An excellent summary of the multiple causes presumed to contribute to the development of PROM. These include biochemical changes, mechanical factors, infection, pH, nutrition, smoking, bleeding, an incompetent cervix, and coitus.
6. Lonky, N. M., and Hayashi, R. N. A proposed mechanism for premature rupture of membranes. *Obstet. Gynecol. Surv.* 43:22, 1988.
   A good review of the different factors currently thought to play an important role in the development of PROM. The potential impact of smoking, infection, and coitus and the balance between proteases and antiproteases are discussed.
7. McGregor, J. A. Prevention of preterm birth: new initiatives based on microbial-host interactions. *Obstet. Gynecol. Surv.* 43:1, 1988.
   An outstanding review of the role of bacteria and the resultant host reaction to infection in relation to PROM. The complex role of prostaglandins is discussed. Potential areas for the future treatment and prevention of PROM are addressed.

Diagnosis
8. Reece, E. A., et al. Amniotic fluid arborization: effect of blood, meconium, and pH alterations. *Obstet. Gynecol.* 64:248, 1984.
   The ability of the fern test to diagnose PROM in the presence of blood meconium and pH alterations was assessed. Ferning was unaffected by meconium or an alteration in the pH, but was absent when blood was mixed in equal amounts with amniotic fluid.
9. Barber, H. R. K. Diagnosis of premature rupture of the membranes (PROM). *Diagn. Gynecol. Obstet.* 4:3, 1982.
   The principal assessment techniques for the diagnosis of PROM are listed by the author in a "cookbook" style. This reference is a handy procedure manual.
10. Eriksen, N. L., et al. Fetal fibronectin: a method for detecting the presence of amniotic fluid. *Obstet. Gynecol.* 80:451, 1992.
    The presence of fetal fibronectin in the posterior fornix is a sensitive way to detect subtle ruptured membranes.
11. O'Keefe, D. F., et al. The accuracy of estimated gestational age based on ultrasound measurement of biparietal diameter in preterm premature rupture of the membranes. *Am. J. Obstet. Gynecol.* 151:309, 1985.

Estimating gestational age using the BPD after PROM occurs is probably inadequate and will likely lead to underestimation. Head circumference or long bone measurements are more accurately correlated with true gestational age.

12. Gembruch, U., and Hansmann, M. Artificial instillation of amniotic fluid as a new technique for the diagnostic evaluation of cases of oligohydramnios. *Prenat. Diagn.* 8:33, 1988.

    The use of ultrasound to direct the transabdominal instillation of electrolyte solution is presented as an approach for diagnosing the cause of severe oligohydramnios. Unsuspected PROM may be found. The ability to obtain fetal fibroblasts for chromosomal analysis is discussed, as well as the major complications of the techniques.

Treatment

13. Moller, M., et al. Rupture of fetal membranes and premature delivery associated with group B streptococci in urine of pregnant women. *Lancet* 1:69, 1984.

    Of 2745 women, there was a greater incidence of PROM and premature delivery occurred more often in those colonized with group B streptococci (based on the findings in urine specimens). In women with PROM, a urine culture for group B streptococci may be indicated.

14. Duff, P., Huff, R. W., and Gibbs, R. S. Management of premature rupture of membranes and unfavorable cervix in term pregnancy. *Obstet. Gynecol.* 63:697, 1984.

    The authors treated 134 patients at term with PROM and an unfavorable cervix either aggressively with induction after 12 hours or by observation. In the intervention group, a longer labor and higher incidence of cesarean birth and intraamniotic infection were noted.

15. Curet, L. B., et al. Association between ruptured membranes, tocolytic therapy, and respiratory distress syndrome. *Am. J. Obstet. Gynecol.* 148:263, 1984.

    The association between PROM, tocolytic therapy, and neonatal RDS was studied in 297 patients. PROM and tocolytic therapy were individually associated with a lower incidence of RDS; however, when both were present in the same patient, the incidence of RDS was actually higher.

16. Moretti, M., and Sibai, B. M. Maternal and perinatal outcome of expected management of premature rupture of membranes in the midtrimester. *Am. J. Obstet. Gynecol.* 159:390, 1988.

    The outcome in 118 patients with PROM at less than 23 weeks' gestation is reviewed. The perinatal survival rate was 13.3 percent, of which approximately two thirds of the offspring were subsequently developing normally. There was one maternal death owing to sepsis.

Complications

17. Nimrod, C., et al. The effect of very prolonged membrane rupture on fetal development. *Am. J. Obstet. Gynecol.* 148:540, 1984.

    In a retrospective study, the findings in 100 patients with PROM for more than 1 week were compared to those in 100 control patients with intact membranes. The incidence of pulmonary hypoplasia was increased when PROM occurred at less than 26 weeks' gestation, and there was a threefold increase in positional deformities.

18. Hardt, N. S., et al. Influence of chorioamnionitis on long-term prognosis in low birth weight infants. *Obstet. Gynecol.* 65:5, 1985.

    The long-term outcome in the infants of mothers who had chorioamnionitis was compared to that in those mothers who did not. The potential advantage of leaving infants in utero after PROM occurs may be offset by the disadvantages posed by chorioamnionitis with respect to future development in the surviving infants.

19. Weitzel, H. K., et al. Clinical aspects of antenatal glucocorticoid treatment for prevention of neonatal respiratory distress syndrome. *J. Perinat. Med.* 15:441, 1987.

    The indications for and contraindications to the use of glucocorticoids are discussed with reference to several key articles on the subject, including a collaborative study. The use of steroids was not believed to be indicated in the setting of

PROM, as there is no clear benefit conferred by them and they may cause the maternal infectious morbidity to double.

20. Roberts, A. B., et al. Fetal breathing movements after preterm premature rupture of membranes. *Obstet. Gynecol.* 164:821, 1991.
A significant reduction in fetal breathing was found to take place during the first 2 weeks after PROM. This finding is hypothesized to play a role in the development of pulmonary hypoplasia when PROM occurs before 24 weeks.

21. Brown, C. L., et al. Cervical dilation: accuracy of visual and digital examinations. *Obstet. Gynecol.* 81:215, 1993.
The findings yielded by visual examination to determine the status of cervical dilatation in patients with PROM correlated well with those from digital examination.

22. Carlan, S. J., et al. Preterm premature rupture of membranes: a randomized study of home versus hospital management. *Obstet. Gynecol.* 81:61, 1993.
Although very few patients with PROM met strict criteria for home management, there was no difference in the perinatal outcome in these patients compared to that observed in association with hospital management.

24. FETAL DEMISE
Garland D. Anderson

In about 1 percent of pregnancies, the mother and the obstetrician are jolted by the realization that the fetus has died in utero. Antepartum fetal demise may occur any time in the course of pregnancy. Early intrauterine death is suspected when the uterus is small for dates and fetal heart tones are not heard. After midpregnancy, loss of viability is often heralded by loss of both subjective fetal activity as well as fetal cardiac activity.

Since the advent of ultrasonography, the confirmation of intrauterine death has become less difficult. A sonogram performed early in pregnancy may show disruption of the gestational sac or an absence of fetal echoes. Later in pregnancy, there is absence of fetal cardiac activity and collapse of the fetus, if a sufficient interval has elapsed since death. A plain x-ray study may show gas in the cardiovascular system, overlapping of the skull bones, or sharp angulation of the spine. If amniocentesis is performed, the fluid obtained is brown and the creatinine phosphokinase level is markedly elevated.

Intrapartum fetal death can occur during labor, with an absence of fetal heart tones, as revealed by scalp electrode recording or ultrasound imaging, confirming the diagnosis. Caution is necessary because the maternal electrocardiogram can be transmitted through the fetus, and any heart activity that is attributed to the fetus must not be synchronous with that of the mother. If there is any question of fetal viability, the presence or absence of fetal heart activity can be determined by real-time ultrasonography.

Management of antepartum fetal death is simplified if the uterus is 14 weeks' size or less, as suction curettage is indicated at this time, although coagulation studies should be performed beforehand. When the uterus is greater than 14 weeks' size, there are several management options: observation only, prostaglandin E_2 vaginal suppositories, intravenous oxytocin, and hysterotomy.

Those who advocate expectant therapy (observation only) realize that 80 percent of the patients will go on to experience spontaneous labor and delivery within 2 to 23 weeks of intrauterine fetal demise. Unfortunately, intrauterine demise represents a great emotional burden for the mother, and this approach to management is unacceptable to most patients. Although it involves great stress, women with fetal deaths may agree to expectant therapy. The key to convincing her is the physician's ability to deal with the couple and not offer delivery immediately in response to the woman's grief. The patient who wants immediate delivery after the diagnosis of fetal demise needs some time to deal with her loss before induction of labor. A 48-hour wait before induction of labor gives the woman time to gather her family together for emotional support. Before induction is begun, what is to be expected should be fully discussed with the woman and her family. For example, they should know that when gestations are less than 24 weeks along, with induction accomplished by prostaglandin E_2 suppositories, the woman will very likely deliver in the labor room. Besides the emotional component, another drawback to observation is the potential for coagulopathy to develop. The woman at risk for this is in her sixteenth week of gestation or greater and has retained a dead fetus for 4 weeks or more. At 5 weeks after fetal demise, there is a 25 percent chance of significant hypofibrinogenemia developing; the subsequent risk increases with the duration of fetal retention.

Hypertonic saline injected intraamniotically has been an effective abortifacient. This method is contraindicated, however, in patients with renal or cardiovascular disease, and its use may increase the risk of a coagulation defect. Intravenous oxytocin has had the widest use for this purpose and is an agent familiar to all obstetricians. Unfortunately, the preterm uterus is relatively insensitive to the effects of oxytocin, even though high dosages (up to 1000 mU/min) have been used. Water intoxication resulting from the antidiuretic effect of oxytocin, uterine rupture, and cardiac arrhythmias has been reported with its use.

Vaginal suppositories containing prostaglandin E_2 (Prostin) have been approved by the Food and Drug Administration (FDA) for use in the patient with intrauterine fetal demise at less than 28 weeks' gestation, and many practitioners use them later in pregnancy. They are easy to administer, and the side effects (nausea, vomiting, diarrhea, and temperature elevation) are transient. The present dosage consists of one half of a 20-mg suppository administered initially and then a full suppository administered every 4 hours until delivery. Delivery will usually occur within 12 to 24 hours, and ripening of the cervix with *Laminaria* or prostaglandin gel (2 mg) may be helpful. Heavy sedation is usually not needed during labor.

The key to successful intervention is an individualized approach. For the patient with a gestation of 14 weeks or less, suction curettage is the treatment of choice. In the second trimester, prostaglandin E_2 vaginal suppositories are usually used. After 28 weeks' gestation, the choice is between intravenous oxytocin and prostaglandin E_2 suppositories. After 36 weeks' gestation, oxytocin induction is almost always used. Hysterotomy is reserved for the unusual patient in whom other options have failed. A special case is the patient who has had a previous cesarean delivery and whose uterus is too large for suction curettage. Use of prostaglandins, hypertonic saline, and oxytocin pose the threat of causing uterine rupture, but if the cesarean birth was performed in the lower segment, labor is usually allowed. An internal-pressure cannula may be placed to monitor uterine contractions. If these conditions cannot be met, hysterotomy is indicated.

Before any mode of therapy is initiated, coagulation studies should be performed. In the rare patient with hypofibrinogenemia, heparin may be indicated if there is no bleeding, and a 1- to 2-day course (1000 units/hr) will increase the fibrinogen concentration to acceptable levels (>200 mg/dl) before attempts to empty the uterus are made. Cryoprecipitate or fresh-frozen plasma is used for the treatment of patients with bleeding hypofibrinogenemia.

Management responsibilities do not cease when the baby has been delivered. Further goals are emotional support for the parents and a search for the cause of the intrauterine death. It is now recognized that the parents experience a grief reaction similar to that occurring with the loss of other family members; thus, there is a definite need for effective bereavement counseling. The stages of grief reaction (shock, anger, questioning, depression, and acceptance) must be resolved by the parents. During delivery, the shock stage is usually dominant. The physician will need to repeat information and explanations. The parents are encouraged to see the baby, and many like a memento of the neonate, such as a photograph or lock of hair. In addition to the grief, there is frequently an element of inappropriate guilt. One or both parents may search at length for something that they did wrong to cause the fetal death. All members of the perinatal team should learn the dynamics of the grief-guilt process, avoid intellectualization, and know the practical aspects involved, such as the proper written forms to use, the arrangements for hospital disposal versus burial, and how to go about requesting postmortem studies. If there is no obvious reason for the baby's death, the parents should be so counseled. Both parents should also be told that the grief process is a normal reaction, and they should discuss their feelings with each other. They should be seen frequently in the office after discharge to see how they are coping with the grief process. The findings from autopsy reports should be discussed at length with both parents as soon as possible after the event. Parents should be encouraged to join support groups.

It is imperative that a cause be sought. Chromosome studies, complete autopsy, total body x-ray films, and full-body photographs should be considered in the evaluation of fetal deaths, when appropriate. Many cases of intrauterine fetal demise are a result of fetal-maternal hemorrhage. This is detected by examining maternal blood for the presence of fetal erythrocytes.

Intrauterine death remains a sad reality. The obstetrician must apply both science and art to ensure safe management of the mother's condition and emotional support for the couple. In subsequent pregnancies, the woman who has suffered a previous intrauterine loss must be considered a high risk. She will need to be seen more frequently and her pregnancy monitored more aggressively.

General
1. Paul, R. H., Gauthier, R. J., and Quilligan, E. J. Clinical fetal monitoring. The usage and relationship to trends in cesarean delivery and perinatal mortality. *Acta Obstet. Gynecol. Scand.* 59:289, 1980.
   The impact of fetal monitoring on the prevention of intrapartum deaths is discussed. An extensive bibliography is available regarding all aspects of this problem.
2. Stierman, E. D. Emotional aspects of perinatal death. *Clin. Obstet. Gynecol.* 30:352, 1987.
   The emotional and psychologic responses of parents who experience fetal death are reviewed.
3. Lake, M. F., et al. Evaluation of a perinatal grief support team. *Am. J. Obstet. Gynecol.* 157:1203, 1987.
   Positive evaluations of a perinatal grief team are presented.
4. Vance, J. C., et al. Early parental responses to sudden infant death, stillbirth or neonatal death. *Med. J. Aust.* 155:292, 1991.
   The authors discuss the initial emotional response of parents to the death of an infant or to a stillbirth.
5. Lemmer, C. M. Parental perceptions of caring following perinatal bereavement. *West. J. Nurs. Res.* 13;475, 1991.
   Parents discuss their perceptions of the events that happen with the death of a fetus or infant.
6. Pauw, M. The social worker's role with a fetal demise or stillbirth. *Health Soc. Work* 16:291, 1991.
   The authors discuss the role the social worker can play in helping parents who have experienced perinatal loss.

Etiology
7. Quinn, P. A., et al. A prospective study of microbial infection in stillbirths and early neonatal death. *Am. J. Obstet. Gynecol.* 151:238, 1985.
   This study illustrates that, particularly in the case of stillbirths that occur for no related cause, infection (most commonly genital Mycoplasma infection) may be associated with the majority of cases.
8. Liban, E., and Salzberger, M. A prospective clinicopathological study of 1108 cases of antenatal fetal death. *Isr. J. Med. Sci.* 12:34, 1976.
   A good review of the etiologic factors contributing to antenatal fetal death.
9. Fay, R. A. Feto-maternal hemorrhage as a cause of fetal morbidity and mortality. *Br. J. Obstet. Gynaecol.* 90:443, 1983.
   A significant number of stillborns may be due to fetal-maternal hemorrhage.

10. Houatta, O., et al. Causes of stillbirth: a clinico-pathological study of 243 patients. *Br. J. Obstet. Gynaecol.* 90:691, 1983.
    The etiology of fetal death is examined in a large number of stillborns.
11. Freeman, R. K., et al. The significance of a previous stillbirth. *Am. J. Obstet. Gynecol.* 151:7, 1985.
    A previous stillbirth is a predictive event when associated with intrauterine growth retardation or hypertension in a current gestation.
12. Branch, D. W. Immunologic disease and fetal death. *Clin. Obstet. Gynecol.* 30: 295, 1987.
    This article presents the immunologic causes of fetal death and includes 124 references.

Diagnosis
13. Barr, M. J. Evaluation of the abortus and stillborn infant. *J. Reprod. Med.* 27:601, 1982.
    Outlines the steps that should be taken in evaluating the abortus or stillborn infant in order to counsel the parents regarding future pregnancies.
14. Woods, D. L., and Draper, R. R. A clinical assessment of stillborn infants. *S. Afr. Med. J.* 57:441, 1980.
    Emphasizes the clinical assessment of stillborn infants. The figures they provide are of assistance in predicting recurrence rates.
15. York, A. C., and Rettenmaier, M. A. An unusual complication of delayed management in the case of fetal death. *Am. J. Obstet. Gynecol.* 150:101, 1984.
    Points out that one of the dangers from delayed management of fetal demise is misdiagnosis of an abdominal pregnancy.
16. Meier, P. R., et al. Perinatal autopsy: its clinical value. *Obstet. Gynecol.* 67:349, 1986.
    The positive value of autopsy in assisting or correcting diagnoses in 139 perinatal deaths is noted.
17. Carey, J. C. Diagnostic evaluation of the stillborn infant. *Clin. Obstet. Gynecol.* 30:342, 1987.
    Describes the evacuative procedures in stillborn infants.

Treatment
18. Southern, E. M., et al. Vaginal prostaglandin E_2 in the management of fetal intrauterine death. *Br. J. Obstet. Gynaecol.* 85:437, 1978.
    Describes results in 709 cases of a missed abortion or intrauterine fetal demise actively managed with prostaglandin E_2 vaginal suppositories.
19. Romero, R., et al. Prolongation of a preterm pregnancy complicated by death of a single twin in utero and disseminated intravascular coagulation. *N. Engl. J. Med.* 310:772, 1984.
    The use of intravenous heparin to reverse disseminated intravascular cogulation allowed the authors to prolong to the time of viability a twin gestation that was complicated by fetal demise.

Complications
20. Graham, M. A., et al. Factors affecting psychological adjustment to a fetal death. *Am. J. Obstet. Gynecol.* 157:254, 1987.
    These authors found that less depression was experienced by women if they were kept informed of problems, received sympathy from medical personnel, and were allowed to see the infant.
21. Taylor, T. B., and Gideon, M. D. Crisis counseling following the death of a baby. *J. Reprod. Med.* 24:208, 1980.
    Very practical advice about effective crisis counseling. A must for those professionals desiring to provide emotional support for the bereaved parents.
22. Callan, N. A., Colmorgen, G. H. C., and Weiner, S. Lung hypoplasia and prolonged preterm ruptured membranes: a case report with implications for possible prenatal ultrasonic diagnosis. *Am. J. Obstet. Gynecol.* 151:756, 1985.

Lung hypoplasia complicating prolonged premature rupture of the membranes is documented by sonographic evidence.

23. Goldenberg, R. L., et al. Pregnancy outcome following a second-trimester loss. *Obstet. Gynecol.* 81:444, 1993.

    Pregnancy loss at 13 to 24 weeks was associated with a 39 percent risk of preterm delivery, a 5 percent risk of stillbirth, and a 6 percent risk of neonatal death in the next pregnancy.

25. SURGERY AND TRAUMA IN PREGNANCY
Rick W. Martin

The evaluation and treatment of the obstetric patient with a disease requiring surgical intervention or one who has sustained recent trauma are modified by the physiologic and anatomic factors related to pregnancy. Accidental injury occurs in approximately 7 percent of pregnant women, and at least 1 percent of parturients will undergo a surgical procedure other than cesarean delivery. This sizable group of patients presents management difficulties for the practitioner who must balance maternal and fetal concerns.

Consideration of the teratogenic effect of drugs and diagnostic procedures predominates in the treatment plans in early gestation. Drug exposure in the 2 weeks after conception results either in an intact fetus or in abortion, the so-called all-or-none principle. The period of organogenesis from week four to twelve (menstrual age) follows. It is during this time that the fetus is most susceptible to damage. For surgical patients, some commonly prescribed analgesics such as codeine should be avoided. Meperidine, morphine, and acetaminophen are acceptable. The antibiotic tetracycline may produce bone and teeth problems in the offspring as well as hepatic toxicity in the mother. Sulfonamides administered in the third trimester may interfere with the protein binding of bilirubin, and kernicterus may result in the newborn. Vaccines that contain live viruses should be avoided in early pregnancy, except when there is a great maternal risk of disease. Toxoids or killed vaccines such as tetanus toxoid, however, can be administered in pregnancy. Most anesthetic agents produce no demonstrable teratogenic effects, although the findings from retrospective studies do point to a higher rate of abortion when anesthesia is given in the first and second trimester. There is the possibility that ionizing radiation at any level may increase the risk of future malignancies in the offspring. Childhood leukemia is particularly worrisome. The teratogenic effects of diagnostic x-ray studies are not detected when the dose to the fetus is low. Currently, a dose of 5 rads (equivalent to that in an intravenous pyelogram) delivered directly to the fetus is considered safe, but abdominal shielding should be used when possible.

Pregnancy alters the nature of the laboratory evaluation in the patient requiring a surgical procedure. Many measurements will reflect the increase in plasma volume, which is 50 percent greater than that in the nonpregnant patient. A white blood cell count less than 15,000/ml is normal. The red blood cell mass is increased by 30 percent, but, secondary to the proportionately greater increase in the plasma volume, the hematocrit falls slightly during pregnancy. The alkaline phosphatase level may be elevated, owing to the placental contribution to this enzyme. The erythrocyte sedimentation rate is mildly elevated. The measurement of thyroid and adrenal hormones is altered by protein binding. The concentrations of most of the clotting factors are elevated in pregnancy. The modest enhanced coagulability increases the risk of thrombosis, especially during and after surgical procedures. The increased respiratory rate and tidal volume lower the partial pressure of carbon dioxide, and thus cause a mild compensated respiratory alkalosis. These respiratory events alter the dosage of anesthetic gases used in pregnancy.

Anatomic variations also change the way in which patients are evaluated. The enlarging uterus is responsible for many of the alterations. In the supine position, vena caval compression may cause hypotension and shortness of breath in the mother and may diminish blood flow to the fetus. The effect is most pronounced during conduction or general anesthesia, unless the gravida is placed in a left lateral tilt position. The obstruction of venous return from the lower extremities is responsible for the edema that many women experience. As the gravid uterus fills the abdomen, the likelihood of esophageal reflux is greater, with an accompanying risk of aspiration of gastric contents. The enlarged uterus also displaces the other organs from their normal position. The appendix is pushed into the right upper quadrant, and the heart is rotated and appears enlarged on a chest roentgenogram. Because the uterus lifts the parietal peritoneum away from the underlying structures, the pain of a small bowel obstruction or appendicitis may be diminished. Ureteral compression at the pelvic brim is more pronounced on the patient's right side, owing to the dextrorotation of the uterus and enlargement of the pelvic vasculature.

Surgical conditions of the maternal abdomen present a difficult challenge for the obstetrician-gynecologist, mainly because of concerns about disturbing the preterm fetus or uterus. Appendicitis is the most common nonobstetric reason for a laparotomy. The most common signs during pregnancy are a vague pain in the right side of the abdomen and anorexia. If the pain felt by the patient when examined in the supine position is reproduced in the same region of the abdomen when the patient is rolled onto her side (Alder's sign), the source of the abdominal discomfort is likely to be extrauterine and possibly caused by appendicitis. If the location of the pain shifts with movement of the uterus, the pain is most likely uterine or adnexal. When laparotomy is performed, a midline incision is recommended during the first trimester. Later in gestation, the incision is usually made over the point of maximal tenderness.

Gallbladder disease is the second-most common surgical condition of pregnancy. Cholecystitis is associated with cholelithiasis in 90 percent of the cases. The hormonal changes that take place in pregnancy are responsible for a decreased contractility of the gallbladder, an elevated biliary cholesterol level, and an increasing gallbladder capacity, which combined predispose to stone formation. Pain, with inspiratory arrest, may be evoked while palpating over the gallbladder (Murphy's sign). Medical therapy consisting of intravenous fluids and nasogastric suction is usually successful, with a positive response within 24 to 48 hours. Surgical intervention is most often implemented in patients when medical management fails, the gallbladder becomes perforated, jaundice arises because of a common duct stone, significant obstruction occurs, or the associated complication of pancreatitis intervenes.

Small-bowel obstruction is encountered usually (1) during months four and five, when the uterus becomes an abdominal organ; (2) during months eight and nine, when the fetal head descends into the pelvis; or (3) during delivery and the puerperium, when there is a sudden change in uterine size that alters the relationship of adhesions and the surrounding bowel. The treatment is surgical. A high index of suspicion is required on the part of the physician to avoid delay and increased mortality.

The presence of a persistent adnexal mass is a cause for concern, owing to the associated risks of an underlying malignancy in approximately 6 percent of such patients. Other risks include the possibility of rupture, torsion, or hemorrhage resulting from such a mass. In the asymptomatic patient, surgical intervention may be postponed until the second trimester, because the chance for adverse effects on pregnancy is less at that time.

Trauma in pregnancy is most commonly incurred in a motor vehicle accident. In fact, automobile collisions are the leading nonobstetric cause of maternal death in the United States. Pregnant women should be encouraged to wear seat belts. The shoulder harness provides the best protection, not only by preventing the mother from being thrown from the automobile but also by distributing the forces of impact over a larger area. When seat belts are not used, the most common cause of maternal death is head trauma associated with expulsion from the automobile. Fetal death is most commonly due to death of the mother. Second in incidence is abruptio placentae. Although delayed abruption has occurred sometimes days after the event, most authors recommend fetal monitoring for 4 hours initially after moderate to severe trauma. Though a positive Kleihauer-Betke test result may indicate maternal-fetal hemorrhage in cases of abruption, clinical correlation is required. A useful adjunct in the evaluation of such patients is paracentesis. Positive findings include the aspiration of grossly bloody fluid, a red blood cell count greater than 100,000/μl, a white blood cell count greater than 500/μl, or an amylase level greater than 175 IU/dl.

The pregnant trauma patient may also be the victim of a stabbing incident or gunshot wound. Especially later in gestation, the enlarged uterus protects other abdominal organs. Although cushioned in amniotic fluid, the fetus can be injured. A projectile may be localized by fetogram or ultrasound. In cases of peritoneal penetration, an exploratory laparotomy is indicated. That portion of the small bowel that is compressed superiorly by the gravid uterus is most likely injured when the projectile enters the upper abdomen.

Thermal injury and electrical shock may adversely affect the pregnancy. Fetal loss is greatest in the setting of first-trimester maternal burns, but later fetal loss depends on the gestational age and the extent of the maternal injury. Even when there does not appear to be an injury from electrical shock, intrauterine growth retardation has been observed in exposed fetuses. Careful follow-up using serial sonography is necessary.

As many as 10 percent of pregnant women may be the victims of physical abuse. It is essential that the practitioner consider this possibility whenever a trauma patient is evaluated. In one series, these women were more likely than control subjects to be divorced or separated, to be of lower socioeconomic status, and to have emotional problems. Many of these women present with chronic psychosomatic complaints. Pregnancy may lead to increased stress and an increase in violent behavior in these families.

In most situations, the well-being of the fetus will parallel that of the patient. Assessment of the fetus when the mother has been traumatized or is to undergo operation is important. Maintenance of the left lateral decubitus position and avoidance of hypotension in the mother are essential to ensuring fetal health. The fetus should be monitored electronically from the outset of the maternal evaluation. Newer technology has enabled the surgeon to monitor the status of the fetus during the surgical procedure, if this is germane to an individual case. Cesarean delivery is not always necessary when exploring the abdomen, and correction of hypovolemia may alleviate an abnormal fetal heart rate. After operation, use of tocolytic drugs should be considered, but they should not be prescribed routinely. Pregnancies complicated by peritonitis or abdominal procedures performed in the third trimester are at greatest risk for preterm labor. Magnesium sulfate, with its fewer cardiovascular effects than the beta-mimetic drugs, is preferred for tocolysis. Adjunctive progesterone therapy is considered when the corpus luteum is removed in early pregnancy.

General
1. Duncan, P. G., et al. Fetal risk of anesthesia and surgery during pregnancy. *Anesthesiology* 64:790, 1986.
   There was no increase in the cases of congenital anomalies in the offspring of women undergoing general anesthesia in the first two trimesters. More spontaneous abortions occurred in the treatment group (relative risk, 1.58).
2. Liu, P. L., et al. Foetal monitoring in parturients undergoing surgery unrelated to pregnancy. *Can. Anaesth. Soc. J.* 32:525, 1985.
   Intraoperative monitoring was feasible in many procedures. Loss of beat-to-beat variability was noted under general anesthesia.
3. Petrikovsky, B. M., and Vintzileos, A. M. Fetal heart rate monitoring during obstetrical operations: a review. *Obstet. Gynecol. Surv.* 43:721, 1988.
   These authors offer a review of the worldwide literature concerning fetal heart rate monitoring during and after obstetric operations. It outlines a clinical management protocol that might be of use to the reader.

Surgical Disorders in Pregnancy
4. Dixon, N. P., Faddis, D. M., and Siberman, H. Aggressive management of cholecystitis during pregnancy. *Am. J. Surg.* 154:292, 1987.

Cholecystitis recurred during pregnancy in 58 percent of the patients. A favorable outcome was achieved when surgery was performed in the second trimester compared to the outcome in patients managed without surgery.

5. Hess, L. W., et al. Adnexal mass occurring with intrauterine pregnancy: report of fifty-four patients requiring laparotomy for definitive management. *Am. J. Obstet. Gynecol.* 158:1029, 1988.
   A malignant tumor was found in 5.9 percent of the cases. Preterm delivery and abortion occurred more frequently in association with emergency surgical intervention than with planned elective celiotomy.

6. Sorensen, V. J., et al. Management of general surgical emergencies in pregnancy. *Am. Surgeon* 56:245, 1990.
   The decision to operate was usually determined by clinical circumstances rather than the results of diagnostic tests.

7. Hansen, G., Toot, P. J., and Lynch, C. O. Subtle ultrasound signs of appendicitis in a pregnant patient. *J. Reprod. Med.* 38:223, 1993.
   A noncompressible appendix with a diameter greater than 6 mm indicates appendicitis in the appropriate clinical setting.

Trauma in Pregnancy

8. Buchsbaum, H. J. Diagnosis and management of abdominal gunshot wounds during pregnancy. *J. Trauma* 15:425, 1975.
   Rarely is the pregnant uterus spared with a gunshot wound to the abdomen late in gestation. Fetal mortality is high in the setting of such injuries.

9. Crosby, W. M. Trauma during pregnancy: maternal and fetal injury. *Obstet. Gynecol. Surv.* 29:683, 1974.
   An excellent review of several aspects of trauma in pregnancy. The author prefers culdocentesis to paracentesis in the evaluation of the pregnant patient.

10. Crosby, W. M. Automotive trauma and the pregnant patient. *Contemp. Ob/Gyn* 8:115, 1976.
    The findings from animal studies reveal the various forces involved in maternal and fetal injury incurred in automobile collisions.

11. Deitch, E. A, et al. Management of burns in pregnant women. *Surg. Gynecol. Obstet.* 161:1, 1985.
    Burns in the first trimester were associated with a high rate of fetal loss. Before 28 weeks, fetal survival was related to maternal survival, but less so after 32 weeks.

12. Higgins, S. D., and Garite, T. J. Late abruptio placenta in trauma patients: implications for fetal monitoring. *Obstet. Gynecol.* 63:10S, 1984.
    Placental abruption occurred 5 days after severe trauma in some patients. Guidelines for monitoring such parturients are given.

13. O'Brien, J. A., et al. Prepartum diagnosis of traumatic fetal-maternal hemorrhage. *Am. J. Perinatol.* 2:214, 1985.
    A test for maternal-fetal hemorrhage is recommended in cases of maternal trauma.

14. Rothenberger, D. A., et al. Diagnostic peritoneal lavage for blunt trauma in pregnant women. *Am. J. Obstet. Gynecol.* 129:479, 1977.
    The technique and criteria for the assessment of peritoneal lavage are discussed.

15. Sakala, E. P., and Kort, D. D. Management of stab wounds of the pregnant uterus: a case report and review of the literature. *Obstet. Gynecol. Surv.* 43:319, 1988.
    Only 19 cases of stab wounds to the pregnant uterus have been reported. The management of such injuries is discussed.

16. Schoenfeld, A., et al. Vehicular trauma in pregnancy: an algorithm for diagnosis and fetal therapy. *Fetal Ther.* 2:51, 1987.
    A useful clinical approach is given for the management of the pregnant trauma patient.

17. Smith, R. J. Avulsion of the nongravid uterus due to pelvic fracture. *South. Med. J.* 82:70, 1989.

The author describes fracture of the pelvis with avulsion of the uterus. Although the patients were not pregnant, a plan was detailed that would also apply during pregnancy.

18. Sandy, E. A., II, and Koerner, M. Self-inflicted gunshot wounds to the pregnant abdomen: report of a case and review of the literature. *Am. J. Perinatol.* 6:30, 1989.
   The maternal mortality from gunshot wounds was low, but fetal wastage was high, ranging from 41 to 71 percent.
19. Pearlman, M. D., and Tintinalli, J. E. Evaluation and treatment of the gravida and fetus following trauma during pregnancy. *Obstet. Gynecol. Clin. North Am.* 18(2):371, 1991.
   An updated overview of the management of trauma in pregnancy is provided.
20. Pearlman, M. D., Tintinalli, J. E., and Lorenz, R. P. A prospective controlled study of outcome after trauma during pregnancy. *Am. J. Obstet. Gynecol.* 162: 1502, 1990.
   Fetal-maternal hemorrhage occurred in 30.6 percent of the pregnancies complicated by trauma, and was more common in the anterior placenta. Electronic fetal monitoring is recommended for 4 hours as a screening tool for adverse perinatal outcome.
21. McFarlane, J., et al. Assessing for abuse during pregnancy. Severity and frequency of injuries and associated entry into prenatal care. *J.A.M.A.* 267(23): 3176, 1992.
   Physical abuse occurred in 17 percent of the pregnancies, and 60 percent of these women reported more than a single episode.
22. Fildes, J., et al. Trauma: the leading cause of maternal death. *J. Trauma* 32(5): 643, 1992.
   Trauma was the leading cause of maternal death observed in this 3-year series from the Cook County medical examiner's office.

26. HYPEREMESIS GRAVIDARUM
Sister Clarice Carroll

Hyperemesis gravidarum is defined as severe vomiting occurring before the twentieth week of gestation. It is a condition that usually necessitates hospitalization and is complicated by weight loss, dehydration, ketonuria, and sometimes by serious psychologic disturbances. It is a complication that can lead to severe maternal nutritional deprivation, and can threaten fetal well-being.

Morning sickness must be distinguished from hyperemesis. Nausea and vomiting are the most common symptoms of early pregnancy, second only to amenorrhea. They can appear within 2 weeks after a missed period and usually diminish by the fourteenth week of gestation in up to 50 percent of pregnant women. These symptoms were described by the Egyptians as early as 2000 B.C. Although a certain degree of nausea and vomiting is to be expected, they are usually the first symptoms of pregnancy and are self-limiting, abating by 12 to 14 weeks' gestation. If the symptoms persist and become more severe, however, fluid and electrolyte imbalance can result. If left untreated, the results can be fatal. If nausea and vomiting are present (particularly if they begin after the twelfth week of pregnancy), a medical or surgical condition may be responsible.

Hyperemesis gravidarum occurs in up to 2 percent of pregnancies, although the diagnosis is not well defined because the diagnostic criteria used differ from one geographic area to another. However, if the vomiting is severe enough to require hospitalization, the diagnosis is usually applied.

Although the cause of hyperemesis remains unclear, the etiologic factors include (1) vitamin B_6 deficiency, owing to a change in protein metabolism; (2) impaired function of the adrenal cortex; (3) hyperthyroidism and excess human chorionic gonadotropin secretion; (4) psychopathologic and emotional factors; (5) alterations in gastrointestinal physiology; (6) a hypersensitivity reaction; and (7) poor nutrition.

The primary clinical manifestation of hyperemesis is frequent and sustained vomiting (usually from 4 to 8 weeks in duration), resulting in significant weight loss and dehydration. Other signs of starvation that gradually develop include metabolic acidosis, ketonuria, hypokalemic alkalosis, oliguria, hemoconcentration, and constipation. In diagnosing and treating hyperemesis, other disorders must be ruled out. Hydatidiform mole, gastroenteritis, multiple gestation, hepatitis, cholecystitis, peptic ulcer, hyperthyroidism, hiatal hernia, gastric carcinoma, and intestinal obstruction may all be mimicked by hyperemesis. Severe forms of hyperemesis involving weight loss of greater than 5 percent of the prepregnancy weight have been associated with poor fetal growth and outcome. Continued vomiting and dehydration can also lead to the formation of brainstem lesions resembling those characteristic of Wernicke's encephalopathy.

The prognosis in these patients is excellent, provided proper treatment is given. The principal underlying treatment of hyperemesis gravidarum is to prevent dehydration and starvation, in addition to handling any psychologic component that may be present. Treatment includes hospitalization in a quiet room (isolation may be required for some patients) and a complete physical examination, including documentation of a verbal history that may be helpful in revealing any emotional problems. Physical and laboratory determinations, such as temperature, pulse, respiration, blood pressure, weight on admission and daily weight, urinalysis, and strict fluid assessment (intake and output), are usually performed. Laboratory evaluation of the electrolyte status, including the potassium, sodium, blood urea nitrogen, glucose, and serum creatinine levels, should be obtained.

In some cases, parenteral nutrition is required to maintain or restore an anabolic state. Parenteral nutrition has improved from its previous regimen of dextrose and sodium chloride to one consisting of either short- or long-term nutritional maintenance, and including the recommended dietary allowances of carbohydrates, amino acids, electrolytes, preparations of fat emulsions, vitamins, and trace elements. The number of calories per day must be determined so that a balance of carbohydrates, fat, and proteins can be administered.

In most cases, gastric rest, gained by not allowing oral intake, is helpful. A nutritional assessment of each patient suffering from hyperemesis must be carried out, as all pregnant women do not have the same nutritional requirements. Simple baseline parameters should include height and weight.

Antiemetics or mild sedatives such as intramuscularly administered promethazine (Phenergan, 25–50 mg) or orally administered phenobarbital (16–32 mg), 1 hour before meals and at bedtime, may also be used. However, because some drugs may have teratogenic effects if given in the first 12 weeks of pregnancy, scrutiny of all medications is wise. Vitamin B complex, vitamin C, and vitamin B_6 (100 mg), added to intravenous solutions, may be useful. Psychiatric consultation is sometimes necessary, and isolation from family and relatives is helpful in some cases.

Some physicians suggest that, when the patient begins to respond to intravenous therapy (as indicated by cessation of vomiting, return of the electrolyte balance to normal, and an increase in urinary output), small sips of water, 1 ounce (30 ml) hourly, can be initiated. As soon as the patient can tolerate food, she should be given small, frequent meals consisting of fairly dry and easily digested high-energy foods in the form of carbohydrates and liquids, such as fruit drinks, tea, and milk. Intravenous therapy should be discontinued as soon as possible, and the diet should progress from liquids to semisolids (e.g., boiled eggs, cooked cereals, toast, and dry crackers) before solids are introduced. Similarly, vitamin, antiemetic, and sedative therapy can be tapered or discontinued.

Moderate activity should gradually be initiated and the patient's weight recorded biweekly. The weight chart, more than any other guide, will document the progress of the patient. In severe cases, the use of total parenteral nutrition is necessary to ensure maternal weight gain. Because the psychologic component can be significant, the patient should be given an opportunity to discuss any problems and should possibly be referred for psychiatric consultation. The patient may be safely discharged from the hospital after the nausea and vomiting have ceased and she begins to gain weight. Continued intensive outpatient follow-up is necessary.

There is little evidence that the patient with hyperemesis gravidarum will deliver a small-for-gestation-age or intrauterine-growth-retarded baby, except in the event of severe hyperemesis. Similarly, there appears to be no increased risk of congenital malformations associated with the condition. Ketonuria, however, should be prevented, because fetal abnormalities are increased if this persists. Maternal complications resulting from persistent vomiting include hemorrhagic retinitis, rupture of the esophagus, aspiration pneumonitis, electrolyte depletion, acid-base disturbance, and dental erosion. Complications of antiemetic therapy include jaundice, irregular jerky movements, and opisthotonos, owing to the administration of phenothiazines. The association of transient hyperthyroidism with hyperemesis gravidarum has been investigated. In this situation, a short course of antithyroid therapy readily reverses the cause of the disease, while resolving the hyperemesis as well.

General
1. Cunningham, F. G., et al. Gastrointestinal Disorders. In *Williams Obstetrics* (19th ed.). Norwalk, CT: Appleton-Century-Crofts, 1993.
   A review of the diagnosis and treatment of nausea and vomiting in pregnancy.
2. Kayuppila, A., Huhtaniemi, I., and Ylikorkala, O. Raised serum human chorionic gonadotrophin concentrations in hyperemesis gravidarum. *Br. Med. J.* 1:1670, 1979.
   An extensive review with 26 references that examines the psychologic, social, and biologic aspects of hyperemesis gravidarum. The effect of body type and psychologic "gain" is emphasized.
3. Kallen, B. Hyperemesis during pregnancy and delivery outcome: a registry study. *Eur. J. Obstet. Gynecol. Reprod. Biol.* 26:291, 1987.
   A study of 3068 pregnancies with the diagnosis of hyperemesis recorded in a Swedish Birth Registry for the years 1973 to 1981.

Etiology
4. DePue, R. H., et al. Hyperemesis gravidarum in relation to estradiol levels, pregnancy outcome, and other maternal factors: a seroepidemiologic study. *Am. J. Obstet. Gynecol.* 156:1137, 1987.
   The findings from an epidemiologic study and a serum hormone study support the hypothesis that elevated estrogen levels early in pregnancy are the major cause of hyperemesis gravidarum.
5. Burrows, G. N., and Ferris, T. F. Nausea and Vomiting of Pregnancy and Hyperemesis Gravidarum. In G. N. Burrows and T. F. Ferris (eds.), *Medical Complications During Pregnancy*. Philadelphia: Saunders, 1988.
   A comprehensive review of the topics of nausea, vomiting, and hyperemesis gravidarum.
6. Mori, M., et al. Morning sickness and thyroid function in normal pregnancy. *Obstet. Gynecol.* 72:355, 1988.
   The authors measured thyroid levels in 132 normal women in early pregnancy and in 20 nonpregnant women. They could not find any correlation between either these levels or the human chorionic gonadotropin titers and the occurrence of hyperemesis.

Diagnosis
7. Samsioe, A. J., Samsioe, G., and Velinder, G. M. Nausea and vomiting in pregnancy—a contribution to its epidemiology. *Obstet. Gynecol. Surv.* 39:424, 1984.
   A study of 244 women with hyperemesis showed that 50 percent of the women experienced nausea and vomiting only in the morning and 36 percent felt sick all day.
8. Juras, N., Banovac, K., and Sekso, M. Increased serum reverse triiodothyronine in patients with hyperemesis gravidarum. *Acta Endocrinol.* 102:284, 1983.
   A study of 33 patients with hyperemesis gravidarum revealed elevated T_3 levels.
9. Levine, M. G., and Esser, D. Total parenteral nutrition for the treatment of se-

vere hyperemesis gravidarum: maternal nutritional effects and fetal outcome. *Obstet. Gynecol.* 72:102, 1988.

This article outlines a clinical management plan that relies principally on psychosocial support and nutritional counseling for the mother.

Treatment

10. Adno, J. Treatment of hyperemesis gravidarum. *S. Afr. Med. J.* 69:110, 1986.
    A local ethnic food that is difficult to regurgitate was used experimentally to treat hyperemesis gravidarum.
11. Rafla, N. Limb deformities associated with prochlorperazine. *Am. J. Obstet. Gynecol.* 156:1557, 1987.
    This author reports on two cases of congenital abnormalities that may have resulted from using an antiemetic only.
12. Long, M. A. D., Simone, S. S., and Tucher, J. J. Outpatient treatment of hyperemesis gravidarum with stimulus control and imagery procedures. *J. Behav. Ther. Exp. Psychiatry* 17:105, 1986.
    A study in which stimulus control and imagery procedures were used to treat patients with hyperemesis.
13. Boyce, R. A. Enteral nutritional in hyperemesis gravidarum: a new development. *J. Am. Diet. Assoc.* 6:733, 1992.
    Enteral nutrition in the treatment of hyperemesis gravidarum is an effective and safe technique.
14. Rayburn, W., et al. Parenteral nutrition in obstetrics and gynecology. *Obstet. Gynecol Surv.* 41:200, 1986.
    A review of the results of parenteral nutrition in the treatment of hyperemesis gravidarum, as observed at the University of Michigan Medical Center.
15. Stellato, T. A., Danziger, L. H., and Burkons, D. Fetal salvage with maternal total parenteral nutrition: the pregnant mother as her own control. *J. Parenter. Enter. Nutr.* 12:412, 1988.
    The authors found that fetal outcome was normal in mothers with severe hyperemesis when total parenteral nutrition was used. Care must be taken in working with such a severely nutritionally depleted patient because total parenteral nutrition also has risks.
16. Walters, W. A. W. The management of nausea and vomiting during pregnancy. *Med. J. Aust.* 147:290, 1987.
    The author provides details on a series of patients with hyperemesis gravidarum who were treated using his clinical approach, consisting of both supportive and therapeutic measures.

Complications

17. Chirino, O., et al. Barogenic rupture of the esophagus associated with hyperemesis gravidarum. *Obstet. Gynecol.* 52:515, 1978.
    Case report of a primigravida suffering from hyperemesis gravidarum.
18. Chatwani, A., and Schartz, R. A severe case of hyperemesis gravidarum. *Am. J. Obstet. Gynecol.* 143:964, 1982.
    Case report of a patient with severe hyperemesis leading to compromised renal and liver function.
19. Park, R. H. Thyroid disease in pregnancy. *Br. Med. J.* 294:647, 1987.
    Hyperthyroidism may develop in patients with hyperemesis gravidarum, but the thyroid disease can persist after the pregnancy.
20. Lao, R. R., Chin, R. K. J., and Chang, A. M. Z. The outcome of hyperemetic pregnancies complicated by transient hyperthyroidism. *Aust. N.Z. J. Obstet. Gynaecol.* 27:99, 1987.
    A study of 39 patients with hyperemesis gravidarum, in 17 of whom transient hyperthyroidism developed. There was no adverse effect on pregnancy outcome.
21. Lao, T. T. H., et al. Transient hyperthyroidism in hyperemesis gravidarum. *J. R. Soc. Med.* 79:613, 1986.
    Case report of a patient with hyperemesis gravidarum and hyperthyroidism who was treated with a short course of antithyroid drugs.

22. Bober, S. A., McGill, A. C., and Tunbridge, W. M. G. Thyroid function in hyperemesis gravidarum. *Acta Endocrinol.* 111:404, 1986.
    A study of 25 patients with hyperemesis gravidarum who exhibited transient hyperthyroidism.
23. Chin, R. K., et al. A longitudinal study of changes in erythrocyte zinc concentration in hyperemesis gravidarum. *Gynecol. Obstet. Invest.* 29:22, 1990.
    Hyperthyroxinemia in patients with hyperemesis gravidarum represents true hyperthyroidism, but is different from classic thyrotoxicosis, in that the elevation in the thyroid hormone levels is transient.

27. INTRAUTERINE GROWTH RETARDATION
Richard O. Davis

Intrauterine growth retardation (IUGR) is a term applied to those infants whose birth weights are much lower than would be expected for their gestational age. These infants may be born prematurely, at term, or post term. Various adjectives have been used to describe these infants: *small for gestational age* (SGA), *malnourished,* and *dysmature.* The baby with IUGR is generally identified by a birth weight that is at or below the tenth percentile for that expected at a given gestational age. Using this criterion, 1 in 10 babies will be so designated. Although there is a marked variability in the "normal" birth weight at any specific gestational age, this definition specifically identifies a group of infants at risk for perinatal morbidity and mortality. In addition, the incidence of neurologic impairment during infancy and childhood appears to be increased in some of these infants. The IUGR infant is also more likely to suffer from congenital anomalies, central nervous system depression, in utero hypoxia, meconium aspiration, cold stress, hypoglycemia, hypocalcemia, hyperviscosity syndrome, respiratory distress, and pulmonary hemorrhage.

If an infant is identified as SGA, various causes may be responsible. Approximately 10 percent of these infants will have chromosomal infections (e.g., rubella, cytomegalovirus, toxoplasmosis, or syphilis). Maternal conditions such as essential hypertension, chronic renal disease, cyanotic heart disease, and the hemoglobinopathies also place the fetus at risk for IUGR. In addition, the maternal nutritional status, socioeconomic level, smoking habits, and use of alcohol and other drugs may adversely affect fetal growth. Studies show that, besides smoking, maternal characteristics that best correlate with IUGR are low prepregnancy weight and weight gain during pregnancy. Placental abnormalities associated with IUGR include nonspecific villositis, chronic abruption, multiple gestation, and placental tumors. Despite these numerous recognized etiologic factors, the cause of IUGR in approximately 50 percent of such babies cannot be clearly identified.

Because the intrauterine fetal weight cannot be easily or accurately measured, and because the gestational age is often not precisely known, the prenatal diagnosis of IUGR presents a formidable obstetric challenge. Some pregnancies at risk for IUGR can be suspected based on the nature of the maternal history and complications. For example, the previous birth of a growth-retarded baby is a strong predictor of risk in subsequent pregnancies. Clinical information, such as maternal weight gain and the serially measured uterine fundal heights, represents a good screening device. Doppler measurements of umbilical and uterine artery waveforms may prove useful in identifying pregnancies at risk for IUGR. If the gestational age can be accurately determined, if normal intrauterine fetal growth patterns are known, and if methods are available to assess fetal growth, normal or altered (increased or decreased) growth can be estimated. However, because the genetic growth potential of any given fetus is unknown, and the range of normal fetal weights vary for a given gestational age, the accurate identification of the fetus with IUGR remains elusive.

There are several factors that are useful in the diagnosis and management of IUGR. For example, an accurate determination of gestational age is of critical importance. Correlation of normal and clearly recalled menstrual data with the findings from a pelvic examination typically found before 12 weeks' gestation and with heart tones, heard by a standard fetoscope by 20 weeks, provides an accurate estimation of gestational age (± 7 days). Ultrasound can be used to enhance and complement the information obtained by these clinical tools. The most accurate method of determining gestational age is to measure the fetal crown-rump lengths between 8 and 12 weeks' gestation (± 5 days). The most commonly used ultrasonic technique for gestational age determination, however, is the measurement of either the biparietal diameter (BPD) or the femur length between 16 and 24 weeks' gestation (± 10 days). In addition to BPD and femur length, the head circumference, abdominal circumference, and other biometric data provide good estimates of gestational age, if performed before the third trimester when there is more variation (± 21 days).

The rate of fetal BPD growth varies as gestation progresses. Normally, the BPD increases by 2 mm per week between 30 and 36 weeks' gestation and by approximately 1.3 mm per week thereafter. The findings from several studies have established that serial BPD measurements can identify whether infants are large, appropriate, or small for gestational age. Because the error in each ultrasonic BPD measurement is approximately 2 mm, serial scans should be spaced at 3-week intervals. Serial values can be compared to "normal" growth curves, and decreasing or arrested BPD growth thereby ascertained. The accuracy of serial scans in identifying the infant who at birth will have manifestations and complications of IUGR varies from 50 to 70 percent. However, most cases of IUGR represent asymmetric growth retardation, and the measurement of the BPD alone may miss those fetuses with such head-sparing effects. Efforts to enhance the ability of ultrasound to diagnose IUGR include measurement of the abdominal circumference, and calculations of the head–abdominal circumference ratio, the femur length–abdominal circumference ratio, and a fetal ponderal index. In addition, oligohydramnios and advanced placental maturation are associated with IUGR. Oligohydramnios, when present, also predisposes to umbilical cord compression, and both may herald fetal deterioration.

Once decreased fetal growth has been diagnosed, obstetric management should be directed at modifying any associated factors that can be changed. For example, nutrition can be improved, cigarette smoking stopped, and alcohol consumption abandoned. Bed rest in the left lateral position augments uterine blood flow and, it is hoped, will thereby improve nutrition of the fetus. Because these fetuses are at risk for suffering uteroplacental respiratory insufficiency, serial nonstress testing or contraction stress testing should be performed to identify its existence. Serial ultrasound examinations to detect oligohydramnios are indicated. A biophysical profile may also be helpful. Serial measurements of the biochemical indicators of placental function, such as the urinary (plasma) estriol or human placental lactogen levels, have been used in the past but are mostly of historic interest.

There are no data to support early delivery of infants with IUGR in the absence of documented fetal uteroplacental insufficiency, as assessed by the aforementioned tests. During either spontaneous or induced labor, a patient with an IUGR fetus should be monitored electronically and observed carefully for evidence of fetal stress. This may take the form of recurrent severe variable or late decelerations with poor short-term variability. The fetoplacental unit with IUGR may not have normal reserve, and in the presence of recurrent hypoxic decelerations unresponsive to treatment (lateral positioning, oxygen, and correction of hypotension or hypovolemia), delivery should be effected safely and expeditiously, most often by cesarean birth. If the amniotic fluid is meconium stained, neonatal meconium aspiration can be minimized by suctioning the oropharynx before delivery of the shoulders and, when indicated, performing endotracheal intubation to clear the trachea after delivery of the fetal body. Cold stress must be avoided, the blood glucose level measured, and the hyperviscosity syndrome and respiratory distress treated if they occur. In addition, these neonates must be evaluated carefully for the presence of congenital anomalies and in utero infections. Therefore, these pregnancies are optimally delivered in a facility that can provide for intensive monitoring during labor and delivery, as well as subsequent care and evaluation in the neonatal period.

The data concerning the subsequent growth and development of these infants should be viewed in light of the heterogeneity of this group of infants as a whole. If infants with chromosomal abnormalities, congenital anomalies, and infections are excluded, the prognosis is generally good for subsequent normal physical development and neurologic outcome. Prevention and treatment of hypoxia during labor and the appropriate management of neonatal problems can decrease the risk of morbidity and mortality in this group of high-risk pregnancies.

General

1. Brenner, W. E., Edelman, D. A., and Hendricks, C. H. A standard of fetal growth for the United States of America. *Am. J. Obstet. Gynecol.* 126:155, 1976.
   The 10th, 25th, 50th, and 75th percentiles of fetal weight were calculated from 8 to 20 menstrual weeks. The derived growth curves are often used for both clinical and investigational purposes.
2. Seeds, J. W. Impaired fetal growth: definition and clinical diagnosis. *Obstet. Gynecol.* 64:303, 1984.
   This landmark article reviews the significance and, clinical definition of impaired fetal growth, and the tests used to diagnose it.
3. Spinnato, J. A., et al. Inaccuracy of Dubowitz gestational age in low birth weight infants. *Obstet. Gynecol.* 63:491, 1984.
   The findings from this study show that, for all infants deemed SGA or IUGR, this may simply result from an error in the neonatal gestational age score (Dubowitz) assigned by the pediatrician. This observation has important clinical implications.
4. Brar, H. S., and Rutherford, S. E. Classification of intrauterine growth retardation. *Semin. Perinatol.* 12:2, 1988.
   This excellent review offers not only a classification for growth retardation but also an anthology on the topic of normal growth. It also contains 125 references.

Etiology

5. Wen, S. W., et al. Intrauterine growth retardation and preterm delivery: prenatal risk factors in an indigent population. *Am. J. Obstet. Gynecol.* 162:213, 1990.
   Prenatally assessed risk factors for low birth weight were investigated in 17,000 indigent women. Smoking, short stature, low weight, and low weight gain showed the greatest correlation to IUGR.
6. Carlson, E. E. Maternal diseases associated with intrauterine growth retardation. *Semin. Perinatol.* 12:17, 1988.
   The various maternal complications categorized by system, and their effect on fetal growth, are detailed in this excellent article. Sixty updated references are listed.
7. Lee, K.-S., et al. Maternal age and incidence of low birth weight at term: a population study. *Am. J. Obstet. Gynecol.* 158:84, 1988.
   Sociodemographic factors and advancing maternal age are associated with a decreased potential for fetal growth and an increased risk of maternal complications that might lead to IUGR.
8. Li, C. Q., et al. The impact on infant birth weight and gestational age of cotinine-validated smoking reduction during pregnancy. *J.A.M.A.* 269:1519, 1993.
   Cotinine-validated smoking reduction rates were positively associated with increased infant birth weight. Women who stopped smoking showed the most improvement in birth weight, but decreasing smoking was also associated with significantly increased birth weight.
9. Econommides, D. L., and Nicolaides, K. Blood glucose and oxygen tension levels in small-for-gestational age fetuses. *Am. J. Obstet. Gynecol.* 160:385, 1989.
   These authors found no significant influence from the maternal-fetal glucose gradient and hypoxia between umbilical venous and arterial samples obtained from SGA babies, indicating that a major cause of hypoglycemia in these neonates is reduced supply rather than increased consumption.

Diagnosis

10. Rosendahl, H., and Rivinen, S. Routine ultrasound screening for early detection of small for gestational age fetuses. *Obstet. Gynecol.* 71:518, 1988.

Real-time ultrasound screening examinations were performed in 3208 unselected singleton pregnancies at 17 and 34 weeks to detect fetuses with IUGR; 4.9 percent were SGA.

11. Vintzileos, A. M., et al. Value of fetal ponderal index in predicting growth retardation. *Obstet. Gynecol.* 67:584, 1984.

    There was relatively poor correlation between fetal and neonatal ponderal indices noted in this study. Although the ponderal index may be useful in ruling out IUGR, it was not very useful in making the diagnosis of IUGR because of the high false-positive rate.

12. Wafsof, S. L., et al. Routine ultrasound screening for antenatal detection of intrauterine growth retardation. *Obstet. Gynecol.* 67:33, 1986.

    An evaluation of 3616 women with early ultrasound confirmation of gestational age was performed. Abdominal circumference proved to be the most sensitive for detecting IUGR; however, the true-positive rate was 44 percent and the true-negative rate was 92 percent.

13. Divon, M. Y., et al. Intrauterine growth retardation—a prospective study of the diagnostic value of real-time sonography combined with umbilical artery flow velocimetry. *Obstet. Gynecol.* 72:611, 1988.

    The best predictor of IUGR was an estimated fetal weight that was less than the tenth percentile for gestational age.

14. Berkowitz, G. D., et al. Sonographic estimation of fetal weight and Doppler analysis of umbilical artery velocimetry in the prediction of intrauterine growth retardation: a prospective study. *Am. J. Obstet. Gynecol.* 158:1149, 1988.

    This is a report on 168 patients at risk for IUGR who were evaluated by Doppler velocimetry studies, and the findings compared with the sonographic prediction of intrauterine growth retardation. The sensitivity of the systolic-diastolic ratio of the umbilical artery was lower than that of the sonographic estimation (55% versus 75%); however, the umbilical artery studies exhibited a higher specificity (92% versus 80%).

15. Pardi, G., et al. Diagnostic value of blood sampling in fetuses with growth retardation. *N. Engl. J. Med.* 328:692, 1993.

    No fetuses with normal heart rates and normal umbilical artery velocimetric readings had hypoxia or acidosis. In those with abnormal fetal heart rate and velocimetry, 64 percent had lactic acidosis, low blood oxygen levels, or low pH values, as determined by fetal umbilical cord sampling.

16. Chervenak, F. A. Diagnosis and management of intrauterine growth retardation. *Female Patient* 13:78, 1988.

    A very practical discussion of the various techniques that one might use, and the time when they should be performed to diagnose IUGR.

Treatment

17. Cox, W. L., et al. Physiology and management of intrauterine growth retardation: a biologic approach with fetal blood sampling. *Am. J. Obstet. Gynecol.* 159:36, 1988.

    The data yielded by fetal blood sampling in 24 cases of IUGR are presented. An elevated white blood cell count (n = 12), mean corpuscular volume (n = 22), and a pH below the normal range (n = 7) were found. Lactic dehydrogenase levels were markedly elevated in most cases, and the glutamyltransferase levels were greatly increased in all but six fetuses.

18. Block, B. S. B., Llanos, A. J., and Creasy, R. K. Responses of the growth-retarded fetus to acute hypoxemia. *Am. J. Obstet. Gynecol.* 148:878, 1984.

    Fetuses who are growth retarded are more likely to suffer acute hypoxemia during labor. Although this study was performed with fetal lambs, it was elegantly controlled and the data would appear to be applicable to humans.

19. Wallace, R. L., Schifrin, B. S., and Paul, R. H. The delivery route for very-low-birth-weight infants. A preliminary report of a randomized, prospective study. *J. Reprod. Med.* 29:736, 1984.

    The delivery route for small babies was studied in this prospective report. The difficulty in accurately diagnosing fetal weight was encountered by the investiga-

tors, but it did not appear that abdominal delivery was advantageous in low-birth-weight babies (< 1500 g).

20. Wallenburg, H. C. S., and Rotmans, N. Prevention of recurrent idiopathic fetal growth retardation by low-dose aspirin and dipyridamole. *Am. J. Obstet. Gynecol.* 157:1230, 1987.

    The article describes a controlled, nonrandomized trial conducted in 24 multigravida women who had had at least two previous pregnancies complicated by IUGR, and who received 1 to 1.6 mg/kg of aspirin and 225 mg of dipyridamole daily from 16 to 34 weeks' gestation. IUGR occurred in 61 percent of the control pregnancies and in 13 percent of the treated pregnancies.

21. McCormick, M. C. The contribution of low birth weight to infant mortality and childhood mortality. *N. Engl. J. Med.* 312:82, 185.

    This article details the effect of low birth weight on subsequent mortality during childhood. It graphically illustrates that babies who are SGA have a proportionately higher risk of dying during childhood, compared with their normal-birth-weight counterparts.

22. Platt, L. D. Genetic factors in intrauterine growth retardation. *Semin. Perinatol.* 12:11, 1988.

    When growth retardation is diagnosed, the possibility of genetic problems should be entertained. The involvement of consultants in the case of a baby who is growth retarded at delivery is an important first step in making the diagnosis of such conditions.

23. Van Zeben-van der Aa, T. M., et al. Morbidity of very low birth weight infants at corrected age of two years in a geographically defined population. Report from project on preterm and small for gestational age infants in the Netherlands. *Lancet* 1:253, 1989.

    In a very homogeneous population with a 97 percent follow-up, a major handicap was found in 4.4 percent of the low-birth-weight infants. This rate is much lower than what has been cited previously for the Netherlands (30%).

24. Low, J. A., et al. Intrauterine growth retardation: a study of long-term morbidity. *Am. J. Obstet. Gynecol.* 142:670, 1982.

    Prospective follow-up study of 76 IUGR children and 88 children with weights appropriate for gestational age. There was no significant difference in the incidence of motor and cognitive handicaps or developmental delay, language developmental delay, and results of vision and hearing tests between the IUGR and control group of children.

VI. FETAL MALPOSITIONS

28. BREECH PRESENTATION
Bryan D. Cowan

Breech presentation is defined as the entrance of the fetal buttocks or the lower extremities into the maternal pelvic inlet. The incidence of term breech presentation varies from 3 to 5 percent, but is almost five times higher among infants weighing less than 2500 g. In defining the orientation of the breech, the denominator is the position of the fetal sacrum within the maternal pelvis; thus, when the sacrum of the fetus is on the right side of the maternal pelvis when viewed cephalad, this is considered a right sacroanterior orientation. The most frequent type of presentation (65%) is a *frank breech*, in which both thighs of the fetus are flexed on the abdomen and both legs are extended over the chest. The *incomplete* or *floating breech*, in which one or both lower extremities of the fetus are extended below the level of the fetal buttocks, accounts for approximately 27 percent of all breech births. The least frequent type (approximately 8%) of presentation is a *complete breech*, in which both thighs of the fetus are flexed onto the abdomen and both legs are flexed at the knee.

In more than half the cases, the cause of breech presentation is not known. During the second and early third trimesters of pregnancy, the ratio of the intrauterine volume to the size of the fetus is large, and this may explain why prematurity is the most commonly observed associated factor of breech presentation. In addition, breech presentation can result from any condition that interferes with the accommodation of the fetus in the uterus. A septate uterus, placenta previa, or uterine myomas also predispose to breech presentations. Other factors favoring breech presentation are fetal malformations, fetopelvic disproportion, multiparity, multiple pregnancy, hydramnios, and hydrocephaly.

To diagnose a breech presentation, Leopold's maneuvers are used to palpate and identify the fetal head in the uterine fundus and the breech in the pelvis. The fetal heart tones are usually best heard above the umbilicus in the breech presentation. Vaginal examination with ruptured membranes can disclose the breech in the pelvis when the fetal anal orifice, which forms a straight line with the ischial tuberosities laterally, is palpated. Another useful landmark in making the differential diagnosis is palpation of the sacrum posterior to the anus. Occasionally on pelvic examination, the breech is confused with a presenting face, shoulder, arm, or anencephalic vertex.

If there is any doubt about the type of fetal presentation, then the diagnosis should be made either sonographically or, classically, by radiographic examination. Additionally, ultrasonography can be used to determine the attitude of the fetal head and to measure the biparietal diameter, thus assisting in the choice of delivery method (vaginal versus abdominal) in some cases.

The accurate diagnosis of breech presentation, especially in the primigravida in the third trimester, is of paramount importance for several reasons. As term approaches, spontaneous conversion to the vertex position is less likely to occur. Although a final decision regarding the method of delivery in a term breech pregnancy should generally not be made until after the onset of labor, the physician should be alert to any complications arising from the presentation per se (i.e., malformations and prolapse of the umbilical cord). External version performed before 36 weeks' gestation has demonstrated promising efficacy, but many fetuses that undergo version spontaneously revert to the breech presentation. External version performed after 36 weeks, however, is permanently successful in approximately 65 percent of the cases. Beta-sympathomimetic–induced uterine relaxation and good fetal reactivity are prerequisites, but the procedure appears to be safe for both the mother and the fetus.

In the past 30 years, the rate of cesarean birth performed for breech delivery has increased. Many physicians recommend abdominal delivery for women with breech presentations of large (> 3800 g) or premature (< 2000 g) infants, women with uterine inertia, and primigravidas. Most studies involving singleton breech presentations have revealed that the route of delivery (vaginal or cesarean) makes no difference in terms of the neonatal mortality in infants weighing more than 2500 g at birth. Cesarean birth, however, is associated with a significantly lower neonatal mortality in those infants with birth weights between 1000 and 2500 g. Operative vaginal manipulation (breech extraction), performed in an attempt to prevent umbilical cord accidents and birth asphyxia, can result in central nervous system injuries (e.g., tentorial tears and intracranial hemorrhages), and thus has generally been abandoned in favor of cesarean delivery.

As early as possible after the patient is admitted to the hospital, the physician must decide whether vaginal delivery or cesarean birth is more appropriate. A useful guide in making this decision has been the "breech scoring index," which attempts to predict the relative safety of vaginal delivery. The final decision regarding the management of the breech birth, however, should be based on careful clinical observation of the patient in labor. X-ray pelvimetry, to evaluate the pelvic capacity, as well as obtaining an anteroposterior view and a lateral view of the abdomen to rule out any evidence of hyperextension of the head, is often performed. Whenever possible, real-time ultrasonography should be performed to rule out the possibility of meningomyelocele, anencephaly, or other malformations that might favor performing cesarean delivery. If an adequate gynecoid pelvis, a well-flexed head (frank or complete breech presentation), and an estimated infant weight that is greater than 2000 g but less than 3500 g are found, labor may be allowed to continue, provided there is progressive cervical dilatation and effacement and normal descent of the presenting part. There should be continuous electronic monitoring of the uterine contractions and fetal heart rate. If the membranes rupture (they are kept intact as long as possible), cord prolapse can occur. Any evidence of acute fetal distress or a prolapsed cord mandates cesarean birth.

A continuous segmental epidural is a good choice for obstetric anesthesia. When regional anesthesia is not available, successful pudendal anesthesia provides good pain relief at the time of delivery of the breech, which is allowed to proceed spontaneously until the umbilicus appears; the obstetrician then gently assists the delivery of the trunk and arms through a liberal episiotomy. The Mauriceau-Smellie-Veit maneuver or the Piper forceps are used to deliver the aftercoming head. In some instances, such as acute fetal distress in a second twin, the fetus must be delivered by breech extraction, provided the pelvis is adequate and the cervix completely dilated. Because breech extraction increases the risk of injury in both the fetus and the mother, it should be performed only when absolutely necessary. Rarely, only partial delivery of the fetal buttocks and thorax occurs, but the head becomes entrapped and the fetus is undeliverable. Using the Zavanelli maneuver, the fetus can often be returned to the vagina (not necessarily the uterus) and safely delivered abdominally. This remarkable treatment seemingly produces little neonatal or maternal morbidity.

In summary, vaginal breech delivery can be carried out in carefully selected patients who make adequate progress and display no signs of fetal compromise. Cesarean delivery should be performed if the clinical circumstances do not favor a vaginal delivery. As data have accumulated, the increased rate of cesarean delivery for breech presentation has been associated with a decreased incidence of perinatal mortality and morbidity, particularly in preterm infants. Nevertheless, the optimal decision in the management of breech presentation should be an individual one and based on clinical grounds.

General
1. Goldenberg, R. L., and Nelson, K. G. The unanticipated breech presentation in labor. *Clin. Obstet. Gynecol.* 27:95, 1984.
   The authors cite 50 references and provide a protocol for the management of both preterm and term breech fetuses whose mothers are in labor.
2. Flanagan, T. A., et al. Management of term breech presentations. *Am. J. Obstet. Gynecol.* 156:1492, 1987.
   This study comprises a review of 716 breech deliveries taking place at 37 or more weeks of gestation. Results confirm that 72 percent of selected patients can be safely delivered vaginally.
3. Ahn, M. O., Cha, K. Y., and Phelan, J. P. The low birth weight infant: is there a preferred route of delivery? *Clin. Perinatol.* 19:411, 1992.
   Although cesarean delivery may be of benefit in the management of the preterm

breech fetus (< 1500 g), there is yet no prospective randomized clinical trial that assesses its use.

Etiology

4. Bingham, P., and Lilford, R. J. Management of the selected term breech presentation: assessment of the risks of selected delivery versus cesarean section for all cases. *Obstet. Gynecol.* 69:965, 1987.
   This review examines the literature published since 1974, and the findings show that the greatest fetal mortality expected from vaginal delivery ranges from 2 to 4 deaths per 1000 live births.
5. Luterkort, M., Persson, P., and Weldner, B. Maternal and fetal factors in breech presentation. *Obstet. Gynecol.* 64:55, 1984.
   This prospective study of 228 breech infants revealed an increased frequency of oligohydramnios, contracted pelvis, and uterine and fetal malformations.

Diagnosis

6. Haberkern, C. M., Smith, D. W., and Jones, K. L. The "breech head" and its relevance. *Am. J. Dis. Child.* 133:154, 1979.
   The authors describe an abnormal head shape, the "breech head," as a factor contributing to birth injury during vaginal delivery of the breech infant.

Treatment

7. Anderson, G., and Strong, C. The premature breech: cesarean section or trial of labour? *J. Med. Ethics* 14:18, 1988.
   The authors discuss the ethics involved in balancing the risk to the mother versus that to the fetus in making obstetric decisions concerning the route of delivery for the preterm breech fetus.
8. Rabinorici, J., et al. Randomized management of the second nonvertex twin: vaginal delivery or cesarean section. *Am. J. Obstet. Gynecol.* 156:52, 1987.
   The authors suggest that the neonatal outcome of the nonvertex twin delivered after 35 weeks of gestation is not affected by the route of delivery.
9. O'Leary, J. Vaginal delivery of the term breech. *Obstet. Gynecol.* 53:341, 1979.
   In a prospective study consisting of 150 term, uncomplicated breech deliveries, the author demonstrates the value of a well-defined management program utilizing the breech score, x-ray pelvimetry, and the Friedman labor curve.
10. Marchick, R. Antepartum external cephalic version with tocolysis: a study of term singleton breech presentations. *Am. J. Obstet. Gynecol.* 158:1339, 1988.
    Successful version occurred in 60 percent of the treated patients. This treatment can reduce the neonatal and maternal morbidity associated with breech presentation.
11. Main, D. M., Main, E. K., and Maurer, M. M. Cesarean section versus vaginal delivery for the breech fetus weighing less than 1,500 grams. *Am. J. Obstet. Gynecol.* 146:580, 1983.
    The authors demonstrated a highly significant increased mortality in breech infants delivered vaginally who weighed between 750 and 1499 g when compared with the mortality noted in infants of the same weight delivered by cesarean section.
12. Watson, W. J., and Benson, W. L. Vaginal delivery for the selected frank breech infant at term. *Obstet. Gynecol.* 64:638, 1984.
    This represents a retrospective review of 254 term breech deliveries. The authors demonstrated that a management program utilizing x-ray pelvimetry, estimated fetal weight, and fetal presentation in labor yielded a favorable outcome.
13. Morrison, J. C., et al. External cephalic version of the breech presentation under tocolysis. *Am. J. Obstet. Gynecol.* 154:900, 1986.
    Version of breech presentation near term significantly reduced the number of breech presentations during labor.
14. Amon, E., Shyken, J. M., and Sibai, B. M. How small is too small and how early is too early? A survey of American obstetricians specializing in high-risk pregnancies. *Am. J. Perinatol.* 9:17, 1992.

Four hundred five maternal-fetal medicine specialists were surveyed to determine their clinical opinions regarding the intrapartum management of the severely preterm fetus requiring delivery. Cesarean section was not performed at less than 24 weeks' gestation, or when the fetal weight was less than 500 g. Ninety percent of the respondents were willing to perform cesarean section in the setting of fetal distress, breech presentation at 26 weeks' gestation, or a fetal weight of 750 g.

Complications

15. Powell, T. G., et al. Cerebral palsy in low-birthweight infants. I. Spastic hemiplegia: association with intrapartum stress. *Dev. Med. Child. Neurol.* 30:11, 1988.
    There was an increased prevalence of spastic hemiplegia in low-birth-weight infants delivered vaginally, suggesting that intrapartum events contributed to the pathogenesis of hemiplegia in some cases.

16. Phelan, J. P., et al. Observations of fetal heart rate characteristics related to external cephalic version and tocolysis. *Am. J. Obstet. Gynecol.* 149:658, 1984.
    Transient fetal heart rate abnormalities were seen in 39 percent of the fetuses after external version. The subsequent fetal outcome appeared to be unrelated to these abnormalities.

17. Sandberg, E. C. The Zavanelli maneuver extended: progression of a revolutionary concept. *Am. J. Obstet. Gynecol.* 158:1347, 1988.
    A report of 15 cases of fetal entrapment in which the infant was returned to the vagina for abdominal delivery. All but one fetus survived, and there were no cases of maternal or fetal trauma.

18. Anderson, G. D., et al. The effect of cesarean section on intraventricular hemorrhage in the preterm infant. *Am. J. Obstet. Gynecol.* 166:1091, 1992.
    Cesarean section performed before the active phase of labor does not change the overall frequency of hemorrhage, but does result in a lower frequency of progression to grade 3 or 4 hemorrhage.

29. NONBREECH ABNORMAL PRESENTATIONS, POSITIONS, AND LIES
James F. McCaul IV

Determination of fetal lie and presentation is essential in the management of labor. Obstetric lie is defined as the relationship between the long axis of the fetus and that of the mother. When the maternal and fetal spines are parallel, the lie is longitudinal; if they are at right angles, the lie is transverse. Axes in between are designated oblique and, owing to their unstable nature, will usually convert to a longitudinal or transverse lie during labor. Longitudinal lies occur in more than 99 percent of laboring patients, and are designated as cephalic or breech, depending on the fetal presentation. The presenting part of the fetus within or closest to the birth canal determines the type of presentation.

In the transverse lie, the fetal head and breech occupy opposite maternal iliac fossae and a shoulder is usually the presenting part. The position is designated as right or left dorsoanterior, dorsoposterior, dorsosuperior, or dorsoinferior. The incidence of a transverse lie ranges from 0.03 to 0.05 percent in the setting of active labor at term in a singleton pregnancy, but the rate is even higher earlier in gestation. A shortened longitudinal uterine axis caused by placental implantation on the dome of the fundus or placenta previa may facilitate this alignment; thus, 10 to 15 percent of transverse lies are associated with a placenta previa or a low-lying placenta. One third occur in grand multiparous women, in whom the incidence is 10 times that in nulliparous women. The lax abdominal wall musculature allows the fetus to fall forward; this interferes with descent and leads to engagement in a transverse lie. Premature labor is also a risk factor. Until 32 weeks, the amniotic cavity is large relative to the fetus; therefore, fetal mobility is increased and transverse lies are more frequent. Likewise, hydramnios increases the probability of a transverse lie occurring at term. A contracted maternal pelvis may also prevent the proper engagement and fixation of the fetal head, and is one of the few conditions in which a longitudinal lie may convert to a transverse lie. Uterine anomalies that widen the bicornuate area also make the transverse diameter more favorable. Lower uterine segment leiomyomata, transverse cesarean section scars, and other pelvic masses may predispose to transverse lie by causing obstruction of the lower uterus. A fetal anomaly or demise may lead to an abnormal lie because of unusual fetal anatomy or flexibility. In twin gestations, 16 percent of the second twins are transverse during labor.

The diagnosis is often based on clinical observations: the transverse diameter of the uterus is greater than expected and the fundal height is inappropriately small for the gestational age. Palpation (Leopold's maneuvers) or a vaginal examination in which the shoulder or arm is palpable can usually confirm the diagnosis. A sonogram, fetogram, or both may provide valuable information when the exact presentation of the fetus is unclear.

The obstetric management of the fetus in a transverse lie depends on the clinical situation; nearly one third of the cases will convert before labor. Many advocate attempting external cephalic version (ECV) when this lie is noted beyond 37 weeks' gestation, but reversion to a transverse lie is common. The success of ECV is increased by the use of tocolytics, but abnormal bleeding, premature rupture of the membranes, and a previously scarred uterus are relative contraindications. When successful, having the patient wear an abdominal binder may prevent spontaneous return to the abnormal lie. Intrapartum ECV (beyond 34 weeks) is successful in 83 percent of the cases of transverse lie, and reduces the need for cesarean delivery by 50 percent in these patients. Attempts to "fix" the presenting part by artificially rupturing the membranes are associated with a high incidence of cord prolapse, and this approach is generally discouraged. In the singleton pregnancy, if ECV fails beyond 39 weeks (or in labor), cesarean delivery is recommended. Internal podalic version may be indicated after ECV has failed in twin pregnancies when the second fetus is transverse and greater than 1500 g. Vaginal delivery is permitted when the conceptus is small and nonviable.

The late hospital arrival of the mother or an inaccurate diagnosis during labor can be responsible for neglected transverse lies. In this setting, the shoulder may become wedged in the pelvic canal and an arm may prolapse into the vagina. If left untreated, the uterus eventually forms a pathologic contraction ring (Bandl's ring) and may rupture. Immediate cesarean section is indicated to avert maternal and fetal death. Uterine rupture, hemorrhage, and infection are all sequelae that must be anticipated and treated aggressively. Fetal risks associated with a transverse lie are prematurity, prolapsed cord, birth injuries, and hypoxia related to manipulative and operative deliveries. Internal podalic version and extraction of a singleton fetus is associated with a corrected neonatal mortality as high as 21 percent and an infant morbidity as high as 33 percent. When cesarean birth is performed, the associated fetal mortality is reduced to approximately 6 percent and the morbidity to approximately 19 percent.

Face presentation represents a malpresentation in which the head is hyperextended with the occiput in contact with the fetal back. This occurs in 1 in 458 deliveries. It is more common in blacks and Eurasians than in whites. Pelvic disproportion, prematurity, multiparity (pendulous abdomen), and macrosomia are the major predisposing factors. On vaginal examination, a face may be confused with a frank breech. In the latter, the anus lies in a straight line with the ischial tuberosities, whereas a face presentation forms a triangle between the fetal mouth and the malar prominences. Palpation of the nose, orbital ridges, frontal sutures, or anterior fontanelle may also aid in the diagnosis. A fetogram or ultrasound may confirm or facilitate the diagnosis.

In a face presentation, the mentobregmatic diameter presents at the pelvic inlet, so engagement occurs much later in labor than it does in the vertex presentation. During internal rotation, the chin should pass under the symphysis pubis. Unless the fetus is unusually small or macerated, vaginal delivery cannot occur in the mentum transverse or posterior positions without internal rotation to the mentum anterior position. Labor may be prolonged, compared with that in a vertex presentation. An increased incidence of abnormal fetal heart rate patterns (up to 53%) has been observed. Fetal scalp electrodes are generally not used, and cesarean delivery should be performed if attempts to rotate the fetus to the mentum anterior position fail or fetal distress occurs. When a face presentation is in the mentum anterior position and the pelvis is adequate, a spontaneous or an outlet forcep vaginal delivery with a generous episiotomy is possible. Overall, 50 to 75 percent of the face presentations can be delivered vaginally, but 80 percent of those in the mentum posterior position require abdominal delivery.

A brow presentation is an unstable malpresentation produced when the fetal head is deflexed so that the orbital ridge and the anterior fontanelle present at the pelvic inlet. Because the occipitomental diameter averages 14 cm, vaginal delivery cannot be accomplished without conversion to either a vertex or face presentation, unless the fetus is very small and the pelvis is large. The incidence of brow presentation is 1 in 1500 deliveries, and predominantly occurs in multiparous whites. The etiology is similar to that for face presentation. A brow presentation is suspected on the basis of vaginal examination findings and is confirmed by x-ray or ultrasound studies. The anterior fontanelle, frontal suture, supraorbital ridge, and root of the nose may be identified on vaginal examination.

In the presence of normal labor and an adequate pelvis, the brow presentation often converts to either a face or vertex presentation. When the brow presentation persists into the second stage of labor, the prognosis is poor for vaginal delivery; a manual attempt to flex and rotate the occiput, either anteriorly or posteriorly, can be made.

Persistent occiput posterior and occiput transverse presentations are seen when the occiput fails to rotate spontaneously to the anterior position prior to delivery. The posterior position is often encountered in the woman with an android or anthropoid pelvis and the occiput transverse position in the woman with a platypelloid pelvis. Most (90%) fetuses in the occiput posterior position undergo spontaneous rotation, followed by an uncomplicated vaginal delivery. However, 5 percent will persist, with a greater predominance among blacks. The second stage of labor is often prolonged in these women, compared with that seen for the occiput anterior position, but the perinatal mortality and morbidity does not differ significantly. The occiput posterior position is confirmed when the small fontanelle is palpated posteriorly. In the event of persistent occiput posterior or transverse positions and a prolonged second stage, manual rotation of the occiput should be attempted. If unsuccessful, the fetus in the occiput posterior position may be delivered as such, utilizing a large episiotomy, forceps, and adequate anesthesia. It is commonly necessary to extend the episiotomy. The Scanzoni maneuver (rotation from the occiput posterior to occiput anterior position) is seldom used except by those experienced with the technique. When the occiput transverse position persists and manual rotation fails, a midforceps rotation may be attempted if the clinician is experienced and there is a roomy pelvis. Abdominal delivery is indicated after a failed forceps trial.

General
1. Cockburn, K. G., and Drake, R. F. Transverse and oblique lie of the fetus. *Aust. N.Z. J. Obstet. Gynecol.* 8:211, 1968.
   This review of 12 years of experience details the incidence, etiology, and maternal and fetal complications of transverse and oblique lies.
2. Cruikshank, D. P., and Cruikshank, J. E. Face and brow presentation: a review. *Clin. Obstet. Gynecol.* 24:333, 1981.
   An excellent review of more than 25 papers discussing the etiology, diagnosis, and appropriate clinical management of face and brow presentations. The authors concluded that (1) the length of labor in face presentations does not differ from that in vertex presentations, (2) the best management is expectant management, (3) oxytocin stimulation of labor is acceptable, (4) outlet forceps delivery is an appropriate method, and (5) face presentation is an indication for intrapartum electronic fetal monitoring.
3. Prevedourakis, C. N. Face presentation: an analysis of 163 cases. *Am. J. Obstet. Gynecol.* 94:1092, 1966.

A large review discussing the incidence, etiology, diagnosis, management, morbidity, and mortality in a patient population from Athens, Greece.
4. Schwartz, Z., et al. Face presentation. *Aust. N.Z. J. Obstet. Gynecol.* 26:172, 1986.
   A review of 51 cases from Israel, focusing on the incidence, etiology, time of diagnosis, and management of labor.

Etiology
5. Duff, P. Diagnosis and management of face presentation. *Obstet. Gynecol.* 57: 105, 1981.
   Discusses the incidence, diagnosis, and possible causes of face presentation, and outlines a management protocol.
6. Floberg, J., et al. Influence of the pelvic outlet capacity on fetal head presentation at delivery. *Acta Obstet. Gynecol. Scand.* 66:127, 1987.
   Using x-ray pelvimetry, this study demonstrated an increased frequency of occiput posterior presentations and lengthened duration of labor with decreasing pelvic outlet capacity.
7. Kawathekay, P., et al. Etiology and trends in the management of transverse lie. *Am. J. Obstet. Gynecol.* 1:39, 1973.
   A discussion of the etiology and trends in management observed in India.
8. Steverson, C. S. Transverse or oblique presentation of the fetus. *Clin. Obstet. Gynecol.* 5:946, 1962.
   An extensive summary of the literature, with emphasis on the etiology, diagnosis, and management.

Diagnosis
9. Jabbar, A., and Meshari, A. Etiology and management of transverse lie. *Int. J. Gynaecol. Obstet.* 18:448, 1980.
   Transverse lie is most often associated with grand multiparity, placenta previa, hydramnios, and a contracted pelvis.
10. Panthaky, R., and Dutta, G. P. Face presentation: a study of 190 cases. *J. Indian Med. Assoc.* 76:126, 1981.
    A review of 190 cases of face presentation seen in an Indian population revealed that most were delivered vaginally, the diagnosis of abnormal presentation in early labor was difficult, and fetal morbidity and mortality were low.

Complications
11. Benedetti, T. J., Lowensohn, R. I., and Truscott, A. M. Face presentation at term. *Obstet. Gynecol.* 55:199, 1980.
    A retrospective study to investigate the possible relationship between intrapartum fetal heart rate abnormalities and face presentation in term infants.
12. Dutta, G. P., and Bhaumik, I. A study of transverse lie: a review of 333 cases. *J. Indian Med. Assoc.* 74:48, 1980.
    A review of the management methods, maternal and neonatal outcome, and demography in 333 cases of transverse lie encountered between 1965 and 1975 in India.
13. Hulet, B., and Platt, L. D. Sinusoidal heart rate pattern and face presentation in a fetus from a postterm pregnancy. *J. Reprod. Med.* 32:211, 1987.
    Case report and brief discussion of abnormal monitor patterns often associated with face presentations.
14. Ingemarsson, E., et al. Influence of occiput posterior position on the fetal heart rate pattern. *Obstet. Gynecol.* 55:301, 1980.
    This study revealed that variable decelerations were significantly more frequent and pronounced in infants presenting in the occiput posterior position than those in control infants.
15. Phelan, J. P., et al. The nonlaboring transverse lie: a management dilemma. *J. Reprod. Med.* 31:184, 1986.
    In a review of patients who did not undergo elective external cephalic version at

37 weeks, the morbidity and mortality was found to be increased, prompting consideration of external cephalic version at 39 weeks and cesarean section in those in whom it is unsuccessful.

Treatment

16. Chervenak, F. A., et al. Intrapartum external version of the second twin. *Obstet. Gynecol.* 62:160, 1983.
    Converting a second twin from a transverse lie to the vertex position may be an alternative to cesarean section or breech extraction.
17. Chervenak, F. A., et al. Intrapartum management of twin gestation. *Obstet. Gynecol.* 65:119, 1985.
    A retrospective review of 362 cases, including 139 vertex-nonvertex presentations, of which 71.2 percent were delivered vaginally. A management scheme is proposed, including the use of intrapartum external cephalic version. Cesarean section is recommended when version is unsuccessful with a fetus weighing less than 2000 g.
18. Pelosi, M. A., et al. The "intra-abdominal version technique" for delivery of transverse lie by low-segment cesarean section. *Am. J. Obstet. Gynecol.* 135:1009, 1985.
    The authors describe a technique of intraabdominal version for delivery of the infant in the transverse lie, to avoid using the classic cesarean delivery and permit the more desirable low transverse cervical cesarean incision to be made.
19. Phelan, J. P., et al. The role of external version in the intrapartum management of the transverse lie presentation. *Am. J. Obstet. Gynecol.* 151:724, 1985.
    External version performed under tocolysis was performed in 12 patients with a transverse lie, with 60 percent going on to deliver vaginally.
20. Phillips, R. D., and Freemen, M. The management of the persistent occiput posterior position. *Obstet. Gynecol.* 43:171, 1974.
    A retrospective study of 552 cases demonstrated that the persistent occiput posterior position does not represent an increased risk factor to the fetus; therefore, premature intervention should be avoided.
21. Rabinovici, J., et al. Randomized management of the second nonvertex twin: vaginal delivery or cesarean section. *Am. J. Obstet. Gynecol.* 156:52, 1987.
    A prospective study of 60 twin deliveries taking place beyond 35 weeks' gestation, with a second twin in a nonvertex presentation. Internal podalic version was used for delivery of the second twin. With the exception of increased maternal morbidity in the cesarean section group, no significant differences were noted.
22. Trofatter, K. F. Twin pregnancy: management of delivery. *Clin. Perinatol.* 15:93, 1988.
    A good summary of twin delivery management, including management of a second twin in the nonvertex presentation. Discusses use of intrapartum external cephalic version with tocolysis and vaginal delivery of the nonvertex second twin if the fetal weight is greater than 1500 g (including the use of internal podalic version). Important exclusions are discussed.
23. Hankins, G. D. V., et al. Transverse lie. *Am. J. Perinatol.* 7:66, 1990.
    In parturients at term who presented in active labor and a transverse lie, the incidence of fetal acidosis and trauma was found to be increased. Active intervention consisting of external version followed by labor induction (or cesarean delivery for version failures) was advocated beyond 38 weeks' gestation.

30. HYDRAMNIOS AND OLIGOHYDRAMNIOS
Richard L. Rosemond

Hydramnios (polyhydramnios) is an excessive amount of amniotic fluid, whereas oligohydramnios is an abnormally low volume of amniotic fluid. The uterus at term contains 800 to 1000 ml of fluid. Volumes greater than 2000 ml or less than 400 ml are abnormal and indicate a pregnancy at risk for adverse outcome.

The incidence of hydramnios ranges from 0.4 to 1.5 percent. The volume of amniotic fluid depends on the relative rates of production from the fetal kidneys and transudation through the fetal skin, versus consumption through the process of fetal swallowing and reabsorption in the lungs. Most explainable causes of hydramnios result from an excess urine production or decreased absorption by the gastrointestinal system. Approximately 20 percent of the cases of hydramnios are associated with congenital malformations. These include (1) central nervous system disorders (52%)—anencephaly; (2) cardiovascular disorders (30%)—arrhythmia, coarctation, and hydrops; (3) gastrointestinal tract disorders (47%)—facial clefts, duodenal atresia, diaphragmatic hernia, and abdominal wall defects; (4) respiratory disorders—cystic adenomatoid malformation and pulmonary sequestration; (5) musculoskeletal defects (19%)—thanatophoric dwarf; and (6) genitourinary anomalies (16%)—uteropelvic junction obstruction and posterior urethral valves. Another 25 percent of the cases of hydramnios are associated with diabetes mellitus. Multiple gestation and isoimmunization each account for 10 percent of the cases; however, the most common cause of hydramnios remains idiopathic (35%).

Chromosomal abnormalities have been reported in the mothers with hydramnios, but at this time there is not enough evidence to support routine karyotype testing in these patients.

Hydramnios should be suspected whenever the uterus is larger than expected for a particular gestational age, there is difficulty palpating the fetus, or the fetal heart tones are difficult to hear with the fetoscope. The volume of amniotic fluid should then be assessed ultrasonographically. There is controversy regarding the best technique to use for confirming the diagnosis. The most common methods are subjective impression, measuring the largest vertical pocket, and calculating an amniotic fluid index. The last technique involves dividing the uterus into four quadrants, using the umbilicus as the center point, and then measuring the largest vertical pocket of each quadrant in centimeters and adding the four values. This index is then compared to a table of normal values, and hydramnios is diagnosed if the index value is greater than the 95th percentile for that gestational age. In sheep models, this was found to be 88 percent accurate, with intraobserver and interobserver errors averaging 1 and 2 cm, respectively.

Maternal complications associated with hydramnios include preterm labor, premature ruptured membranes, maternal discomfort, and respiratory compromise. The incidence of these complications is even greater when the evolution of the hydramnios is acute (days) rather than chronic (weeks).

The treatment of hydramnios should be directed at the underlying cause, when this is known. Correction of a fetal arrhythmia or improvement in maternal glycemic control are examples of directed therapy. When a specific cause is not identified, generally no treatment is indicated unless maternal complications develop. Treatment is either surgical or medical. Surgical therapy consists of amniocentesis, with removal of sometimes tremendous quantities of amniotic fluid. Care is taken not to decompress the uterine cavity so rapidly as to cause an abruption. From personal experience, removal of 1000 ml of fluid over 10 to 15 minutes seems safe. This procedure can be repeated many times; however, each additional procedure carries an additional risk of precipitating preterm labor, premature ruptured membranes, abruption, and amnionitis. In addition, maternal discomfort and the cost of the procedure should be considered.

Medical therapy consists of the administration of indomethacin (25 mg orally every 6 hours). The mechanism of action appears to be a decrease in urine output and a subsequent decrease in the amniotic fluid volume. It has the added benefit of being an effective tocolytic agent; however, there are risks and contraindications to consider. Indomethacin should not be given to any woman beyond 34 weeks' gestation, as the risk of attendant fetal ductal constriction increases after this time. Similarly, fetuses should be screened for any kind of ductal-dependent heart defect prior to administration. The fluid volume usually decreases steadily when this approach to treatment is used, but it may be several days or even weeks before the desired level is reached. Monitoring during this time should include weekly fluid volume assessment and Doppler evaluation of ductal flow.

Multiple gestation can pose a unique problem to the obstetrician, in that hydramnios of one twin can exist simultaneously with oligohydramnios of the other. This represents the "stuck twin" phenomenon, and may reflect the twin-twin transfusion syndrome. Although this generally carries a poor prognosis, one study revealed favorable outcomes following serial therapeutic amniocentesis.

In summary, patients identified with hydramnios should undergo a careful anatomic ultrasound examination to detect any structural abnormalities and rule out macrosomia. The diabetes mellitus status of the patient should be assessed, and treatment instituted if a cause is found or if maternal complications warrant.

Oligohydramnios may be suspected when the size of the uterus is less than that expected for a particular gestational age, when there is evidence of fetal crowding, or when variable decelerations appear during fetal monitoring. The diagnosis is confirmed by ultrasound. Again, oligohydramnios can be determined either by a subjective assessment of the fluid volume, or by an objective one, using the fifth percentile of the amniotic fluid index as the cutoff.

Oligohydramnios occurs in approximately 4 percent of pregnancies. The most common causes include ruptured membranes, intrauterine growth retardation (IUGR), postdates syndrome, and fetal anomalies. The presence of oligohydramnios together with ruptured membranes may be associated with a decreased latency period and an increased risk of infection; however, this is not necessarily an indication for delivery. As the placental blood flow to an IUGR fetus decreases, the blood in the fetus is shunted away from the kidneys and urine output decreases. The presence of oligohydramnios, therefore, is a marker for the more severe forms of IUGR. Abnormal Doppler flow measurements of the umbilical and uterine system may identify the fetus at greater risk for an adverse outcome in this scenario. If oligohydramnios occurs early in the pregnancy, or otherwise there is no explanation for the decreased placental function, chromosome analysis should be considered. The development of oligohydramnios in the postdate pregnancy is an indication for delivery. Fetal anomalies known to cause oligohydramnios include renal obstruction or agenesis. The absence of fetal kidneys is called Potter's syndrome, and results in typical facies and skeletal malformations as well as lung hypoplasia. This is a fatal condition. When there is urinary obstruction and subsequent oligohydramnios, delivery may be indicated, except in the very premature fetus, who might benefit from an in utero shunt procedure.

The fetus in an environment of oligohydramnios is at risk for cord compression and subsequent demise. Patients who present in labor with significant variable decelerations have been treated with amnioinfusion, with resolution of the variable decelerations in some cases. Amnioinfusion is performed by placement of an intrauterine pressure catheter and infusion of 500 ml of warmed normal saline or lactated Ringer's solution, followed by continuous infusion at a rate of 100 to 200 ml/hr. Overdistention of the uterus must be avoided. This technique has also been used to decrease the incidence of meconium aspiration syndrome. Amnioinfusion has also been used to improve visualization for the anatomic evaluation of a fetus with oligohydramnios.

In summary, when oligohydramnios is present, ruptured membranes and fetal anomalies need to be ruled out. If IUGR is found, aggressive monitoring should be instituted, including Doppler flow studies. Finally, oligohydramnios in the postdate pregnancy should be considered an indication for delivery.

General
1. Cardwell, M. S. Polyhydramnios: a review. *Obstet. Gynecol. Surv.* 42:612, 1987.
   An excellent review of the subject of polyhydramnios. More than 40 references are offered.
2. Boylan, P., and Parisi, V. An overview of hydramnios. *Semin. Perinatol.* 10:136, 1986.
   A fine overview of the definition of as well as outcome from hydramnios states.
3. Peipert, J. F., and Donnenfeld, A. E. Oligohydramnios: a review. *Obstet. Gynecol. Surv.* 46:325, 1991.

A comprehensive review of the topic of oligohydramnios covering diagnosis, prognosis, and management, and including over 150 references.

Etiology

4. Furlong, L. A., et al. Pregnancy outcome following ultrasound diagnosis of fetal urinary tract anomalies and/or oligohydramnios. *Fetal Ther.* 1:134, 1986.
   The contribution of fetal urinary tract abnormalities to the diagnosis of oligohydramnios is demonstrated in this excellent report.
5. Landy, H. J., Isada, N. B., and Larsen, J. W., Jr. Genetic implications of idiopathic hydramnios. *Am. J. Obstet. Gynecol.* 157:114, 1987.
   Hydramnios is often associated with chromosomal abnormalities.
6. Hendrix, S. K., et al. Diagnosis of polyhydramnios in early gestation: indication for prenatal diagnosis? *Prenat. Diagn.* 11:649, 1991.
   Of 138 cases of polyhydramnios, there were seven involving chromosomal abnormalities; all were associated with other ultrasound findings. The authors doubt the need for amniocentesis after the diagnosis of early polyhydramnios.
7. Hickok, D. E., et al. Unexplained second trimester oligohydramnios: a clinical pathologic study. *Am. J. Perinatol.* 6:8, 1989.
   The authors emphasize the importance of oligohydramnios in the absence of fetal malformations as a cause of adverse pregnancy outcome. Hypoplastic lungs as well as cord accidents were more common.
8. Kirshon, B. Fetal urine output in hydramnios. *Obstet. Gynecol.* 73:240, 1989.
   Fetal urine output in patients with hydramnios may be the result of polyuria in the hyperperfused twin.

Diagnosis

9. Quetel, T. A., et al. Amnioinfusion: an aid in the ultrasonic evaluation of severe oligohydramnios in pregnancy. *Am. J. Obstet. Gynecol.* 167:333, 1992.
   The diagnostic capability was improved in 13 patients who presented with early oligohydramnios by the transabdominal infusion of warmed saline and indigocarmine dye.
10. Phelan, J. P., et al. Amniotic fluid index measurements during pregnancy. *J. Reprod. Med.* 32:601, 1987.
    The technique for quantitative assessment of amniotic fluid volume is detailed in this report.
11. Moore, T. R. Superiority of the four-quadrant sum over the single deepest pocket technique in ultrasonic identification of abnormal amniotic fluid volumes. *Am. J. Obstet. Gynecol.* 163:762, 1990.
    Maximum vertical pocket measurements failed to identify 58 percent of the cases of oligohydramnios identified by the amniotic fluid index.
12. Lombardi, S. J., Rosemond, R. L., and Ball, R. Umbilical artery velocimetry as a predictor of adverse outcome in pregnancies complicated by oligohydramnios. *Obstet. Gynecol.* 74:338, 1989.
    The findings from umbilical Doppler flow studies were found to be predictive of an adverse outcome in patients with unexplained oligohydramnios.

Treatment

13. Sivan, E., et al. The role of amnioinfusion in current obstetric care. *Obstet. Gynecol. Surv.* 47:80, 1992.
    An up-to-date review of the technique of, indications for, and outcome from amnioinfusion.
14. Elliott, J. P., Urig, M. A., and Clewell, W. H. Aggressive therapeutic amniocentesis for treatment of twin-twin transfusion syndrome. *Obstet. Gynecol.* 77:537, 1991.
    Reports on 17 cases of twin-twin transfusion, with a remarkable 79 percent perinatal survival.
15. Moise, K. J. Indomethacin therapy in the treatment of symptomatic polyhydramnios. *Clin. Obstet. Gynecol.* 34:310, 1991.
    Summarizes the experience to date on this subject. Indomethacin treatment was

successful in 36 of 38 cases, with attainment of normal fluid volume in 4 to 20 days.

16. Hendrix, S. K., et al. Oligohydramnios associated with prostaglandin synthetase inhibitors in preterm labor. *Br. J. Obstet. Gynaecol.* 97:312, 1990.
   Oligohydramnios occurred in 70 percent of the patients treated with indomethacin. All cases resolved after discontinuation of the medication.

Complications

17. Lawrence, S., and Rosenfeld, C. R. Fetal pulmonary development and abnormalities of amniotic fluid volume. *Semin. Perinatol.* 10:142, 1986.
   Reviews the pathophysiologic characteristics of lung hypoplasia in the setting of oligohydramnios. Includes data from both animal and human studies.

18. Vintzileos, A. M., et al. Degree of oligohydramnios and pregnancy outcome in patients with premature rupture of the membranes. *Obstet. Gynecol.* 66: 162, 198.
   These authors showed that oligohydramnios, occurring after premature rupture of membranes that lasted for more than several days, was correlated with a poor outcome in the fetus.

19. Major, C. A., and Kitzmiller, J. L. Perinatal survival with expectant management of midtrimester rupture of membranes. *Am. J. Obstet. Gynecol.* 163:838, 1990.
   A report documenting improved perinatal survival rates as neonatal care has become more sophisticated. This report gives survival statistics that can be used in counseling patients.

20. Roussis, P., Rosemond R. L., and Glass, C. Preterm premature rupture of membranes: detection of infection. *Am. J. Obstet. Gynecol.* 165:1099, 1991.
   The authors described the predictive ability of a daily modified biophysical profile to detect subclinical infection in patients with premature rupture of the membranes.

VII. LABOR AND DELIVERY

31. ANALGESIA AND ANESTHESIA FOR LABOR AND DELIVERY
L. Wayne Hess and James J. Sowash

The use of medications during the intrapartum period must be carefully assessed because they may potentiate the physiologic effects of pregnancy in the mother and may adversely affect the fetus. It is important to carry out antepartum and intrapartum risk assessment to detect maternal and fetal complications before introducing other variables such as analgesia and anesthesia. Although there is a move toward a more family oriented and natural approach to the birth process, many patients elect to receive analgesia or anesthesia during labor and delivery. The type of analgesia or anesthesia can be selected only after the history, physical findings, obstetric conditions, and desires of the patient are evaluated in the context of the practices and philosophy of the obstetrician and anesthesiologist. Although many patients and physicians prefer regional anesthesia, systemic analgesics are the primary form of pain relief used in the practice of obstetrics in the United States, and most of this analgesia is provided by obstetricians.

Almost every drug used for analgesia in the mother during labor crosses the placenta and can affect the fetus. Most analgesic agents are small in molecular weight (<1000), are lipid soluble, and have a high pKa, thus allowing for easy transit across the placenta. Narcotic agents, principally meperidine (Demerol), are the most common type of analgesic administered during pregnancy. In most cases, meperidine, given in 25- to 50-mg increments every 2 to 4 hours, is sufficient for pain relief during labor and has little effect on the baby other than decreasing the beat-to-beat variability of the fetal heart. At these dosage levels, if the fetus is depressed at birth, invariably it is not due to the analgesic. Although neurobehavioral changes have been associated with meperidine usage, these effects are self-limited and have no long-term consequences. Additionally, some have interdicted meperidine just before parturition because of the risk of fetal depression. However, most agree that the drug should not be withheld because the patient is going to deliver within the next 1 to 2 hours.

Regional anesthesia is used more today in obstetrics than ever before. The use of segmental epidural blocks has gained wide popularity in the United States. Epidural analgesia using the amide derivative drugs (lidocaine and bupivacaine) may selectively block uterine pain during labor and has the advantage of also being able to render satisfactory anesthesia for delivery. Complications include inadvertent entry into the spinal canal and hypotension. Paresthesia, an infrequent complication, usually occurs with the ester-based local anesthetics (2-chloroprocaine). Direct toxicity with high-percentage bupivacaine (0.75%) has been observed after epidural anesthesia. In addition, many obstetricians believe that the use of conduction anesthesia prolongs labor and leads to an increased incidence of fetuses in the transverse (vertex) position and the subsequent need for midforceps rotation or cesarean section. The adverse effects on the mother and fetus in this setting, however, are far outweighed by the benefits of this type of anesthesia.

Psychoprophylaxis (prepared childbirth) has also gained wide acceptance in this country as a method of analgesia in labor and, if successful, is very rewarding for the parturient and her support person. If unsuccessful, small doses of analgesic agents can be administered, and this permits the parturient to still actively participate in the birth process. It is necessary to tailor psychoprophylaxis to each patient, rather than to enforce a rigid protocol of analgesia versus no analgesia, because hyperventilation with resultant hypocapnia and epinephrine release may result in fetal hypoxia directly related to natural childbirth.

Sedatives and hypnotics are now used infrequently in labor and delivery suites. Barbiturate usage, at least during the active intrapartum phase of labor, is almost entirely limited to the induction of general anesthesia for cesarean birth. For vaginal deliveries, these agents are best avoided because they are ineffective analgesic agents and there are disadvantages associated with their use in both the mother and fetus.

151

The Duke inhaler, the intermittent administration of anesthetic gases such as methoxyflurane or nitrous oxide, and "twilight sleep" (morphine and scopolamine) are not popular, and are now considered inadvisable for use in intrapartum analgesia. Once popular narcotic analgesics such as alphaprodine (Nisentil) and anileridine (Leritine) are no longer marketed in the United States. Other marketed narcotics such as fentanyl (Sublimaze), sufentanil (Sufenta), codeine, buprenorphine (Buprenex), oxymorphone (Numorphan), and hydromorphone (Dilaudid) are not approved by the Food and Drug Administration nor are they recommended by the manufacturer for use as intrapartum analgesics.

Anesthesia for vaginal delivery may include low spinal (saddle block) anesthesia. This method provides good relaxation for a forceps delivery, if this proves necessary. Hypotension is the principal problem that may arise, and must be prevented by ensuring adequate hydration and wedging the patient to prevent development of the supine hypotensive syndrome. The use of local agents such as lidocaine provides analgesia to the episiotomy site and allows for episiotomy repair. Pudendal anesthesia is also frequently used, but carries a high degree of partial effects even in the best hands.

Anesthesia for cesarean delivery can be accomplished by general or regional means. Regional anesthesia includes the epidural or spinal techniques. For cesarean birth, regional anesthesia up to the T10 dermatome is the objective. For both regional techniques, hypotension is the principal danger, but it can be prevented by maintaining adequate hydration and by wedging (tilting) the patient to prevent the supine hypotension syndrome from developing. Balanced endotracheal anesthesia utilizing rapid induction, in which intravenous barbiturates and a muscle relaxant are given, is equally efficacious for providing anesthesia in abdominal deliveries. If the patient's case is uncomplicated, the team gathered for the procedure (anesthesiologists, pediatrician, and obstetrician) can usually allow the patient to choose the method of anesthesia. In complicated cases, the obstetric anesthesiologist in consultation with the perinatologist and neonatologist should decide the best method of anesthesia for delivery.

The use of new agents (such as the endorphins or peridural morphine) is investigational at this time, but holds promise for the future. Other analgesic and anesthesia techniques include hypnosis and acupuncture. These techniques, although demonstrated effective in some studies, have not generally been accepted by the medical community. Additionally, patient-controlled analgesia is becoming increasingly popular for labor analgesia.

General

1. Shnider, S. M., and Levinson, G. *Anesthesia for Obstetrics* (3rd ed.). Baltimore: Williams & Wilkins, 1992.
   A comprehensive text dealing with obstetric physiology and pharmacology, analgesia and anesthesia for routine and complicated vaginal and abdominal deliveries, complications of obstetric anesthesia, and fetal and neonatal effects of analgesia and anesthesia.
2. Ostheimer, G. W. Obstetric analgesia and anesthesia I and II. *Clin. Anesthesiol.* 4:1, 1986.
   A comprehensive review of all aspects of obstetric analgesia and anesthesia.
3. Gibbs, C. P., et al. Obstetric anesthesia: a national survey. *Anesthesiology* 65:298, 1986.
   This article reviews trends in obstetric anesthesia and analgesia observed in hospitals in the United States.
4. Pasternak, G. W. Multiple morphine and enkephalin receptors and the relief of pain. *J.A.M.A.* 259:1362, 1988.
   An excellent review of the physiology of narcotics.
5. Pitcock, C. D., and Clark, R. B. From Fanny to Fernand: the development of consumerism in pain control during the birth process. *Am. J. Obstet. Gynecol.* 167:581, 1992.
   An excellent review of patient's views concerning analgesia options during labor.

6. Hughes, S. C. Analgesia methods during labour and delivery. *Can. J. Anaesth.* 39:R18, 1992.
   An excellent review of all methods of analgesia for use in the laboring patient.
7. Faure, E. A. The pain of parturition. *Semin. Perinatol.* 15:342, 1991.
   A general review of the physiology of pain during labor.
8. Harris, A. P., and Michitsch, R. U. Anesthesia and analgesia for labor. *Curr. Opin. Obstet. Gynecol.* 4:813, 1992.
   A complete review of analgesia and anesthesia for labor.
9. Samuels, P. Advances in anesthesia and pharmacology in the puerperium. *Curr. Opin. Obstet. Gynecol.* 3:773, 1991.
   An excellent review of the pharmacology of labor analgesia.

Parenteral Analgesia
10. Kuhnert, B. R., et al. Disposition of meperidine and normeperidine following multiple doses during labor. I. Fetus and neonate. *Am. J. Obstet. Gynecol.* 151:410, 1985.
    The administration of multiple doses of meperidine with a long drug-to-delivery interval results in the accumulation of normeperidine in fetal tissues and subsequent neonatal depression.
11. McIntosh, D. G., and Rayburn, W. F. Patient controlled analgesia in obstetrics and gynecology. *Obstet. Gynecol.* 78:1129, 1991.
    A general review of patient-controlled analgesia.
12. Dan, U., et al. Intravenous pethidine and nalbuphine during labor: a prospective double-blind comparative study. *Gynecol. Obstet. Invest.* 32:39, 1991.
    A comparison of Demerol and Nubain for analgesia.
13. Hughes, S. C. Analgesia methods during labour and delivery. *Can. J. Anaesth.* 39:R18, 1992.
    An excellent review of analgesia for labor.
14. Berg, T. G., and Rayburn, W. F. Effects of analgesia on labor. *Clin. Obstet. Gynecol.* 35:457, 1992.
    A review of the possible risks of analgesia during labor.
15. Coalson, D. W., and Glosten, B. Alternatives to epidural analgesia. *Semin. Perinatol.* 15:375, 1991.
    A view of analgesia that excludes the regional techniques.

Regional Analgesia and Anesthesia
16. Swayze, C. R., et al. Efficacy of subarachnoid meperidine for labor analgesia. *Reg. Anesth.* 16:309, 1991.
    An evaluation of intrathecal Demerol during labor.
17. Abboud, T. K., et al. Continuous infusion epidural analgesia in parturient receiving bupivacaine, chloroprocaine, or lidocaine—maternal, fetal, and neonatal effects. *Anesth. Analg.* 63:421, 1984.
    Continuous epidural anesthesia was achieved with bupivacaine, chloroprocaine, or lidocaine. Those receiving bupivacaine exhibited a higher incidence of fetal heart decelerations. All the methods were associated with good maternal analgesia, excellent neonatal outcome, and normal laboratory values.
18. Saini, C. S., et al. Effect of general and spinal anesthesia on neuro-behavioral responses in cesarean babies. *Indian Pediatr.* 29:621, 1992.
    This describes the fetal effects of regional anesthesia.
19. Eddleston, J. M., et al. Comparison of the maternal and fetal effects associated with intermittent or continuous infusion of extradural analgesia. *Br. J. Anaesth.* 69:154, 1992.
    There are minimal fetal effects associated with epidural anesthesia.
20. Parker, R. K., and White, P. F. Epidural patient-controlled analgesia: an alternative to intravenous patient-controlled analgesia for pain relief after cesarean delivery. *Anesth. Analg.* 75:245, 1992.
    Patient-controlled analgesia leads to improved patient acceptance and satisfaction.

21. Kumar, A., et al. Spinal anesthesia with lidocaine 2% for caesarean section. *Can. J. Anaesth.* 39:915, 1992.
    Examines the safety and efficacy of spinal anesthesia for cesarean section.
22. Curran, M. J. Options for labor analgesia: techniques of epidural and spinal analgesia. *Semin. Perinatol.* 15:348, 1991.
    A general review of the regional methods used to achieve analgesia for labor.
23. Thorp, J. A., et al. Epidural analgesia and cesarean section for dystocia: risk factors in nulliparas. *Am. J. Perinatol.* 8:402, 1991.
    When regional analgesia is used during labor, this does appear to increase the risk of operative delivery.
24. Goins, J. R. Experience with mepivacaine paracervical block *in an obstetric private practice. Am. J. Obstet. Gynecol.* 167:342, 1992.
    Introduction of a paracervical block during labor appears beneficial and is associated with minimal risks.

Psychologic Analgesia
25. Skibsted, L., and Lange, A. P. The need for pain relief in uncomplicated delivery ward. *Pain* 48:183, 1992.
    Psychosocial influences modify the pain of labor.
26. Bernat, S. H., et al. Biofeedback assisted relaxation to reduce stress in labor. *J. Obstet. Gynecol. Neonatal Nurs.* 21:295, 1992.
    A review of the various relaxation techniques to decrease the pain of labor.

General Anesthesia
27. Yam, I., and Rubin, A. P. Emergency caesarean section. *Br. J. Hosp. Med.* 48:244, 1992.
    The methods of anesthesia for emergency delivery are reviewed.
28. Dick, W., et al. General anesthesia versus epidural anesthesia for primary caesarean section—a comparative study. *Eur. J. Anaesthesiol.* 9:15, 1992.
    The comparative risks of general versus regional anesthesia during labor are analyzed.
29. Marx, G. F., and Katsnelson, T. The introduction of nitrous oxide analgesia into obstetrics. *Obstet. Gynecol.* 80:715, 1992.
    Historic review of balanced anesthesia in labor.
30. Pedersen, J. E., Fernandes, A., and Christensen, M. Halothane 2% for caesarean section. *Eur. J. Anaesthesiol.* 9:319, 1992.
    Halothane appears to be a safe agent for cesarean section anesthesia.
31. Finster, M., et al. Obstetric anesthesia. *Minerva Anestesiol.* 58:853, 1992.
    A review of general anesthesia in labor.

Complications
32. AAP Committee on Drugs. In Collaboration with the ACOG Committee on Obstetrics. Effect of medication during labor and delivery on infant. *Maternal Fetal Medicine* March 1985.
    The American Academy of Pediatrics and American College of Obstetricians and Gynecologists prepared this joint statement concerning the use of drugs in pregnancy and the effects of medication on the infant.

New Techniques
33. Bundse, P., and Ericson, K. Pain relief in labor by transcutaneous electrical nerve stimulation. *Acta Obstet. Gynecol. Scand.* 61:1, 1982.
    The use of transcutaneous electrical nerve stimulation to achieve pain relief was tested in 15 parturients. Good pain relief was experienced by these women, with no adverse effect on either the mother or newborn.
34. Naulty, J. S., et al. Epidural butorphanol-bupivacaine for analgesia during labor and delivery. *Anesthesiology* 65:A369, 1986.
    Epidural butorphanol provides excellent analgesia with a minimum of side effects.
35. Chestnut, D. H., et al. Continuous infusion epidural analgesia during labor. A

randomized, double-blind comparison of 0.0625 percent bupivacaine/0.0002 percent fentanyl versus 0.125 percent bupivacaine. *Anesthesiology* 68:754, 1988. *Both of these methods of analgesia appear equally effective.*

32. FORCEPS AND VACUUM EXTRACTION
Richard L. Rosemond and Rudolph P. Fedrizzi

The American College of Obstetricians and Gynecologists has defined the following categories of forceps operations. An *outlet forceps delivery* is one in which (1) the skull is visible at the introitus without separating the labia, (2) the fetal skull has reached the pelvic floor, (3) the sagittal sutures are in the anteroposterior position, and (4) the fetal head is at or on the perineum. According to this definition, rotation cannot exceed 45 degrees. The application of forceps when the leading point of the skull is at the +2 station or more, but other criteria for outlet forceps extraction are not met, is termed a low-forceps delivery. The low-forceps delivery has two subdivisions: (1) rotation 45 degrees or less (e.g., left occiput anterior to occiput anterior and left occiput posterior to occiput posterior), and (2) rotation more than 45 degrees. The application of forceps when the head is engaged but the leading point of the skull is above the +2 station is called a *midforceps delivery*. Under unusual circumstances, such as the sudden onset of severe fetal or maternal compromise, application of forceps above the +2 station but below or equal to the zero station may be attempted while simultaneously initiating preparation for cesarean delivery in the event that the forceps maneuver is unsuccessful. Forceps should not be applied to an unengaged head or when the cervix has not completely dilated.

The forceps instrument is described in terms of its design with special reference to the blade (solid or fenestrated), the pelvic curve (straight or curved), the cephalic curve (wide or narrow), the shanks (separate or overlapping), the lock (English or sliding), and the handle. There are many different models of forceps from which to choose, and each has its own particular application. The Simpson, Elliott, and Tucker-McLean instruments are classic outlet forceps. The latter two are used primarily for the unmolded head, with the difference being that the blade on the Elliott forceps is fenestrated and the blade of the Tucker-McLean forceps is not. Simpson forceps are preferred for the larger molded head. Specialized forceps such as the Kielland and Barton are used primarily for rotation. The Kielland has an absent pelvic curve, and the resulting rotational motion is much like the action of a key in a lock. The Barton forceps are used to deliver the head through a platypelloid pelvis. Piper forceps are used for the aftercoming head in a breech delivery.

The indication for the use of forceps should be clearly documented in the patient's chart. Accepted indications include the presence of maternal diseases (cardiac, cerebrovascular, or pulmonary), which may worsen with prolonged pushing or maternal exhaustion, or an inability to push effectively secondary to excessive analgesia or lack of cooperation. Fetal indications include fetal distress, malposition, asynclitism, and deflexion. Another indication is a prolonged second stage, which is defined as greater than 2 hours in the nulliparous patient and greater than 1 hour in the parous patient. An additional hour is added if conduction anesthesia is used. However, before an operative vaginal delivery is attempted because of a prolonged second stage, the operator must be sure that cephalopelvic disproportion is not present. There is hardly a worse scenario than to forcibly deliver the head and have a shoulder dystocia occur.

Prerequisites for applying forceps include (1) complete cervical dilatation, (2) ruptured membranes, (3) an engaged head, (4) known fetal position, (5) adequate analgesia, (6) assessment of the maternal pelvis–fetal size relationship, (7) capability for performing a cesarean section, (8) empty bladder and rectum, and (9) the presence of an experienced operator. Deviations from these requirements can result in a poor outcome.

Controversy regarding the safety of forceps-assisted delivery persists to the present time. However, a large study conducted by the Collaborative Perinatal Project involving approximately 30,000 babies, all undergoing periodic examinations for up to 4 years, failed to reveal any evidence that forceps operations increased the hazard of neonatal death or were associated with subsequent neurologic impairment of the neonates. Another large retrospective study from Israel revealed no physical or cognitive differences at 17 years of age among those born by instrumental vaginal, spontaneous vaginal, or cesarean section delivery. Conflicting data also surround midforceps delivery. This problem exists because some forceps operations are easy, whereas others are difficult; and a fair comparison cannot be made between the two. Regardless, persisting in attempts to effect vaginal delivery when it is obviously difficult may lead to unfavorable results. The maternal pelvic tissue is more frequently injured during these types of deliveries.

Over the past decade, there has been a decline in the frequency of forceps-assisted vaginal delivery and a reluctance to use midforceps extraction. According to a recent survey of residency programs, 14 percent do not even teach the techniques of midforceps delivery. This is alarming, for every obstetrician has been in a situation where fetal distress is present and a cesarean delivery is not immediately possible. A skillful forceps delivery in this scenario can be lifesaving.

Whereas forceps have been used in obstetrics for over four centuries, the *vacuum extractor* has been in use for only four decades. This device consists of a metal or plastic cup through which a vacuum suction is created after application to the fetal head. Traction is then applied during contractions. The force of suction should not exceed 0.8 kg/cm^2.

A definitive study comparing vacuum extraction to forceps delivery has not been carried out, although relevant data do suggest that vacuum extraction is associated with decreased maternal morbidity. Other advantages include its ease of application and the need for less anesthesia. The vacuum extractor can also be applied without decreasing the station of the head. It takes up very little space in the vagina, and does not cause deflexion of the head. It can also be used in special circumstances such as when fetal distress occurs in a second vertex twin when the station precludes the use of forceps, or for delivery of the fetal head through the uterine incision during a cesarean section.

Disadvantages include causing increased scalp trauma to the fetus and an increased failure-to-deliver rate. Fortunately, most of the trauma is mild in nature and rarely clinically serious. The artificial caput (chignon) that is created usually resolves within several hours, but may persist for 1 to 2 days. More important complications include subgaleal and retinal hemorrhages.

The indications for vacuum extraction are the same as those for forceps delivery. It is contraindicated for face or brow and breech presentations, if there is a suspected fetal coagulation defect, and if fetal scalp blood sampling has been done.

Many find the use of this device frustrating because there are no clear standards for its use. For example, how many "pulls" can be safely attempted, how many times can the device "pop off" the fetal head before the procedure should be abandoned, and what is the safe total time limit to effect delivery? These are questions that need to be addressed in the literature.

In summary, the same indications and requirements that pertain to forceps deliveries apply to the use of the vacuum extractor. Obstetricians need to be trained in the use of both modalities, and selection should be based on individual patient needs and circumstances. Every operator has his or her own preference, and there is something to be said for using an instrument with which one is comfortable; however, this should not be an excuse for a lack of skill in the full range of operative vaginal delivery techniques.

General
1. ACOG Committee on Obstetrics: Maternal and Fetal Medicine. Obstetric Forceps. *ACOG Committee Opinion* No. 71, August 1989.
   The entire classification of forceps has been revised to include new definitions for outlet-, low-, and midforceps procedures.

2. Dennen, P. C. *Dennen's Forceps Deliveries* (3rd ed.). Philadelphia: Davis, 1989.
   A well-illustrated, readable primer on the history, instruments, and techniques of forceps use.
3. Laufe, L. E., and Berkus, M. D. *Assisted Vaginal Delivery.* New York: McGraw-Hill, 1992.
   With an emphasis on forceps delivery, this authoritative book reviews all instrumented-assisted vaginal delivery techniques.
4. Ramin, S. M., et al. Survey of forceps delivery in North America in 1990. *Obstet. Gynecol.* 81:307, 1993.
   Compares the current use of forceps with the findings from a previous survey conducted in 1981.

Techniques/Indications
5. Boehm, F. H. Vacuum extraction during cesarean section. *South. Med. J.* 78:1502, 1985.
   The author describes the use of the vacuum extractor during cesarean section to facilitate the delivery of the presenting vertex.
6. Boyd, M. E., et al. Failed forceps. *Obstet. Gynecol.* 68:779, 1986.
   This large investigation (more than 6000 patients) assessed the reasons for failed forceps deliveries and noted that birth trauma was not increased in the setting of mid-forceps delivery, when it was successful.
7. Broekhuizen, F. F., et al. Vacuum extraction versus forceps delivery: indications and complications, 1979 to 1984. *Obstet. Gynecol.* 69:338, 1987.
   This retrospective study revealed that both modalities have their respective roles in contemporary obstetric practice.
8. Chow, S. L. S., et al. Rotational delivery with Kielland's forceps. *Med. J. Aust.* 146:616, 1987.
   The authors describe the results from a large study examining the use of the Kielland forceps. There was a 7.6 percent incidence of birth trauma associated with difficult forceps deliveries. The avoidance of pitfalls in these types of cases is emphasized.
9. Dell, D. L., Sightler, S. E., and Plauche, W. C. Soft cup vacuum extraction: a comparison of outlet delivery. *Obstet. Gynecol.* 66:624, 1985.
   One hundred patients were randomly assigned to undergo a forceps delivery, a Silastic vacuum extraction delivery, or delivery using the Mityvac vacuum extractor. All three instruments were considered effective for outlet delivery.
10. Schifrin, B. S. Polemics in perinatology: disengaging forceps. *J. Perinatol.* 8:242, 1988.
   The author's comments regarding forceps are set in a practical manner; this is a must-read article for persons who use forceps.
11. Williams, M. C., et al. A randomized comparison of assisted vaginal delivery by obstetric forceps and polyethylene vacuum cup. *Obstet. Gynecol.* 78:789, 1991.
   This prospective, randomized study revealed no significant differences in the safety or efficacy between these two modalities in a population undergoing predominantly low-pelvic assisted delivery.
12. Yeomans, E. R., and Hankins, G. D. V. Operative vaginal delivery in the 1990's. *Clin. Obstet. Gynecol.* 35:487, 1992.
   The authors provide contemporary guidelines for the proper conduct of instrumental delivery, including both forceps and vacuum extraction.

Complications
13. Punnonen, R., et al. Fetal and maternal effects of forceps and vacuum extraction. *Br. J. Obstet. Gynaecol.* 93:1132, 1986.
   In this large series, vacuum extraction and forceps delivery were compared, and there was a reduced incidence of low Apgar scores and a reduced amount of birth trauma associated with the latter.
14. Robertson, P. A., Laros, R. K., and Zhao, R. Neonatal and maternal outcome in

low-pelvic and midpelvic operative deliveries. *Am. J. Obstet. Gynecol.* 162:1436, 1990.

A retrospective analysis utilizing the updated American College of Obstetricians and Gynecelogists classifications of operative vaginal deliveries, which cautions against the use of midforceps or midvacuum delivery unless the maternal benefit is balanced carefully with the fetal risk.

15. Seidman, D. S., et al. Long-term effects of vacuum and forceps deliveries. *Lancet* 337:1583, 1991.

A retrospective review of more than 2600 instrumental vaginal deliveries compared to spontaneous vaginal delivery and cesarean section revealed no evidence of physical or cognitive impairment at 17 years of age associated with instrumental delivery.

33. CESAREAN BIRTH

Frank H. Boehm and Cornelia R. Graves

Cesarean birth is the delivery of an infant through an incision made in the abdominal and uterine walls. It has become the most commonly performed hospital-based operative procedure in the United States, accounting for approximately 25 percent of live births. Although cesarean delivery with the expectation of survival of both the mother and the fetus was proposed in the late 18th century and the first operation was performed in the early 19th century, the technique was not widely used until the 1920s. Improved surgical and anesthesia skills, antibiotic coverage, aseptic techniques, and blood availability have decreased the risks of this procedure. However, cesarean birth still poses a much greater risk to the mother, with a maternal mortality rate of 20 per 100,000 in the United States, compared with a maternal mortality rate of 2.5 per 100,000 for vaginal delivery. Indications for performing a primary cesarean section include dystocia (29%), breech or other abnormal presentation (15%), fetal distress (5%), and other maternal and fetal indications (45%).

Types of uterine incisions used in cesarean section are the low cervical (transverse or vertical) and the classic. Currently, a low-transverse incision is employed in more than 90 percent of the cesarean births. Low-cervical incisions are made into the portion of the uterus that is less muscular than other portions. This allows the physician to remove the infant through an area of the uterus that is less likely to rupture during subsequent pregnancies, more likely to heal without significant complications, and usually more hemostatic during the procedure. The low-vertical incision is usually employed in cases of breech or other malpresentation. The classic uterine incision is made in the upper active uterine segment. Although this incision allows for rapid uterine entry, possible complications include increased blood loss and a greater risk of uterine rupture before or during labor in a subsequent pregnancy.

Extraperitoneal cesarean section was first described by Frank in 1907. Before the availability of antibiotics, this technique was employed to minimize the occurrence of peritonitis. This procedure is still occasionally used to diminish the degree of serious postoperative infections when severe amnionitis is present at the time of delivery. However, with the increased availability and efficacy of antibiotic therapy, there is some controversy over whether this procedure is still needed.

A cesarean hysterectomy is a hysterectomy performed at the time of cesarean delivery, and it is usually an emergency procedure. The indications for emergency cesarean hysterectomy include placenta accreta (45%), uterine atony (20%), bleeding (15%), uterine rupture (10%), placenta percreta (5%), large leiomyoma (3%), and infection (1%). Elective cesarean hysterectomy as a means to achieve sterilization is generally regarded as carrying excessive risks because of the increased operative morbidity involved. Although cesarean hysterectomy is a more difficult operation, in experienced hands, it has been shown to be safe and may play an important role in the overall management of obstetrics patients in selected instances.

Elective cesarean sections are the major source of iatrogenic prematurity in the United States. Some studies have indicated that 1 to 20 percent of the cases of hyaline membrane disease (HMD) are the product of elective delivery. When some type of abdominal delivery must be performed before maturity, it is imperative to document, confirm, or be assured of fetal pulmonary maturity. This may be ascertained by early ultrasound (the first trimester is best for dating), reliable dates for the last menstrual period, quickening movements, auscultation of fetal heart tones with the fetoscope at 20 weeks, or early uterine examinations. Delivery no earlier than 39 weeks is advised by the American College of Obstetricians and Gynecologists. If the patient has diabetes during pregnancy, or dating cannot be firmly established, amniocentesis is recommended to confirm lung maturity by means of a series of lung phospholipid studies.

The anesthesia for cesarean birth is usually divided into two categories: a balanced general technique and regional blocks. Regional blocks usually make use of either the spinal or epidural technique. Regional anesthesia provides pain control, with minimal risk of aspiration in the patient. The advantage of epidural over spinal anesthesia is that the former provides a continuous dosage of anesthetic, thereby freeing the surgeon from concerns about the length of the operation. It can also be used for postoperative pain management. General anesthesia is frequently used in emergency situations. The major disadvantages of general anesthesia are the risk of aspiration and possible neonatal suppression. The advantages include its reliability, expeditious induction, and the avoidance of hypotension.

Regardless of the technique, it is important that the anesthesiologist be experienced in dealing with the physiologic changes in pregnancy and be aware of the fetal considerations.

For the past decade, rising cesarean section rates have been the subject of much attention from the medical and lay communities. In 1965, the cesarean birth rate in the United States was 4.5 per 100 births; by 1988, it had risen to 24.7 per 100 births. As approximately 25 percent of the cesarean sections in this country are repeat procedures, vaginal births after cesarean section (VBAC) have become increasingly supported by the medical community. The success rate for VBAC has been reported to range from about 60 percent for patients who underwent previous cesarean delivery because of pelvic dystocia to more than 70 percent for patients who had undergone cesarean delivery because of nonrecurring conditions, such as breech or fetal distress.

The advantages of vaginal birth include decreased maternal and neonatal morbidity, as well as decreased hospital time for both the mother and baby. The use of oxytocin or epidural anesthesia is not contraindicated in the setting of VBAC. A trial of labor should be recommended for all women in whom a nonclassic incision was made. The risk of uterine rupture, for which the dictum "once a cesarean section, always a cesarean section" was once invoked, is approximately 0.5 percent. Prenatal education regarding the risks and benefits, access to banked blood and anesthesia, as well as the capability for rapid cesarean delivery are recommended prerequisites for the trial of labor.

Although the incidence of maternal morbidity has decreased significantly with cesarean section, it is still between 8 and 12 times higher than that for a vaginal birth. The postoperative febrile morbidity associated with cesarean birth, depending on whether it is performed electively or during labor with ruptured membranes, ranges from 10 to 50 percent, but is markedly decreased with vaginal delivery (1–3%). Prophylactic antibiotic coverage can reduce the frequency of postoperative infection by 50 percent in high-risk patients. Risk factors for postoperative infection include maternal obesity, operation duration of more than 1 hour, blood loss of more than 800 ml, ruptured membranes, multiple examinations, internal pressure monitoring, and general anesthesia. This increase in maternal morbidity, along with a prolonged hospital stay, adds to the cost of health care, which are of concern to both the patient and the public.

While the cesarean section rates have increased, the incidence of cerebral palsy has remained constant. Although some studies implicate fetal monitoring as a reason for the overall increase in the number of cesarean sections performed, there are also data to indicate that fetal monitoring is not responsible. Changes in the management of breech presentation, a reluctance to perform difficult forceps deliveries, and a more aggressive approach to the high-risk obstetric patient, combined with the increased safety of the procedure and the changing medicolegal climate, have all contributed significantly to the increase in the number of cesarean births.

Risks to the fetus resulting from cesarean birth, including neonatal depression caused by anesthesia, incisional trauma to the fetus while entering the uterus, fetal blood loss while traversing an underlying placenta, and injury to the fetus during extraction procedures, as well as an increased likelihood of transient respiratory distress syndrome, are increased versus those in infants delivered vaginally.

General

1. Taffel, S. M., et al. 1989 U.S. cesarean section rate studies—VBAC rate rises to nearly one in five. *Birth* 18:2, 1991.
   The findings from this study suggest that the 25-year rise in the cesarean section rate may have plateaued as the vaginal birth rate has increased.

2. Porreco, R. P. High cesarean section rate: a new perspective. *Obstet. Gynecol.* 65:307, 1985.
   Using specific management criteria for common abdominal delivery indications, a primary cesarean birth rate of 5.7 percent was revealed; the Apgar scores and neonatal mortality did not differ from those cited for other studies with higher cesarean rates.

3. Beguin, E. A. Vaginal birth after cesarean section: what are the risks? *Female Patient* 13:16, 1988.
   An excellent general reference that summarizes the place of VBAC in the obstetrician's armamentarium. Recommendations for use are given.

4. Fraser, W., et al. Temporal variation in rates of cesarean section for dystocia: does "convenience" play a role? *Am. J. Obstet. Gynecol.* 156:300, 1987.
   The authors found that more cesarean sections were performed in the evening after office hours, but that this timing of cesarean birth did not have an overall effect on cesarean birth rates.

5. Shiono, P. H., et al. Recent trends in cesarean birth and trial of labor rates in the United States. *J.A.M.A.* 257:494, 1987.
   An excellent general reference regarding the number of cesarean births and the reasons why they are performed.

6. Ophir, E., et al. Trial of labor following cesarean section: dilemma. *Obstet. Gynecol. Surv.* 44:19, 1988.
   This fine article boasts 49 references covering all aspects of this very complicated subject. The authors' conclusions allow the clinician to more effectively manage patients undergoing VBAC.

7. Leveno, K. J., Cunningham, F. G., and Pritchard, J. A. Cesarean section: The House of Horne revisited. *Am. J. Obstet. Gynecol.* 160:78, 1989.
   The authors note that, although the cesarean birth rate is higher in the United States than it is in Ireland, the similar perinatal mortality rates are accounted for by the fact that U.S. hospitals have almost a five times greater low-birth-weight rate. When the populations are equalized, the increase in the cesarean section rate appears to be associated with a benefit to the infant.

Etiology

8. Rosen, M. G., et al. NIH consensus development statement on cesarean childbirth. *Obstet. Gynecol.* 57:537, 1981.
   The findings from a 2-year study conducted as the basis for a consensus development statement on cesarean section prepared by the National Institutes of Health are summarized in this article. It is must reading for all those interested in the increase in the rate of cesarean sections in our society.

9. Rosen, M. B., and Chik, L. The effect of delivery route on outcome in breech presentation. *Am. J. Obstet. Gynecol.* 149:909, 1984.
   No significant association was found between outcome and birth route, except in the footling breech, if the infant was alive at the start of labor and had no major abnormalities.

10. Oshan, A. F., et al. Cesarean birth and neonatal mortality in very low birth weight infants. *Obstet. Gynecol.* 64:267, 1984.
    After adjustment for birth weight, presentation, and the place of birth, cesarean birth was not associated with a decreased mortality rate in very-low-birth-weight infants.

11. Phelan, J. P. Delivery following cesarean section and perinatal mortality. *Am. J. Perinatol.* 6:95, 2089.
    This is a nice editorial that sums up well the experience with VBAC. A good narrative of the experience is also included.

12. Phelan, J. P., et al. Twice a cesarean, always a cesarean? *Obstet. Gynecol.* 73:161, 1989.
    In an effort to increase the number of VBACs, the authors looked at the records of more than 6250 women who had had cesarean sections. Of these, 1088 had had two previous cesarean sections and underwent a trial of labor, with 69 percent delivering vaginally. They also believed that the use of oxytocin is integral to a successful VBAC rate.

13. Gould, J., Davey, B., and Stafford, R. Socioeconomic differences in rates of cesarean section. *N. Engl. J. Med.* 321:233, 1989.
    Several reports suggest that the rate of cesarean section is increased in direct proportion to the patient's socioeconomic status.

Diagnosis

14. Read, J. A. The scheduling of repeat cesarean section operations: prospective management protocol experience. *Am. J. Obstet. Gynecol.* 151:557, 1985.
    In a controlled environment (Army Medical Corps), a protocol for delineating previous cesarean sections with good dates was used to schedule delivery without the need for amniocentesis or labor onset. Almost half the patients managed by this method delivered electively without problems in the mother or the baby.

15. Gilstrap, L. C., III, Hauth, J. C., and Toussaint, S. Cesarean section: changing incidence and indications. *Obstet. Gynecol.* 63:205, 1984.
    Meticulous monitoring and rapid responses to dystocia and fetal distress may help decrease the incidence of primary cesarean section.

16. Lonky, N. M., Worthen, N., and Ross, M. G. Prediction of cesarean section scars with ultrasound imaging during pregnancy. *J. Ultrasound Med.* 8:15, 1089.
    The authors used ultrasound to examine 47 women who had undergone previous cesarean sections. Scars were visualized well in 28 percent; this may be helpful in patients with an unknown incision who are considering vaginal birth after a cesarean.

Treatment

17. Ayers, J. W. T., and Morley, G. W. Surgical incision for cesarean section. *Obstet. Gynecol.* 70:706, 1987.
    The authors assess the operative morbidity in relation to the abdominal incision. They conclude that, as long as the incision is adequate, the type of incision does not play a role in the morbidity of either the mother or the baby.

18. Flamm, B. L., et al. Oxytocin during labor after previous cesarean section: results of a multicenter study. *Obstet. Gynecol.* 70:709, 1987.
    This large series consisting of 776 patients demonstrates that it is wise to use oxytocin in patients who have had previous cesarean births.

19. Flamm, B. L., et al. Vaginal birth after cesarean section: results of a multicenter study. *Am. J. Obstet. Gynecol.* 158:1079, 1988.
    This is the largest series to date of patients undergoing labor after previous cesarean birth (4929 patients); the authors did not discover a single maternal or perinatal death that was related to uterine scar rupture.

20. Phelan, J. P., et al. Vaginal birth after cesarean. *Am. J. Obstet. Gynecol.* 157:1510, 1987.
    This report on a large series of patients undergoing vaginal birth after cesarean section notes that the benefits to the patient associated with a trial of labor out-

weigh the risks. The policy of "once a cesarean section, always a cesarean section" should be abandoned.

21. Haynes, D. M., and Martin, B. J. Cesarean hysterectomy: a twenty-five year review. *Am. J. Obstet. Gynecol.* 134:393, 1979.
    This 25-year review of 149 cesarean hysterectomies suggests that cesarean hysterectomy should remain a part of the obstetrician's repertoire, but that it may not be advisable for strictly elective indications.
22. ACOG-AAP. Guidelines for Vaginal Delivery After a Previous Cesarean Birth. In *Perinatal Guidelines* (3rd ed.). Washington, D.C.: American College of Obstetricians and Gynecologists, 1992.
    These American College of Obstetricians and Gynecologists and American Academy of Pediatrics guidelines for vaginal delivery after a previous cesarean section have been updated and emphasize the benefits of a vaginal delivery after a previous cesarean section, as well as the need for each hospital to develop its own protocol for management.

Complications
23. Gibbs, R. S., Blanco, J. D., and St. Clain, P. J. A case-control study of wound abscess after cesarean delivery. *Obstet. Gynecol.* 62:498, 1983.
    An excellent review of the complications associated with wound abscess.
24. Duff, P. Pathophysiology and management of postcesarean endomyometritis. *Obstet. Gynecol.* 67:269, 1986.
    This article describes the pathophysiology and management of postcesarean endomyometritis and is an excellent review of the subject.
25. Emmons, S. L., et al. Development of wound infections among women undergoing cesarean section. *Obstet. Gynecol.* 72:559, 1988.
    In more than 1000 women undergoing cesarean birth, wound infections were most often due to Staphylococcus aureus, *and the attack rate was not related to prolonged labor or other factors during labor.*
26. Stanco, L. M., et al. Emergency peripartum hysterectomy and associated risk factors. *Am. J. Obstet. Gynecol.* 168:879, 1993.
    A review of 123 cases of emergency cesarean hysterectomy encountered in a large university center during 1985 to 1990.

34. FAILURE TO PROGRESS IN LABOR
Rick W. Martin

The term *labor* refers to the progressive dilatation of the uterine cervix in the presence of repetitive uterine contractions. *Failure to progress* refers to the lack of progressive cervical dilatation or descent of the fetal head. There are three stages of labor. The first stage of labor begins with the onset of labor and lasts to the time of full cervical dilatation. The second stage of labor follows, and continues until delivery of the infant. The period after delivery of the infant until delivery of the placenta is the third stage of labor. The first stage of labor can be depicted graphically. If time is plotted on the abscissa and cervical dilatation on the ordinate, two phases are described, latent and active. The active phase of labor is further divided into the acceleration phase, which is the phase with a maximum slope, and the deceleration phase. Active labor usually begins when the cervix is dilated 3 to 4 cm and the rate of cervical dilatation is also notably increased from the latent phase. Abnormal labor patterns have been characterized by Friedman. A prolonged latent phase lasts more than 20 hours in the nulligravida and 14 hours in the multipara. There are also protraction disorders of dilatation (<1.2 cm/hr, nulligravida; <1.5 cm/hr, multigravida) and descent (change in station <1 cm/hr in the nulligravida and <2 cm/hr in the multipara in the second stage of labor). Arrest of dilatation is deemed to occur when cervical dilatation has ceased for more than 2 hours. Arrest of descent occurs after a 1-hour interval.

Arrest of cervical dilatation may be primary or secondary. A prolonged latent phase is often treated with a therapeutic rest, in which the mother is given sedation with morphine or meperidine. When the mother awakens from the sedation, the contractions will either have subsided, indicating that the patient was not in true labor, or the contractions will resume in a more effective manner. X-ray pelvimetry is rarely used today to assess pelvic size, but the pelvis should be assessed clinically. A clinical estimation of fetal weight should also be obtained. Although an ultrasound-derived estimation of fetal weight is somewhat inaccurate, ultrasonography may be performed to help identify an extremely large fetus or a fetal anomaly that might interfere with normal cervical dilatation. One simple method for determining the adequacy of the pelvis for vaginal delivery is the Müller-Hillis maneuver, which consists of exerting pressure on the fundus while performing a vaginal examination. An impression of easy downward movement of the presenting part suggests that the pelvis is adequate. Once the active phase of labor is reached and failure to progress has occurred, many authors prefer to rupture the membranes and insert an intrauterine pressure catheter for better evaluation of uterine activity. Although there is a wide range of uterine activity that is considered adequate, contractions of at least 50 mm Hg occurring every 2 to 3 minutes and lasting 45 to 60 seconds are desirable.

Cephalopelvic disproportion is responsible for the arrest disorder in as many as 50 percent of the women, and these women require cesarean section for delivery. If it is the labor that is judged inadequate, gentle augmentation with an oxytocin infusion is recommended. An interval of 40 to 60 minutes after initiating an oxytocin infusion is required for a steady-state concentration to be reached. Oxytocin is administered in a balanced-salt solution via a controlled-infusion device. Careful monitoring of the fetal heartbeat is advised, and the oxytocin infusion is discontinued if any signs of fetal distress appear. The patient must also be observed for possible uterine hyperstimulation. The infusion is increased by 1 to 2 mU/min over a 30-minute interval until an adequate labor pattern is established. The findings from early studies suggested that perinatal morbidity was higher when the second stage of labor exceeded 2 hours. With the availability of fetal monitoring, a longer time is now allowable, as long as the fetal heart rate remains satisfactory. The effects of epidural anesthesia may lengthen the second stage of labor, and the use of forceps for delivery to shorten the second stage is also increased in this setting.

In attempts to lower a rising cesarean section rate that may exceed 20 percent, investigators in Europe have adopted a strategy of active management of labor. Once labor is diagnosed, the longest acceptable interval to delivery is considered to be 12 hours. When hourly examinations document a rate of progress of less than 1 cm per hour, an oxytocin infusion is begun. Amniotomy was also performed at an earlier time in labor. Using this policy, a cesarean rate of 4.8 percent was achieved.

In summary, the appropriate management of arrest or protraction disorders of labor requires careful attention to the progress of labor. Cervicographic analysis is often helpful for this purpose. Assessment of fetal size, pelvic dimensions and uterine forces is necessary to achieve an optimal outcome for both the mother and the baby.

1. Lopez-Zeno, J. A., et al. A controlled trial of the program for the active management of labor. *N. Engl. J. Med.* 326:450, 1992.
   An active plan for the management of labor consisting of early amniotomy and a higher rate of oxytocin infusion increased the rate of vaginal delivery without increasing maternal and neonatal morbidity.
2. Dystocia. *ACOG Tech. Bull.* No. 137, December 1989.
   An excellent review of the stages of labor and approaches to the management of failure to progress.
3. Induction and augmentation of labor. *ACOG Tech. Bull.* No. 157, July 1991.
   General guidelines are given for the use of oxytocin.
4. O'Driscoll, K., Foley, M., and MacDonald, D. Active management of labor as an alternative to cesarean section for dystocia. *Obstet. Gynecol.* 63:485, 1984.

A cesarean section rate of 4.8 percent was achieved at the National Maternity Hospital in Dublin through the active management of labor.

5. Seitchick, J., and Castillo, M. Oxytocin augmentation of dysfunctional labor: I. Clinical data. *Am. J. Obstet. Gynecol.* 144:899, 1982.
   The authors recommend that the oxytocin infusion be increased by 1 mU/min at intervals of not less than 30 minutes. This regimen was effective, and hyperstimulation was avoided in most cases.

6. Friedman, E. A. Normal and Dysfunctional Labor. In W. R. Cohen, D. B. Acker, and E. A. Friedman (eds.), *Management of Labor* (2nd ed.). Rockville, MD: Aspen Publishers, 1989.
   An excellent overview of normal and dysfunctional labor.

7. Bishop, E. H. Pelvic scoring for elective induction. *Obstet. Gynecol.* 24:260, 1964.
   A scoring system is presented to evaluate patients for elective induction based on different variables determined by vaginal examination.

8. Piper, J. M., Bolling, D. R., and Newton, E. R. The second stage of labor: factors influencing duration. *Am. J. Obstet. Gynecol.* 165:976, 1991.
   A prolonged second stage of labor was associated with the use of epidural anesthesia, a prolonged active-phase duration, lower maternal parity, excess maternal weight gain, and increasing fetal weight.

9. Bottoms, S. F., Hirsch, V. J., and Sokol, R. J. Medical management of arrest disorders of labor: a current overview. *Am. J. Obstet. Gynecol.* 156:939, 1987.
   With medical management, arrest disorders were not associated with an increased risk of adverse perinatal outcome.

10. Whittels, B. Does epidural anesthesia affect the course of labor and delivery? *Semin. Perinatol.* 15:358, 1991.
    A review of the various techniques of epidural anesthesia and their effect on the course of labor is presented.

11. Johnson, N., Johnson, V. A., and Gupta, J. K. Maternal positions during labor. *Obstet. Gynecol. Surv.* 46:428, 1991.
    An interesting overview of the effect of maternal position on the fetus and labor progress.

12. Balas, E. A., et al. A computer method for visual presentation and programmed evaluation of labor. *Obstet. Gynecol.* 78:419, 1991.
    A computer-generated display of labor curves facilitated interpretation of labor progress.

13. Morgan, M. A., and Thurnau, G. R. Efficacy of the fetal-pelvic index in nulliparous women at high risk for fetal-pelvic disproportion. *Am. J. Obstet. Gynecol.* 166:810, 1992.
    A combination of the ultrasonography-derived estimation of fetal weight with x-ray pelvimetry findings was utilized to develop a fetal-pelvic index.

14. Johnson, J. W. C., Longmate, J. A., and Frentzen, B. Excessive maternal weight and pregnancy outcome. *Am. J. Obstet. Gynecol.* 167:353, 1992.
    An increased maternal weight gain in pregnancy resulted in a higher frequency of fetal macrosomia with an associated increase in the cesarean section rate.

15. Chelmow, D., and Laros, R. K. Maternal and neonatal outcomes after oxytocin augmentation in patients undergoing a trial of labor after prior cesarean delivery. *Obstet. Gynecol.* 80:966, 1992.
    The findings from this retrospective analysis support the use of oxytocin and epidural anesthesia to augment labor after a prior cesarean section.

16. Rosen, M. G., et al. Abnormal labor and infant brain damage. *Obstet. Gynecol.* 80:961, 1992.
    A diagnosis of failure to progress was not associated with increased neurologic abnormalities in infants. Neither the method of delivery nor the use of oxytocin were factors in the etiology of infant brain damage.

17. Satin, A. J., et al. High- versus low-dose oxytocin for labor stimulation. *Obstet. Gynecol.* 80:111, 1992.
    High-dose oxytocin therapy to augment ineffective labor minimized the number of cesarean sections for dystocia but increased the cesarean rate for fetal distress.

18. Thorp, P. J. A., et al. Epidural analgesia and cesarean section for dystocia: risk factors in nulliparas. *Am. J. Perinatol.* 8:402, 1991.
    Epidural analgesia may lead to an increase in cesarean sections performed for dystocia in nulliparas.

35. CEPHALOPELVIC DISPROPORTION
Baha M. Sibai

Normal labor is characterized by the progressive effacement and dilatation of the cervix, associated with descent of the fetal presenting part. During the cervical changes that begin either during or before the latent phase of labor, the cervix undergoes significant biochemical changes in the ground substance structure, reticulum, and water content. The rate of dilatation accelerates rapidly during the active phase, is complete by the end of the first stage, and depends on uterine contractions of adequate intensity and frequency. Descent of the fetal head begins during the last 2 weeks of gestation in about 80 percent of primigravidas, is maximal during the deceleration phase of labor, and depends on uterine contractions, maternal pelvic capacity, and fetal factors.

Most labors progress in a normal fashion, leading to spontaneous vaginal delivery, but a small percentage manifest abnormal patterns of progress, in the form of protraction or arrest of dilatation, descent, or both, as measured by the Friedman labor curve or partogram. This dystocia represents a potential adverse effect on the fetus and mother. Consequently, it is prudent for all obstetric providers to recognize these abnormal patterns as early as possible, so that an orderly, systematic plan of management can be undertaken.

Cephalopelvic disproportion (CPD) is defined as the inability of the presenting part of the fetal head to pass through the maternal pelvis. CPD is responsible for most abnormal labor patterns if uterine activity, as measured by intrauterine pressure monitoring, is adequate. It occurs in about 1 to 3 percent of all primigravidas and in 30 percent of those who have a protracted active phase of dilatation or descent, while about 50 percent of these parturients have an arrest of descent. CPD is categorized into two sets of factors: (1) maternal factors, which include the size and shape of the bony pelvis as well as soft tissue resistance, and (2) fetal factors, which include size, presentation, position, and moldability of the fetal head. Clinical evaluation of pelvic capacity can be performed by digital examination during the first antepartum visit, and typing of the pelvis should be carried out according to the Caldwell-Moloy classification (i.e., gynecoid, android, anthropoid, or platypelloid). Attention must be directed to the diagonal conjugate, the inclination of the pelvic side walls, the prominence of the ischial spines, the shape of the sacrum, and the angle of the suprapubic arch. About 85 percent of the patients will have a clinically adequate pelvic capacity; 1 percent will have a clearly inadequate pelvis; and the remainder will have a "borderline" pelvis. The following findings indicate a possible contracted pelvis: (1) ability to touch the sacral promontory with the index finger; (2) significant convergence of the side walls; (3) forward inclination of a straight sacrum; (4) sharp ischial spines with a narrow interspinous diameter; (5) a narrow suprapubic arch; (6) a congenital sacral abnormality; (7) a history of difficult labor; (8) maternal disease, such as rickets or polio, and trauma; and (9) adolescent pregnancy. Digital pelvimetry should be repeated during the intrapartum period, with attention paid to the fetal-pelvic relationship, so that the pelvic capacity can be gauged against the presenting fetal part.

The presence of abnormal progress in labor (dystocia) may be the first evidence of pelvic inadequacy. Because about 45 percent of patients who experience secondary arrest of dilatation or descent, or both, have CPD, careful evaluation is mandatory before labor stimulation is utilized. Ultrasound imaging and x-ray pelvimetry to determine the fetal head size are used by some to compare pelvic capacity with the fetal vertex, but there is much controversy regarding the benefits of such techniques. Some clinicians believe that the benefits may far outweigh the theoretical risk from radiation exposure, whereas the majority believe that the knowledge imparted by these tests may not be helpful in clinical management.

Maternal risks associated with CPD include abnormal thinning of the lower uterine segment with possible uterine rupture, pressure necrosis of the bladder, pelvic lacerations associated with instrument delivery, postpartum hemorrhage, and increased postpartum uterine infections. Fetal risks include fetal distress (10%), cord prolapse, intracranial hemorrhage, skull fracture, and long-term neurologic abnormalities.

Proper management of CPD involves early recognition during labor, identification of the cause, and prompt institution of therapy. A good initial history and physical examination, with a high index of suspicion in those with predisposing factors, is a most important initial step. Attention should be given to the position and presentation of the fetal head, as noted during a combined abdominal and pelvic examination, with special emphasis on the thrust of the fetal head into the birth canal during contractions or when applying fundal pressure (the Müller-Hillis maneuver). In many cases, particularly in primigravidas, the active management of labor, which includes early amniotomy, use of oxytocin in the latent phase, and aggressive treatment of arrest or protraction disorders, may help in preventing the need for cesarean delivery previously deemed to be due to CPD. On the other hand, the identification of dystocia, which assumes the form of protraction or arrest disorders, should be a warning sign of CPD. Dystocia is usually best detected by frequent assessment during labor and the use of a labor graph or partogram in each pregnancy.

The association of documented CPD with abnormal patterns of progress, in the form of arrest of dilatation or descent, is an indication for cesarean birth without any further trial of labor. The use of oxytocin (Pitocin) stimulation or midforceps procedures in the presence of probable CPD or arrest patterns of labor is usually unsuccessful. In other cases of borderline CPD with dystocia or in patients with inadequate labor, oxytocin stimulation may be indicated. Recent reports emphasize the importance of aggressively managed labor, with oxytocin stimulation an alternative to performing an abdominal delivery in those with borderline CPD. In addition, the use of an intrauterine catheter and pressure-curve integrator to measure uterine activity, coupled with a specific computer-defined goal of contractile activity, has made it much safer to use oxytocin stimulation in cases of borderline CPD. Once CPD is diagnosed, cesarean delivery is the treatment of choice.

General
1. Bowes, W. A. Clinical Aspects of Normal and Abnormal Labor. In R. K. Creasy and R. Resnik (eds.), *Maternal-Fetal Medicine: Principles and Practice.* Philadelphia: Saunders, 1989.
   The physiology and normal progress of labor are detailed. Abnormal forms of labor during the first and second stage are described, and the diagnosis and management of these abnormalities are detailed.
2. Induction and augmentation of labor. *ACOG Tech. Bull.* No. 157, November 1991.
   Details the indications for and contraindications to induction of labor and the methods used for oxytocin administration; new dosage schedules are recommended.

Etiology
3. Fairlie, F. M., et al. An analysis of uterine activity in spontaneous labour using a microcomputer. *Br. J. Obstet. Gynaecol.* 95:57, 1988.
   A significant parity-related difference in the contraction frequency was observed in the first stage but not in the second stage (higher activity in the nulliparous). Epidural analgesia did not appear to influence uterine activity in the first stage but was associated with a lower mean active pressure, contraction frequency, and intensity in the second stage.

4. Fisk, N. M., and Shweni, P. M. Labor outcome of juvenile primipara in a population with a high incidence of contracted pelvis. *Int. J. Gynecol. Obstet.* 28:5, 1989.

   The authors compare the labor outcome in primiparous women younger than 17 years of age with that observed in the normal population. There was no difference in the rate of cesarean birth in this population, but the incidence of operative delivery, low birth weight, and perinatal mortality was higher among the adolescents.

5. Thurnau, G. R., et al. Evaluation of the fetal-pelvic relationship. *Clin. Obstet. Gynecol.* 35:570, 1992.

   This review provides a historical and analytic approach to the study of fetal-pelvic relationships. In addition, methods of evaluating the fetal-pelvic relationship, as well as current concepts on this subject, are described.

6. Dystocia. *ACOG Tech. Bull.* No. 137, December 1989.

   The etiology, diagnosis, and management of dystocia are summarized in detail.

7. Harbert, G. M., Jr. Assessment of uterine contractility and activity. *Clin. Obstet. Gynecol.* 35:546, 1992.

   The physiology as well as the methods of measuring uterine contractility and activity are detailed. Abnormal forms of uterine contractility leading to dysfunctional patterns of labor during the first and second stage are reviewed and the clinical management of these patterns is described.

Diagnosis

8. O'Brien, W. F., and Cefalo, R. C. Evaluation of x-ray pelvimetry and abnormal labor. *Clin. Obstet. Gynecol.* 25:157, 1982.

   The authors review the history, anatomic basis, and current systems of x-ray pelvimetry. The risks and benefits are also summarized. They conclude that the use of intrapartum x-ray pelvimetry does not lead to an improved perinatal outcome, and its potential risks outweigh its benefits.

9. Yamazaki, H., and Uchida, K. A mathematical approach to problems of cephalopelvic disproportion of the pelvic inlet. *Am. J. Obstet. Gynecol.* 147:25, 1983.

   The authors describe a mathematical formula to calculate a pelvic index based on a calculation of the ratio between an area of the pelvic inlet plane and a cross-area of the fetal skull. They suggest that this index may serve as a guide to the proper management of labor in patients with CPD.

10. Raman, S., et al. A comparative study of x-ray pelvimetry and CT pelvimetry. *Aust. N.Z. J. Obstet. Gynaecol.* 31:217, 1991.

    The results of conventional erect lateral x-ray pelvimetry were compared to those yielded by computed tomagraphic (CT) pelvimetry in 24 patients who had a cesarean section for various obstetric reasons. The risks and benefits are also summarized. The authors conclude that CT pelvimetry is preferred and should be performed postpartum in nulliparous women who were delivered by cesarean section for CPD or who had difficult forceps delivery.

11. Morgan, M. A., and Thurnau, G. R. Efficacy of the fetal-pelvic index in nulliparous women at high risk for fetal-pelvic disproportion. *Am. J. Obstet. Gynecol.* 166:810, 1992.

    The fetal-pelvic index and two other methods of identifying fetal-pelvic disproportion (estimated fetal weight >4000 g derived from ultrasound measurement and Mengert's index) were compared with respect to the clinical outcome as well as the accuracy of predicting the presence of CPD in 137 nulliparous women at high risk for CPD. The authors found the fetal-pelvic index to be more efficacious than ultrasonography or x-ray pelvimetry in determining the presence or absence of CPD.

Treatment

12. Chazotte, C., and Cohen W. R. Drug use selection for latent-phase labor. *Contemp. Ob/Gyn* 30:73, 1987.

    Many drugs are available for influencing contractility and relieving pain during the latent phase of labor. This report reviews the benefits and side effects of the various drugs during this stage.

13. Bottoms, S. F., Hirsch, V. J., and Sokkol, J. Medical management of arrest disorders of labor: current overviews. *Am. J. Obstet. Gynecol.* 156:935, 1987.
This report analyzes the management and outcome in 5399 births selected to rule out risks clearly not caused by abnormal labor. Arrest disorders occurred in 11 percent, and medical management was used in 96 percent of these cases. Fifty percent of the patients in this group delivered without oxytocin stimultion, and only 21 percent in this group required cesarean section.

14. Satin, A. J., et al. Factors affecting the dose response to oxytocin for labor stimulation. *Am. J. Obstet. Gynecol.* 166:1260, 1992.
The authors used a computerized database to determine the obstetric variables affecting the dose response to oxytocin for labor stimulation in 1773 pregnancies. They found that gestational age, parity, and cervical dilatation influenced the pregnancy response to oxytocin. However, they found considerable variability in the response to oxytocin, suggesting that these risk factors were not useful in predicting the dose response to oxytocin for labor stimulation.

15. Muller, P. R., et al. A prospective randomized clinical trial comparing two oxytocin induction protocols. *Am. J. Obstet. Gynecol.* 167:373, 1992.
One hundred fifty-one women were randomized into one of two oxytocin induction protocols. One protocol consisted of the gradual increase in the dose of 1 to 2 mU/ min at 30-minute intervals (n = 76) and the other protocol consisted of doubling the rate of oxytocin administration every 40 minutes (n = 75). The authors found that induction with larger dose increments resulted in a shorter time until adequate labor was achieved, without an associated increase in uterine hyperstimulation or poor neonatal outcome. However, the larger-dose protocol was associated with a higher frequency of altered fetal heart rate changes during induction.

16. Owen, J., and Hauth, J. C. Oxytocin for the induction or augmentation of labor. *Clin. Obstet. Gynecol.* 35:464, 1992.
Details the methods of oxytocin administration; new dosage schedules are compared; and recommendations for induction and augmentation of labor are made.

17. Lopez-Zeno, J. A., et al. A controlled trial of a program for the active management of labor. *N. Engl. J Med.* 326:450, 1992.
The authors describe a program for labor management that consists of early amniotomy plus administering oxytocin at an initial rate of 6 mU/ min, which is subsequently increased by 6 mU/min every 15 minutes (to a maximum of 36 mU/ min) until there are seven contractions every 15 minutes. This program reduced the incidence of dystocia and increased the rate of vaginal delivery without increasing maternal or neonatal morbidity.

Complications

18. Seitchik, J., Holden, A. E. C., and Castillo, M. Amniotomy and oxytocin treatment of functional dystocia and route of delivery. *Am. J. Obstet. Gynecol.* 155:585, 1986.
The authors describe the details of clinical management in 101 nulliparous patients with functional dystocia who underwent amniotomy and were treated with oxytocin in the first stage of labor. Sixty-eight delivered vaginally, and 33 were delivered by cesarean section.

19. Saunders, N. G., et al. Neonatal and maternal morbidity in relation to the length of the second stage of labour. *Br. J. Obstet. Gynaecol.* 99:381, 1992.
Maternal and neonatal morbidity were correlated to the duration of the second stage of labor in 25,069 women who gave birth to an infant of at least 37 weeks' gestation after the spontaneous onset of labor. The risks of both postpartum hemorrhage and maternal infection were increased in relation to an increased second stage of labor. In contrast, the duration of the second stage of labor was not associated with a poor neonatal outcome. The authors conclude that second-stage labors of up to 3 hours' duration are not associated with fetal risks.

20. Cahill, D., et al. Does oxytocin augmentation increase perinatal risk in primigravid labor? *Am. J. Obstet. Gynecol.* 166:847, 1992.
The occurrence of adverse maternal and perinatal outcomes was analyzed in

30,874 primigravid term deliveries in which high-dose oxytocin augmentation was used. The authors conclude that high-dose oxytocin stimulation to correct dystocia is safe for both the mother and fetus.

36. FETAL DISTRESS IN THE INTRAPARTUM PERIOD
Rick W. Martin

Although the term *fetal distress* is used to describe a variety of fetal situations, most physicians associate this phrase with fetal asphyxia. *Asphyxia* generally refers to fetal hypoxia and metabolic acidosis. Because of the decreased uterine blood flow during contractions, labor is associated with a relative fetal hypoxia. Usually this is tolerated well by the normal fetus, and fetal heart rate monitoring is the most widely used method to evaluate fetal status in labor. The fetal heart rate may be determined by simple auscultation with a fetoscope or by electronic monitoring. If auscultation is chosen, low-risk patients are monitored every 30 minutes during the active phase of labor and at least every 15 minutes in the second stage of labor. The intervals are decreased for high-risk patients, with auscultation performed every 15 minutes in the active phase of labor and every 5 minutes in the second stage of labor. The findings from current studies indicate that there is little difference in outcome regardless of whether electronic monitoring or auscultation is used, though many busy obstetric services find they cannot perform auscultation according to the standards just described.

The normal fetal heart rate varies between 120 and 160 beats per minute, although rates slightly above and below this may be considered normal in the absence of ominous patterns. Accelerations of the fetal heart during contractions are generally considered to be a reassuring pattern. The short-term fetal heart rate variability (beat-to-beat) usually varies between 3 and 7 beats per minute. Loss of short-term variability may suggest fetal hypoxia, but other factors may also be responsible, such as the fetal sleep state or the effect of drugs administered to the mother.

Certain periodic changes in the fetal heart rate have been observed in association with uterine contractions. There are three classic types of changes: early, variable, and late decelerations. Early decelerations usually mirror the effect of uterine contraction on the fetal heart rate tracing, with the heart rate returning to baseline as the contraction is completed. Fetal head compression with descent into the birth canal is the usual explanation for this phenomenon. Variable decelerations occur at different times in association with uterine contractions. In these, there is a more rapid decrease in the rate and a quicker return to the baseline, and they are thought to be due to compression of the umbilical cord, as might occur in the presence of a nuchal cord or cord compression in the setting of oligohydramnios. Although mild variable decelerations are tolerated well, more severe ones may result in fetal acidosis. When the fetal heart rate pattern is symmetrical with the uterine contraction but returns to baseline only after completion of the contraction, this is deemed a late deceleration. Repetitive late decelerations may be associated with fetal distress approximately 50 percent of the time. A more ominous pattern is late decelerations in the presence of decreased beat-to-beat variability.

Certain measures may improve the fetal status if the fetal heart rate is abnormal. If oxytocic agents are being administered, they should be discontinued. Maternal hydration may improve intervillous perfusion and administering oxygen to the mother may enhance placental gas exchange. In addition, the mother should be placed in the lateral decubitus position to improve uterine blood flow. If the ominous fetal heart rate pattern is corrected, then further observation is indicated. In the presence of a nonreassuring fetal heart rate pattern, the physician must decide between immediate delivery by cesarean section or further observation. Because of the high false-positive rate observed for fetal heart rate monitoring, some physicians elect to perform fetal scalp pH sampling in this situation. This procedure is technically cumbersome, but values greater than 7.25 pH would permit further observation. A scalp blood pH of less than 7.20 is generally an indication for medical or surgical intervention.

At the time of delivery, the infant may have a low Apgar score, but this does not necessarily correlate with fetal acidosis. This is especially true in the preterm infant. Some recommend obtaining umbilical cord arterial blood gas measurements to better determine the neonatal status. Using the term *birth asphyxia* to refer to the diagnosis is not recommended, as it is an imprecise term. For a possible neurologic deficit to be associated with perinatal asphyxia, the following criteria should be met: (1) profound umbilical artery acidemia (pH <7.0); (2) an Apgar score of less than 3 after 5 minutes; (3) neonatal neurologic sequelae such as seizures; and (4) multiorgan system dysfunction, which may include cardiovascular, gastrointestinal, pulmonary, or renal difficulties.

General
1. Parer, J. T., and Livingston, E. G. What is fetal distress? *Am. J. Obstet. Gynecol.* 162:1421, 1990.
   An excellent discussion of the fetal response to asphyxia.
2. Sandmire, H. F. Whither electronic fetal monitoring? *Obstet. Gynecol.* 76:1130, 1990.
   A protocol for auscultation of the fetal heart rate is presented, and some of the problems with electronic fetal monitoring are also reviewed.
3. Intrapartum Fetal Heart Rate Monitoring. *ACOG Tech. Bull.* No. 132, September 1989.
   Current practices in intrapartum fetal heart rate monitoring are reviewed.
4. Sykes, G. S., et al. Do Apgar scores indicate asphyxia? *Lancet* 1:494, 1982.
   Only 19 percent of the babies with a 5-minute Apgar score less than 7 had severe acidosis.
5. Petrie, R. H. Intrapartum Fetal Evaluation. In S. G. Gabbe, J. R. Niebyl, and J. L. Simpson (eds.), *Obstetrics: Normal and Problem Pregnancies.* New York: Churchill Livingstone, 1991.
   Good summary of fetal heart rate monitoring, along with some discussion of the underlying physiology.
6. Morrison, J. C., et al. Intrapartum fetal heart rate assessment: monitoring by auscultation or electronic means. *Am. J. Obstet. Gynecol.* 168:63, 1993.
   Auscultation performed in accordance with standard recommendations is not feasible on a busy obstetric service.
7. Quirk, J. G., and Miller, F. C. FHR tracing characteristics that jeopardize the diagnosis of fetal well-being. *Clin. Obstet. Gynecol.* 29:12, 1986.
   Excellent review of available information on intrapartum fetal monitoring as it relates to perinatal death and fetal acid-base status.

Acid-Base Evaluation
8. Low, J. A., et al. The prediction of intrapartum fetal metabolic acidosis by fetal heart rate monitoring. *Am. J. Obstet. Gynecol.* 139:299, 1981.
   The probability of fetal metabolic acidosis was 48 percent in the presence of late decelerations.
9. Assessment of Fetal and Newborn Acid-Base Status. *ACOG Tech. Bull.* No. 127, April 1989.
   The types of acidemia and the interpretation of umbilical cord gas values are reviewed. Umbilical artery pH values of less than 7.0 more realistically reflect clinically significant acidosis.
10. Perkins, R. P. Perinatal observations in a high-risk population managed without intrapartum fetal pH studies. *Am. J. Obstet. Gynecol.* 149:327, 1984.
    Intrapartum fetal scalp blood pH studies were not utilized in this institution. The rates of stillbirth, operative intervention, and neonatal compromise did not appear to be increased over those observed in institutions using this method.
11. Clark, S. L., Gimobsky, M. L., and Miller, M. C. Fetal heart rate response to scalp blood sampling. *Am. J. Obstet. Gynecol.* 144:706, 1982.

Fetal heart rate accelerations in response to scalp blood sampling were associated with a scalp pH greater than 7.20.

12. Goldenberg, R. L., Huddleston, J. F., and Nelson, K. G. Apgar scores and umbilical arterial pH in preterm newborn infants. *Am. J. Obstet. Gynecol.* 149:651, 1984.
    In preterm infants, little correlation between the Apgar score and the umbilical cord pH was observed.

13. Page, F. O., et al. Correlation of neonatal acid-base status with Apgar scores and fetal heart rate tracings. *Am. J. Obstet. Gynecol.* 154:1306, 1986.
    The combination of fetal heart rate monitoring, cord blood pH, and Apgar assessment was better than any one technique alone in predicting fetal status after delivery.

14. Small, M. L., et al. Continuous tissue pH monitoring in the term fetus. *Am. J. Obstet. Gynecol.* 161:323, 1989.
    A system for the continuous monitoring of tissue pH in the fetus was evaluated. A poor correlation was shown between capillary pH and tissue pH.

Neonatal Outcome

15. Fetal and Neonatal Neurologic Injury. *ACOG Tech. Bull.* No. 163, January 1992.
    Approximately 10 percent of the cases of cerebral palsy in term infants are associated with perinatal asphyxia.

16. Rosen, M. G., and Hobel, C. J. Prenatal and perinatal factors associated with brain disorders. *Obstet. Gynecol.* 68:416, 1986.
    The various causes of mental retardation and brain disorders are reviewed.

17. Low, J. A., et al. Intrapartum fetal hypoxia: a study of long-term morbidity. *Am. J. Obstet. Gynecol.* 145:129, 1983.
    There was no significant difference in the pattern of motor and cognitive handicaps or developmental delay in children who suffered hypoxia during the intrapartum period versus that in controls.

37. DELIVERY OF THE SMALL AND LARGE INFANT
Bruce A. Harris, Jr.

Fetal size is often erroneously estimated. The most reliable method of determining fetal weight today is by ultrasound. Nevertheless, errors of the order of 8 to 10 percent are seen, even for these modern techniques, and, clinically, the findings may not be helpful in practice situations.

The first priority in the care of the small fetus is to prevent delivery, if reasonably possible. However, this chapter deals with the management of premature labor when attempts at prevention have been unsuccessful. The small infant may be premature, growth retarded, or both, and its condition is often very fragile. Careful estimation of fetal weight, based on ultrasound findings, clinical history, developmental milestones, and other measures, should be carried out. The previous birth of a low-birth-weight infant to the same mother is associated with significantly smaller than normal newborn measurements in the current pregnancy. Labor should be conducted near a nursery capable of providing sophisticated intensive care, as infants delivered in such a setting fare better than those who are transferred after birth. Therefore, parturients at risk of premature labor or with suspected growth-retarded infants should be transferred to a tertiary-care facility for delivery, if possible.

Intraventricular hemorrhage is common in tiny babies. If hypoxia occurs, the blood flow to the brain will increase two to four times. Hypoxia also impairs cerebral circulatory autoregulation, such that cerebral blood flow becomes excessive. The periventricular capillary matrix then breaks down, and intraventricular hemorrhage ensues.

Electronic fetal monitoring should be utilized during labor in women with small fetuses to facilitate the early detection of hypoxia and acidosis, which in turn may result in hypoperfusion of the lungs, gastrointestinal tract, and kidneys, as well as direct damage to the brain. Hypoperfusion of the lungs may cause diminished surfactant production, with an attendant increased likelihood of respiratory distress syndrome. Growth-retarded infants are especially at risk for suffering hypoxia during labor. Therefore, if vaginal delivery is elected, the obstetrician should be prepared to intervene surgically in the event of recurrent, significant (late or severe variable, or both) decelerations of the fetal heart rate, significant loss of fetal heart rate variability, or both. Severe variable decelerations are commonly seen late in the labor of women with small fetuses, and may represent not only pressure on the umbilical cord but also compression of the fetal thorax. These factors may constitute an ominous sign if the fetal heart rate variability is diminished, the fetal heart rate returns slowly to the baseline rate, or there is "overshoot" of the baseline. Labor involving such infants should be conducted in an area where cesarean delivery can be performed rapidly and with adequate nursing as well as support personnel present. Low birth weight has been reported to be associated with lower intelligence scores that persist through adolescence. Therefore, the greatest vigilance must be exercised in labors involving small infants, so that changes stemming from undue hypoxia do not occur.

Small singleton infants presenting by the vertex may be delivered vaginally. Although cesarean delivery of the tiny (600–1000 g) infant in the vertex presentation has been advocated, the recent literature indicates that the outcome from vaginal delivery is in no way inferior. Forceps may be used, but spontaneous delivery is recommended in many cases. If the membranes can be preserved, gentle delivery of the tiny infant "in caul" (i.e., within an intact bag of waters) may offer increased protection. The mother of the tiny fetus should be observed carefully during labor and taken to the delivery room in sufficient time to permit a controlled delivery. Appropriate pediatric personnel should be present at all such deliveries.

A breech presentation of the small infant is an especially difficult situation. In this event, the vertex is proportionately larger than the rest of the infant, compared to that in the term baby. The body and extremities may be delivered before the cervix is dilated sufficiently to permit the passage of the head. The resulting dystocia, together with umbilical cord compression, may precipitate severe hypoxia. Subsequent efforts of the obstetricians may then cause severe trauma to the infant's neck, brachial plexus, or both. Labor with a breech presentation is frequently associated with cord complications, uterine inertia, and infection. The findings from most studies indicate the perinatal morbidity and mortality are substantially greater in the small breech infant delivered vaginally, and, for this reason, such an infant estimated to weigh 1500 g or less is best delivered by cesarean section.

When the delivery of premature or growth-retarded infants involves twins, slightly different considerations apply. If the first twin presents as a breech, the management is the same as that for a singleton birth, and cesarean delivery is usually performed. If the first twin has delivered as a vertex and the second twin is in a breech or transverse presentation, extraction of the second twin may be performed, provided the operator is experienced and an anesthesiologist is on hand who is skilled in the administration of anesthesia that produces maximal uterine relaxation, such as halothane. External version may be performed under ultrasound control. Otherwise, cesarean section is recommended for the delivery of both twins. Ultrasonic evaluation of both biparietal diameters is advisable to ascertain whether the second twin's head is substantially larger than the first twin's. Twin deliveries should take place in the operating room, with a complete operating team standing by, including anesthesiology personnel and scrub nurses. The latter should be scrubbed and gowned, and the surgical instrument pack should be open and ready for use.

If both twins present by the vertex and the first twin is delivered vaginally, vaginal delivery may reasonably be expected for the second twin. A scalp electrode should be placed on the second twin, if possible, to permit close observation of its condition. If fetal distress develops, if labor is not effectual despite the intravenous administration of oxytocin, or if mechanical dystocia is encountered, cesarean delivery should take place immediately.

Anesthesia and analgesia should be used sparingly in the labor and delivery of mothers with small infants. Systemic agents may cause neonatal depression if used in large doses. On the other hand, sedatives may depress fetal brain metabolism and maternal catecholamine secretion, thus increasing uteroplacental blood flow while reducing the fetal oxygen requirement. I believe that epidural anesthesia for labor, possibly supplemented by pudendal block for delivery, if needed, confers the best prognosis for the infant.

If cesarean delivery is to be performed, the uterine incision must be large enough to permit easy delivery of the small fetus. If the lower uterine segment is poorly developed, attempts to perform a low transverse cesarean section may result in a difficult delivery, with consequent trauma to the infant. Accordingly, most cesarean deliveries of small infants should be carried out using a generous low vertical incision, which often extends well up into the upper uterine segment. This is particularly important if the fetus is a breech or transverse lie.

Perinatal morbidity and mortality, as well as maternal adverse effects, are increased in association with the macrosomic (>4000–4500 g) fetus. Large fetuses are more commonly male and are often associated with postdate pregnancies or maternal diabetes. Estimation of fetal weight is very difficult in the large fetus, and it is best to ask the mother (if she is a multipara) for her own estimate of the fetal weight. A recent study has shown that the birth weights predicted at term by parous women are as accurate as clinical or sonographic-based estimates of fetal weight. The second stage of labor tends to be prolonged and the likelihood of shoulder dystocia is increased in the setting of large-birth-weight infants. Mechanical dystocia of all kinds is also more common. Breech delivery is associated with an increased incidence of prolonged labor, intrapartum asphyxia, and mechanical dystocia. The added risk of fetal macrosomia makes vaginal delivery unacceptable, if the macrosomia is known in advance. For all these reasons, the macrosomic fetus in breech presentation is usually delivered by cesarean section.

The progress of labor may be slow with the large fetus, even in the vertex presentation. Slow descent often suggests subsequent shoulder dystocia. If midpelvic arrest occurs, cesarean delivery should be strongly considered. Shoulder dystocia is most likely to arise in the presence of fetal macrosomia, maternal obesity, maternal diabetes (especially the less severe varieties), and a history of previous infants weighing more than 4000 g. Shoulder dystocia is best treated by being prevented. A vertex in the midpelvis after a second stage of 2 hours or more in a primigravida (or 1 hour or more in a multigravida) is a danger signal. The accoucheur must now anticipate the possibility of a difficult delivery of the shoulders. Midforceps delivery or midpelvic vacuum extraction of the vertex of a large fetus may sometimes result in shoulder dystocia because the shoulders have not had sufficient opportunity to mold into the midpelvis. For this reason, spontaneous delivery, or an easy low-forceps delivery after a substantial amount of vertex protrudes from the outlet, is preferable to a midforceps delivery. One must remember that, after a long labor with a large fetus, the vertex may appear to protrude from the outlet. However, what the attendant sees may actually only be edematous scalp; the bony vertex may still be at an unacceptably high station for instrumental delivery.

If shoulder dystocia does occur, the following sequence of maneuvers should take place: The patient's legs should be removed from the stirrups and the thighs completely flexed upon the abdomen. This causes the symphysis to rotate backward, thereby increasing the pelvic diameter, and this may unlock the anterior shoulder. At the same time, firm suprapubic (not fundal) pressure should be applied to the anterior shoulder. Gentle downward traction (so as not to injure the brachial plexus) should now deliver the anterior shoulder. If the anterior shoulder cannot be thus disengaged, a large mediolateral episiotomy or an episioproctotomy should be performed. The posterior shoulder should be pushed toward the infant's chest, so that the thorax rotates. This frequently disengages one shoulder. Rotation of the shoulders and not the head is essential, because twisting the head while the shoulders are locked may fracture the neck or injure the brachial plexus. If the shoulders are still undelivered, a hand can be introduced posteriorly and pressure applied in the antecubital fossa of the posterior arm. As the elbow flexes, the forearm and hand are drawn across the baby's chest and out of the vaginal opening. This will disengage the posterior shoulder. If it is necessary to deliver the posterior arm, the operator should be prepared for fracture of the humerus, clavicle, or both. These bones will heal speedily, usually without residual deformity. These fractures appear to be an acceptable price to pay for the delivery of a living child without neurologic injury. If all other means fail, the head may be taken into the palm of the operator's hand and flexed. It is then replaced within the vagina, to the level of the spines (general anesthesia may be required for this procedure). Cesarean delivery is then performed. This procedure has been called the *Zavanelli maneuver*. Should the Zavanelli maneuver fail, as a last resort, the patient should be placed on the operating table with her legs separated and flexed. A low transverse incision is then made in the uterus. The anterior shoulder will pop into the incision, freeing the posterior shoulder, which can then be delivered from below using extraction of the posterior arm by an obstetrician positioned between the patient's legs. Once the posterior arm has been delivered, the rest of the vaginal delivery can be accomplished with relative ease.

Delivery of the large infant is best conducted using moderate amounts of systemic analgesia during labor. Supplementation with the inhalation of nitrous oxide (50%) with oxygen (50%) is desirable at delivery. It is important that the mother retain sufficient natural expulsive powers so that she is able to bring her head down to the perineum. In this way, difficult forceps operations may be avoided. Regional anesthesia, despite its many benefits, may be associated with an inadequate propulsive force.

General

1. Phillips, J. B., III, et al. Characteristics, mortality, and outcome of higher-birth weight infants who require intensive care. *Am. J. Obstet. Gynecol.* 149:875, 1984.
   This excellent article details the common diagnoses in normal-sized to macrosomic infants who were admitted to neonatal intensive care units because of pulmonary disease, asphyxia, congenital malformations, diabetic mothers, hematologic disease, or infection.
2. Moore, T. R., and Resnik, R. Special problems of VLBW infants. *Contemp. Ob/Gyn* 23:175, 1984.
   A comprehensive review.
3. Harris, B. A. Shoulder dystocia. *Clin. Obstet. Gynecol.* 27:106, 1984.
   A review of shoulder dystocia: causes, methods of prevention, and treatment.

Diagnosis

4. Morgan, M. A., and Thurmau, G. R. Efficacy of the fetal-pelvic index for delivery of neonates weighing 4000 grams or greater: a preliminary report. *Am. J. Obstet. Gynecol.* 158:1133, 1988.
   The fetal-pelvic index is an accurate method of predicting the absence or presence of fetal-pelvic disproportion in patients delivering neonates weighing 4000 g or more.
5. Pielet, B. W., et al. Ultrasonic prediction of birth weight in preterm fetuses. *Am. J. Obstet. Gynecol.* 157:411, 1987.
   The ultrasonic prediction of birth weight showed an error of 8 to 10 percent.
6. Deter, R. L., et al. Development of individual growth curve standards for estimates of fetal weight. *J. Clin. Ultrasound* 16:215, 1988.
   Random errors of 10 to 13 percent for infants with weights below 200 g and 6 to 8 percent for infants with weights above 2000 g were noted.
7. Athey, P. A., et al. *Ultrasound in Obstetrics and Gynecology* (2nd ed.). St. Louis: Mosby, 1985.
   Standard methods for determining fetal weight using ultrasound.
8. Mondanlou, H. D., et al. Large-for-gestational-age neonates: anthropometric reasons for shoulder dystocia. *Obstet. Gynecol.* 60:417, 1982.
   In the fetus, a chest-to-head circumference difference of 4.8 cm should be considered a possible indication of impending shoulder dystocia.
9. Landon, M. B., Mintz, M. C., and Gabbe, S. G. Sonographic evaluation of fetal abdominal growth: prediction of the large-for-gestational-age infant in pregnancies complicated by diabetes mellitus. *Am. J. Obstet. Gynecol.* 160:115, 1989.

Serial ultrasonography performed during the third trimester may document the onset of accelerated fetal growth in diabetic pregnancies.

10. Goldenberg, R. L., et al. The influence of previous low birth weight on birth weight, gestational age, and anthropometric measurements in the current pregnancy. *Obstet. Gynecol.* 79:276, 1992.
The previous birth of a low-birth-weight infant is associated with significantly smaller anthropometric measurements in the current fetus.

11. Chauhan, S. P., et al. Intrapartum clinical, sonographic, and parous patients' estimates of newborn birth weight. *Obstet. Gynecol.* 79:956, 1992.
Maternal estimates of birth weight were comparable to those made by the clinician or those based on sonographic measurement.

12. Johnson, J. W., Longmate, J. A., and Irentzen, D. Excessive maternal weight and pregnancy outcome. *Am. J. Obstet. Gynecol.* 167:353, 1992.
Increased maternal weight gain in pregnancy results in a higher frequency of fetal macrosomia, which in turn leads to major maternal and fetal complications.

Treatment

13. Harris, B. A., et al. In utero versus neonatal transport of high-risk perinates: a comparison. *Obstet. Gynecol.* 57:496, 1981.
The infant transported to the tertiary-care facility before delivery has a better prognosis than the infant transported after delivery.

14. Kitchen, W., et al. Caesarean section or vaginal delivery at 24 to 28 weeks' gestation: comparison of survival and neonatal and two-year morbidity. *Obstet. Gynecol.* 66:149, 1985.
Little evidence supports the routine delivery of infants of borderline viability by cesarean section, except for recognized obstetric indications.

15. Olshan, A. F., et al. Cesarean birth and neonatal mortality in very low birth weight infants. *Obstet. Gynecol.* 64:267, 1984.
Recent decreases in neonatal mortality among very low-birth-weight infants seem to be unrelated to the increased use of cesarean delivery.

16. Acker, D. B., et al. Risk factors for shoulder dystocia in the average-weight infant. *Obstet. Gynecol.* 67:614, 1986.
When low-forceps delivery is undertaken in a patient with a labor complication, shoulder dystocia should be anticipated. Shoulder dystocia is more likely when the course of labor is characterized by arrest disorders.

17. O'Leary, J. A., et al. Option for shoulder dystocia: cephalic replacement. *Contemp. Ob/Gyn* 27:157, 1986.
This article describes the procedure of cephalic replacement for shoulder dystocia.

18. Gonik, B., Stringer, C. A., and Held, B. An alternate maneuver for management of shoulder dystocia. *Am. J. Obstet. Gynecol.* 145:882, 1983.
Exaggerated flexion of the mother's thighs may free a trapped anterior shoulder.

19. Seidman, D. S., Laor, A., and Gale, R. Birth weight and intellectual performance in late adolescence. *Obstet. Gynecol.* 79:543, 1992.
Children with low birth weights exhibit low intelligence scores that persist through adolescence.

20. Grerg, P. C., et al. The effect of presentation and mode of delivery on neonatal outcome in the second twin. *Am. J. Obstet. Gynecol.* 167:901, 1992.
This paper does not support the use of routine cesarean delivery for twins of any birth weight when the second twin in nonvertex.

21. O'Leary, J. A., and Cuva, A. Abdominal rescue after failed cephalic replacement. *Obstet. Gynecol.* 80:514, 1992.
Persistent failed cephalic replacement can be successfully resolved with a hysterotomy using a low transverse incision.

Complications

22. Levine, M. G., et al. Birth trauma: incidence and predisposing factors. *Obstet. Gynecol.* 63:792, 1984.
The etiology of birth trauma to macrosomic infants is detailed.

23. Mondanlou, H. D., et al. Macrosomia—maternal, fetal, and neonatal implications. *Obstet. Gynecol.* 55:420, 1980.
    The birth of macrosomic infants was positively correlated with maleness, multiparity, diabetes, and prior macrosomia. Ten percent of macrosomic infants need to be admitted to the neonatal intensive care unit.
24. Strauss, A., et al. Perinatal events and intraventricular/subependymal hemorrhage in the very low-birth-weight infant. *Am. J. Obstet. Gynecol.* 151:1022, 1985.
    The presence or absence of labor, fetal presentation, and the route of delivery do not play a role in intraventricular hemorrhage.
25. Low, J. A., et al. Maternal, fetal and newborn complications associated with newborn intracranial hemorrhage. *Am. J. Obstet. Gynecol.* 154:345, 1986.
    Intraventricular hemorrhage is poorly associated with maternal medical and obstetric complications and with labor and delivery characteristics.
26. Archer, D. B., et al. Risk factors for Erb-Duchenne palsy. *Obstet. Gynecol.* 71:389, 1988.
    One in six infants of diabetic gravidas who sustained shoulder dystocia suffered Erb-Duchenne palsy. This adverse outcome was more commonly observed in connection with deliveries performed by recently graduated (<4-years' postresidency) obstetricians than by senior clinicians, though this latter group also delivered infants who were affected.

VIII. PUERPERIUM

38. LACTATION AND LACTATION SUPPRESSION
Harriette L. Hampton

Prolactin is the key hormone controlling milk production. The entire process of lactogenesis, however, requires multiple hormonal interactions that affect the development of both the ductal and alveolar cells as well as modulate the nutritional content of milk. Growth of the epithelium comprising the duct system depends on estrogen, which is synergized by the presence of growth hormone, prolactin, and cortisol. Development of the lobular alveolar system requires both estrogen and progesterone in the presence of prolactin. The synthesis of milk protein and fat is regulated principally by prolactin and facilitated by insulin and cortisol.

Although estrogen and progesterone act to stimulate mammary development, these hormones inhibit the formation of milk during pregnancy, thereby reserving milk production for the postpartum state. High levels of estrogen and progesterone block prolactin action on the mammary target cells through antagonism of prolactin receptors. After delivery, estrogen and progesterone levels fall rapidly. This precipitous decline in the circulating hormone levels results in unopposed autoregulatory increases in the mammary prolactin receptor content. As prolactin receptors become abundant in glandular mammary tissue, milk production (lactogenesis) begins and is usually apparent 3 to 4 days postpartum.

While the initiation of lactation depends on sex steroids and trophic hormone stimulation, its maintenance depends on unique neuroendocrine responses to mechanical stimulation of the nipple during suckling. Sensory signals originating in the nipple during stimulation are conveyed in a somatic afferent spinohypothalamic pathway via the periventricular and supraoptic nuclei of the hypothalamus. This neuronal system controls the release of oxytocin and prolactin. The myoepithelial cells contract the mammary alveolar duct and eject milk in response to oxytocin stimulation. Maternal-fetal play or the anticipation of feeding by the mother can produce an episodic release of oxytocin, clearly illustrating the involvement of higher centers in the neuroendocrine control of oxytocin secretion.

In addition to the oxytocin release that occurs with nursing, there is a prompt and dramatic release of prolactin that is temporally associated with, but independent of, the episodic oxytocin release. The transient increase in prolactin secretion is usually sufficient to maintain an adequate supply of milk for the infant until the next feeding time. In the first postpartum week, prolactin levels in breast-feeding women decline from pregnant levels of 200 to 300 ng/ml to approximately 100 ng/ml. The prolactin levels are then sustained at 40 to 50 ng/ml for the next 2 to 3 months, with transient 10- to 20-fold increases in the serum concentrations during suckling. In the first 3 to 4 months after birth, the basal prolactin levels fall to normal, but suckling still produces episodic releases, which are essential for continued milk production.

The composition of human milk has been analyzed extensively. Physiochemically, milk is an isotonic emulsion of fat and water. Mature human milk contains 3 to 5 percent fat, 0.8 to 1.2 percent protein, 6.8 to 7.2 percent carbohydrates, and 0.2 percent mineral constituents. The energy content is 60 to 75 kilocalories per 100 ml. Colostrum, the secretory product of the breast before the initiation of lactogenesis, contains more protein and less carbohydrate than mature milk. The major proteins in milk are caseins, alpha-lactalbumin, lactoferrin, immunoglobulin A (IgA), lysozyme, and serum albumin. All vitamins, except vitamin K, are present in human milk, but in variable amounts. Human milk contains a low concentration of iron, although this iron is absorbed more readily than that from cow's milk. The immunologic advantage afforded by breast milk is not found in other milk sources. The immunoglobulins (especially secretory IgA), lactoferrin, and lysozyme found in breast milk are able to protect the neonate against infections.

The nutritional status of the mother during lactation is important. For each 20 calories of milk produced, the mother who breast-feeds must consume 30 calories. A dietary caloric requirement of approximately 600 additional calories per day is observed in women who maintain their body weight while lactating. The energy cost of lactation is met in most, however, by the mobilization of fat stores laid down during pregnancy. Recommended daily dietary increases for lactation consist of a 20-gm increase in protein, a 20 percent increment in all vitamins and minerals except folic acid, which should be increased by 50 percent, and a 33 percent elevation in the intake of calcium, phosphorus, and magnesium. Continuation of prenatal vitamin and iron supplementation usually meets these requirements.

Breast-feeding is not an instinctive art. A nurse or other practitioner is invaluable in helping the new mother position the baby and in offering support and encouragement. The most common problems encountered in breast-feeding are nipple soreness and engorgement, particularly in the early days of nursing. Reassurance from the physician that it is common and temporary is essential to the breast-feeding mother. Persistent nipple soreness does not result from the duration of breast-feeding but from an improper grasp of the nipple and areola. Allowing the nipples to air-dry after nursing can be of benefit when nipples are painful or cracking. The application of plain anhydrous lanolin may help, as long as moisture is not trapped beneath the ointment.

Engorgement of the breast involves lymphatic and vascular congestion as well as an accumulation of milk in the ductal system. The best management of engorgement, of course, is prevention, which can be most easily accomplished by having the infant nurse in an early, unscheduled, and frequent fashion. Treatment includes proper bra support and the application of cold packs after nursing. If the baby is nursing poorly, the problem should be addressed through manual pumping of the breast. The temporary use of analgesics may be necessary for some women.

Less frequent breast-feeding problems include an impaired let-down reflex and a poor milk supply. Virtually any woman can produce milk, but, if she cannot release it, production will not continue. The let-down reflex depends on the pituitary release of oxytocin. Signs and symptoms of let-down include sensations ranging from a sense of tightening or pressure to a pronounced "pins and needles" feeling in the nipple. The most powerful trigger for this surge of oxytocin is the infant suckling. Like most reflexes mediated by the hypothalamus, the let-down reflex is inhibited most commonly by psychologic factors. The treatment of impaired let-down includes increased maternal rest, comfort, privacy, and removal of distractions. If this is unsuccessful, a trial of synthetic oxytocin (Syntocinon, available as a nasal spray) has proved useful for some women.

Milk supply is determined by a simple supply-and-demand feedback loop. Problems of insufficient milk production are primarily related to inadequate frequency or length of feedings, provided that nutrition is adequate. Once again, the availability of a support person is of critical importance for mothers who are breast-feeding, should problems arise.

The question of contraception during lactation is important. The contraceptive effect of breast-feeding alone has been observed in third world settings. A mother who is breast-feeding exclusively has only a 1 in 1250 chance of ovulating during the first 9 weeks postpartum. After this time, however, ovulation occurs more often and is unpredictable, prompting the need for reliable contraception. Barrier contraception has no contraindications, and the intrauterine device is acceptable for the multigravid, breast-feeding mother who is aware of the risks involved. Steroidal contraceptives appear to have little or no effect on milk composition, but the combined oral contraceptive may have an adverse effect on breast milk production. The degree to which lactation is suppressed relates to the dosage and timing of therapy. The minidose progestin-only pill and injectable progestin do not adversely affect breast milk production.

As a general rule, it should be assumed that any drug ingested by a nursing mother may be present in breast milk at 1 to 2 percent of the maternal dosage. The excretion of a drug in breast milk is increased for pharmacologic agents with any of the following properties: low molecular weight, high lipid solubility, low protein binding, small volumes of distribution, and a long half-life. Metabolism of the drug by the neonate depends on the infant's stage of development. The current literature should be reviewed before administering any drug to breast-feeding patients. Relative contraindications must be considered in light of the risk-benefit relationship.

Suppression of lactation can be achieved in the postpartum period in approximately 60 percent of patients by mechanical compression and avoidance of nipple stimulation. Pharmacologic measures to suppress lactation were attempted as early as 1940. A variety of estrogens and androgens have been administered with variable success rates. In 1980, bromocriptine (Parlodel), a dopamine receptor agonist, was marketed for the prevention of physiologic lactation. Both oral and injectable depot forms of Parlodel are now commercially available. There are episodic reports of hypertension, cerebrovascular accidents, seizures, and myocardial dysfunction, with and without the concomitant use of sympathomimetics. Parlodel therapy should be discontinued if hypertension; severe, progressive, or unremitting headache; or central nervous system toxicity develops. Parlodel remains the only pharmacologic agent approved for lactation suppression.

General

1. Ogle, K. S., and Alfano, M. A. Common problems of initiating breast-feeding. *Postgrad. Med.* 82:159, 1987.
   A thoughtful review of the management of common problems encountered in breast-feeding.
2. Vance, M. L., Evans, W. S., and Thorner, M. O. Bromocriptine. *Ann. Intern. Med.* 100:78, 1984.
   A comprehensive review of the pharmacologic and therapeutic uses of bromocriptine, including the suppression of physiologic lactation.
3. Shingleton, W. W., and McCarty, K. S., Jr. What you should know about breast pathology. *Contemp. Ob/Gyn* 29:90, 1987.
   A practical look at breast pathology, containing a nice section on the major hormonal influences on the breast as well as the clinical correlates of histologic changes in the breast that may occur during or before pregnancy.
4. Whitehead, R. G. Nutritional aspects of human lactation. *Lancet* 1:167, 1983.
   An excellent comprehensive report, although brief, in which the dietary role of breast milk is detailed.

Etiology

5. Yen, S. C., and Jaffe, R. B. *Reproductive Endocrinology* (2nd ed.). Philadelphia: Saunders, 1986. Pp. 240–252.
   The composition of breast milk is detailed in this superlative report.
6. Darr, M. S., and Taylor, R. B. A practical guide to drugs in breast milk. *Female Patient* 13:42, 1988.
   A simple but comprehensive guide for the clinician and patient regarding the effects of drugs on breast milk.
7. Neifert, M. R., and Seacat, J. M. How to help patients breastfeed successfully. *Contemp. Ob/Gyn* (special issue) April 1987; 85–108.
   Using excellent visual aids, details how to assist patients in breast feeding.
8. Bauchner, J., Leventhal, J. M., and Shapiro, E. D. Studies of breast-feeding and infections. How good is the evidence? *J.A.M.A.* 256:887, 1986.
   An excellent compilation of 20 studies, meeting stringent methodologic standards, that examined the association between breast-feeding and infections in the neonate. The authors found that breast-feeding conferred minimal protection in nursing mothers from industrialized countries.

Diagnosis

9. Feller, W. F. Steps in evaluation of a breast mass. *Contemp. Ob/Gyn* 32:11, 1988.
   How to evaluate a breast mass and how to diagnose breast masses in pregnancy are discussed.
10. Scialli, A. R., and Fabro, S. What drugs are safe during nursing? *Contemp. Ob/Gyn* 22:211, 1984.

This excellent article details how to determine which drugs are safe for mothers who are nursing.

11. Bergevin, U., Dougherty, C., and Kramer, M. S. Do infant formula samples shorten the duration of breast-feeding? *Lancet* 1:1148, 1983.
    The results from this large and elegant study indicate that, when babies are fed infant formula, this may shorten the duration of breast-feeding and may indeed hasten the age when they are given solid food.

Treatment

12. Ford, K., and Labbok, M. Contraceptive usage during lactation in the United States: an update. *Am. J. Public Health* 77:79, 1987.
    Barrier method contraception was found to be preferred in a survey of breast-feeding women conducted in the United States.

13. West, C. P. The acceptability of a progestin-only contraceptive during breastfeeding. *Contraception* 27:563, 1983.
    Use of the progestin-only pill did not adversely affect either breast milk production or the infant.

14. Shiparo, A. G., and Thomas, L. Efficacy of bromocriptine versus binders as inhibitors of postpartum lactation. *South. Med. J.* 77:719, 1984.
    The use of breast binders was compared to bromocriptine therapy in 50 postpartum patients. Bromocriptine was more successful in suppressing breast problems but the side effects were higher; thus, the dosage was reduced from 2.5 to 1.25 mg twice a day, which is the currently recommended clinical dosage.

15. Defoort, P., et al. Bromocriptine in an injectable form for puerperal lactation suppression: comparison with estrandron prolongatum. *Obstet. Gynecol.* 70:866, 1987.
    Bromocriptine (injectable) was compared to estrandron. Both appeared to suppress lactation adequately.

16. Kremer, J. Lactation inhibition by a single injection of a new depot-bromocriptine. *Br. J. Obstet. Gynaecol.* 97:527, 1990.
    Encouraging results from the depot administration of Parlodel are reported.

17. Koetsawang, S. The effects of contraceptive methods on the quality and quantity of breast milk. *Int. J. Gynecol. Obstet.* 25:115, 1987.
    An excellent review of the third world experience with contraceptive agents in the postpartum period.

18. Dunson, T. R., et al. A multicenter clinical trial of progestin-only oral contraceptive in lactating women. *Contraception* 47:23, 1993.
    Progestin-only oral contraceptive pills were effective for postpartum breast-feeding women.

Complications

19. Katz, M., et al. Puerperal hypertension, stroke, and seizures after suppression of lactation with bromocriptine. *Obstet. Gynecol.* 66:822, 1985.
    Two cases of cerebrovascular events that occurred after the use of bromocriptine are presented.

20. Yaffe, S. J. Drugs and the nursing mother. *Female Patient* 9:19, 1984.
    In this well-detailed report, a compendium of drugs is presented that are contraindicated in the breast-feeding mother. It also depicts nicely the pharmacologic principles at work in the secretion of drugs in breast milk.

21. Tchabo, J.-G., and Stay, E. J. Gravidic macromastia: case report. *Am. J. Obstet. Gynecol.* 160:88, 1989.
    The authors describe a rare condition called gravidic macromastia, *in which the breasts become engorged as a result of marked hormonal influence. Medical therapy with dihydroprogesterone is recommended first, followed by surgical intervention if the former proves unsuccessful.*

22. Kulig, K. Bromocriptine-associated headache: possible life-threatening sympathomimetic interaction. *Obstet. Gynecol.* 78:941, 1991.
    Cases involving a sympathomimetic interaction with Parlodel are reported.

23. Deutinger, M., and Deutinger, J. Breast feeding after aesthetic mammary opera-

tions and cardiac operations through horizontal submammary skin incision. *Surg. Gynecol. Obstet.* 176:267, 1993.

Postpartum women who had undergone an aesthetic mammary operation were able to breast-feed their infants.

39. POSTPARTUM HEMORRHAGE
Baha M. Sibai

Postpartum hemorrhage (PPH) is a serious complication of pregnancy and the puerperium that may result in serious maternal morbidity, and is a leading cause of maternal mortality in several countries. Defined as a blood loss exceeding 500 ml, the exact incidence is difficult to determine because the clinical estimation of blood loss during delivery is inaccurate by as much as 50 percent, compared to the actual loss that can be determined after delivery. When measured correctly, the mean blood loss during vaginal delivery and postpartum in one large series was found to be 505 ml, with 39 percent of the patients losing more than this. About 4 percent of the patients lose more than 1000 ml, although the actual incidence of PPH severe enough to cause hemorrhagic shock is less than 1 percent. The bleeding is usually continuous but may be slow or brisk, depending on the cause. PPH is considered early if it occurs during the first 24 hours postpartum, and late if it develops after this time.

Uterine atony is the cause of early PPH in approximately 90 percent of the cases; genital tract lacerations, including uterine, cervical, vaginal, and perineal lacerations account for 6 percent; and retained placental fragments are responsible in 3 to 4 percent of the cases. The last accounts for most cases of late PPH, but routine exploration of the uterus after delivery can eliminate 90 percent of these. Other infrequent causes include uterine inversion and blood dyscrasias, such as von Willebrand's disease, factor VII deficiency, thrombotic thrombocytopenic purpura, and acquired coagulation problems associated with amniotic fluid embolism or abruptio placentae after fetal demise. The risk of PPH is increased if any of the following factors are present: (1) overdistention of the uterus owing to hydramnios, multiple pregnancy, or a macrosomic fetus; (2) high parity; (3) prolonged difficult labor, especially after oxytocin induction; (4) history of previous PPH; (5) preeclampsia; or (6) precipitous labor. Other correlates include general anesthesia, abnormal placentation such as placenta previa or accreta, abruptio placentae, and a succinate placental lobe, as well as operative delivery using either instrumentation or version and extraction.

The steps to be taken in the management of PPH include early recognition, aggressive correction of hypovolemia, and control of the specific bleeding sites. Patients with predisposing factors should be monitored closely, and blood should be available at the time of delivery. Universal therapy for all patients should include prompt blood and volume replacement, maintenance of good urinary output, and serial monitoring of the patient's vital signs, hematocrit, and central venous pressure. After the initial steps have been implemented, the patient should be examined under general anesthesia, with systematic exploration of the genital tract to identify the cause of bleeding.

The classic management of uterine atony consists of the mechanical stimulation of uterine contractions by means of firm, but not vigorous, massage of the uterus through the abdomen and concomitant bimanual compression of the elevated, anteverted uterus. These measures should be performed in conjunction with the simultaneous administration of oxytocic agents in amounts sufficient to initiate and maintain uterine contractility. Mechanical maneuvers to stop the attendant bleeding include digital compression of the uterine arteries in the paracervical area and compression of the descending aorta against the maternal spine.

Oxytocin should be given by continuous intravenous administration in a dosage as high as 20 to 30 units/500 ml of Ringer's lactate solution. It should never be given as a bolus because hypertension, myocardial arrhythmias, and cardiac arrest may occur. The simultaneous intramuscular administration of 0.2 mg of methylergonovine may be used in those who are normotensive if the uterus fails to respond to oxytocin. If the aforementioned measures fail to control the bleeding resulting from uterine atony within 15 minutes, other potent ecbolic agents such as prostaglandins may be used. The intramuscular administration of 0.25 mg of 15-methyl PGF_2 (a prostaglandin F_2 analogue) has been shown in several studies to be very effective in controlling PPH secondary to uterine atony when it is unresponsive to conventional methods. The drug can be injected directly into the myometrium or can be given intramuscularly. Some of the side effects reported include nausea, vomiting, diarrhea, pyrexia, and acute hypertension, with the last usually seen in preeclamptic patients. Prostaglandin E_2 has also been used, both intravenously and as vaginal suppositories, to treat severe cases of PPH even in preeclamptic patients.

If all the aforementioned measures fail to control the bleeding resulting from uterine atony, other recommended methods of treatment include the instillation of heated solutions into the uterus, intrauterine packing, or surgical intervention, although the efficacy of intrauterine packing remains controversial. Some consider it a valuable procedure for uterine atony, whereas others believe it is unphysiologic and ineffective, contributes to further bleeding, predisposes to infection, and may delay definitive treatment by obscuring the amount of blood loss. Most do agree, however, that intrauterine packing can be used as a temporary measure in preparation for surgical management, and, occasionally, it may be a lifesaving or uterus-preserving measure. Surgical intervention may include laparotomy with these options: ligation of the uterine arteries, ovarian blood supply, or hypogastric arteries, or total or subtotal hysterectomy, depending on the condition of the parturient as well as the desire to preserve fertility. The selective arterial infusion of antidiuretic hormone (Pitressin), embolization, or both, may be used to control life-threatening PPH in some cases when laparotomy is not possible.

Retained fragments of the placenta can be removed digitally once the proper cleavage plane is found by means of manual exploration just after delivery. This can be facilitated by the use of placental forceps to grasp fragments and a piece of gauze spread out over the gloved fingers to remove small fragments and adherent placental membranes. Occasionally, curettage of the uterus may be necessary using a large blunt curette. The diagnosis of placenta accreta should be suspected in the absence of a cleavage plane and inability to remove placental fragments. Treatment usually requires hysterectomy, although intrauterine packing has been used successfully in some cases.

Vaginal and cervical lacerations are usually the result of the use of instruments at delivery, but may also result from precipitous spontaneous delivery. The most common sites for cervical lacerations are at the 3 and 9 o'clock positions. Control of bleeding is usually achieved by simple suture repair after larger vessels are isolated and tied individually. Deep lacerations should be closed in layers to avoid hematoma formation, and the repair should start above the apex of the laceration. Vaginal packing may be helpful in preventing venous oozing or bleeding from varicosities.

Laceration of the lower uterine segment or rupture of the uterus should be suspected following difficult midforceps operations, internal uterine manipulation, and hyperstimulation (oxytocin), as well as in the setting of vaginal delivery after previous cesarean section. Bleeding resulting from uterine rupture may be internal, and the diagnosis can be confirmed by digital exploration of the uterus. Treatment of uterine rupture includes laparotomy, with the options comprising repair of the laceration, as well as total or subtotal hysterectomy, depending on the type, extent, and site of laceration, as well as the patient's condition and the desire to preserve the uterus.

Acute puerperal inversion of the uterus is a rare cause of PPH and one that is usually associated with excessive fundal pressure, strong traction on the umbilical cord, grand multiparity, placenta accreta, and uterine atony. Classic symptoms include shock, hemorrhage, and pain. If the diagnosis is made early and general anesthesia is available, manual replacement is possible in most cases. Applying constant slow pressure, Trendelenburg positioning, and filling the vagina with warm sterile saline solution may also be helpful in restoring the organ to its correct position.

The incidence of late PPH is about 1 in 1000 deliveries, with most cases occurring between the sixth and tenth day after delivery. Frequent causes are subinvolution of the uterus and retained placental fragments. Other causes include endometritis and withdrawal bleeding from estrogens. Many of these patients can be managed conservatively with ecbolic agents, especially if placental inspection and uterine exploration are done routinely at the time of delivery. The use of curettage along with the simultaneous administration of oxytocin is necessary in about 65 percent of the patients, but may be associated with potential complications, such as uterine perforation and an increased incidence of Asherman's syndrome.

The potential complications of PPH include postpartum infection, anemia, transfusion hepatitis, Sheehan's syndrome, and Asherman's syndrome, especially if curettage was part of the management. Sheehan's syndrome, or acute pituitary necrosis, occurs in a small number of patients after severe PPH, and is associated most commonly with prolonged shock and secondary ischemic necrosis of the anterior pituitary gland. Prolactin-secreting cells are the first to be affected by anterior pituitary ischemia; hence, the diagnosis should be suspected early in the absence of lactation. Treatment consists of hormonal replacement.

In summary, the best management of PPH is prevention but, when it occurs, good clinical acumen in combination with treatment is called for.

General
1. Hayashi, R. Obstetric Hemorrhage and Hypovolemic Shock. In S. L. Clark, et al. (eds.), *Critical Care in Obstetrics*. Philadelphia: Blackwell Scientific, 1991.
   The pathophysiologic causes of hemorrhagic shock are listed, and a step-by-step approach to the management of obstetric hemorrhage is discussed.
2. Harris, B. A. Acute puerperal inversion of the uterus. *Clin. Obstet. Gynecol.* 27:134, 1984.
   The etiology, incidence classification, clinical course, and treatment of postpartum uterine inversion are summarized.

Etiology
3. Benedetti, T. J. Obstetric Hemorrhage. In S. G. Gabbe, J. R. Niebyl, and J. L. Simpson (eds.), *Obstetrics, Normal and Problem Pregnancies*. New York: Churchill Livingstone, 1991.
   The various causes of postpartum hemorrhage are listed, and a step-by-step approach to the management of obstetric hemorrhage is discussed.
4. Hayashi, R. H. Heading off disaster in postpartum hemorrhage. *Contemp. Ob/Gyn* 20:91, 1982.
   Definition, incidence, and the various factors associated with postpartum hemorrhage are reviewed. The author also describes a step-by-step approach for managing patients with postpartum hemorrhage stemming from uterine atony.
5. Brar, H. S., et al. Acute puerperal uterine inversion. New approaches to management. *J. Reprod. Med.* 34:173, 1989.
   A retrospective review of 56 patients with uterine inversion is presented in this article. Patients who received oxytocin were at high risk for inversion. Magnesium sulfate or the beta-mimetics were acceptable alternatives to general anesthesia in relaxing the uterus.

Diagnosis
6. Herbert, W. N. P., and Cefalo, R. C. Management of postpartum hemorrhage. *Clin. Obstet. Gynecol.* 27:139, 1984.
   The etiology, predisposing factors, and management of postpartum hemorrhage are summarized.
7. Watson, P., Besch, N., and Bowes, W. A. Management of acute and subacute puerperal inversion of the uterus. *Obstet. Gynecol.* 55:12, 1980.
   Eighteen cases of puerperal inversion of the uterus were studied. The most com-

mon signs were hemorrhage (94%) and shock (39%). Treatment regimens are summarized.

Treatment

8. Magil, B. PGF$_2$ for postpartum hemorrhage—how well does it work? *Contemp. Ob/Gyn* 23:111, 1984.
   Physicians who have participated in clinical trials of PGF$_2$ report their findings. The dosage and number of doses needed, the clinical efficacy, and the side effects are detailed. Definitions and the factors associated with postpartum hemorrhage are also discussed.

9. Garite, T. J., and Buttino, L., Jr. The use of 15-methyl F$_2$ α prostaglandin (prostin 15M) for the control of postpartum hemorrhage. *Am. J. Perinatol.* 3:241, 1986.
   Describes the use of prostin 15M in 26 patients with postpartum hemorrhage who did not respond to conventional treatment, including fundal massage plus oxytocin and methylergonovine. All patients had uterine atony. The success rate was 84.6 percent (22 patients responded). Two patients underwent hysterectomy because of placenta accreta, one patient required dilatation and curettage, and one patient underwent bilateral uterine artery ligation. The mean number of doses given was 2.2 (range, one to seven doses).

10. Hayashi, R. H., Castillo, M. S., and Noah, M. L. Management of severe postpartum hemorrhage with an F$_2$ analogue. *Obstet. Gynecol.* 63:806, 1984.
    Fifty-one patients with postpartum hemorrhage unresponsive to conventional therapy were studied. The use of intramuscular PGF$_2$ analogue in the management of these patients is detailed.

11. Gaye, H., Gough, J. D., and Gillmer, M. D. G. Control of persistent primary postpartum hemorrhage due to uterine atony with intravenous prostaglandin E$_2$ case report. *Br. J. Obstet. Gynaecol.* 90:280, 1983.
    Describes the successful use of PGE$_2$, given intravenously, in a patient with intractable primary postpartum hemorrhage stemming from uterine atony.

12. Gunning, J. E. For controlling intractable hemorrhage: The gravity suit. *Contemp. Ob/Gyn* 22:23, 1983.
    The gravity suit can be a lifesaving measure in some patients with severe postpartum hemorrhagic shock. A detailed description of how and when to use the suit is presented.

13. Hestler, J. D. Postpartum hemorrhage and reevaluation of uterine packing. *Obstet. Gynecol.* 45:501, 1975.
    Reports on 153 patients with postpartum hemorrhage. Uterine packing, surgical intervention, and conservative management are compared.

14. Malviya, V. K., and Deppe, G. Control of intraoperative hemorrhage in gynecology with the use of fibrin glue. *Obstet. Gynecol.* 73:284, 1989.
    The authors describe the use of fibrin glue in three patients. They believe that, if used in conjunction with good surgical technique, it would decrease the need for blood transfusions.

Treatment

15. Gilbert, W. M., et al. Angiographic embolization in the management of hemorrhagic complications of pregnancy. *Am. J. Obstet. Gynecol.* 166:493, 1992.
    Use of this procedure in the management of 109 women with pregnancy-related hemorrhage is described, including three cases due to postcesarean bleeding, four stemming from vaginal wall hematomas, two due to cervical pregnancies, and one due to postpartum bleeding. The procedure was successful in all cases and the average duration of the procedure was 167 minutes. The authors conclude that angiographic embolization is effective for controlling postpartum hemorrhage in hemodynamically stable patients.

16. Altabef, K. M., et al. Intravenous nitroglycerin for uterine relaxation of an inverted uterus. *Am. J. Obstet. Gynecol.* 166:1237, 1992.
    Nitroglycerin (50–100 mg), given intravenously, was used to promote uterine relaxation and thus permit replacement of a tightly contracted, inverted uterus. The

relaxation accomplished with this drug was rapid, effective, and without adverse side effects.

Complications

17. Visscher, J. C., and Visscher, R. D. Early and Late Postpartum Hemorrhage. In J. J. Sciarra (ed.), *Gynecology and Obstetrics,* Vol. 2. Hagerstown, MD: Harper & Row, 1980.
    A most complete reference to the causes of both early and late postpartum hemorrhage. The steps taken to prevent this complication are discussed.
18. Feinberg, B. B., et al. Angiographic embolization in the management of late postpartum hemorrhage. A case report. *J. Reprod. Med.* 32:929, 1987.
    Bilateral selective embolization of the internal iliac arteries was used to control late recurrent postpartum hemorrhage. The authors recommend using this procedure as a means of preserving fertility.
19. Weckstein, L. H., Masserman, J. S. H., and Garite, T. J. Placenta accreta: a problem of increasing clinical significance. *Obstet. Gynecol.* 69:480, 1987.
    The case of a woman with placenta previa and accreta is described. The risk factors, incidence, and recommendations for management are discussed.
20. DeSimone, C. A., et al. Intravenous nitroglycerin aids manual extraction of a retained placenta. *Anesthesiology* 73:787, 1990.
    The authors describe the use of intravenous nitroglycerin in 22 patients who required uterine relaxation for manual removal of the placenta. The method was successful in all cases, and there were no maternal side effects.
21. Duggan, P. M., et al. Intractable postpartum hemorrhage managed by angiographic embolization: case report and review. *Aust. N.Z. J. Obstet. Gynaecol.* 31:229, 1991.
    A comprehensive review of the use of this technique to control intractable postpartum hemorrhage. The technique of angiographic embolization and the risks involved are detailed.

40. PUERPERAL INFECTIONS
Michel E. Rivlin

Postpartum febrile morbidity is defined as a temperature of 100.4°F (38°C) occurring in any 2 of the first 10 days after delivery, exclusive of the first 24 hours. Sources of infection in the puerperal period consist of genital tract infection (endometritis), urinary tract infection, breast infection, anesthetic complications, wound infections (including episiotomy), and septic thrombophlebitis. The overall rate of postpartum infection is estimated to range from one to eight percent, and sepsis remains an important, albeit rare, cause of maternal death in the United States.

The most common cause of puerperal fever is genital tract infection, usually of the uterus, generally referred to as *endomyometritis.* Cesarean section is the major predisposing clinical factor for pelvic infection, the risk being five to ten times greater after cesarean section than after vaginal birth. Electively scheduled operations are associated with lower infection rates than are emergency procedures. The risk is much higher after prolonged labor or rupture of the membranes, or both, and after numerous manual cervical examinations, as well as in women who are affected by any of the factors usually associated with postoperative infection—low socioeconomic status, obesity, anemia. Endometritis is most often a mixed infection with aerobic and anaerobic bacteria from the genital tract. The aerobic organisms commonly found include gram-negative bacteria such as *Escherichia coli.* Gram-positive aerobes include group B streptococci. Identification of this particular organism is important because the infant is then at risk for sepsis. In the same way, group A streptococci may cause epidemic infection, and these patients should be isolated. *Staphylococcus aureus* is uncommon but is usually penicillin resistant. The important anaerobes include *Bacteroides fragilis* and *B. bivius,* as well as the anaerobic streptococci (*Peptococcus* and *Peptostreptococcus*) and *Clostridium* species. Genital *Mycoplasma* organisms and *Chlamydia trachomatis* have been implicated; however, many of these patients respond to standard antibiotic regimens, which, in theory, would not cover these organisms.

Diagnosis is based on a clinical picture consisting of fever, malaise, abdominal pain, uterine tenderness, and purulent or foul lochia. The laboratory investigation includes blood count, urinalysis, as well as aerobic and anaerobic blood plus uterine cultures. After vaginal delivery, responses to antibiotic therapy with penicillin plus an aminoglycoside are usually excellent. The few nonresponders probably have anaerobic sepsis, and usually respond to the addition of an appropriate antibiotic such as clindamycin, metronidazole, or chloramphenicol. When endometritis develops after cesarean section, the response is not as good; therefore, initial therapy with clindamycin or high-dose aqueous penicillin combined with gentamicin is recommended and provides better results. Enterococcus (*Streptococcus faecalis*) is the only common isolate that is resistant to the combination of clindamycin and gentamicin, but it does respond to the addition of a penicillin ("triple therapy"). Clindamycin can have serious side effects, including diarrhea in two to six percent of patients and, rarely, precipitates pseudomembranous colitis. Aminoglycoside therapy may lead to nephrotoxicity or ototoxicity, and therapeutic levels are difficult to achieve in obstetric patients with standard doses, thus adding to the expense of treatment the costs of performing "peak and trough" measurements. Therefore, milder cases are often treated with single agents, reserving the use of multiple agents for more severe infections. The new penicillins and cephalosporins have few side effects and are associated with high cure rates. The monobactams (aztreonam) possess specific gram-negative activity and cause fewer side effects than the aminoglycosides, which they may be substituted for. The widespread use of prophylactic antibiotics, usually cephalosporins, has spawned an increase in enterococcal infections; thus, antibiotics active against these organisms (penicillins) should be used when infection occurs in a patient who has received cephalosporins for either therapeutic or prophylactic purposes.

In the postpartum septic patient whose condition is worsening despite appropriate antibiotic therapy, an infected nidus must be sought, both using clinical measures and ultrasound or computed tomographic imaging, as indicated. Possible sites of infection include retained products of conception, pelvic hematomas, pelvic abscess, wound infection, and septic pelvic vein thrombosis. Hematomas and abscesses may be amenable to open or closed drainage, or their clinical course may be followed to resolution with serial imaging studies.

Up to ten percent of lactating women experience mastitis, or breast infection. Usually it is preceded by a clogged duct, unrelieved engorgement, or a cracked nipple; a teething infant and an ill-fitting bra are also predisposing events. Symptoms include a flulike syndrome consisting of generalized myalgia, malaise, and fever, with focal pain and a wedge of erythema in the affected breast. Culture of the milk can distinguish between infection and an inflammatory, noninfectious process or clogged duct. Mastitic milk contains greater than 10^6/ml of white blood cells and more than 10^3/ml of bacterial colonies. The organisms are usually penicillin-resistant *S. aureus* or *epidermidis,* and appropriate antibiotics include dicloxacillin, a cephalosporin, or erythromycin taken orally for 7 to 10 days. Adjunctive measures include ice packs, breast support, and analgesics. Nursing on both breasts should continue, although, if too painful, gentle use of a breast pump may be preferred. Infants do not seem to suffer any adverse effects from suckling an infected breast, unless an abscess develops. Unusually when an abscess forms, incision and drainage with appropriate intravenous antibiotics is necessary.

The obstetric predisposition to urinary tract infection (UTI) continues into the puerperium. Symptoms consisting of frequent urination, dysuria, back pain, fever, and costovertebral angle tenderness suggest the diagnosis, which is confirmed by the demonstration of pyuria and by culture. Although traditionally colonies exceeding 10^5/ml were considered significant, it is now thought that the finding of greater than 10^2/ml is more specific and sensitive in symptomatic patients. Generally, *E. coli* is isolated in this setting, although other gram-negative aerobic bacilli and enterococci may be found. Because it is possible for bacteremia to develop in the setting of pyelonephritis, hospital admission with the parenteral administration of antibiotics is indicated, generally ampicillin or a cephalosporin initially with an aminoglycoside added if septic shock develops or if a resistant organism is suspected. Anesthetic complications may arise after general anesthesia administered for cesarean section, and atelectasis and pulmonary infections may present with fever after delivery. Rarely, transvaginal pudendal blocks may be complicated by the formation of a deep-seated abscess behind the psoas or beneath the gluteus muscles. Drainage is required for these serious infections. Infections related to conduction anesthesia are extremely rare.

Wound infection occurs in about 10 percent of patients who undergo cesarean section. A wound is defined as "infected" if there is a pus discharge and as "possibly infected" if either inflammation or serous discharge is present. The risk factors are the same as those associated with intrauterine infections. Early onset infections (within the first 48 hours) are usually caused by a single pathogen, commonly group A or B streptococcus or *Clostridium perfringens*. There may be spreading cellulitis, and aggressive therapy with extensive debridement of necrotic tissue may be required to prevent necrotizing fasciitis. Penicillin is the antibiotic of choice for clostridia and group A streptococci infection. Late-onset infections (4–8 days after operation) are much more common, and these infections are usually polymicrobial. Opening the wound to allow drainage, together with the institution of broad-spectrum antibiotic therapy, is generally successful in controlling the infection. The possibility of dehiscence or necrotizing fasciitis must be kept in mind. Episiotomy infections are generally simple to treat, and treatment consisting of opening, exploring, and allowing the perineal wound to drain is usually sufficient. Antibiotics are indicated if group A streptococci are present or if cellulitis is marked. The incision should be allowed to heal by granulation. If resuture is necessary, this should be delayed until the field is infection free (generally several weeks later). Rare, potentially fatal cases of necrotizing fasciitis have occurred, requiring early extensive resection of necrotic tissue together with intensive supportive and antibiotic therapy.

Septic pelvic thrombophlebitis occurs once in 2000 spontaneous vaginal deliveries, and is approximately 10 to 20 times more frequent after cesarean section. Organisms spread within thrombosed veins, and, from these foci, septic thromboemboli may result in the formation of pulmonary emboli and metastatic abscesses, with intermittent septicemia. Anaerobic bacteria are commonly implicated. The most characteristic presentation is a fever of unknown origin, with no demonstrable focus, that is complicating a pelvic infection and not responding to complete antibiotic coverage. Clinical evaluation includes blood gas determinations, chest x-ray studies, and a lung scan if pulmonary emboli are suspected. Ultrasound, computed tomography, or nuclear magnetic resonance imaging may reveal the blood clot; however, the heparin challenge test is probably the most practical approach. Rapid lysis of the fever within 48 hours indicates that the disease is probably present. Therapy consists of antibiotic coverage and anticoagulation (heparin for 5 to 7 days, then warfarin for 30 days more). Rarely, heparin failure requires operative intervention consisting of the ligation of the involved veins or the placement of an inferior vena cava filter.

General

1. Soper, D. E. Postpartum endometritis. Pathophysiology and prevention. *J. Reprod. Med.* 33:97, 1988.
    Endomyometritis may spread to the adnexa, broad ligaments, peritoneal cavity, and pelvic veins, causing pelvic abscesses, peritonitis, or septic pelvic thrombophlebitis.
2. Fortunato, S. J., and Dodson, M. G. Therapeutic considerations in postpartum endometritis. *J. Reprod. Med.* 33:101, 1988.
    Early and more severe patterns of onset, especially with evidence of septic shock,

suggest less common infections, particularly Streptococcus pyogenes, Escherichia coli, *and* Clostridium welchii.

Etiology

3. Hohnson, S. R., et al. Maternal obesity and pregnancy. *Surg. Gynecol. Obstet.* 164:431, 1987.
   In obese women undergoing cesarean section, there was an increased incidence of blood loss exceeding 1 L, operating time longer than 2 hours, and postoperative wound infection.
4. Hoyme, U. B., Kiviat, N., and Eschenbach, D. A. Microbiology and treatment of late postpartum endometritis. *Obstet. Gynecol.* 68:226, 1986.
   Endometritis occurring 7 to 42 days after delivery may be related to retained products of conception and to infections with Chlamydia *or genital* mycoplasma *organisms. Erythromycin therapy was successful in 10 of the 13 women followed in this study.*
5. Walmer, D., Walmer, K. R., and Gibbs, R. S. Enterococci in post-cesarean endometritis. *Obstet. Gynecol.* 71:159, 1988.
   In the National Nosocomial Infection System report on obstetric bacteremias, staphylococci were the most common infecting orgamism (20.4%), anaerobes were the next most common (12.2%), followed by E. coli *(8.2%), and thereafter the "breakthrough" organism enterococci (6.1%).*
6. Newton, E. R., Prihoda, T. J., and Gibbs, R. S. A clinical and microbiologic analysis of risk factors for puerperal endometritis. *Obstet. Gynecol.* 75:402, 1990.
   Cesarean delivery and the detection of certain organisms, such as bacterial vaginosis or high-virulence organisms, predict the presence of endometritis. Clinical variables may be facilitators rather than predictors of endometritis.
7. Watts, D. H., et al. Bacterial vaginosis as a risk factor for post-cesarean endometritis. *Obstet. Gynecol.* 75:52, 1990.
   At the time of endometritis, anaerobes and Gardnerella *were isolated more frequently from the endometrium among patients with bacterial vaginosis than among those with a normal gram-stained specimen. Bacterial vaginosis may be an important risk factor for postcesarean endometritis.*
8. Chang, P. L., and Newton, E. R. Predictors of antibiotic prophylactic failure in post-cesarean endometritis. *Obstet. Gynecol.* 80:117, 1992.
   The number of vaginal examinations was the single predictor of prophylactic antibiotic failure.
9. Seo, K., et al. Preterm birth is associated with increased risk of maternal and neonatal infection. *Obstet. Gynecol.* 79:75, 1992.
   Among the women delivered by cesarean section, the incidence of postpartum endometritis was higher in those with preterm rupture of membranes than in those with term rupture of membranes.
10. Olsen, C. G., and Gordon, R. E., Jr. Breast disorders in nursing mothers. *Am. Fam. Physician* 41:1509, 1990.
    Mastitis develops in approximately 2.5 percent of nursing women, usually between 2 and 5 weeks after delivery.

Diagnosis

11. Awadalla, S. G., Perkins, R. P., and Mercer, L. J. Significance of endometrial cultures performed at cesarean section. *Obstet. Gynecol.* 68:220, 1986.
    Staphylococcus aureus is occasionally found, usually in diabetics or patients with cervical lacerations, an episiotomy, or other trauma. The infection is clinically similar to that caused by anaerobes.
12. Duff, P., et al. Endometrial culture techniques in puerperal patients. *Obstet. Gynecol.* 61:217, 1983.
    The most satisfactory culture procedure was brush biopsy or lavage performed through a double-lumen catheter.
13. Lev-Toaff, A. S., et al. Diagnostic imaging in puerperal febrile morbidity. *Obstet. Gynecol.* 78:50, 1991.
    Only two of 31 patients with refractory puerperal febrile morbidity had negative

imaging studies. Sonography is the usual initial modality, with computed tomography the usual backup and magnetic resonance imaging used only occasionally.

Treatment

14. Soper, D. E., Brockwell, N. J., and Dalton H. P. The importance of wound infection in antibiotic failures in the therapy of postpartum endometritis. *Surg. Gynecol. Obstet.* 174:265, 1992.

Close correlation between endometrial and wound cultures suggests a frequent relationship. Wound infection should be suspected if the patient is still febrile 48 hours or more after antibiotics were commenced.

15. Pastorek, J. G., II, and Sanders, C. V., Jr. Antibiotic therapy for postcesarean endomyometritis. *Rev. Infect. Dis.* 9:S752, 1991.

The widespread clinical use of a drug predicts its eventual ineffectiveness as bacterial resistance emerges.

16. Faro, S., et al. Comparative efficacy and safety of mezlocillin, cefoxitin, and clindamycin plus gentamicin in postpartum endometritis. *Obstet. Gynecol.* 69:760, 1987.

Single-agent therapy using the newer broad-spectrum beta-lactam drugs (e.g., semisynthetic penicillins, cefotaxime, moxalactam, and clavulanic acid [Timentin]) appears to be as effective clinically as "gold-standard" therapy.

17. Pastorek, J. G., II, Ragan, F. A. Jr., and Phelan, M. Tobramycin dosing in the puerperal patient. *J. Reprod. Med.* 32:343, 1987.

Puerperal patients require much higher aminoglycoside dosages than usual, so that serum levels must be monitored for therapeutic reasons rather than for toxicity. The authors suggest replacing the aminoglycoside with one of the new monobactams (aztreonam), which has a wide range of activity, minimal toxicity, and similar efficacy.

18. Dinsmoor, M. J., Newton, E. R., and Gibbs, R. S. A randomized, double-blind, placebo-controlled trial of oral antibiotic therapy following intravenous antibiotic therapy for postpartum endometritis. *Obstet. Gynecol.* 77:60, 1991.

Oral antibiotic therapy is unnecessary after successful intravenous antibiotic therapy for endometritis.

19. Karstrup, S., et al. Ultrasonically guided percutaneous drainage of breast abscesses. *Acta Radiol.* 31:157, 1990.

This avoided the need for surgical drainage, and three of the four patients continued nursing during and after the period of treatment.

Complications

20. Cruse, P. E., and Foord, R. Epidemiology of wound infection. A 10-year prospective study of 62,930 wounds. *Surg. Clin. North Am.* 60:27, 1980.

The infection rate for clean wounds was 1.7 percent; for clean-contaminated wounds, 8.8 percent; for contaminated wounds, 17.5 percent; and for dirty wounds, 30 percent.

21. Dodson, M. K., Magann, E. F., and Meeks, G. R. A randomized comparison of secondary closure and secondary intention in patients with superficial wound dehiscence. *Obstet. Gynecol.* 80:321, 1992.

Secondary closure of a superficial wound dehiscence is superior to healing by secondary intention.

22. Ramin, S. M., et al. Early repair of episiotomy dehiscence associated with infection. *Am. J. Obstet. Gynecol.* 167:1104, 1992.

Successful early repairs were accomplished in 32 of 34 patients.

23. Ammari, N. N., et al. Postpartum necrotizing fasciitis: case report. *Br. J. Obstet. Gynaecol.* 93:82, 1986.

The pathognomonic feature is subcutaneous necrosis. A moderate-to-severe systemic toxic reaction is usually associated. It is essential to make an early diagnosis followed almost immediately by surgical debridement to healthy margins.

24. Rivlin, M. E., and Hunt, J. A. Surgical management of diffuse peritonitis complicating obstetric/gynecologic infections. *Obstet. Gynecol.* 67:652, 1986.

Severe infections resistant to medical therapy are rare but require timely surgical intervention to prevent serious morbidity and even mortality.

25. Cohen, M. B., et al. Septic pelvic thrombophlebitis: an update. *Obstet. Gynecol.* 62:83, 1983.

    A clinical response after the addition of heparin to the antibiotic regimen provides presumptive evidence of the diagnosis. Operative ligation of the ovarian veins is rarely necessary.

26. Rosenberg, J. M., et al. *Clostridium difficile* colitis in surgical patients. *Am. J. Surg.* 147:486, 1984.

    Features of significant antibiotic-associated pseudomembranous colitis include watery diarrhea, cramps, fever, leukocytosis, and rectal bleeding.

27. Pearlman, M., and Faro, S. Obstetric septic shock: a pathophysiologic basis for management. *Clin. Obstet. Gynecol.* 33:482, 1990.

    Life-threatening complications of uncontrolled sepsis include septicemia, septic shock, adult respiratory distress syndrome, and multiple-organ failure.

41. DEEP VEIN THROMBOSIS AND PULMONARY EMBOLISM
Baha M. Sibai

Deep vein thrombosis (DVT) is an infrequent but serious complication of pregnancy because of the ultimate risk of pulmonary embolism and potential fatal outcome. The incidence of DVT ranges from 0.5 to 1.0 per 1000 pregnancies during the antepartum period, increasing fivefold postpartum. If untreated, 16 percent of the patients will suffer a pulmonary embolism, which carries a 10 to 15 percent mortality rate. If adequately treated, however, pulmonary embolism occurs in less than 5 percent, with a mortality rate of less than 1 percent.

Pregnancy is considered a state of hypercoagulopathy owing to the progressive increase in the levels of all plasma coagulation factors (except XI and XIII). There is also a decrease in the fibrinolytic activity because of a reduction in the level of the circulating plasminogen activator. At the same time, there is progressive venous stasis because of venous dilatation and elevated capacitance, as well as increased pressure on the pelvic vessels. This combined effect of hypercoagulability and venous stasis appears to be responsible for the greater risk of thromboembolism present during pregnancy. This risk is further accentuated by the following individual factors: (1) cesarean birth, (2) instrumental vaginal delivery, (3) increased maternal age, (4) suppression of lactation by estrogens, (5) sickle cell disease, (6) prior history of thrombophlebitis, (7) maternal cardiac disease, (8) prolonged immobilization, (9) obesity, (10) maternal infection, and (11) chronic venous insufficiency.

The diagnosis of DVT during the antepartum period is usually made on the basis of certain clinical signs and symptoms, identified by nonspecific, noninvasive techniques. Diagnostic x-ray and radiosotope studies are potentially harmful to the fetus and are not performed. Symptoms include swelling, muscle pain, and tenderness, as well as a positive Homans' sign and Lowenberg's test. Unfortunately, reliance on these findings alone will result in an incorrect diagnosis (false positive or false negative) in 50 percent of the cases. Moreover, it is important that DVT be differentiated from superficial inflammation of the vein, as the treatment and prognosis of this problem are radically different.

Investigations using venography have revealed that about half of the patients with DVT exhibit no clinical signs, whereas the venographic findings are normal in 45 percent of those with clinical signs. Clinical diagnosis is most reliable in the presence of significant thrombosis in a tense, swollen extremity, with attendant pain and tenderness that extend to the thigh. Noninvasive techniques such as the Doppler ultrasonic velocity flow detector and impedance plethysmography can be helpful in detecting major venous obstruction (mainstream occlusive thrombi from the popliteal vein to the vena cava and large clots below the knee), but are unreliable for identifying minor venous thrombosis in the calf muscle area (sural and tibial veins). The overall accuracy of these tests is about 80 to 95 percent. The special advantages of these techniques are that they can be used as screening techniques, performed serially, and potentially used for day-to-day follow-up studies. Thermography is another noninvasive technique that is potentially useful for detecting calf vein and femoral vein thrombosis. This technique has an accuracy of 90 percent, compared to that of contrast-enhanced phlebography. Ascending contrast-enhanced phlebography can also be used in the evaluation of the patient with suspected DVT, and is the most sensitive and reliable of all tests for its detection. It can be used during pregnancy, but its disadvantages are that it is invasive and carries a moderate degree of risk, and hence should not be used as a screening procedure. The fibrinogen uptake test (using iodine 125–labeled fibrinogen) is of value in diagnosing lower extremity venous thrombosis and is most valuable in screening patients with risk factors during the postpartum period. This test should not be used in patients who are breast-feeding or pregnant.

The diagnosis of pulmonary embolism depends on the clinical history and course, physical findings, appropriate laboratory test findings, and results of specific procedures. The signs, symptoms, and laboratory data are often nonspecific, however, as nearly 50 percent of the cases arise without a prior diagnosis of thrombophlebitis having been made. The most common findings are dyspnea, tachypnea, chest pain, hemoptysis, and tachycardia. An arterial oxygen tension (PaO_2) of less than 80 mm Hg in room air in conjunction with a positive lung scan is a useful finding in confirming the diagnosis. Both anteroposterior and lateral scans should be obtained to reduce the likelihood of false-negative results. If positive, the scan reveals a lung perfusion defect but does not delineate the cause. Pulmonary arteriography remains the most specific and reliable diagnostic procedure for the definitive diagnosis of pulmonary embolism. These techniques are used during gestation because of the serious nature of a pulmonary embolism, but they do have significant risks for both the fetus and the mother.

Symptomatic treatment in the form of bed rest, elevation of the affected extremity, the application of moist heat, and the wearing of elastic stockings may be helpful in managing DVT. Anticoagulant therapy consisting of either heparin or warfarin, however, is the definitive mode of treatment for DVT, with or without pulmonary embolism. Heparin is the drug of choice in the antepartum period because it does not cross the placenta owing to its large molecular size and negative charge. The usual regimen of heparin is a loading dose of 5000 units, followed by a continuous intravenous maintenance dose of 1000 units/hr.

Many also use a loading dose of 20,000 units if a pulmonary embolus is suspected. Adjustment of the maintenance dose should be based on a prolonged Lee-White clotting time or a partial thromboplastin time that is twice the normal value.

Intravenous heparin therapy should be continued for about 7 to 10 days after the resolution of all symptoms. Following this regimen, the patient is switched to receiving low-dose heparin injections, usually 5000 to 10,000 units every 12 hours. The heparin therapy is continued throughout pregnancy and for 6 to 12 weeks postpartum, administered either by the subcutaneous route or by intravenous injections through an implanted Teflon intravenous catheter. Heparin may be discontinued at the time of labor and resumed immediately postpartum, but many continue its use even through operative deliveries without undue hemorrhage occurring. Oral warfarin sodium can be used in the postpartum period but is difficult to regulate, with frequent prothrombin time assessment necessary for follow-up care. In addition, warfarin is a small molecule that readily crosses the placenta, and there is an inherent risk of its producing congenital anomalies if given during the first trimester. If used later in pregnancy, it can cause fetal anticoagulation, leading to fetal or neonatal hemorrhage as well as placental abruption. On the other hand, prolonged heparin therapy in pregnancy can cause bone demineralization and may lead to spinal fractures. Another serious side effect of heparin use is the possible development of thrombocytopenia, which usually occurs within 1 to 2 weeks after the initiation of therapy. Hence, patients treated with heparin should have serial platelet counts.

Pulmonary embolism constitutes a serious life-threatening situation that requires immediate aggressive management. Medical management consists of intravenous heparin therapy, the same as that for DVT except for a larger loading dose, and intravenous treatment should be maintained for a minimum of 2 weeks. After this regimen, either intermittent heparin is given or oral warfarin is used, as outlined previously. Supportive therapy in the form of oxygen therapy to keep the maternal PaO_2 above 70 mm Hg, bronchodilators, maternal sedation, and the immediate management of shock or congestive heart failure are of equal importance. If an embolism develops postpartum, anticoagulation should be continued for 3 to 6 months following initial therapy. Surgical intervention should be reserved for patients with massive embolization, those whose embolism recurs despite adequate medical therapy, and parturients in whom anticoagulation is contraindicated.

Septic pelvic thrombophlebitis is usually a complication of postpartum, postabortal, or postoperative pelvic infections. The clinical picture includes persistent spiking fever, with or without chills, and tachycardia—all in spite of adequate antibiotic therapy. The pelvic examination findings may be normal, and the diagnosis is made on the basis of the clinical response to a trial of heparin therapy. The treatment of choice is intravenous heparin and antibiotics maintained for a minimum of 7 days.

The use of "minidoses" of heparin for prophylaxis has been reported to decrease the incidence of DVT and fatal pulmonary emboli in patients undergoing major surgical procedures. In standard regimens, 5000 units are given subcutaneously 2 hours before operation, to be repeated every 8 to 12 hours postoperatively until the patient is fully ambulatory. This small dose acts by enhancing the action of antithrombin factor III, which inhibits the activation of factor X. Unfortunately, little is known about its use in pregnancy, but it may be helpful in patients with high-risk factors, such as previous thromboembolic disease and massive obesity and when DVT develops early in the antepartum period. More data, however, are needed to document its effectiveness during pregnancy.

General
1. Sipes, S. L., and Weiner, C. P. Venous thromboembolic disease in pregnancy. *Semin. Perinatol.* 14:103, 1990.
   This comprehensive article details the pathogenesis, risk factors, prophylaxis, and management of thromboembolic disease.
2. Thromboembolic Risk Factors (THRIFT) Consensus Group. Risk of and prophylaxis for venous thromboembolism in hospital patients. *Br. Med. J.* 305:567, 1992.
   Reports the findings from a consensus conference held in Great Britain. It describes the groups at risk for venous thromboembolism, and the incidence and outcome according to a classification that categorizes a patient as low, moderate, or high risk. Prophylaxis is recommended for patients requiring a gynecologic operation, either during pregnancy or in the puerperium.

Etiology
3. Vorherr, H. Puerperium: Maternal Involution Changes and Management of Puerperal Problems and Complications. In J. J. Sciarra (ed.), *Gynecology and Obstetrics,* Vol. 2. Hagarstown, MD: Harper & Row, 1985.
   The etiologic and associative factors related to thrombophlebitis that develops after pregnancy are discussed.
4. Colditz, G. A., Tuden, R. L., and Oster, G. Rates of venous thrombosis after general surgery: combined results of randomised clinical trials. *Lancet* 2:143, 1986.
   Data from 45 trials of prophylactic methods to decrease the occurrence of DVT after surgical procedures were compared in this elegant meta-analysis. Most of the studies revealed a clear difference between the rate of DVT in the control group and that in the various treatment groups. The results suggest that combined therapy may be most beneficial.

5. Esmon, C. T. The regulation of natural anticoagulant pathways. *Science* 235: 1348, 1987.
   An excellent and up-to-date summary of the natural anticoagulant pathways.
6. Tengborn, L., et al. Recurrent thromboembolism in pregnancy and puerperium. Is there a need for thromboprophylaxis? *Am. J. Obstet. Gynecol.* 160:90, 1989.
   The authors compared the effects of heparin prophylaxis versus no prophylaxis in patients during a pregnancy that followed a thromboembolic episode. The frequency of recurrent thrombosis was approximately half that seen in those who did not receive treatment.

Diagnosis
7. Didolkar, S. M., Koontz, C., and Schimberg, P. I. Phleborheography in pregnancy. *Obstet. Gynecol.* 61:363, 1983.
   The authors compared the phleborheographic findings in 48 asymptomatic pregnant patients studied during the second or third trimesters or immediately postpartum to the normal phleborheographic findings in nonpregnant patients. This study indicated that both chronic and acute venous obstruction are absent during normal pregnancy.
8. Sandler, D. A., et al. Diagnosis of deep-vein thrombosis: comparison of clinical evaluation, ultrasound, plethysmography, and venoscan with x-ray venogram. *Lancet* 2:716, 1984.
   Of multiple devices available for the diagnosis of DVT, only the x-ray venogram proved suitable for definitive diagnosis, while the venoscan (fibrinogen scintigraphy) was found to be suitable only as a screening device.
9. Lensing, A. W. A., et al. Detection of deep-vein thrombosis by real-time B-mode ultrasonography. *N. Engl. J. Med.* 320:342, 1989.
   The authors give details on 220 consecutive patients with suspected DVT diagnosed by B-mode ultrasonography. They believe it to be a highly accurate, simple, and objective noninvasive method of diagnosis, particularly in proximal vein areas.
10. White, R. H., et al. Diagnosis of deep-vein thrombosis using duplex ultrasound. *Ann. Intern. Med.* III:297, 1989.
    The authors reviewed all published studies comparing duplex ultrasound with venography in the diagnosis of DVT. The sensitivity of duplex ultrasound in detecting proximal thrombi ranged from 92 to 95 percent (average, 93%), and the specificity ranged from 97 to 100 percent (94.8%).

Treatment
11. Bergquist, A., Bergquist, D., and Hallbook, T. Deep vein thrombosis during pregnancy. A prospective study. *Acta Obstet. Gynecol. Scand.* 62:443, 1983.
    Seventeen women with DVT occurring during pregnancy were studied prospectively. The diagnosis made using noninvasive techniques and confirmed by phlebography. The patients were treated with heparin during pregnancy. The authors recommend that the diagnosis of DVT should be verified objectively before the institution of treatment.
12. Turpie, A. G. G., et al. Double-blind randomised trial of Org 10172 low-molecular-weight heparinoid in prevention of deep-vein thrombosis in thrombotic stroke. *Lancet* 1:523, 1987.
    Prophylaxis using low-molecular-weight heparin (heparinoids) was carried out in patients who were bedridden. Patients given heparin prophylactically responded better than did the control group in terms of the rate of DVT, and there was only one complication.
13. Hahn, C. L. A. Pulsatile heparin administration in pregnancy: a new approach. *Am. J. Obstet. Gynecol.* 155:283, 1986.
    Fifteen women used a portable infusion pump to administer heparin, either subcutaneously or intravenously, for up to 25 weeks. Patient acceptability of the pump was excellent, and there were no untoward events.
14. Turner, G. M., Cole, S. E., and Brooks, J.H. The efficacy of graduated compres-

sion stocking in the prevention of deep vein thrombosis after major gynaecological surgery. *Br. J. Obstet. Gynaecol.* 91:588, 1984.

Patients at risk for DVT were treated with a graduated compression stocking, and the occurrence of thromboembolic complications was less than that seen in the patients not wearing the stockings.

15. Turpie, A. G. G., et al. Randomised comparison of two intensities of oral anticoagulant therapy after tissue heart valve replacement. *Lancet* 1:1242, 1988.

Two intensities of treatment were used in patients receiving oral anticoagulants; the hemorrhagic complications associated with the standard regimen were more than twice more frequent than those seen for the treatment consisting of smaller doses of anticoagulants.

16. Dahlman, T. C., et al. Thrombosis prophylaxis in pregnancy with use of subcutaneous heparin adjusted by monitoring heparin concentration in plasma. *Am. J. Obstet. Gynecol.* 161:420, 1989.

Twenty-six pregnant women were given heparin prophylactically because of previous thromboembolic complications. The amount of heparin was adjusted to keep plasma levels at about 0.1 IU/ml, measured in the form of antifactor XA activity. The average dose of heparin used was 16,400 IU/24 hr or 225 IU/kg of body weight. This method was not associated with adverse effects on either the platelet count or on the amount of blood loss at delivery. None of the patients suffered spinal fractures resulting from osteoporosis. The authors concluded that a heparin dosage of about 240 IU/kg-hr, divided into two doses (7500–10,000 IU twice daily), is appropriate in most pregnant patients.

17. Porreco, R. P., McDuffie, R. S., Jr., and Peck, S. D. Fixed mini-dose warfarin for prophylaxis of thromboembolic diseaes in pregnancy: a safe alternative for the fetus? *Obstet. Gynecol.* 81:806, 1993.

Warfarin, 1 mg daily, was given in the third trimester of pregnancy. Fetal cord blood samples were obtained at 33, 36, and 38 weeks. No fetal coagulation abnormalities were detected.

Complications

18. DeSwiet, M., et al. Prolonged heparin therapy in pregnancy causes bone demineralization. *Br. J. Obstet. Gynaecol.* 90:1129, 1983.

The authors studied the relationship between osteoporosis and prolonged heparin therapy in 20 patients who received subcutaneous heparin during pregnancy and postpartum. The findings indicated that prophylactic heparin therapy in pregnancy is associated with bone demineralization that is dose related.

19. Landefeld, C. S., et al. Identification and preliminary validation of predictors of major bleeding in hospitalized patients starting anticoagulant therapy. *Am. J. Med.* 82:703, 1987.

In this large study involving 617 patients on long-term anticoagulant therapy, the most common site of bleeding was in the gastrointestinal tract. A prediction profile of the risks for bleeding complications was detailed by the authors and included old age, a very elevated prothrombin time or partial thromboplastin time, liver dysfunction, and multiorgan disease.

20. Floyd, R. C., et al. Administration of heparin by subcutaneous infusion with a programmable pump. *Am. J. Obstet. Gynecol.* 165:931, 1991.

The use of a programmable automated subcutaneous heparin infusion pump in conjunction with weekly home nursing visits was studied in eight pregnant women requiring such therapy during pregnancy. Eight well-matched women who received intermittent subcutaneous heparin prophylaxis served as the control group. The coagulation achieved in women receiving heparin by means of a pump was better (20.6 versus 10.4 seconds above control) than that in those receiving intermittent heparin injections. There were no maternal complications resulting from use of the pump, and the pump was better received by patients than was the intermittent injection technique.

21. Dahlman, T. C. Osteoporotic fractures and the recurrence of thromboembolism during pregnancy and the puerperium in 184 women undergoing thromboprophylaxis with heparin. *Am. J. Obstet. Gynecol.* 168:1265, 1993.

One hundred eighty-four women received prophylactic heparin treatment during pregnancy. Vertebral fractures occurred in 2.2 percent and 2.7 percent of the women had recurrent thromboembolic problems.

42. POSTPARTUM DEPRESSION
Joseph P. Bruner and Frank H. Boehm

One of the most significant events in a woman's life is childbearing. In terms of the physiologic and psychologic changes involved, it may surpass those of menarche and menopause. The appearance of a variety of psychologic reactions in the postpartum period, therefore, is not unusual. The most common of these is the so-called maternity blues, which occurs in 50 to 70 percent of women after childbirth. The incidence of true postpartum depression ranges from 10 to 15 percent, while puerperal psychosis, including major postpartum depression and postpartum psychotic depression, occurs in only 0.14 to 0.26 percent of women postpartum.

Mild depression after delivery is quite common and, upon close questioning, most patients admit to experiencing some form of the "blues" in the postpartum period. Considering the psychologic and physiologic changes that take place during pregnancy, along with the extreme excitement evoked by the labor and delivery process, it is to be expected that a woman will often experience an emotional letdown postpartum. After returning home from the hospital, she is alone with her new baby and the realities of caring for her infant. The telephone calls, visitors, and attention she received in the hospital have diminished, and most women describe a feeling of isolation that is clinically much like mild depression. Although definitions of the disorder vary, "postpartum blues" are manifested by tearfulness, despondency, anxiety, and confusion. The clinical symptoms are typically transient, appearing within 3 to 4 days after delivery and resolving in less than 2 weeks. Although most patients handle this stressful transition without significant or serious depression arising, certain women suffer true postpartum depression, requiring extensive treatment and follow-up.

During the early postpartum period, the signs and symptoms of "maternity blues" and true postpartum depression are similar and may be difficult to distinguish. Should "postpartum blues" either persist or worsen, however, the possibility of true depression or even postpartum psychosis must be carefully watched for. The appearance of suicidal ideations, hallucinations, or delusions is especially concerning, and dictates the need for prompt psychiatric consultation for consideration of inpatient care. Although certain symptoms are common to all of the postpartum depressive disorders, it may be misleading to think of them as progressively more severe stages of the same psychologic disturbance.

Although the etiology of postpartum depression is not known, there are three general elements that may play an important role. Although there is no proof that the massive physiologic changes of pregnancy bring about postpartum depression, most authors believe that biologic changes may contribute to its development. The postpartum patient has just come through a very stressful period of labor and delivery, which may include blood loss, anesthesia, surgery, and often substantial discomfort. Postpartum levels of steroid and peptide hormones fall rapidly. Finally, recent evidence suggests a link between neurotransmitter or thyroid dysfunction and depressive symptomatology.

A second theory, or element, is that of an underlying psychiatric disorder that the pregnancy brings out. Studies to determine the effect of antecedent psychologic status on the subsequent development of postpartum depression, however, have been frustrating. In one study of 60 pregnant women, none of the women with the poorest premorbid personality function developed serious psychiatric illness during the early postpartum period. Another study of 198 cases of serious psychiatric disorders arising during pregnancy revealed that 46 percent of the patients had a history of preexisting psychiatric problems, 22 percent of the illnesses began during the pregnancy, and a psychiatric disorder arose in the postpartum period in 32 percent. Of the last group, only half of the cases were detected before hospital discharge. The occurrence of postpartum psychosis is most closely correlated with the severity of previous psychiatric disorders and with a previous psychotic episode occurring just before pregnancy.

In a third theory, negative social factors are thought to play a role. The newborn infant may represent a significant financial burden for the mother and family, and may impose an added emotional problem on an already unstable marriage. A patient who is involved in her own career may find the added burden of childrearing creates an ever-increasing dilemma. Women who become distressed postpartum report less spousal support and more stressful life events than do women who are not depressed, confirming the concept that the perception of adequate social support mitigates the harmful effects of stress.

Although biologic, physiologic, and sociologic factors cannot be definitely linked to the etiology of postpartum depression, they may, singularly or in concert, play a role in its eventual evolution. Postpartum depression knows no socioeconomic boundaries and may lead to considerable problems for any puerperal patients.

There is no known way to prevent either postpartum "blues" or true depression, but early diagnosis and treatment are important, so the health-care provider should (1) maintain a high level of suspicion; (2) when indicated, alert the husband and family to the problem; (3) help ease the patient's insomnia by prescribing a mild sedative; and (4) be flexible in scheduling postpartum follow-up, seeing the patient as early as 1 to 2 weeks after discharge rather than waiting the usual 6 weeks for the first postpartum visit. The health-care provider should be willing to spend more time with the patient, explaining the process of childbearing to her and her husband in the hope of reducing the stress. In patients who still have ambivalent feelings about the infant at the time of labor and delivery, enhanced parent-infant interactions may be of help. This is accomplished through close physical contact between the mother and child, beginning immediately after delivery and continuing throughout the hospitalization.

Except for the relatively mild "maternity blues," the mainstay of treatment is pharmacotherapy consisting of standard antidepressants, neuroleptics, and lithium, as dictated by the severity and particular subset of symptoms manifested. In cases in which the response to drugs is poor, electroconvulsive therapy may reduce the need for prolonged hospitalization. Because the recurrence risk may be as high as 25 percent in subsequent pregnancies, treatment may be initiated in the immediate postpartum period for some patients. Equally important, however, is having the patient become involved in proper psychiatric therapy and take advantage of other support services, most of which can be done on an outpatient basis. With early diagnosis and therapy, the prognosis for this condition is usually good. The investigators in one study of 21 patients with puerperal psychosis concluded that the prognosis in the setting of spontaneous recovery is excellent. Even patients who require active intervention can be expected to do well, although follow-up in the children of women who suffer postpartum psychosis has revealed that behavioral disturbances occur in some. However, the existence of multiple intervening variables makes the findings from such studies difficult to interpret. The best predictor of successful therapy is the presence of adequate support both in the family and from health-care providers.

General
1. Watson, J. P., et al. Psychiatric disorders in pregnancy and the first postnatal year. *Br. J. Psychiatry* 144:453, 1984.
   Most cases of an affective disorder were associated with a previous psychiatric history or reaction to stressful events, including childbirth itself.
2. Kendell, R. E. Emotional and physical factors in the genesis of puerperal mental disorders. *J. Psychosom. Res.* 29:3, 1985.
   Excellent review article of past and current literature.
3. Wrate, R. M., et al. Postnatal depression and child development. *Br. J. Psychiatry* 146:622, 1985.
   Those children whose mothers had postpartum depressive symptoms and in-

creased anxiety about child welfare exhibited more behavioral disturbances than those children whose mothers experienced either no depression or severe depression. Findings suggest that more than one intervening variable contributes to outcome.

4. Youngs, D. D., and Lucas, M. J. Postpartum depression: hormonal versus alternative perspectives. In D. D. Youngs and J. Ehrhardt (eds.), *Psychosomatic Obstetrics and Gynecology.* Norwalk, CT: Appleton-Century-Crofts, 1980.

   This chapter, which is an excellent review on the subject of postpartum depression, discusses biologic and psychologic factors.

5. Hatherley, L. I., et al. Psychiatric disorders in obstetrics. *Med. J. Aust.* 2:399, 1979.

   The rate of puerperal psychosis cited in this article is 2.4 per 1000 and the incidence of psychiatric problems throughout pregnancy is as high as 7.2 cases per 1000.

Etiology

6. Handley, S. L., et al. Tryptophan, cortisol and puerperal mood. *Br. J. Psychiatry* 136:498, 1980.

   This article suggests that tryptophan, a neurotransmitter precursor, is implicated in the psychologic changes that take place postpartum.

7. Gard, P. R., et al. A multivariate investigation of postpartum mood disturbance. *Br. J. Psychiatry* 145:567, 1987.

   In a study of 52 women, the authors were able to discriminate between "blues" and depression using statistical analyses. The two are only weakly related and are associated with separate and independent causative factors.

8. Gennaro, S. Postpartal anxiety and depression in mothers of term and preterm infants. *Nursing Res.* 37:82, 1988.

   The mothers of preterm infants exhibited more anxiety and depression initially than did the mothers of term infants, but the differences did not persist over time. Acute anxiety does not necessarily predispose to the development of long-term postpartum depression.

9. Nemeroff, C. B., et al. Antithyroid antibodies in depressed patients. *Am. J. Psychiatry* 142:840, 1985.

   Elevated levels of antimicrosomal and antithyroglobulin antithyroid antibodies were detected in a sample of nonpregnant euthyroid psychiatric inpatients with prominent depressive symptoms.

10. Smith, R., et al. Mood changes, obstetric experience and alterations in plasma cortisol, beta-endorphin and corticotrophin releasing hormone during pregnancy and the puerperium. *J. Psychiatr. Res.* 34:53, 1990.

    The finding from this prospective study of 97 primiparous Australian women suggest that, although antenatal mood states were primarily determined by obstetric events, a significant association exists between maternal postnatal mood states and serum levels of beta-endorphin.

11. O'Hara, M. W., et al. Prospective study of postpartum blues. *Arch. Gen. Psychiatry* 48:801, 1991.

    Potential biologic and psychosocial causative factors responsible for the postpartum blues were examined in a prospective study of 182 women. Women experiencing postpartum depression reported more stressful life events and less support from their spouses after delivery.

12. Beck, C. T. Teetering on the edge: a substantive theory of postpartum depression. *Nurs. Res.* 42:42, 1993.

    Postpartum depression was analyzed in a group of women over an 18-month period. Loss of control was revealed to be the main psychologic problem.

Diagnosis

13. Hans, A. Postpartum assessment: the psychological component. *J.O.G.N.* 15:49, 1986.

    Presents a comprehensive approach to the assessment of postpartum adaptation during the short hospital stays currently in vogue. May help in the early identification of problems.

14. Frank, E., et al. Pregnancy-related affective episodes among women with recurrent depression. *Am. J. Psychiatry* 144:288, 1987.
    The observations in this article confirm those from other reports that women with recurrent episodes of postpartum affective disorders tend to be younger at first onset, are less emotionally stable, and are found to be more severely depressed at the baseline examination.

15. Affonso, D. D., et al. A standardized interview that differentiates pregnancy and postpartum symptoms from perinatal clinical depression. *Birth* 17:121, 1990.
    In a prospective longitudinal study of 202 primigravidas, three standardized clinical tools were modified to differentiate pregnancy and postpartum symptoms from those of depression.

16. Brockington, I. F., et al. The clinical picture of the depressed form of puerperal psychosis. *J. Affect. Disord.* 15:29, 1988.
    In this study, 104 patients admitted for postpartum psychoses were studied over a 5-year period. In general, patients who become depressed after delivery have a form of puerperal psychosis, but show less anger and more animation than other depressed patients.

Treatment

17. Munoz, R. A. Postpartum psychosis as a discrete entity. *J. Clin. Psychiatry* 46:182, 1985.
    Defines three categories of postpartum depressive disorders: "blues," nonpsychotic depression, and postpartum psychosis. The severity of symptoms and the nature of effective therapy differ somewhat for each.

18. Robinson, G. E., and Stewart, D. E. Postpartum psychiatric disorders. *Can. Med. Assoc. J.* 134:31, 1986.
    Antidepressants, major tranquilizers, and lithium may be prescribed according to the nature of the symptoms if the disorder lasts longer than 2 weeks or is disabling.

19. Mortola, J. F. The use of psychotropic agents in pregnancy and lactation. *Psychiatr. Clin. North Am.* 12:69, 1989.
    A systematic review of the pharmacodynamics, indications, and concerns governing the use of neuroleptics, antidepressants, antimanics, and benzodiazepines during pregnancy and lactation.

20. Theesen, K., Alderson, M., and Hill, W. Caring for the depressed obstetric patient. *Contemp. Ob/Gyn* 33:123, 1989.
    A very clinically oriented article offering a list of antidepressants most commonly used to treat this problem.

Complications

21. Zuckerman, B. S., and Beardslee, W. F. Maternal depression: a concern for pediatricians. *Pediatrics* 79:110, 1987.
    The effects of maternal depression on growth patterns, behavioral development, accidents, and childhood illnesses are discussed.

22. Misri, S., and Sivertx, K. Tricyclic drugs in pregnancy and lactation: a preliminary report. *Int. J. Psychiatry Med.* 21:151, 1991.
    In this report of women treated with tricyclic antidepressants before and during pregnancy and lactation, there were no fetal malformations and no unusual complications of labor and delivery. There were only short-term withdrawal symptoms in the neonate. No adverse effects on breast-fed infants were noted. All of the lactating mothers who refused tricyclic antidepressants suffered exacerbation of their symptoms.

23. Meltzer, E. S., and Kumar, R. Puerperal mental illness, clinical features and classification: a study of 142 mother-and-baby admission. *Br. J. Psychiatry* 147:647, 1985.
    The majority of patients were classified as having affective disorders. One third

had relatively minor disorders that would probably have responded well to out-patient management if adequate supportive services had been available.

24. O'Hara, M. W. Social support, life events, and depression during pregnancy and the puerperium. *Arch. Gen. Psychiatry* 43:569, 1986.
   Prepartum and postpartum depression may actually be different entities in some women. Women who were depressed prepartum reported less spousal support and more confidant support. Women who were depressed postpartum reported less spousal support and more stressful life events than did nondepressed women.

25. Marks, M. N., et al. Contribution of psychological and social factors to psychotic and non-psychotic illness was predicted by a severe life event. *J. Affect. Disord.* 29:253, 1992.
   Recurrence of psychosis postpartum was predicted by a psychiatric history, a recent psychiatric admission, and the presence of marital difficulties.

IX. ADVANCES IN OBSTETRICS

43. ANTEPARTUM DIAGNOSIS OF FETAL ANOMALIES
L. Wayne Hess, Darla B. Hess, and Linda C. Buchheit

Three to five percent of all liveborn infants have a significant congenital anomaly at birth. Most such infants are delivered of mothers with no known risk factors for a fetal malformation. The general public believes that most birth defects occur because of exposure during pregnancy to teratogenic drugs, chemicals, x-rays, or viruses. However, contrary to these public assumptions, the available scientific data reveal that, of all birth defects, only 2 percent are due to exposure to these teratogens; 98 percent occur secondary to random mutations, the expression of lethal genes in the parents, autosomal or multifactorial genetic expression, aneuploidy, and so on. This tremendous public confusion has substantially increased the difficult challenge obstetricians face when a malformed infant is delivered. Therefore, the obstetrician has an increased responsibility to detect fetal anomalies in those gravidas at risk.

The prevention of fetal anomalies has been increasingly emphasized by the American College of Obstetricians and Gynecologists (ACOG). All women of childbearing age are encouraged to undergo preconceptional evaluation and counseling. A careful past medical, family, and genetic history should be taken from all women of childbearing age. Other information, such as maternal and paternal age, ethnic background, type of employment, occupational exposures, family pets, as well as cigarette, alcohol, and drug use, should be obtained. In addition, immunity to rubella should be ascertained. These preconception measures should allow the health-care provider to determine which obstetric patients are at risk for fetal anomalies, and therefore provide appropriate therapy, counseling, and fetal evaluation. Additionally, preconceptional folic acid supplementation may be considered to minimize the risk of a fetal neural tube defect (NTD) developing.

In most European countries, sonographic screening is recommended for all pregnancies. In this country, ultrasonography is routinely utilized only for selected indications during pregnancy. The availability of real-time ultrasonography in the office practice of obstetrics, on the other hand, has led to an increase in the frequency with which antepartal fetal anomalies are detected in the low-risk gravida. ACOG, however, has advised physicians who do not have special expertise in prenatal diagnosis to limit the office sonographic evaluation in these selected gravidas to a "basic" examination, which should include (1) the fetal number, (2) fetal presentation, (3) documentation of fetal life, (4) placental localization, (5) amniotic fluid volume, (6) gestational dating, (7) detection and evaluation of pelvic masses, and (8) survey of fetal anatomy for gross malformations. If this basic examination reveals a suspected fetal abnormality, the patient should be referred to a center where a physician with expertise in prenatal diagnosis can perform a "targeted" fetal ultrasonographic examination.

Historic screening of all gravidas for risk factors for congenital anomalies is now a standard part of practice in the United States. In addition, serum alpha-fetoprotein (AFP) or "triple test" screening should be offered to all patients between 15 and 17 weeks' gestation. For those patients with any positive test finding for anomalies, testing by means of a targeted sonographic examination, midtrimester amniocentesis, fetal echocardiography, cordocentesis, and so on is carried out, in addition to definitive counseling. These tests must be completed in time (usually by 22 weeks' gestation) to allow the patient the option of pregnancy termination if she desires. These tests should be performed by individuals and laboratories experienced in prenatal diagnosis.

The antenatal diagnosis of NTDs has received increasing public attention. The background risk for NTDs in the United States is 1 to 2 per 1000 live births. Most NTDs occur in patients with no known predisposing risk factors. The recurrence risk for these defects follows the typical polygenic pattern, with a risk of 3 to 5 percent if one primary relative has the disease, 5 to 7 percent if two primary relatives have the disease, and so on. In those women with no risk factors but who have two verified serum AFP values greater than 2.5 multiples of the median, there is a 10 percent risk for NTDs. These patients are offered targeted fetal ultrasonographic evaluation and genetic amniocentesis. The targeted sonographic evaluation in these patients includes measurement of the inner and outer orbital diameter; evaluation of the ventricular atrium; measurement of the cerebellar dimensions; longitudinal, sagittal, and transverse evaluation of the fetal spinal column; exclusion of the "lemon" and "banana" signs, and so on. Amniotic fluid obtained during midtrimester amniocentesis in these women is generally evaluated, and this includes determination of the AFP content and fetal karyotype. If the amniotic AFP content is evaluated, the fluid is also tested for acetylcholinesterase to confirm an NTD. If an NTD is detected, the option of pregnancy termination should be available to the patient.

At 18 to 20 weeks' gestation, gravidas at risk for fetal anomalies should undergo a targeted fetal sonographic evaluation. This examination should be performed by a physician with special training and experience in targeted sonography. Careful fetal biometry with measurement of the appropriate fetal organs and biometric ratios should allow the detection of 60 to 70 percent of all fetuses with anomalies. Targeted sonography is 90 to 95 percent accurate in identifying the nature of lesions that are specifically assessed.

Gravidas at risk for fetal cardiac anomalies should undergo fetal echocardiography. This examination is generally performed jointly by a maternal-fetal medicine specialist and a cardiologist. The two-dimensional examination of the fetal heart should include four-chamber, left ventricular outflow tract, right ventricular outflow tract, and aortic and ductal arch views of the fetal heart. Color-flow mapping of the fetal heart allows the detection of unusual turbulence patterns. These areas can then be evaluated by either pulsed or continuous-wave Doppler. The doppler velocities across the valves will allow diagnosis of stenotic and regurgitant lesions.

M-mode fetal echocardiography should permit the accurate diagnosis of most fetal cardiac dysrhythmias. At times Doppler may be a helpful adjunct. If an anatomic anomaly of the fetal heart is detected, determination of the fetal karyotype is indicated, as aneuploidy exists in 30 percent of these fetuses. A fetus with a dysrhythmia has the following risks for a structural anomaly of the heart: supraventricular tachycardia, 10 percent; ventricular dysrhythmia, 1 to 2 percent; and complete heart block, 50 to 60 percent. Fetal supraventricular tachycardia (with no other fetal anomalies) is usually treated with maternal digoxin (with the goal of achieving a maternal serum level of 2 ng/ml) or verapamil (80 mg orally three times a day). If the digoxin fails to convert the dysrhythmia and verapamil is added as a second agent, the digoxin dose is reduced by 50 percent to prevent toxicity. A maternal 12-lead electrocardiogram should be obtained and her electrolyte pattern assessed to confirm that these are normal before therapy is begun. Fetal ventricular dysrhythmias rarely require therapy. The finding of congenital heart block should prompt an evaluation for lupus erythematosus or other connective tissue disease in the mother (antinuclear antibody and Rho antibody, also known as anti-SSA antibody). Infants with complete heart block frequently require transvenous cardiac pacing after delivery.

Other techniques for prenatal diagnosis that are available at selected centers in the United States include embryoscopy, chorionic villus sampling (vaginal and abdominal), genetic amniocentesis (first or second trimester), fetal organ biopsy, and cordocentesis (percutaneous umbilical blood sampling). Cordocentesis appears to be the most promising of these techniques. Since its introduction by Daffos in 1985, it has enjoyed a rapid gain in popularity worldwide. This technique is capable of such diverse applications as fetal blood karyotyping, measurement of immunoglobulin M titers (to detect congenital infections), enzyme analysis, ABO grouping, determination of the Rh and other antigen status, hematocrit measurement, and assessment of the acid-base status. This technique carries a 1 to 2 percent risk of causing fetal loss. It may be used for second- or third-trimester diagnosis.

The advent of the polymerase chain reaction (PCR), DNA probes, and other exciting molecular genetics techniques has substantially increased the prenatal diagnostic ability. Mitochondrial and nontraditional genetics (uniparental disomy) are also expanding the prenatal diagnostic horizons. Analysis of fetal cells in the maternal circulation may also soon allow prenatal diagnosis by noninvasive means.

In summary, all gravidas at risk should be screened for anomalies prior to 22 weeks' gestation. If an anomaly is detected before this time, the options of either pregnancy termination or informed continuation of the pregnancy are available to the patient. Those gravidas with anomalies first detected in the late second or third trimesters should be referred to a physician with expertise in prenatal diagnosis. Prenatal diagnosis in these fetuses will permit optimal planning for the timing, method, and place of delivery.

General

1. Chervenak, F. A., Isaacson, G., and Campbell, S. *Ultrasound in Obstetrics and Gynecology*. Boston: Little, Brown, 1993.
   A comprehensive text of prenatal diagnosis.
2. Simpson, J. L., and Golbus, M. S. *Genetics in Obstetrics and Gynecology*. Philadelphia: Saunders, 1992.
   A basic text of genetics for obstetrics and gynecology.
3. Ultrasound in Pregnancy. *ACOG Tech. Bull.* No. 116, May 1988.
   An updated publication details the ACOG's recommendations concerning the use of ultrasound in pregnancy.
4. Romero, R., et al. *Prenatal Diagnosis of Congenital Anomalies*. Norwalk, CT: Appleton & Lange, 1988.
   This reference is a good comprehensive text for the clinician as it concerns fetal malformations. It also contains a fine treatment section for each fetal malformation.
5. Jones, K. L. *Smith's Recognizable Patterns of Human Malformations*. Philadelphia: Saunders, 1988.
   This excellent text is the most up-to-date and complete reference on all fetal anomalies. All aspects of each of the fetal malformations diagnosed after birth are listed in separate categories.
6. Reed, K. L., Anderson, C. F., and Shenker, L. *Fetal Echocardiography: An Atlas*. New York: Liss, 1988.
   This atlas of fetal echocardiography offers anatomic correlation with each etiologic cause of congenital heart disease.
7. Devore, G. R., Brar, H. S., and Platt, L. D. Doppler ultrasound in the fetus: a review of current applications. *J. Clin. Ultrasound* 15:687, 1987.
   The use of Doppler ultrasound to diagnose fetal anomalies during pregnancy is recommended, and suggested treatment modalities for various fetal anomalies are given. The article also reviews all aspects of the fetal Doppler evaluation.
8. Winter, R. M., et al. *The Malformed Fetus and Stillbirth: A Diagnostic Approach*. New York: Wiley, 1988.
   A successful approach toward the application of diagnostic ultrasound in the evaluation of suspected fetal malformations. It also includes a section on how to handle the diagnostic dilemmas that arise after fetal death.
9. Bo, W. J., et al. *Basic Atlas of Cross Sectional Anatomy*. Philadelphia: Saunders, 1980.
   This is the best reference for an understanding of the anatomic relationships that will correlate with the ultrasound images obtained by the clinician. The use of cross-sectional anatomy is also helpful in clinical situations in which fetal anomalies are suspected.

Diagnostic Techniques

10. Cardoza, J. D., Goldstein, R. B., Filly, R. A. Exclusion of fetal ventriculomegaly with a single measurement: the width of the lateral ventricular atrium. *Radiology* 169:711, 1988.
    A review with the intention to improve the accuracy of the diagnosis of ventriculomegaly.
11. Bombard, T., and Rigdon, D. T. Prospective pilot evaluation of early (11–14 weeks' gestation) amniocentesis in 75 patients. *Mil. Med.* 157:339, 1992.
    A review of first-trimester genetic amniocentesis.

12. Lippman, A., et al. Canadian multicentre randomized clinical trial of chorion villus sampling and amniocentesis. Final report. *Prenat. Diagn.* 12:385, 1992.
    The Canadian chorionic villus sampling trial.
13. Pergament, E., et al. The risk and efficacy of chorionic villus sampling in multiple gestations. *Prenat. Diagn.* 12:377, 1992.
    First-trimester prenatal diagnosis in twins.
14. Perry, K. G., Jr., et al. Cordocentesis (funipuncture) by maternal-fetal fellows: the learning curve. *Fetal Diagn. Ther.* 6:87, 1991.
    A review of the risks of cordocentesis.
15. Hess, L. W., et al. Fetal echocardiography. *Obstet. Gynecol. Clin. North Am.* 17:41, 1990.
    A comprehensive review of fetal echocardiography.
16. Satish, J. Prenatal genetics in laboratory medicine. A cytogeneticist's perspective. *Clin. Lab. Med.* 12:493, 1992.
    Importance of laboratory findings to prenatal diagnosis.
17. Maddalena, A., Bick, D. P., and Schulman, J. D. Molecular diagnosis of genetic disease. *J. Reprod. Med.* 37:437, 1992.
    A review of molecular methods of prenatal diagnosis.
18. Larsen, J. W., Jr. Diagnosis of abnormalities of the human fetus during the first, second, and third trimesters. *Teratology* 46:23, 1992.
    A comprehensive review of all prenatal diagnostic techniques.
19. Chambers, H. M. The perinatal autopsy: a contemporary approach. *Pathology* 24:45, 1992.
    Contemporary approach to the fetal or neonatal autopsy.
20. Jackson, L. G., et al. A randomized comparison of transcervical and transabdominal chorionic-villus sampling. The U.S. National Institute of Child Health and Human Development Chorionic-Villus Sampling and Amniocentesis Study Group. *N. Engl. J. Med.* 327:594, 1992.
    The American experience with chorionic villus sampling.
21. Cutting, G. R., and Antonarakis, S. E. Prenatal diagnosis and carrier detection by DNA analysis. *Pediatr. Rev.* 13:138, 1992.
    DNA analysis for prenatal diagnosis.
22. Reece, E. A. Embryoscopy: new developments in prenatal medicine. *Curr. Opin. Obstet. Gynecol.* 4:447, 1992.
    A review of the applications of embryoscopy for making prenatal diagnosis.
23. Stoll, C., et al. Evaluation of prenatal diagnosis by a registry of congenital anomalies. *Prenat. Diagn.* 12:263, 1992.
    A critical assessment of the accuracy of prenatal diagnostic techniques.
24. Chueh, J., and Golbus, M. S. The search for fetal cells in the maternal circulation. *J. Perinat. Med.* 19:411, 1992.
    An exciting potential future diagnostic technique.
25. Cooper, D. N., and Schmidtke, J. Molecular genetic approaches to the analysis and diagnosis of human inherited disease: an overview. *Ann. Med.* 24:29, 1992.
    The field of molecular genetics in review.
26. Wald, N. J., and Kennard, A. Prenatal biochemical screening for Down's syndrome and neural tube defects. *Curr. Opin. Obstet. Gynecol.* 4:302, 1992.
    A comprehensive review of the biochemical screening done to detect fetal anomalies.
27. Neilson, J. P. Prenatal diagnosis in multiple pregnancies. *Curr. Opin. Obstet. Gynecol.* 4:280, 1992.
    A comprehensive review of the aspects of prenatal diagnosis.
28. Lescale, K. B., Eddleman, K. A., and Chervenak, F. A. Prenatal diagnosis of structural anomalies. *Curr. Opin. Obstet. Gynecol.* 4:249, 1992.
    A comprehensive review of the various aspects of prenatal diagnosis.
29. Hill, L. M. New ultrasound observations of fetal anomalies in the second trimester. *Curr. Opin. Radiol.* 4:93, 1992.
    A review of recent developments in ultrasound.
30. Anderson, R. H. Simplifying the understanding of congenital malformations of the heart. *Int. J. Cardiol.* 32:131, 1991.

A comprehensive review of fetal cardiac malformations.
31. Golbus, M. S., et al. Selective termination of multiple gestations. *Am. J. Med. Genet.* 31:339, 1988.
    A possible option for multiple gestations.
32. Ruitenbeek, W., et al. The use of chorionic villi in prenatal diagnosis of mitochondriopathies. *J. Inherit. Metab. Dis.* 15:303, 1992.
    A new diagnostic technique in the field of nontraditional genetics.
33. Canick, J. A., and Knight, G. J. Multiple-marker screening for fetal Down syndrome. *Contemp. Ob/Gyn* 36:3, 1992.
    The accuracy and limitations of triple-screen prenatal testing are described.
34. Wilson, G. N. Human congenital anomalies: application of new genetic tools and concepts. *Semin. Perinatol.* 16:385, 1992.
    An excellent review of the application of new genetic diagnostic techniques.
35. Jackson, J. G., et al. Weighing the advantages CVS confers. *Contemp. Ob/Gyn* 38:107, 1993.
    A general review of chorionic villus sampling.
36. D'Alton, M. E., and DeCherney, A. H. Prenatal diagnosis. *N. Engl. J. Med.* 328:114, 1993.
    A Current Concepts article from the New England Journal of Medicine.

Prognosis and Therapy
37. Mateau, T. M., et al. The psychological effects of false-positive results in prenatal screening for fetal abnormality: a prospective study. *Prenat. Diagn.* 12:205, 1992.
    This describes the maternal stress incurred as the result of incorrect prenatal diagnosis.
38. Smythe, J. F., Copel, J. A., and Kleinman, C. S. Outcome of prenatally detected cardiac malformations. *Am. J. Cardiol.* 69:1471, 1992.
    A multicenter review of the various aspects of the prenatal detection of cardiac malformations.
39. Simpson, J. L., et al. Vitamins, folic acid and neural tube defects: comments on investigations in the United States. *Prenat. Diagn.* 11:641, 1991.
    A possible method to prevent NTDs is described.
40. Northern Regional Survey Steering Group. Fetal abnormality: an audit of its recognition and management. *Arch. Dis. Child.* 67:770, 1992.
    A general review of the management involved.
41. Evans, M. I., Johnson, M. P., and Holzgreve, W. Fetal therapy: the next generation. *Women's Health Issues* 1:31, 1990.
    Potential new fetal therapies are described.
42. Karson, E. M., Polvino, W., and Anderson, W. F. Prospects for human gene therapy. *J. Reprod. Med.* 37:508, 1992.
    Practical recommendations for gene therapy are offered.

44. GENETIC COUNSELING

Joseph P. Bruner

The 2 to 3 percent incidence of serious birth defects found at delivery in the general population has remained unchanged for decades. As advances are made in the treatment of other obstetric and newborn complications, however, genetic disorders play a proportionately larger role in neonatal morbidity and mortality. Genetic counseling, therefore, is becoming more important in the practice of modern obstetrics, and the physician providing health care to pregnant women must understand the basics of such prenatal counseling. Genetic counseling addresses two major areas: hereditary and environmental disorders. The hereditary category includes those mendelian disorders inherited in an autosomal dominant, autosomal recessive, or X-linked recessive fashion, as well as polygenic or multifactorial and chromosomal aberrations. Environmental factors encompass exposure to viruses, radiation, and drugs, including alcohol and tobacco.

General counseling begins with the performance of screening procedures to identify those individuals at greater risk of producing offspring with genetic abnormalities than the population at large. This identification process requires a thorough family and reproductive history, as well as information regarding possible exposure to various environmental factors. Counseling is best carried out when both parents are involved and when the needs of both parents are identified. The timing of the counseling session is of critical importance, because some interventions, such as folate administration or glycemic control, should be carried out before conception occurs, whereas others, such as maternal serum alpha-fetoprotein (MSAFP) determinations or triple screening, must be timed for 15 to 18 weeks of gestation.

Counseling is the process that opens the lines of communication between the health-care provider and the patient for the purpose of disseminating accurate and reliable information, thereby allowing the patient and her partner to make fundamental decisions about the pregnancy. The objective of genetic counseling is to provide information, assist in the decision-making process and adjustment to the problem at hand, and ultimately to decrease the incidence of genetic defects at birth.

Adequate genetic counseling requires that the abnormality of concern be clearly defined and that the information presented to the parents be accurate and timely. A thorough family history (pedigree) and physical examination, combined with various investigative procedures, are necessary to establish an accurate diagnosis. The risks, benefits, and failures of each diagnostic procedure, such as amniocentesis and ultrasound, should be explained in an honest and noncoercive manner. Accurate data dissemination and a description of the full range of alternatives must be presented to the couple. Confidentiality is of the utmost importance, as is the development of a trusting relationship between the health-care provider and patient. It is essential to follow up on each couple who receives counseling.

Women delivering after the age of 35 years constitute one of the largest categories of patients requiring counseling during the prenatal period. The risk of delivering an infant with trisomy 21, or Down syndrome, increases in direct proportion to maternal age, reaching 1 in 365 pregnancies at age 35 years and 1 in 12 pregnancies at age 49. Besides this age-related risk, couples who have had a previous infant with Down syndrome face a recurrence risk in future pregnancies of approximately 1 percent, regardless of maternal age. Couples in whom one parent has a known chromosomal rearrangement, such as a balanced translocation, are also at risk for giving birth to a child with a chromosomal aberration, and are candidates for counseling or prenatal diagnosis, or both.

One of the most common methods of genetic screening is high-resolution ultrasound imaging of the fetus using transvaginal or, more commonly, transabdominal transducers. A fetal femur length less than 91 percent of that expected for the gestational age, a nuchal skin fold thickness greater than 5 mm, or both findings, noted between 15 and 20 weeks' gestation, are associated with Down syndrome; the finding of a posterior nuchal cystic hygroma has been linked to Turner's syndrome; and cardiac defects and overlapping digits in the hand reportedly occur in 100 percent of the fetuses with trisomy 13 or 18. These findings, however, are considered too nonspecific for making a reliable diagnosis of fetal aneuploidy, and invasive testing after appropriate counseling is required to establish the diagnosis.

Another common indication for genetic counseling is the patient at risk for delivering a child with a neural tube defect (NTD). NTDs are among the most common birth defects in humans. These anomalies, which include spina bifida, anencephaly, and encephalocele, occur in approximately 1 per 1000 births in the United States. However, delivery of one child with an NTD is associated with a 2 to 3 percent recurrence risk in a future pregnancy.

MSAFP testing is performed at 15 to 18 weeks' gestation. Abnormally elevated values, usually defined as those greater than 2.5 multiples of the median for the appropriate gestational age, may identify NTDs, as well as ventral wall malformations and other fetal anomalies, and should prompt further investigation by means of ultrasound imaging. Approximately 90 percent of the structural fetal anomalies can be detected by an experienced ultrasonographer. Although ultrasound scanning should identify all cases of anencephaly, amniotic fluid assays for alpha fetoprotein and acetylcholinesterase may identify an additional 5 percent of small NTDs undetectable by current high-resolution imaging techniques. Unexplained elevated MSAFP values, presumably due to fetomaternal hemorrhage secondary to abnormal placentation, have been associated with other pregnancy complications, such as preterm labor, intrauterine growth retardation, and stillbirth. Low MSAFP values, when corrected for maternal age, race, and the presence of diabetes mellitus, have been associated with age-independent Down syndrome. Universal screening with the measurement of MSAFP levels in pregnancy may detect up to 20 percent of the cases of Down syndrome in women younger than 35 years at delivery. Use of the triple screen to detect abnormally low values of serum estriol and abnormally elevated levels of human chorionic gonadotropin, in addition to the MSAFP measurement, may identify up to 60 percent of the cases of Down syndrome in this low-risk population.

In 1991, the Medical Research Council Vitamin Study Group reported that the daily intake of 4 mg of folic acid periconceptually prevented 71 percent of the NTDs in women with one affected offspring. In September 1992, the U.S. Public Health Service recommended that all women attempting pregnancy take the recommended daily allowance (0.4 mg) of folate during pregnancy for 1 month before conception and for at least 3 months after conception. Women at risk for delivering an infant with NTDs because of the previous delivery of such an infant should be cautioned against achieving 4 mg/day of folic acid by ingesting several prenatal vitamins, as this practice may expose them to toxic levels of other vitamins (e.g., vitamin A). Since folic acid supplementation cannot be expected to prevent all NTDs, prophylaxis does not preclude MSAFP or ultrasound testing later in pregnancy.

Since 1952 an increasing number of diseases, known as inborn errors of metabolism, have been determined to be secondary to an abnormality in a fetal metabolic process. Most of these disorders are inherited in an autosomal recessive or X-linked fashion. Detection of the approximately 100 inborn errors currently amenable to prenatal diagnosis is generally performed by enzyme activity assay of cultured amniotic fluid cells or of placental villi obtained by chorionic villus sampling (CVS). One notable exception is phenylketonuria (PKU), which is diagnosed with newer molecular techniques.

Although several mendelian disorders can also be diagnosed by enzymatic determination, DNA analysis for diagnosis can now be performed on any nucleated cell. Duchenne muscular dystrophy, hemophilia, sickle cell disease, adult-onset polycystic kidney disease, and Huntington's chorea are only a few of the disorders detectable in utero by recently developed molecular techniques.

Invasive testing is now possible throughout gestation through the use of transcervical or transabdominal CVS, early amniocentesis, midtrimester amniocentesis, and cordocentesis. Couples should be informed that genetic amniocentesis performed at 15 to 16 weeks' gestation is associated with an approximately 0.5 percent incidence of spontaneous abortion. The risk may be slightly higher in the setting of early amniocentesis, performed between 12 and 14 weeks. Amniocentesis should be performed under ultrasonic guidance to minimize the risk of maternal and fetal injury. Thorough screening with ultrasound is necessary before the procedure to rule out the presence of fetal anomalies, twins, and fetal death, and to accurately ascertain the gestational age. Those women who are Rh negative with Rh-positive partners should receive Rh immunoglobulin after any invasive procedure to prevent maternal sensitization.

Although amniocentesis has provided the means for the early detection of many chromosomal and metabolic disorders, one drawback has been the need to wait until the second trimester before performing it. Long-term culture of retrieved amniocytes may require an additional 2 to 3 weeks before the results are available. This long waiting period contributes to mounting patient anxiety. Moreover, if a fetal abnormality is detected, the option of pregnancy termination is often less acceptable due to the advanced gestational age and the increased maternal risk involved. Finally, effective fetal therapy may depend on early diagnosis followed by the prompt initiation of treatment. For these reasons, interest in the first-trimester diagnosis of fetal anomalies has increased markedly over the past several years. CVS is one method that makes this possible. It consists of a placental biopsy performed under ultrasound guidance at 9 to 12 weeks' gestation. Because the chorionic material obtained in this procedure is genetically identical to that of the fetus, it can be subjected to the same chromosomal, metabolic, and DNA analyses possible with amniocentesis, except for alpha-fetoprotein testing. However, the studies are performed directly on fetal-derived tissue, which permits results to be available within a few days, rather than the weeks necessary for amniotic fluid studies. Although the risk involved depends to some degree on operator experience, CVS compares favorably to amniocentesis in terms of safety. A large multicenter trial revealed the procedure loss rate of CVS to be slightly greater than that seen for amniocentesis, but the difference did not reach statistical significance. Recent reports of fetal limb malformations following CVS have caused concern about developmental risks, but the procedure has been shown to be a comparably safe alternative to genetic amniocentesis. Appropriate counseling, an expert operator, and an experienced laboratory are mandatory components of a CVS program.

Cordocentesis is a new invasive technique that allows the in utero diagnosis of a wide range of fetal disorders. Also known as *percutaneous umbilical blood sampling* (PUBS), cordocentesis consists of the fine-needle aspiration of fetal blood using high-resolution ultrasound guidance. Because the most common aspiration site is a blood vessel in the umbilical cord, cordocentesis is technically feasible only after about 18 to 20 weeks' gestation. In a review of over 5000 cases, the National PUBS Registry has determined the fetal loss rate to be only 1.15 percent per procedure.

The cytogenetic analysis of lymphocytes obtained from fetal blood yields a fetal karyotype in 2 days or less. Use of cordocentesis for rapid karyotyping enables the physician and patient to work together to quickly formulate optimal management strategies.

Armed with a basic knowledge of genetic screening and counseling and with appropriate information concerning the risk factors, health-care providers can play a crucial role in the overall management of reproductive-aged women at genetic risk. Although it is not necessary that each provider be expert in genetic counseling, each clinician does have responsibility to recognize the potential for genetic disorders and to provide the means of obtaining accurate counseling and testing for his or her patients.

Counseling
1. Harper, P. S. *Practical Genetic Counseling.* Oxford: Butterworth-Heinemann, 1991.
   A useful introductory guide for clinicians involved in advising patients and their families about inherited diseases. The first part of the book describes the basic principles of genetic disorders. The second section discusses the genetic risks for a variety of different disorders.
2. Brucker, M. C., and MacMullen, N. J. Chorionic villus sampling: counseling your patient. *Nurse Pract.* 12:34, 1987.
   Presents a good overview of the information needed to adequately counsel patients regarding the risks and benefits of CVS.
3. Ekwo, E. E., et al. Factors influencing maternal estimates of genetic risk. *Am. J. Med. Genet.* 20:419, 1985.
   Less than half of the women who agreed to undergo amniocentesis remembered the risks quoted them of delivering an affected child. Neither a knowledge of genetics nor the general educational level were correlated with the ability to remember the odds.
4. Elkins, T. E., et al. Attitudes of mothers of children with Down's syndrome concerning amniocentesis, abortion, and prenatal counseling techniques. *Obstet. Gynecol.* 68:181, 1986.
   The importance of not anticipating patient values in providing genetic information is stressed. Even among women who previously delivered children with Down

syndrome and who chose to undergo amniocentesis in the subsequent pregnancy, only half did so with the intent to abort an abnormal fetus.

5. Sorenson, J. R., and Wertz, D. C. Couple agreement before and after genetic counseling. *Am. J. Med. Genet.* 25:549, 1986.

   Counseling was not found to alter disagreements between spouses regarding their concerns and reproductive plans, but did promote agreement about risk interpretation and the identification of problems associated with raising an affected child.

6. Wertz, D. C., and Sorenson, J. R. Client reactions to genetic counseling: self-reports of influence. *Clin. Genetics* 30:494, 1986.

   Clients reported that counseling was beneficial in helping them make decisions. Evidence indicated that counseling did not supplant clients' personal values but did assist in clarifying their decisions.

Genetic Diagnosis

7. Driscoll, M. C., et al. Prenatal diagnosis of sickle hemoglobinopathies: the experience of the Columbia University Comprehensive Center for Sickle Cell Disease. *Am. J. Hum. Genet.* 40:548, 1987.

   The authors report on the effectiveness of prenatal testing of fetuses at risk using molecular methods. Although the ability of amniocentesis to detect affected fetuses is high, the efficiency of the screening depends on the early identification of at-risk couples and on the accuracy of counseling.

8. Simpson, J. L. What causes chromosomal abnormalities and gene mutations? *Contemp. Ob/Gyn* 17:99, 1981.

   This article present a basic approach to identifying chromosomal abnormalities resulting from a variety of sources. Practical recommendations for patient counseling are given.

9. Antonarakis, S. E. Diagnosis of genetic disorders at the DNA level. *N. Engl. J. Med.* 320:153, 1989.

   This presents a comprehensive update on the diagnostic techniques, based on an understanding of the biochemical mechanics of molecular genetics. This article contains several illustrative examples as well as 139 references.

10. Asch, D. A., et al. Reporting the results of cystic fibrosis carrier screening. *Am. J. Obstet. Gynecol.* 168:1, 1993.

    Five mutations of the cystic fibrosis gene constitute about 85 percent of the alleles. The authors recommend only one partner be tested.

Ultrasound

11. Romero, R., et al. *Prenatal diagnosis of congenital anomalies.* Norwalk, CT: Appleton & Lange, 1988.

    This text provided the first encyclopedic approach to the diagnosis and therapy of fetal congenital anomalies. Well organized and comprehensive, each section can be read in less than 10 minutes.

12. Nyberg, D. A., Mahony, B. S., and Pretorius, D. H. *Diagnostic Ultrasound and Fetal Anomalies: Text and Atlas.* Chicago: Yearbook Medical Publishers, 1990.

    Another superbly organized encyclopedic approach to prenatal diagnosis and therapy. Richly endowed with photographs.

13. Seeds, J. S., and Azizkhan, R. G. *Congenital Malformations: Antenatal Diagnosis, Perinatal Management, and Counseling.* Rockville, MD: Aspen Publishers, 1990.

    An easy-to-understand primer describing the ultrasound diagnosis and management of fetal anomalies.

Alpha-Fetoprotein: Neural Tube and Other Defects

14. Alpha-Fetoprotein. *ACOG Tech. Bull.* No. 154, April 1991.

    An unusually thorough yet succinct discussion of the physiology of alpha-fetoprotein, the maternal screening involved, and the recommended clinical management of abnormally high and low values.

15. Merkatz, I. R., et al. An association between low maternal serum alpha-fetoprotein and fetal chromosomal abnormalities. *Am. J. Obstet. Gynecol.* 148:886, 1984.

Forty-one women who delivered infants with autosomal trisomy were found to have MSAFP levels significantly lower than those observed in a group of normal matched control subjects.

16. Haddow, J. E., et al. Prenatal screening for Down's syndrome with use of maternal serum markers. *N. Engl. J. Med.* 327:588, 1992.
    Measuring the serum alpha-fetoprotein, chorionic gonadotropin, and estriol levels proved to be more effective in screening for fetal Down syndrome than measuring the MSAFP levels alone. Using the triple screen, the rate of detection of Down syndrome among 25,207 pregnant women and adolescents was 58 percent.

17. Committee on Obstetrics; Maternal and Fetal Medicine. Folic acid for the prevention of recurrent neural tube defects. *ACOG Committee Opinion* No. 120, March 1993.
    The periconceptual administration of 4 mg of folic acid daily is recommended for the prevention of recurrent NTDs among women with one affected child, while 0.4 mg daily is recommended to prevent the initial occurrence.

18. Cheng, E. Y., et al. A prospective evaluation of a second-trimester screening test for fetal Down syndrome using maternal serum alpha-fetoprotein, hCG, and unconjugated estriol. *Obstet. Gynecol.* 81:72, 1993.
    Use of a triple-screen procedure to detect Down syndrome was found to have a sensitivity of 91 percent and a specificity of 94 percent.

Amniocentesis

19. Prevention of D isoimmunization. *ACOG Tech. Bull.* No. 147, October 1990.
    Indications for the use of anti-Rh immunoglobulin are detailed.

20. Elejalde, B. R., Elejalde, M. M., and Acuna, J. M. Prospective study of amniocentesis performed between weeks 9 and 16 gestation: its feasibility, risks, complications and use in prenatal diagnosis. *Am. J. Med. Genet.* 35:188, 1990.
    Although the outcome from amniocentesis performed between the ninth and the fourteenth weeks of gestation is similar to that when amniocentesis is performed between the fifteenth and sixteenth weeks, early amniocentesis is associated with higher rates of fetal losses and amniotic fluid leakage, more confined cytogenetic abnormalities, and an increased number of patients who have their procedure postponed.

21. Tabor, A., et al. Randomized controlled trial of genetic amniocentesis in 4606 low-risk women. *Lancet* 1:1287, 1986.
    The outcome of pregnancy after amniocentesis was studied in a randomized controlled trial of 4606 women, aged 25 to 34 years, without a known risk of genetic disease.

Chorionic Villus Sampling

22. Rhoads, G. G., et al. The safety and efficacy of chorionic villus sampling for early prenatal diagnosis of cytogenetic abnormalities. *N. Engl. J. Med.* 320:609, 1989.
    In this seven-center study, the safety and efficacy of CVS in 2278 women compared favorably to those observed for midtrimester genetic amniocentesis.

23. Canadian Collaborative CVS—Amniocentesis Clinical Trial Group. Multicentre randomized clinical trial of chorion villus sampling and amniocentesis: First report. *Lancet* 1:1, 1989.
    A must-read article for those interested in CVS because this is the largest study to date conducted in North America. Almost 3000 women underwent CVS, and, compared to amniocentesis, there was an increased propensity for women to have late perinatal mortality, usually beyond 28 weeks. The difference in the overall perinatal loss rate was 2.4 percent higher for CVS.

24. NICHD Collaborative CVS Study Group. Transcervical and transabdominal CVS are comparably safe procedures for first trimester prenatal diagnosis: preliminary analysis. *Am. J. Hum. Genet.* 47:A278, 1990.
    In this eight-center prospective trial, 2353 women who were randomized in the first trimester to undergo either transcervical or transabdominal CVS demonstrated no difference in the rate of successful sampling, required number of insertions, spontaneous abortion, or total pregnancy loss.

25. Holzgreve, W., et al. Safety of placental biopsy in the second and third trimester. *N. Engl. J. Med.* 317:1159, 1987.

No immediate or late complications were identified in 73 women undergoing transabdominal placental biopsy between 15 and 37 weeks of pregnancy. The authors conclude that transabdominal CVS is a promising approach to rapid fetal karyotyping, with direct-preparation results available the same day.

Cordocentesis
26. Tipton, R. E., et al. Rapid chromosome analysis with the use of spontaneously dividing cells derived from umbilical cord blood (fetal and neonatal). *Am. J. Obstet. Gynecol.* 161:1546, 1989.

The authors describe an accurate and reproducible method for producing high-quality metaphases within 24 hours in fetal blood obtained by PUBS.

45. ANTEPARTUM ASSESSMENT OF FETAL WELL-BEING
Rick W. Martin

The average perinatal mortality rate in the United States is approximately 13 per 1000 live births. In certain high-risk populations, this number may increase to 30 to 40 per 1000 live births. There are now several tests available that can assess fetal status, and thus their use may lead to a substantially reduced perinatal mortality. Not all physicians agree on the method of testing that is best nor on which patients should be tested; however, some of the indications for antepartum fetal testing include maternal hypertension, maternal diabetes mellitus, oligohydramnios, intrauterine growth retardation, postdates pregnancy, multiple gestation, isoimmunization, maternal renal disease, maternal collagen vascular disease, maternal heart disorders, a previous unexplained fetal demise, or decreased fetal movement as perceived by the mother. Although various chemical tests, such as estriol and human placental lactogen determinations, have been utilized in the past, monitoring of the fetal heart rate and other biophysical parameters give a more immediate result and have become more popular in recent times.

The knowledge that fetal heart rate decelerations in association with uterine contractions predicted fetal morbidity served as the basis for the development of the oxytocin challenge test in the 1970s. In this test, a baseline fetal heart rate tracing is obtained for 15 to 20 minutes with an ultrasound transducer and uterine activity is measured with a tocodynamometer. At least three contractions within a 10-minute period are required. These contractions may be spontaneous or they may be induced by oxytocin administered by intravenous infusion. More recently, nipple stimulation has been used to induce uterine contractions. The advent of nipple stimulation has reduced the time needed to perform a contraction stress test (CST) as well as the expense of the test.

The interpretation of the CST findings falls into five categories: negative, a tracing with no late decelerations; positive, late decelerations follow over half the contractions; suspicious, intermittent labor or variable decelerations; unsatisfactory, fewer than three contractions occurring within 10 minutes or the tracing was of poor quality; and hyperstimulation, there were decelerations but they may have been due to excessive uterine activity. Most physicians do not perform CSTs in patients who are at risk for preterm labor or when placenta previa is suspected.

Because accelerations of the fetal heart rate with contractions were noted to be associated with a favorable fetal outcome, the nonstress test (NST) was developed. The NST involves a 20-minute period of fetal heart rate observation. The tracing is deemed reactive if two accelerations of 15 beats per minute which last 15 seconds are noted. Should the tracing be nonreactive, an additional 20 minutes of observation is carried out to allow for possible fetal sleep-wake cycles. Although the presence of mild variable decelerations is not necessarily associated with an adverse perinatal outcome, this may indicate the need for ultrasound examination to look for oligohy-dramnios. A nonreactive NST may also be more common early in the third trimester, but, by 32 weeks' gestation, the incidence of nonreactive tests should be comparable to that seen at term. NSTs may be performed on a weekly basis, though some authors recommend more frequent testing, especially in the setting of conditions such as in-trauterine growth retardation or maternal diabetes. To shorten the time required to obtain a reactive NST, vibroacoustic stimulation using an artificial larynx has been employed. When a reactive NST is obtained through the use of vibroacoustic stimu-lation, this appears to be as reassuring of fetal well-being as that obtained with the nonstimulated NST. In approximately 1 to 2 percent of the cases, significant fetal bradycardia may be noted when the artificial larynx is applied.

The fetal biophysical profile (BPP) may sometimes be used to minimize the number of false-positive NST and CST results. The BPP consists of a NST combined with 30 minutes of ultrasound observation. Two points are awarded for each component of the BPP, as follows: a reactive NST; one or more episodes of fetal breathing of 30 seconds or more; three or more discrete limb movements; one or more episodes of extension of an extremity with return deflection indicating fetal tone; and a quan-titative amniotic fluid volume assessment of a 1-cm pocket or more. A score of 8 or 10 is considered normal and scores below 4 are considered abnormal.

Doppler velocimetry takes advantage of the frequency shift that takes place when a sound wave strikes a moving object. This has been helpful in examining various measures of volumetric flow. Either continuous or pulse Doppler velocimetry has been utilized to evaluate the fetal condition. There are certain methodologic problems involved, but measurement of the systolic to diastolic (S/D) ratio is most widely used, with higher values indicating a greater resistance to flow. This method has been of particular use in the evaluation of hypertensive pregnancies and suspected intra-uterine growth retardation. By 30 weeks' gestation, the S/D ratio in the umbilical artery should be below 3, and the ratio falls with increasing gestational age.

Some physicians attempt to evaluate fetal acid-base status more directly. Umbili-cal cord pH values and lactic acid measurements may be obtained by directly sam-pling the umbilical cord under ultrasound guidance. This more invasive procedure may be associated with fetal complications, but it may be indicated in certain in-stances, especially when fetal blood is being obtained for other reasons, such as for determination of Rh isoimmunization or for genetic studies.

There are many unanswered questions concerning the topic of antepartum fetal surveillance. In general, fetal testing should begin once viability has been reached and the physician ordering such tests should be prepared to act on the results. Most begin fetal testing at 32 weeks' gestation in high-risk pregnancies; however, for cer-tain maternal conditions, testing could begin much earlier. The risk of stillbirth occurring within 1 week of a reassuring test result is low, no matter which test is employed, after correcting for congenital anomalies. Ultimate fetal mortality rates of 1.4 per 1000 for the NST, 0.6 per 1000 for the BPP, and 0.0 per 1000 for the CST, when findings indicate fetal well-being, attest to the worth of the tests.

General
1. Gabbe, S. G. Antepartum Fetal Evaluation. In S. G. Gabbe, J. R. Niebyl, and J. L. Simpson (eds.), *Obstetrics: Normal and Problem Pregnancies.* New York: Churchill Livingstone, 1991.
   Methods of antepartum fetal evaluation are reviewed, as well as the associated issues of perinatal mortality.
2. Moore, T. R., and Piacquadio, K. A prospective evaluation of fetal movement screening to reduce the incidence of antepartum fetal death. *Am. J. Obstet. Gy-necol.* 160:1075, 1989.
   A count-to-10 with fetal movement screening program led to a reduction in the fetal mortality rate in low-risk patients.
3. Smith, C. V. Antepartum fetal surveillance in the preterm fetus. *Clin. Perinatol.* 19:437, 1992.
   Due to immaturity of the fetal nervous system, alternative methods such as the BPP and Doppler examination may help in identifying a compromised fetus.

4. Patrick, J. The physiological basis for fetal assessment. *Semin. Perinatol.* 13:403, 1989.
Fetal tests are based on observations of normal fetal behavior and results should be interpreted with caution between 20 and 30 weeks' gestation.
5. Antepartum fetal surveillance. *ACOG Tech. Bull.* No. 107, August 1987.
Currently accepted methods of fetal evaluation are presented, including procedures for performing the individual tests.

Nonstress Test and Contraction Stress Test
6. Devoe, L. D., et al. A prospective comparative study of the extended nonstress test and the nipple stimulation contraction stress test. *Am. J. Obstet. Gynecol.* 157:531, 1987.
Both the extended NST and nipple-stimulation CST provided excellent methods for fetal surveillance.
7. Druzin, M. L., and Foodim, J. Effect of maternal glucose ingestion compared with maternal water ingestion on the nonstress test. *Obstet. Gynecol.* 67:425, 1986.
There was no significant difference in the mean time of reactivity when maternal water and glucose ingestion were compared.
8. Zimmer, Z., and Divon, M. Y. Fetal vibroacoustic stimulation. *Obstet. Gynecol.* 81:451, 1993.
The safety of vibroacoustic stimulation and its ability to elicit fetal heart rate accelerations are reviewed.
9. Platt, L. V., et al. Fifteen years of experience with antepartum fetal testing. *Am. J. Obstet. Gynecol.* 156:1509, 1987.
The authors discussed the results seen in over 16,000 patients undergoing antepartum fetal assessment and the evolution of protocols within their institution.
10. Owen, J., et al. A comparison of perinatal outcome in patients undergoing contraction stress testing performed by nipple stimulation versus spontaneously occurring contractions. *Am. J. Obstet. Gynecol.* 160:1081, 1989.
The perinatal effects of nipple stimulation and spontaneous contraction CSTs were compared. The fetal death rates were 4.9 and 8.6 per 1000 live births for the nipple stimulation and spontaneous contraction groups, respectively.
11. Smith, C. V., et al. Fetal death following antepartum fetal heart rate testing: a review of 65 cases. *Obstet. Gynecol.* 70:18, 1987.
The most common autopsy findings were meconium aspiration, perinatal infection, and abnormal umbilical cord position.
12. Ray, M., et al. Clinical experience with the oxytocin challenge test. *Am. J. Obstet. Gynecol.* 114:1, 1972.
The initial experience with the oxytocin challenge test is presented.
13. Freeman, R. K., Anderson, G., and Dorchester, W. A prospective multi-institutional study of antepartum fetal heart rate monitoring. II. Contraction stress test versus nonstress test for primary surveillance. *Am. J. Obstet. Gynecol.* 143:778, 1982.
The antenatal death rate was found to be eight times higher when the NST was used as the primary surveillance test, versus the rate noted for the CST.

Ultrasound and Doppler
14. Manning, F. A. The fetal biophysical score: current status. *Obstet. Gynecol. Clin. North Am.* 17:147, 1990.
The concept of the BPP is presented and recommendations are provided for its use in clinical management.
15. American College of Obstetricians and Gynecologists. Utility of antepartum fetal Doppler for estimating umbilical and uterine artery flow. *ACOG Committee Opin.* No. 116, November 1992.
Currently, Doppler velocimetry remains an investigational tool in this setting.
16. Vintzileos, A. M., et al. The use and misuse of fetal biophysical profile. *Am. J. Obstet. Gynecol.* 156:527, 1987.
Frequent errors of interpretation are described, and a protocol for antepartum fetal evaluation that makes use of the BPP is suggested.

17. Vintzileos, A. M., et al. The relationships among fetal biophysical profile, umbilical cord pH, and Apgar scores. *Am. J. Obstet. Gynecol.* 157:627, 1987.
The first manifestations of fetal acidosis are a nonreactive NST and loss of fetal breathing. With advanced fetal acidemia, fetal movements and tone are compromised.
18. Hendricks, S. K., et al. Doppler umbilical artery waveform indices—normal values from 14 to 42 weeks. *Am. J. Obstet. Gynecol.* 161:761, 1989.
The normal declines in the Pourcelot index and S/D ratio are demonstrated in this report on 590 Doppler studies.

46. LABORATORY TESTS OF FETAL LUNG MATURITY
Neil S. Whitworth

During the twenty-fifth to twenty-sixth week of gestation, the fetal pulmonary alveolar epithelium begins to differentiate into type I and type II pneumocytes. The type II pneumocytes synthesize a surface active material (surfactant), which is both stored and then secreted in the form of lamellar bodies. There is a modest but progressive increase in surfactant output beginning at week 26. This is followed by a striking increase at week 34, which continues until delivery of the fetus. Pulmonary surfactant consists largely of phospholipids (80–90%), with phosphatidylcholine the major active component (60–70%), together with lesser quantities of phosphatidylglycerol ([PG] 5–10%) and other phospholipids.

The primary function of pulmonary surfactant is to maintain a low, stable surface tension (<10 dyn/cm^2) at the alveolar air-liquid interface. This action lowers the pressure needed to inflate the lungs and decreases the likelihood of alveolar collapse. A deficiency of surfactant at the time of birth is usually a result of preterm delivery before the surfactant production pathways are fully developed. It is also thought to be associated with certain maternal-fetal disorders that interfere with surfactant synthesis, even in the term infant. In either case, surfactant deficiency is the principal etiologic factor responsible for the neonatal respiratory distress syndrome (RDS). RDS affects 10 to 15 percent of the infants weighing less than 2500 g at birth, and it remains the leading cause of morbidity and mortality in preterm neonates. For this reason, developing laboratory tests for determining the status of fetal lung maturity (FLM) has been the object of considerable research and these tests continue to play an important role in the management of obstetric delivery.

Virtually all laboratory tests for FLM are based on the analysis of various constituents and characteristics of amniotic fluid. This is thought to constitute an accurate and practical approach to estimating the status of pulmonary surfactant, as (1) lamellar bodies are carried into amniotic fluid by fetal respiratory movements, and (2) amniotic fluid specimens are relatively accessible to amniocentesis or vaginal collection in the case of ruptured membranes. Although numerous tests for FLM have been developed, the analytic principles underlying these tests cause the tests to fall into one of two general categories: (1) those based on the biochemical analysis of amniotic fluid phospholipids, such as the lecithin-sphingomyelin (L/S) ratio and the PG content, and (2) those based on measurement of the biophysical characteristics of amniotic fluid, such as the optical density and surfactant activity.

Recommendations for the appropriate clinical use of FLM tests have been derived from the literally hundreds of published studies that have evaluated and compared the predictive accuracy of these tests. There are, however, several methodologic features of these studies (particularly the earlier investigations) that render these comparisons less than ideal. RDS, the ultimate end-point when it comes to evaluating test performance, has not always been clearly defined and RDS criteria may vary from study to study. At times, important variables that can affect the incidence of RDS have not been well controlled, for example, gestational age, fetal sex, and mode of delivery. Amniotic fluid specimens contaminated with blood or meconium are frequently excluded from analysis. However, because these contaminants can occur in up to 20 percent of the specimens, this exclusion likely introduces substantial patient sample bias. Patient demographics and obstetric risk factors are often insufficiently considered. In particular, evidence indicates that the results yielded by FLM test validation studies conducted in relatively normal term pregnancies do not generalize well to the high-risk obstetric populations encountered at tertiary-care facilities. Studies of new methods to predict FLM generally suffer from verification bias. This is because the new test is usually compared to the L/S ratio, and elective delivery will rarely be allowed if the ratio indicates immaturity. Results that show immaturity are therefore less likely to be verified than those that show maturity. Despite these limitations, several aspects of FLM test performance are well established, and these tests can aid the obstetrician in situations requiring an estimate of RDS risk.

Although introduced over 20 years ago, the L/S ratio remains the most widely used test of FLM and it is the standard to which newer tests of FLM are compared. The test uses thin-layer chromatography (TLC) to isolate the amniotic fluid phospholipids, and the analytes are then quantified by densitometry or planimetry. The test results may be less reliable if the specimen is contaminated with blood or meconium. The test takes about 3 hours to perform, it is technically difficult, and it requires a well-trained, experienced test operator. For this reason, the means for determining the L/S ratio are rarely available on an around-the-clock basis. Because of test difficulty and many procedural variations, L/S ratio results are highly variable between laboratories. In recent surveys of L/S ratio proficiency testing conducted by the College of American Pathologists, the percent coefficient of variation between laboratories was found to be as high as 40 percent. As a result, it was suggested that each laboratory establish its own L/S ratio reference values for FLM, rather than rely on the widely published "textbook" value of 2.0:1. Despite these drawbacks, the L/S ratio represents one of the most accurate FLM tests available. If the L/S ratio shows maturity, the probability of RDS occurring in an infant delivered at that time is very low (1–3%). Earlier studies had suggested that the mature predictive value ([PV_{Mat}], or the percentage of mature test results that correctly predict lung maturity) of the L/S ratio was less accurate in certain classes of diabetic pregnancies. However, the findings from more recent investigations indicate that the customary FLM reference values are valid for diabetic populations. The immature predictive value ([PV_{Imm}], or the percentage of immature test results that correctly predict RDS) of the L/S ratio is considerably lower than the PV_{Mat}, and is usually reported to be about 50 percent. Although most concern has been focused on minimizing the falsely mature FLM test result, to avoid the consequences of a neonate with RDS, the high rate of falsely immature results seen for the L/S ratio is not inconsequential. This is particularly true for those high-risk obstetric situations in which it may be desirable to deliver the fetus as soon as possible.

The other amniotic fluid phospholipid frequently measured as a test of FLM is PG. Originally the test methodology used two-dimensional TLC, which is even more laborious than the L/S ratio procedure. This test has largely been replaced by a commercially available immunoagglutination test for PG (AmnioStat-FLM; Irvine Sci. Santa Ana, CA). The results of this newer test correlate highly with the TLC procedure, and 0.5 μg/ml is set as the PG concentration indicative of FLM. The test turnaround time is relatively fast (less than 30 minutes) and the procedure is simple to perform. However, the manufacturer does caution that the test results may be unreliable if there is more than moderate blood or meconium contamination. The presence of PG in amniotic fluid is a very accurate marker for FLM, and the PV_{Mat} for this test is often reported to range from 98 to 100 percent. The absence of PG, however, is not an accurate predictor of RDS, as the PV_{Imm} is only about 30 percent. This is due to the fact that substantial amounts of PG do not appear in amniotic fluid until 36 to 37 weeks of gestation, and up to 25 percent of term mature amniotic fluid specimens do not exhibit PG. Other amniotic fluid phospholipids, combinations of phospholipids, and even hormones have been measured to serve as tests for FLM, but none has achieved the widespread use of the L/S ratio and PG measurement.

Many of the other rapid tests of FLM rely on the biophysical characteristics of amniotic fluid rather than on its chemical makeup. One of the most well known of these tests is the surfactant foam test (shake test). The shake test depends on the capacity of fetal pulmonary surfactant to produce stable foam in the presence of a graded series of ethanol dilutions. A commercial form of the test is available, the Lumadex Foam Stability Index, or FSI (Beckman Instruments, Brea, CA), which simplifies measurement and provides semiquantitative results. A Lumadex FSI of 0.47 or greater is considered to indicate lung maturity. In addition to its foaming properties, mature amniotic fluid exhibits a characteristic opalescence, which is due in part to the increasing concentration of surfactant-containing lamellar bodies. This property can be quantified by measuring the optical density (OD) of the sample at a wavelength of 650 nm, and is the basis for the OD 650 test of FLM. One of the few tests of FLM not measuring some aspect of surfactant activity is the Nile blue–staining fetal fat cell (FFC) test. These lipid-containing cells are thought to be derived from the fetal sebaceous glands, whose development correlates highly with fetal pulmonary development. Lung maturity is indicated when the amniotic fluid concentration of fat-staining cells exceeds 10 percent. All three of these tests take less than 30 minutes to perform and do not require great technical expertise. The reliability of the shake and OD 650 tests is subject to the effects of blood and meconium contamination and also the potential dilutional effects associated with oligohydramnios or polyhydramnios. The FFC test, on the other hand, can tolerate relatively large amounts of meconium and blood in the amniotic fluid sample. When the results of any one of these tests indicate lung maturity, the attendant incidence of RDS is rare (1–3%). Like the PG test, however, an immature test result is unreliable, with the PV_{Imm} reported to be as low as 10 percent and usually not much higher than 30 percent.

Of the newer tests of FLM, two look particularly promising. The lamellar body–density test is a variant of the OD 650 test and uses an electronic cell counter to directly determine the concentration of amniotic fluid lamellar bodies. The second procedure, the TDx FLM test (Abbott Lab., Abbott Park, IL), is a modification of the older microviscosity test, and is a commercial system that employs a fluorescence polarization method to measure the amniotic fluid surfactant phospholipid-to-albumin ratio. The automated equipment required for these procedures is widely available in hospital laboratories and is simple to operate. The tests can be performed rapidly with a degree of precision higher than that of the L/S ratio, and the results appear to correlate well with the results of other tests of FLM. The PV_{Mat} of these procedures is reported to be comparable to that of other FLM tests (97–99%). The PV_{Imm}, although substantially lower, is not yet well documented, as studies of these newer tests inherently suffer from verification bias.

Several factors should be considered when adopting a strategy of FLM testing. The utility of FLM testing is very dependent on gestational age. There is little benefit in terms of patient management to testing at or beyond 37 weeks of gestation because the incidence of RDS is very low at this time (<1%). Furthermore, a test result showing immaturity at this stage is likely to be false, and may cause the obstetrician to delay an otherwise appropriate delivery. Similarly, FLM testing at week 30 or less is generally not useful because the likelihood of RDS is so high (≥60%) that it is often just as effective to assume that RDS will occur if delivery takes place at this time. As a result, FLM testing is most useful during the intermediate stages (weeks 32 to 35), when conditions prevail that may threaten either the mother or the fetus, for example, preterm labor, premature rupture of membranes, situations necessitating labor induction or cesarean section, and poorly documented gestational age. The clinician should also keep in mind that, although the PV_{Mat} of all FLM tests is highly accurate (97–99%), a price is paid for this accuracy in the form of a high falsely immature rate. The PV_{Imm} for the L/S ratio is only 50 percent and is even lower for many other tests (≤30%). A final consideration is the logistics of test performance. The L/S ratio, although the most accurate measure of FLM, is a lengthy test and may not be available during evenings or weekends, making it probable that the physician will wait several hours or longer for a test result. As an alternative, the rapid tests of FLM at least offer an accurate PV_{Mat} and the test turn-around time can be less than 30 minutes.

Given these considerations, a sequential protocol can provide an efficient scheme for FLM testing. Begin FLM testing with any of the simple, rapid tests (e.g., the shake test, AmnioStat-FLM or TDx FLM). The result will be quickly available and, if it shows maturity, the result is highly reliable and can be acted on. If the test shows immaturity, the result is not reliable and testing must therefore proceed to the more accurate, but difficult, L/S ratio. An L/S ratio showing maturity indicates that the risk for RDS is minimal. If the L/S ratio shows immaturity, the risk for RDS is approximately 50 percent.

The extent to which new developments, such as fetal ultrasound assessment or RDS therapy with exogenous surfactant, may alter the nature of obstetric management and FLM testing is not yet established. The protocol just described can, however, provide the clinician with a rapid and cost-effective means of evaluating FLM.

General
1. Amenta, J. S., Brocher, S. C., and Serenko-Aber, A. L. Comparing different statistical methods for evaluating diagnostic effectiveness of clinical tests: respiratory distress syndrome as a model. *Clin. Chem.* 34:273, 1988.
   Discusses the appropriate statistical procedures for evaluating FLM tests and establishing FLM reference values.
2. Bourbon, J. R., and Farrell, P. M. Fetal lung development in the diabetic pregnancy. *Pediatr. Res.* 19:253, 1985.
   Reviews the influence of maternal diabetes on fetal lung development and the incidence of RDS.
3. Chapman, J. F., and Herbert, W. N. Current methods for evaluating fetal lung maturity. *Lab. Med.* 17:597, 1986.
   Discusses the biochemical and biophysical tests of FLM.
4. Dubin, S. B. Assessment of fetal lung maturity: in search of the Holy Grail. *Clin. Chem.* 36:1867, 1990.
   Discusses the problems associated with developing accurate FLM tests and testing strategies.
5. Dubin, S. B. The laboratory assessment of fetal lung maturity. *Am. J. Clin. Pathol.* 97:836, 1992.
   A comprehensive review of the utility of several laboratory tests in predicting FLM.
6. Roberts, W. E., and Morrison, J. C. Pharmacologic induction of fetal lung maturity. *Clin. Obstet. Gynecol.* 34:319, 1991.
   Reviews the use of glucocorticoids and exogenous surfactant for the antenatal induction of FLM and the postnatal treatment of RDS.
7. Scarpelli, E. M. *Pulmonary Physiology: Fetus, Newborn, Child, and Adolescent* (2nd ed.). Philadelphia: Lea & Febiger, 1990.
   Comprehensive presentation of the topic of fetal pulmonary physiology.
8. Schreiner, R. L., and Bradburn, N. C. Newborns with acute respiratory distress: Diagnosis and management. *Pediatr. Rev.* 9:279, 1988.
   Reviews the etiology, diagnosis, and management of neonatal RDS.

Laboratory Analysis
9. Amenta, J. S., Brocher, S. C., and Serenko-Aber, A. L. Evaluating the clinical effectiveness of amniotic fluid assays in predicting respiratory distress syndrome in the neonate. *Clin. Chem.* 33:647, 1987.
   Uses stepwise discriminant function analysis to evaluate the clinical effectiveness of phospholipid tests of FLM.
10. Ashwood, E. R., et al. Lamellar body counts for rapid fetal lung maturity testing. *Obstet. Gynecol.* 81:619, 1993.
    The results from this 3-year prospective study indicate that the lamellar body density test is a useful and rapid screening test for FLM.
11. Ashwood, E. R., Palmer, S. E., and Lenke, R. R. Rapid fetal lung maturity testing: Commercial versus NBD-phosphatidylcholine assay. *Obstet. Gynecol.* 80:1048, 1992.
    The rapid TDx FLM test performance correlates highly with that of the more laborious L/S ratio.
12. Dubin, S. B. Characterization of amniotic fluid lamellar bodies by resistive-pulse

counting: relationship to measures of fetal lung maturity. *Clin. Chem.* 35:612, 1989.
First description of the use of resistive-pulse counting of amniotic fluid lamellar body concentration as an FLM test.

13. Garite, T. J., Freeman, R. K., and Nageotte, M. P. Fetal maturity cascade: a rapid and cost-effective method for fetal lung maturity testing. *Obstet. Gynecol.* 67:619, 1986.
Shows that a sequential test protocol combining rapid FLM tests with the L/S ratio can provide timely test results with a cost savings of 30 percent.

14. Gluck, L., et al. Diagnosis of the respiratory distress syndrome by amniocentesis. *Am. J. Obstet. Gynecol.* 109:440, 1971.
The original paper describing the clinical utility of the L/S ratio in predicting RDS.

15. Hunink, M. G., et al. Testing for fetal pulmonary maturity: ROC analysis involving covariates, verification bias, and combination testing. *Med. Decis. Making* 10:201, 1990.
Demonstrates the effect of verification bias on FLM test validation studies.

16. Kjos, S. L., et al. Prevalence and etiology of respiratory distress in infants of diabetic mothers: predictive value of fetal lung maturation tests. *Am. J. Obstet. Gynecol.* 163:898, 1990.
The L/S ratio, PG, and the OD 650 test were used to predict FLM in a population of 526 diabetic mothers. The results suggest that the conventional test cutoff values are valid for diabetic patients.

17. Morrison, J. C., et al. Nile blue staining of cells in amniotic fluid for fetal maturity: part II. in complicated obstetric cases. *Obstet. Gynecol.* 44:362, 1974.
Demonstrates that the Nile blue–staining FFC test accurately predicts FLM.

18. Oulton, M., Fraser, M., and Robinson, S. Correlation of absorbance at 650 nm with the presence of phosphatidylglycerol in amniotic fluid. *J. Reprod. Med.* 35:402, 1990.
The OD 650 test is a useful rapid screening test for the initial evaluation of FLM.

19. Ragosch, V., et al. Prediction of RDS by amniotic fluid analysis: a comparison of the prognostic value of traditional and recent methods. *J. Perinat. Med.* 20:351, 1992.
Compares test performance of the L/S ratio, AmnioStat-FLM PG test, and TDx FLM test. The PV$_{Mat}$ for all tests was high and the falsely immature rate was lowest for the L/S ratio.

20. Richardson, D. K., et al. Diagnostic tests in obstetrics: a method for improved evaluation. *Am. J. Obstet. Gynecol.* 152:613, 1985.
Uses receiver operating characteristic curve analysis to suggest that the L/S ratio is a more accurate predictor of RDS than the Lumadex FSI or OD 650 test.

21. Sher, G., and Statland, B. E. Assessment of fetal pulmonary maturity by the Lumadex foam stability index test. *Obstet. Gynecol.* 61:444, 1983.
The authors present their observations from the initial validation study of the Lumadex-FSI test of FLM.

22. Statland, B. E., and Sher, G. Reliability of amniotic fluid surfactant measurements. *Am. J. Clin. Pathol.* 83:382, 1985.
There is high interlaboratory variability in the L/S ratio results.

23. Steinfeld, J. D., et al. The utility of the TDx test in the assessment of fetal lung maturity. *Obstet. Gynecol.* 79:460, 1992.
TDx FLM test performance was improved by the adoption of less conservative FLM reference values.

24. Towers, C. V., and Garite, T. J. Evaluation of the new Amniostat-FLM test for the detection of phosphatidylglycerol in contaminated fluids. *Am. J. Obstet. Gynecol.* 160:298, 1989.
Evaluates the performance of the second-generation ultrasensitive AmnioStat-FLM test for PG. The results indicate good concordance with the chromatographic PG procedure.

GYNECOLOGY

X. GENERAL GYNECOLOGY

47. UTERINE FIBROIDS
Abraham Rubin

Fibroids (myomas, fibromyomas, and leiomyomas) are the most common benign tumors of the female genital tract. They usually occur in the uterus but can also be found in the round ligament, the ovary, and, rarely, in the labia majora. These growths are solid tumors but may undergo degeneration, and even liquefaction, sometimes producing softening of the tumors.

Degenerations, which may be hyaline, cystic, carneous, or fatty, are usually due to diminished blood supply when the tumor becomes large. Red degeneration (or necrobiosis) may occur during pregnancy or postpartum, and it has been encountered in menopause. It is due to venous obstruction producing intense congestion and necrosis. Malignant (sarcomatous) change is a rare complication in the menopausal woman.

Uterine fibroids may be either submucous (growing into the cavity), intramural, or subserous (bulging into the peritoneal cavity). This last type may develop a pedicle, become attached to other structures (usually the omentum), and obtain extra blood supply from these areas. Knowing the anatomic site of the myomas is important with regard to the symptomatology, complications, and management. Little has been documented regarding their etiology. It has been established that they are more common, grow more extensively, and occur at a younger age in the black population. They are somehow associated with infertility (either as a possible cause or effect), and appear to be related to hormonal influences. They may get larger during pregnancy and with estrogen administration. However, the prolonged use of oral contraceptives effectively reduces the risk of developing fibroids by 30 percent after 10 years. Use of birth control pills does not lead to an increased risk of developing fibroids. These tumors diminish in size postmenopausally and may regrow or recur after surgical removal. They can be extremely large, irregular, and multiple, yet remain benign. They have been found in patients as young as 11 years of age.

Pathologically, fibroids are distinguished by their definitive pseudocapsule and whorled macroscopic appearance on cross section. *Leiomyoma* is the correct term for these tumors, because they arise from a single smooth muscle cell. Deposits of calcium, after long-standing degeneration, account for the tumor's gritty texture on cutting and the typical stippled appearance seen on x-ray films.

The most frequent presenting feature is menorrhagia (75% of the patients), and it is the resultant anemia that may cause the patient to seek medical attention. Infertility, dysmenorrhea (usually of the congestive type), and the presence of an abdominal mass account for most of the other symptoms. Acute episodes, such as retention of urine owing to sudden enlargement and impaction in the cul-de-sac, are occasionally encountered. Metrorrhagia may also occur. A large number of patients harbor symptomless fibroids that are identified only during routine vaginal or general medical examinations. Autopsy shows that 20 percent of women older than 30 years have symptomless fibroids, and 50 percent of the patients with symptoms present before age 35 years.

The majority of signs and symptoms that occur in women with fibroids are due to the submucous fibroids, and include dysmenorrhea, menorrhagia (resulting from an increased bleeding surface area), metrorrhagia, and intermittent pain. The submucous fibroid can become pedunculated and can be delivered through the cervix. The surface of the exposed tumor can become eroded and septic, and can produce marked metrorrhagia, which will bring the patient to the hospital. Submucous fibroids may also induce abortion, stemming from interference with placentation, or postpartum hemorrhage, resulting from incomplete placental separation. However, the spontaneous abortion rate associated with fibroids is overall not greater than that for the general population. Patients with large fibroids do more frequently deliver prematurely. The size, number, and location of the fibroids do not influence pregnancy outcome, and the overall mode of delivery does not differ from that of patients who have no fibroids. The incidence of fibroids is 0.3 to 2.5 per 100 live births.

Intramural fibroids cause the fewest problems, and produce symptoms only because of their size. The mechanism whereby they affect fertility has not yet been elucidated. They are most likely the result, rather than the cause, of sterility.

Subserous fibroids are usually asymptomatic unless they are very large or pedunculated. The pedunculated ones may cause some peritoneal irritation or, rarely, if very mobile, undergo torsion. Even extremely large fibroid uteri seldom produce more than slight mechanical obstruction or anatomical deviation of the ureters. Edema of the legs and increased varicosities in the extremities may also be noted with large tumors.

In the postmenopausal woman, sudden enlargement (with or without pain) can indicate either cystic or sarcomatous degeneration. The latter occurs in fewer than 0.5 percent of the patients.

Leiomyosarcomas occur postmenopausally. The average age of presentation is 55 years and they are more common in the black population. The incidence is unrelated to parity. The most common presenting symptom is vaginal bleeding. The tumor is nonencapsulated and consists of a bulging, homogeneous, grayish white, soft pultaceous mass in which the whorled appearance has disappeared.

This malignancy must not be confused with cellular leiomyomas, which are fibroid tumors that exhibit increased cellularity and closely opposed nuclei microscopically. They display a low mitotic count compared to that of sarcomas, with little or no anaplasia, and have a propensity to enlarge rapidly during pregnancy.

The benign metastasizing leiomyoma is a condition in which uterine myomas are found together with pulmonary nodules composed of well-differentiated, benign smooth muscle. It is probably related to the dissemination of intravenous leiomyomas, which is the presence of well-differentiated smooth muscle in the lumina of uterine and pelvic veins. Microscopically, wormlike cords of tumor can be seen extending from the myometrium into veins of the broad ligament. There is no inclination toward extravascular invasion. The clinical symptoms consist of vaginal bleeding and, infrequently, abdominal enlargement.

Leiomyomatosis peritonealis disseminata is a rare pathologic entity. In it, multiple, 1- to 2-cm, raised, white nodules are seen on the peritoneal surface, including the liver and bowel. These are often associated with large uterine leiomyomas. They are grossly indistinguishable from a disseminated malignant tumor, but are benign, both microscopically and in their clinical behavior. The condition is metaplastic rather than metastatic in its pathogenesis.

The diagnosis of myomas is usually based on clinical findings. Bimanual pelvic examination reveals a characteristically firm-to-hard, irregularly shaped, enlarged uterus. Abdominal x-ray studies may show the soft tissue tumor and the possible presence of calcification, which appears as concentric white rings. Ultrasound may also be helpful, as it can confirm that the tumors are not extrauterine masses. Magnetic resonance imaging is valuable in differentiating myomas from adenomyomas. Dilated pelvic veins are absent in the setting of adenomyomas. Intravenous pyelography may show evidence of pressure effects on the ureters, and should be included in the evaluation. Panoramic hysteroscopy can be used to effectively diagnose submucous and pedunculated tumors. The differential diagnosis includes ovarian tumors, chronic tuboovarian abscess, hydrosalpinx, uterine sarcoma, and adenomyosis.

The management of myomas depends primarily on the patient's age, parity, and symptoms, as well as her desire for future pregnancies. As a rule, a total abdominal hysterectomy (a vaginal hysterectomy may be performed if feasible) is the procedure of choice in the older patient for whom fertility is not a factor.

The treatment of leiomyosarcomas is total abdominal hysterectomy and bilateral salpingo-oophorectomy. The 5-year survival rate is only 20.7 percent. The pelvis is the most common initial site for metastases, with the peritoneum and lung next in frequency.

In the younger patient, small submucous fibroids may be removed by curettage after cervical dilatation (*Laminaria* is an effective dilator) or with polyp forceps under hysteroscopic vision. When the fibroid has become pedunculated and presents through the cervix, the tumor may be twisted off or the pedicle cut at the base. This is followed by immediate curettage or hysteroscopic review, if the cervix is not dilated more than 1 cm, to make sure that there are no small residual fibroid polyps.

Hysterosalpingography may reveal whether submucous fibroids are present and establish the patency, or otherwise, of the fallopian tubes. Laparoscopy may be done before definitive surgical intervention to determine whether myomectomy or hysterectomy is indicated. The final decision usually depends on the condition of the tubes.

Myomectomy is performed when there is tubal patency or when tuboplasty is possible, when the uterus is not too large (not more than 20 weeks' gestational size), and when the fibroids are not too numerous. Small subserous or pedunculated subserous fibroids may be evaporated by laser performed via laparoscopy. The long-term administration of long-acting gonadotropin-releasing hormone (GnRH) agonists by injection given monthly (3.75 mg) may reduce the tumor's size by 40 to 60 percent after 2 to 6 months of therapy. Probably 3 months is sufficient before attempting surgical removal. Rapid regrowth occurs when treatment ceases. Side effects of agonist treatment include hot flashes, dry vagina, acne, seborrhea, and, rarely, hoarseness and loss of libido. GnRH analogues have potent antiestrogenic and antiprogestogenic properties. GnRH injection causes the uterine volume and tumor size to decrease, thereby making laparoscopic or vaginal hysterectomy feasible. It also promotes restoration of blood volume in anemic patients. Ultrasound documentation of the volume status is useful. The main complications of myomectomy are hemorrhage at operation and postoperative sepsis. Prophylactic antibiotics should be administered in all patients undergoing myomectomies. The disadvantage of resecting the fibroids only is that there is a 10 percent recurrence rate. With young patients, 50 percent will conceive in the first 2 years after myomectomy if there are no other infertility factors. The pregnancy rates in women older than 35 years are only 5 to 10 percent.

Asymptomatic myomas, when the uterus is less than 12 weeks' gestational size and not palpable suprapubically, may be treated expectantly. Two or three examinations annually will indicate whether they are dormant or enlarging. The rare acute red degeneration that occurs in pregnancy responds to pain relief and antipyretic treatment. Obstructed labor owing to fibroids is extremely rare, and requires cesarean section for delivery. The fibroids shrink rapidly postpartum, and surgical treatment should be delayed for at least 6 weeks after delivery.

Review
1. Buttram, V. C., Jr., et al. Uterine leiomyomata. Etiology, symptomatology and management. *Fertil. Steril.* 36:433, 1981.
   A good overview of various aspects of leiomyomata and their possible causes.
2. Howkins, J., and Stallworthy, J. Abdominal Myomectomy. In *Bonney's Gynecological Surgery* (8th ed.). London: Balliere-Tindall, 1974.
   A clear, concise, well-illustrated, step-by-step approach to myomectomy. It remains the standard text for the abdominal approach to fibroids.
3. Glavind, K., et al. Uterine myoma in pregnancy. *Acta Obstet. Gynecol. Scand.* 69:617, 1990.
   Good review of the effects of pregnancy on fibroids.
4. Fedele, L., et al. Diffuse uterine leiomyomatosis. *Acta Eur. Fertil.* 13:125, 1982.
   A detailed review and discussion of this interesting pathogenesis of leiomyomas.
5. Adamson, G. D. Treatment of uterine fibroids. Current findings with gonadotropin releasing hormone agonists. *Am. J. Obstet. Gynecol.* 143:6, 1982.
   The benefits of reducing uterine size and fibroid volume preoperatively are discussed.

Etiology
6. Soules, M.R., et al. Leiomyomas. Steroid receptor content. Variations within normal menstrual cycles. *Am. J. Obstet. Gynecol.* 143:6, 1982.
   The number of estrogen receptors is significantly greater in fibroids then in normal myometrium.
7. Chandrasekhar, Y., et al. Insulin-like growth factor I & II binding in human myometrium and leiomyomas. *Am. J. Obstet. Gynecol.* 166:64, 1992.

The number of insulin-like growth factor I (but not II) receptors is increased in leiomyomata compared to myometrium. This may therefore play a role in the generation and growth of the tumor.

8. Milwidsky, A., et al. Glycogen metabolism of normal human myometrium and leiomyoma—possible hormonal control. *Gynecol. Obstet. Invest.* 15:147, 1983.
   A hormonal basis for myomatous growth.

Diagnosis
9. Weinstein, D., et al. Hysterography before and after myomectomy. *A.J.R.* 129: 899, 1977.
   The value of preoperative hysterography in confirming the diagnosis and localization of myomas is stressed.
10. Samuelson, S., and Ovall, S. J. The value of laparoscopy in the differential diagnosis between uterine fibromyomata and adnexal tumors. *Acta Obstet. Gynecol. Scand.* 49:175, 1970.
    Laparoscopy may be indicated for the evaluation of subserous fibroids.
11. Gross, B. H., et al. Sonographic features of leiomyomas. Analysis of 41 problem cases. *J. Ultrasound Med.* 2:401, 1983.
    A detailed picture of the sonographic appearances of fibroids.
12. Tada, S., et al. Computed tomographic features of uterine myoma. *J. Comput. Assist. Tomogr.* 5:866, 1981.
    Appearance of fibroids on computed tomographic scans.
13. Mark, A. S., et al. Adenomyosis and leiomyoma: differential diagnosis with MR imaging. *Radiology* 163:527, 1987.
    Leiomyomas can be differentiated from adenomyosis using magnetic resonance imaging, which can be difficult with other techniques.
14. La Sela, G. B., et al. Panoramic diagnostic microhysteroscopy. Analysis of results obtained from 976 outpatients. *Acta Obstet. Gynecol. Scand.* 141:91, 1987.
    Excellent review of the use of hysteroscopy for the diagnosis of submucous fibroids.

Problems with Pregnancy and Contraceptive Pills
15. Treissman, D. A., et al. Epidural use of morphine in managing the pain of carneous degeneration of a uterine leiomyoma during pregnancy. *Can. Med. Assoc. J.* 126:505, 1982.
    Novel therapy for this painful condition.
16. Davis, J. L., et al. Uterine leiomyomas in pregnancy. A prospective study. *Obstet. Gynecol.* 75:41, 1990.
    The size of fibroids had no influence on pregnancy status.
17. Payne, P., et al. Uterine fibromyomata and secondary polycythaemia. *J. Obstet. Gynaecol. Br. Commonw.* 76:845, 1989.
    Fibroids may secrete erythropoietin, resulting in secondary polycythemia. This may account for the absence of anemia in patients with documented menorrhagia.
18. Rubin, A., and Ford, J. A. Uterine fibromyomata in urban blacks. A preliminary survey of the relationship between symptomatology, blood pressure and haemoglobin levels. *S. Afr. Med. J.* 48:2060, 1974.
    An association between fibroids and hypertension has been sought, because the two conditions frequently coexist. This relationship is probably only statistical, however, as both disorders are very common in black patients.
19. Maheux, R., et al. Use of intranasal luteinizing hormone releasing hormone agonist in uterine leiomyomas. *Fertil. Steril.* 47:229, 1987.
    Fewer side effects occur when this agent is used intranasally, and there is a marked reduction in size.
20. Burton, C. A., et al. Surgical management of leiomyomata during pregnancy. *Obstet. Gynecol.* 74:707, 1989.
    Leiomyomata may require surgical treatment because of symptoms or an uncertain diagnosis. Surgical treatment is safe in selected cases.

Management
21. Hutchins, F. Z., Jr. Myomectomy after selective preoperative treatment with a gonadotropin releasing hormone analog. *J. Reprod. Med.* 37:699, 1992.

This article describes the effective and safe preoperative management to reduce the size of tumor and thus decrease the morbidity associated with the procedure.

22. Schlaff, W. D., et al. A placebo-controlled trial of a depot gonadotropin-releasing hormone analogue (leuprolide) in the treatment of uterine leiomyomata. *Obstet. Gynecol.* 74:707, 1989.
    Uterine size and myomata were reduced with this treatment. Symptoms disappeared during therapy, and even 6 months after the therapy has remained so.
23. Dubiuisson, J. B., et al. Myomectomy by laparoscopy: a preliminary report of 43 cases. *Fertil. Steril.* 56:827, 1991.
    A report on 43 patients who underwent removal of 92 myomata. No patients required laparotomy or transfusions.
24. Berkeley, A. S., et al. Abdominal myomectomy and subsequent fertility. *Surg. Gynecol. Obstet.* 156:319, 1983.
    A reminder of the positive effects of myomectomy.
25. Neuwirth, R. S. Hysteroscopic management of symptomatic submucous fibroids. *Obstet. Gynecol.* 62:509, 1983.
    A relatively easy and effective way of removing small submucous fibroids under direct visualization per vaginam.
26. Indman, P. D. Hysteroscopic treatment of menorrhagia associated with uterine leiomyomas. *Obstet. Gynecol.* 81:716, 1993.
    Of 51 women treated, three subsequently required hysterectomy.
27. Reyniak, J. V., et al. Microsurgical laser technique for abdominal myomectomy. *Microsurgery* 8:92, 1987.
    Laser treatment can effectively vaporize small fibroids.
28. Friedman, A. J., and Haas, S. T. Should uterine size be an indication for surgical intervention in women with myomas? *Am. J. Obstet. Gynecol.* 168:751, 1993.
    The authors argue against the routine removal of asymptomatic fibroid uteri based on the size of the uterus exceeding that of a 12-week gestation.

---

48. PROLAPSE

Michel E. Rivlin

Weakness of the pelvic supporting structures may allow the pelvic organs to descend into the vagina. This process is termed *genital prolapse*. Descent of the anterior vaginal wall with protrusion of the bladder is called a *cystocele*. If the urethra sags as well, this is a *cystourethrocele*. A protrusion of the rectum through the posterior vaginal wall is termed a *rectocele*; it is frequently found in association with a herniation of intestine through the cul-de-sac, termed an *enterocele*. The degree of descent of the uterus varies and is deemed first degree if the cervix reaches the introitus, second degree if the cervix protrudes through the introitus, and third degree if the entire uterus protrudes. One or more forms of uterovaginal prolapse may exist in an individual patient.

The fixed, unyielding support of the pelvic organs is derived from the pelvic bones, while the major soft tissue support is afforded by the muscular pelvic floor. This latter is formed by the levator muscles (pubococcygeus, iliococcygeus, and ischiococcygeus). The more superficial perineal muscles and the urogenital diaphragm also provide some limited muscular support, although they are much less important than the levators in this regard. In addition to the pelvic floor muscles, certain connective tissues, called the *endopelvic fascia*, play a vital role in pelvic organ support. These include the paired uterosacral ligaments, passing from the cervix to the sacrum, and lateral thickenings in the base of the broad ligament, called *transverse cervical, cardinal*, or *Mackenrodt's ligaments*, which suspend the cervix and upper vagina from the pelvic side walls. The anterior and posterior vaginal walls are also supported by the pubocervical and rectovaginal fascia, respectively.

Prolapse is almost always a result of damage to the pelvic supporting structures incurred during childbirth, and is often aggravated by the lack of estrogen in menopause. As in any other hernial conditions, obesity, chronic cough, constipation, and occupations involving much standing and lifting may be contributory factors. Under normal conditions and in the erect position, the levator plate (central tendon of the levator muscles) lies in the horizontal plane; the uterus, vagina, and rectum all lie parallel to the plate, with the latter two structures lying in the hollow of the sacrum. When intraabdominal pressure increases, all three structures are forced against the levator plate, which contracts to support them. In addition, contraction of the levator, particularly the crura (i.e., the puborectalis and pubococcygeus), narrows the urogenital and anal hiatus. If structural or functional impairment of the levator occurs, the crura fail to narrow the pelvic hiatus and the levator sags and assumes a position that is inclined from the horizontal. Increased intraabdominal pressure results in a tendency for the uterus and vagina to slide down the inclined plane through the widened and elongated pelvic hiatus.

Mild to moderate pelvic relaxation is often associated with stress urinary incontinence (SUI). Poor transmission of abdominal pressure to the urethra is the main pathophysiologic reason for SUI. With the loss of anatomic support to the bladder base, the urethrovesical junction descends with the Valsalva maneuver and is no longer in the intraabdominal pressure domain. With the anatomic displacement of the urethrovesical junction and proximal urethra outside of its normal intrapelvic location above the urogenital diaphragm, any abdominal pressure increase is well transmitted to the bladder but is poorly transmitted to the urethra, and this results in the formation of a pressure gradient across to the urethrovesical junction and an involuntary loss of urine. Substantial SUI is usually associated with demonstrable defects in anterior vaginal wall support, most often with concurrent defects in uterine and posterior vaginal wall support. Other symptoms of prolapse include a feeling of "bulging in the vagina" or a "dragging feeling." Rarely, when prolapse is marked, it may be necessary to apply digital pressure to allow micturition or defecation. Residual urine, owing to incomplete emptying of a cystocele, may be a source of urinary tract infections (UTIs). There may be dyspareunia owing to the "vaginal bulge," or the patient may complain of feeling "too large." Backache that is most painful on arising and abates during the day is likely to be orthopedic in origin. If it is absent on arising, worsens during the day, and is relieved by lying down, the traction caused by genital prolapse may be the problem. In major degrees of prolapse, the protruding cervix and vagina may ulcerate, with consequent bleeding and discharge.

Prolapse is diagnosed on the basis of findings revealed by pelvic examination, which should be carried out in both the lithotomy and standing positions. The anterior and posterior vaginal walls are examined separately for the presence of descent with straining, as is the cervix. When primary damage involves the upper suspensory system, the cervix or vaginal vault will appear first, followed by any cystocele and rectocele. In cases of primary damage to the lower supportive system, the order is reversed. SUI is assessed if present. The size and position of the uterus are outlined on bimanual examination; the uterus is usually axial or retroverted with prolapse. It is not uncommon for the cervix to be well supported and for vaginal wall prolapse to result in elongation of the supravaginal cervix. Particular care must be taken to assess levator muscle tone and to determine whether there is an enterocele. A urine culture should be performed for every patient. Many patients with no urinary complaints may become incontinent when the prolapse is reduced, and this must be taken into account when planning surgical correction. Uroflowmetry and measurement of residual urine may help identify the patients at risk. The cystometrogram also identifies underlying detrusor instability or a hypotonic bladder. Multichannel pressure testing and fluoroscopy can comprehensively define the function of the lower urinary tract, but are not universally available. If third-degree descensus is present, an intravenous pyelogram is required, because ureteric obstruction is common in major instances of prolapse.

Medical treatment of prolapse is confined to patients with mild forms, especially young women in the first few months after childbirth. Conservative therapy includes pelvic floor exercises, weight loss, control of cough, and management of constipation. In older women, estrogen therapy may improve the condition of the vaginal mucosa and relieve minor symptoms. All these measures are also useful in preparing patients for surgical repair.

Vaginal pessaries have a place as a temporary measure after childbirth, during pregnancy, or in patients for whom surgical treatment is contraindicated. This last group includes aged and medically debilitated women for whom the operative risk appears too great, as well as those who refuse the procedure. Pessaries are usually made of plastic in the shape of a ring and are placed in a fashion similar to that of the contraceptive diaphragm. Pessaries should be cleaned and reinserted every few months because, if neglected, they may cause vaginal ulceration. A modern pessary should cause less trouble than a dental plate.

Conservative measures are usually insufficient in all but the mildest cases of prolapse. Surgical correction is usually required as the definitive therapy, but, because prolapse is seldom a health hazard, surgical repair should not be recommended unless the symptoms warrant the operative risk. Urinary and local vaginal infections or ulcerations must be cleared up before the operation. In planning the procedure, the patient's attitude toward future pregnancy, the presence or absence of SUI, and the importance of coital activity to the individual must be considered in detail.

Because the favored procedure for the treatment of uterine descent is a vaginal hysterectomy with support of the vaginal vault by the transverse cervical and uterosacral ligaments, it is fortunate that most patients who require it are older. If an enterocele is present, the peritoneal sac is excised and closed, and the uterosacral ligaments are approximated in the midline to prevent further herniation. In most cases, this procedure is followed by anterior vaginal wall repair (colporrhaphy), with particular attention to support of the urethrovesical angle if SUI is a problem. If there is a rectocele and a deficient perineum, posterior vaginal wall repair and restoration of the perineal body (colpoperineorrhaphy) complete the procedure.

For those women who desire further pregnancies, surgical treatment can be delayed. If this is not possible, modified repairs can be performed, although these are much less likely to be successful. If these patients become pregnant, delivery should be by cesarean section; otherwise, the repair is likely to break down at the time of delivery. In older women in whom intercourse is no longer a factor, a stronger repair is possible, as less attention needs to be given to maintaining a functional vagina.

Postoperative care is chiefly directed at urinary function and the relief of pain associated with the posterior repair. Hemorrhage and infection are the major postoperative complications, but the incidence of infection is much reduced by the administration of perioperative prophylactic antibiotics, especially in premenopausal patients.

Long-term postoperative complications include dyspareunia and vault prolapse. Dyspareunia may be relieved by vaginal dilatation and estrogen therapy. Vault prolapse is usually due to failure of the enterocele repair. Several operative procedures, by both abdominal and vaginal routes, have been used to alleviate this difficult surgical problem, but no completely satisfactory method has yet been developed.

Reviews
1. Nichols, D. H. Surgery for pelvic floor disorders. *Surg. Clin. North Am.* 71:927, 1991.
   Important goals of reconstructive surgical treatment include upward relocation of the vesicourethral junction to a point where it is once again under the influence of intraabdominal pressure, as well as restoration of normal vaginal depth and axis.
2. Harris, T. A., and Bent, A. E. Genital prolapse with and without urinary incontinence. *J. Reprod. Med.* 35:792, 1990.
   Prolapse may involve damage to the cardinal and uterosacral ligament complex, the urogenital diaphragm, including its pubourethral components, the pelvic diaphragm, and the perineal body. A basic surgical rule is to overrepair the primary site of damage to reduce the chance of recurrence.

Anatomy
3. Berglas, B., and Rubin, I.C. Study of the supportive structures of the uterus by levator myography. *Surg. Gynecol. Obstet.* 97:677, 1953.

These researchers believe that the levator muscles form a flat plate supporting the vagina and uterus, and that the levator plate responds to changes in intraabdominal pressure.
4. Dickins, A. Uterine ligaments and the treatment of prolapse. *J. R. Soc. Med.* 77:353, 1984.
   Reviews the debate regarding the roles of the suspensory support (cardinal ligament complex) and the support from below (levator ani–urogenital diaphragm) in maintaining the position of the pelvic viscera.
5. Peters, W. A., III, and Thornton, W. N., Jr. Surgical anatomy of the perirectal fascia: a gynecologic perspective. *Obstet. Gynecol. Surv.* 42:605, 1987.
   The only true fascia in the pelvis overlies the levator ani, piriformis, and obturator internus muscles. However, the fibroareolar tissue that accompanies the major blood vessels to the urinary, genital, and intestinal tracts is termed visceral fascia, or ligaments, and divides the retroperitoneum into the avascular spaces, which are so important in the performance of pelvic operations.

Etiology
6. Bayatpour, M., et al. Neonatal genital prolapse. *Pediatrics* 90:465, 1992.
   Genital prolapse may occur in normal infants or can be associated with neurologic defects, including meningomyelocele and spina bifida occulta.
7. El-Shaaly, H. A., and el-Sherif, A. K. Is the benign joint hypermobility syndrome benign? *Clin. Rheumatol.* 10:302, 1991.
   Connective tissue disorders with lax tissue, such as Marfan's syndrome, and neurogenic disorders, such as multiple sclerosis, may be associated with pelvic relaxation.
8. Wiskind, A. K., Creighton, S. M., and Stanton, S. L. The incidence of genital prolapse after the Burch colposuspension. *Am. J. Obstet. Gynecol.* 167:399, 1992.
   Thirty-five of 131 patients required surgical treatment for prolapse after the Burch procedure. It is unclear whether the prolapse was due to operative disruption of the vaginal axis or to an intrinsic weakness of the pelvic floor.

Diagnosis
9. Beecham, C. T. Classification of vaginal relaxation. *Am. J. Obstet. Gynecol.* 136:956, 1980.
   The article offers a suggested classification of the various components of vaginal relaxation, as no general agreement exists at this time.
10. Rosenzweig, B. A., et al. Prevalence of abnormal urodynamic test results in continent women with severe genitourinary prolapse. *Obstet. Gynecol.* 79:539, 1992.
    Reduction of the prolapse with a pessary before surgical repair may identify some patients with genuine SUI previously masked by the prolapse.
11. Kelvin, F. M., et al. Pelvic prolapse: assessment with evacuation proctography (defecography). *Radiology* 184:547, 1992.
    This method contributes to surgical planning by identifying clinically unsuspected enteroceles, sigmoidoceles, and coexistent disorders of rectal evacuation.
12. Creighton, S. M., Pearce, J. M., and Stanton, S. L. Perineal video-ultrasonography in the assessment of vaginal prolapse: early observations. *Br. J. Obstet. Gynaecol.* 99:310, 1992.
    Movement of the whole pelvic floor can be demonstrated using this method. All measurements taken were found to be reproducible.
13. Yang, A., et al. Pelvic floor descent in women: dynamic evaluation with fast MR imaging and cinematic display. *Radiology* 179:25, 1991.
    Quantification of the pelvic descent process may be of value in surgical planning and postoperative follow-up.

Medical Therapy
14. Elia, G., and Bergman, A. Pelvic muscle exercises: When do they work? *Obstet. Gynecol.* 81:283, 1993.
    The Kegel exercise program involves isometric contractions of the muscles of the

pelvic diaphragm. An effective regimen consists of 15 consecutive strong contractions lasting 3 seconds each and performed six times daily.

15. Zeitlin, M. P., and Lebherz, T. B. Pessaries in the geriatric patient. *J. Am. Geriatr. Soc.* 40:635, 1992.
    A plastic ring, a rubber doughnut, or an inflatable pessary may be used in the elderly patient. To retain a pessary comfortably, the patient must have some strength in the pelvic diaphragm measured at the levator "sling"—the hiatus at which the levator ani crosses the sides of the vagina.

Surgical Procedures

16. Shaw, W. F. The treatment of prolapsus uteri, with special reference to the Manchester operation of colporrhaphy. *Am. J. Obstet. Gynecol.* 26:667, 1933.
    The Fothergill or Manchester procedure, consisting of anterior repair with cervical amputation, has been largely replaced by vaginal hysterectomy with repair.

17. Langmade, C. F., Oliver, J. A., Jr., and White, J. S. Cooper ligament support of vaginal vault prolapse, twenty-eight years later. *Am. J. Obstet. Gynecol.* 131:132, 1978.
    Gynecologists have suspended the vagina from the rectus fascia, the pubis, the sacrum, and Cooper's ligaments.

18. Ahranjani, M., et al. Neugebauer–Le Fort operation for vaginal prolapse. *J. Reprod. Med.* 37:959, 1992.
    Obliterates the central portion of the vagina, leaving lateral channels for drainage. Can be performed under local anesthesia in very debilitated patients, but is seldom required in modern practice.

19. Langmade, C. J., and Oliver, J. A., Jr. Partial colpocleisis. *Am. J. Obstet. Gynecol.* 154:1200, 1986.
    For older, debilitated patients not requiring a functional vagina, avoiding scarring between the anterior and posterior walls prevents the SUI often reported after complete colpocleisis.

20. Nichols, D. H. Types of enterocele and principles underlying choice of operation for repair. *Obstet. Gynecol.* 40:257, 1972.
    The types of enteroceles covered include congenital (persistent sac), pulsion (plus eversion of the vaginal wall), traction (plus cystocele and rectocele pulling the vault into eversion), and iatrogenic (anterior or posterior to the vagina).

21. McCall, M. L. Posterior culdoplasty. *Obstet. Gynecol.* 10:595, 1957.
    Culdoplasty, consisting of the narrowing or obliteration of the cul-de-sac of Douglas, can be performed by either a vaginal or an abdominal approach for the prophylaxis or therapy of enterocele. Commonly used procedures, are, in general, modifications of the techniques introduced by Moschcowitz, Halban, and McCall.

22. Beck, R. P., McCormick, S., and Nordstrom, L. A 25-year experience with 519 anterior colporrhaphy procedures. *Obstet. Gynecol.* 78:1011, 1991.
    The cure rate achieved for the treatment of genuine SUI in 194 patients increased from 75 to 94 percent when a Kelly-Kennedy technique was modified to include a vaginal retropubic urethropexy.

23. Nichols, D. H. Posterior colporrhaphy and perineorrhaphy: Separate and distinct operations. *Am. J. Obstet. Gynecol.* 164:714, 1991.
    Discusses the preoperative assessment of defects in the support of the posterior vaginal wall and describes the important steps required for successful, surgical reconstruction.

24. Shull, B. L., and Baden, W. F. A six-year experience with paravaginal defect repair for stress urinary incontinence. *Am. J. Obstet. Gynecol.* 160:1432, 1989.
    This describes a technique intended specifically for the repair of lateral detachment of the vagina with resultant cystocele and SUI. Excellent results were obtained in selected patients.

25. Cruikshank, S. H. Sacrospinous fixation—should this be performed at the time of vaginal hysterectomy? *Am. J. Obstet. Gynecol.* 164:1072, 1991.
    In selected high-risk patients, sacrospinous fixation should be performed as an adjunct to other steps taken to prevent posthysterectomy prolapse.

26. Nichols, D. H. Fertility retention in the patient with genital prolapse. *Am. J. Obstet. Gynecol.* 164:1155, 1991.
   There are several treatments from which to choose for the repair of symptomatic prolapse in the patient who wishes to retain fertility.
27. Allahbadia, G. N. Obstetric performance following conservative surgery for pelvic relaxation. *Int. J. Gynaecol. Obstet.* 38:293, 1992.
   Less than 2 percent of the cases of prolapse occur in nulliparous women.

Vaginal Inversion
28. DeLancey, J. O. L. Anatomic aspects of vaginal eversion after hysterectomy. *Am. J. Obstet. Gynecol.* 166:1717, 1992.
   The author states that the "paracolpium" supports the vagina in the same way that the "parametrium" supports the uterus. Postulates that trauma to the paracolpium results in vaginal eversions.
29. Snyder, T. E., and Krantz, K. E. Abdominal-retroperitoneal sacral colpopexy for the correction of vaginal prolapse. *Obstet. Gynecol.* 77:944, 1991.
   Satisfactory correction of prolapse with maintenance of vaginal patency was achieved in 93 percent of the 147 patients treated.
30. Heinonen, P. K. Transvaginal sacrospinous colpopexy for vaginal vault and complete genital prolapse in aged women. *Acta Obstet. Gynecol. Scand.* 71:377, 1992.
   The coccygeus muscle and sacrospinous ligament are the same fibromuscular structure. In suspending the prolapsed vagina from the ligament, great care must be taken to avoid injury to the pudendal nerve and vessels laterally and the sciatic nerve and inferior gluteal vessels superiorly.

49. STRESS INCONTINENCE
Mendley A. Wulfsohn

Stress urinary incontinence (SUI) can be defined as an involuntary loss of urine from an intact urethra that occurs without any conscious desire to void and as the result of a rise in intraabdominal pressure. It is by far the most common cause of urinary incontinence in the female. Minor degrees of SUI may occur in at least 50 percent of nulliparous women, though only 1 percent of all patients requiring surgical correction are nulliparous. Pregnancy and childbirth undoubtedly play a role in the causation of SUI in susceptible subjects by damaging the supports of the bladder neck and urethra. SUI is four times as common in Caucasians as in blacks, but the reason for this is uncertain.

The following are the five mechanisms responsible for continence: (1) The bladder neck, or internal sphincter, consists of smooth muscle derived from the detrusor muscle fibers. (2) The distal sphincter, which is a smooth muscle sphincter that surrounds the middle and lower portion of the urethra, is relatively weak in the female. Both smooth muscle sphincters are innervated by alpha-adrenergic receptors. (3) The external sphincter is a striated muscle that surrounds the middle third of the urethra and acts together with the pelvic floor musculature. Reflex contractions of these muscles, occurring with sudden rises in abdominal pressure, tend to prevent SUI. Damage to this external sphincter mechanism is therefore important in the pathogenesis of SUI. (4) The resilience and elasticity of the epithelium lining the urethra play a small additional role in continence. This is important in elderly patients with a lack of estrogen and atrophic changes in the distal urethral epithelium. (5) The upper third of the urethra lies above the pelvic diaphragm, and thus is intraabdominal. This ensures that any rise in intraabdominal pressure is transmitted to both the bladder and the upper urethra simultaneously. Prolapse of the upper urethra below the pelvic floor therefore eliminates this mechanism.

Patients with grade I SUI complain of a transient leaking of urine with sudden increases of intraabdominal pressure, such as during coughing, sneezing, or exertion during sporting activities. Incontinence does not occur while at rest in bed. In grade II SUI, the symptoms are more severe, with incontinence occurring with lesser degrees of exertion, such as walking, standing up from a sitting position, or even sitting up in bed. Grade III SUI is so severe that there is almost continuous leaking while the person is erect or with virtually any movement while lying down. About 5 to 10 percent of patients also have incidental urinary tract infection (UTI) that requires control.

The general physical examination should be directed toward the detection of neurologic disease, chronic respiratory conditions, large bowel disorders, and the presence of a pelvic mass. Signs of senile atrophy should be observed, and the appearance and size of the urethral meatus should be noted. The presence and extent of descent of the anterior vaginal wall are noted when the patient coughs or strains. At the same time, cystocele, rectocele, and uterine prolapse are sought. The patient should be examined when the bladder is comfortably full. SUI can be demonstrated when the patient is coughing. Failing this, the table may be tilted downward 45 degrees. If this technique fails, she can be tested while in the erect position with a receiver between the thighs.

The Marshall (Bonney) test consists of the digital elevation of the vagina on either side of the bladder neck, which prevents demonstrable stress incontinence. This is an unreliable test, however, because only the slightest compression of the urethra itself will prevent all forms of incontinence. The Q-tip test is performed by inserting a lubricated Q-tip into the urethra. Anterior rotation of the Q-tip with straining indicates prolapse of the bladder base. Cystoscopy and urethroscopy should be performed to rule out any other bladder disorder. Renal ultrasound imaging should be done before any surgical procedure.

SUI must be distinguished from other forms of incontinence, such as true incontinence caused by diverse pathology (e.g., pelvic fracture, irradiation, and surgical trauma). Urinary fistulas in the vagina usually produce a constant dribbling incontinence, but a small fistula may cause leakage only during stress. Rarely, an ectopic ureteral opening into the female genital tract presents with pseudostress incontinence. Chronic urinary retention may also present with stress as well as overflow incontinence. Urgency incontinence is usually readily distinguishable based on a careful history, but there is a select group of patients with bladder instability whose symptoms and signs are indistinguishable from those of SUI. Urgency incontinence must be confirmed by urodynamic evaluation, as surgical treatment in this type of patient is likely to have a poor outcome. "Giggle incontinence" is an inborn abnormality in which a detrusor contraction is initiated by laughter.

The anatomy of the bladder outlet can be demonstrated radiologically by filling the bladder with contrast material via a catheter. Fluoroscopy is then performed and x-ray studies are taken with the patient in the erect position. Observations are made with the patient at rest, while coughing and straining, and during voiding. In type 0 and I SUI, the base of the bladder is situated at or above the upper border of the pubic symphysis at rest, and the vesical neck is closed. During stress, the bladder neck opens and descends less than 2 cm. In type 0, actual leakage cannot be demonstrated, although normally it is present. In type I, the incontinence is visualized. The bladder base has a similar appearance at rest in type II A, but, when the patient strains, the vesical neck opens and descends below the lower border of the symphysis. Because the distal urethra is fixed, descent of the bladder base results in flattening of the posterior vesicourethral angle. With progressive prolapse, the urethra comes to lie horizontally and the angle may exceed 180 degrees. However, loss of the posterior vesicourethral angle is *not* the cause of SUI, but reflects the anatomic deformity, which is a cystourethrocele. In type II B SUI, the bladder base is below the lower border of the pubic symphysis at rest. During stress, further descent may or may not take place, but the urethra opens and incontinence ensues. Type III is the most severe variety of SUI and often occurs after previous failed surgery. The position of the bladder base varies, but, universally, the bladder neck and proximal urethra are open at rest and leaking occurs with minimal stress (e.g., by gravity).

It is important to carry out a filling cystometrogram with water, using simultaneous rectal (intraabdominal) and intravesical pressures to detect detrusor instability.

By measuring both pressures, it is possible by subtraction to determine the true detrusor pressure and to record uninhibited bladder contractions. Instability is defined as any reflex contraction of 15 cm of water or more that cannot be inhibited by the patient. In some cases, unstable contractions may be initiated by coughing or by changing to the erect posture (postural hyperreflexia). When a significant bladder contraction occurs immediately after coughing, the symptoms closely resemble those of true SUI. A considerable number of women with SUI also complain of urinary urgency, and about 16 percent have urodynamically demonstrable detrusor instability. This condition is not a contraindication to the surgical correction of proven true SUI, as instability will resolve 80 percent of the time after operation. Bladder instability may develop in a small number of patients de novo postoperatively.

The urethral pressure profile is obtained by measuring the pressure along the length of the urethra. The maximal closing pressure and functional length of the urethra are generally reduced in patients with SUI. The urethral pressure profile study is important for detecting severely decompensated urethral musculature, usually as a result of scarring from previous repeated surgical treatment. These patients will have a very low maximum closing pressure.

Conservative therapy can be tried in mild cases of SUI. Pelvic floor exercises and faradic stimulation of the perineal muscles are occasionally successful. Alpha-adrenergic receptor stimulants may be tried to increase tone in the bladder neck and urethral smooth muscle. Oral or vaginal doses of conjugated estrogen may be helpful in elderly patients with atrophic vaginitis. Incontinence associated with detrusor hyperreflexia requires treatment with anticholinergic agents or detrusor relaxants. UTI must be cleared. Surgical treatment should be offered to patients who have significant SUI. In the elderly, vaginal pessaries may adequately control SUI. The periurethral insertion of Teflon or collagen may be successful in 70 to 80 percent of the cases.

Numerous operations have been designed for the cure of SUI, but controversy exists as to which type of operation is best suited for which type and grade of defect. Undoubtedly, the first operation should be the best operation, because subsequent repairs become progressively more difficult and achieve a lower success rate. There are four main groups of operations in common use today, all of which are aimed at the restoration of normal anatomy, elongation of the urethra, and fixation of the bladder neck: (1) Anterior vaginal repairs that are aimed at correcting the defective pelvic floor and buttressing the bladder neck with sutures apposing the pubocervical fascia (Kelly plication). The low success rates associated with this procedure have been largely responsible for eliminating its use. (2) Retropubic vesicourethropexy procedures (Marshall-Marchetti and Burch) entail the placement of sutures between the paraurethral and paravesical tissues and the pubic bones, thereby elevating and fixating the bladder neck. (3) In endoscopic vesical neck suspension operations (the Stamey, Raz, and Gittes), the area of the bladder neck is elevated by the placement of heavy polypropylene sutures on either side using special needles. These sutures are passed suprapubically and tied down to the rectus fascia. During the operation, cystoscopy is performed to confirm the correct position of the suspension sutures. Both vesicourethropexy and endoscopic suspension procedures have a high success rate (90—95%) for types 0 to II SUI. (4) Sling operations are usually required for the treatment of type III SUI. Materials that can be used are rectus fascia, fascia lata, and prosthetic material. Rarely, it becomes necessary to insert an artificial urinary sphincter, although the complication rate is extremely high if there have been multiple previous operations. When all else has failed, urinary diversion may be the last resort for managing intractable incontinence.

Reviews
1. Varner, R. E., and Sparks, J. M. Surgery for stress urinary incontinence. *Surg. Clin. North Am.* 71:1111, 1991.
   Updated review of pathogenesis and management. Conservative and surgical approaches to management are reviewed.
2. Lam, T. C., and Hadley, H. R. Surgical procedures for uncomplicated ("routine") female stress incontinence. *Urol. Clin. North Am.* 18:327, 1991.

A review of the surgical options. The authors prefer the Burch or needle suspension procedures. They emphasize the importance of not interfering with the delicate mechanism of the urethra, but explain the necessity of using its vaginal wall as a firm support for the bladder neck.

Etiology and Pathogenesis

3. McGuide, E. Urethral sphincter mechanism. *Urol. Clin. North Am.* 6:39, 1979.
   The physiology of continence. Inferior and posterior displacement of the urethra into the vagina during stress results in transient incontinence.
4. Thind, P., Lose, G., and Colstrup, H. Initial urethral pressure increased during stress episodes in genuine stress incontinent women. *Br. J. Urol.* 69:137, 1992.
   Bladder and urethral pressures are measured simultaneously with a double-microtip transducer catheter. Findings suggest the presence of a defective active closure mechanism in urinary bladder incontinence (UBI).
5. Staski, D. R., et al. The pathophysiology of stress incontinence. *Urol. Clin. North Am.* 12:271, 1985.
   Review of the anatomy and physiology of stress and other forms of incontinence.

Diagnostic Studies

6. Viktrup, L., et al. The symptoms of stress incontinence caused by pregnancy or delivery in primiparas. *Obstet. Gynecol.* 79:945, 1992.
   Stress incontinence occurs as a natural consequence of pregnancy in 32 percent of primiparas. Persistent UBI occurs in only 1 percent. The importance of obstetric factors as an etiologic agent is unclear.
7. Weprin, S. A., and Zuspan, F. P. The standing cystometrogram. *Am. J. Obstet. Gynecol.* 138:369, 1980.
   This discusses the diagnosis and management of incontinence secondary to detrusor hyperreflexia. Sixteen percent of the patients with SUI have detrusor hyperreflexia.
8. Gordon, D., et al. Comparison of ultrasound and lateral chain urethrocystography in the determination of bladder neck descent. *Am. J. Obstet. Gynecol.* 160:182, 1989.
   Diagnostic procedures include urethroscopy, urodynamics, cystometry, urethral closure pressure profiles, uroflowmetry, electromyography of the pelvic floor, radiologic procedures, and ultrasound.
9. Migliorini, G. D., and Glenning, P. P. Bonney's test—fact or fiction? *Br. J. Obstet. Gynaecol.* 94:157, 1987.
   This study invalidates the Bonney test by objectively demonstrating that the test restores continence by directly obstructing the urethra and urethrovesical junction.
10. Bhatia, N. N., and Bergman, A. Pessary tests in women with urinary incontinence. *Obstet. Gynecol.* 65:220, 1985.
    The authors found that use of a pessary differentiated patients with bladder instability from those with SUI caused by correctable anatomic defects.
11. Low, J. A., Mauger, G. M., and Draovic, J. Diagnosis of the unstable detrusor: comparison of an incremental and continuous infusion technique. *Obstet. Gynecol.* 65:99, 1985.
    The diagnosis of an unstable detrusor depends on the demonstration of one or more involuntary detrusor contractions in the absence of evidence of organic neurologic disease. Diagnosis is achieved by performing cystometry, a method that measures the pressure/volume relationship of the bladder.
12. Walters, M. D., and Diaz, K. Q-tip test: a study of continent and incontinent women. *Obstet. Gynecol.* 70:208, 1987.
    The Q-tip test has limited value in predicting the specific cause of incontinence.
13. Blaivas, J. G., and Olsson, C. A. Stress incontinence: classification and surgical approach. *J. Urol.* 139:727, 1988.
    A videourodynamic study led to the formulation of a modified classification for SUI based on the nature of vesical neck descent and the integrity of the intrinsic sphincteric mechanisms.

Therapy

14. Marshall, V. F., Marchetti, A. A., and Krantz, K. E. The correction of stress incontinence by simple vesicourethral suspension. *Surg. Gynecol. Obstet.* 88: 509, 1949.
    In this procedure, sutures appose paraurethral tissues and the bladder neck to the back of the pubis.
15. Barnett, R. M. The modern Kelly plication. *Obstet. Gynecol.* 34:667, 1969.
    In this anterior vaginal approach, plicating sutures are placed at the bladder neck.
16. Karram, M. M., and Bhatia, N. N. Management of coexistent stress and urge urinary incontinence. *Obstet. Gynecol.* 73:4, 1989.
    The authors recommend initial medical management with various combinations of oxybutynin, imipramine, and estrogen.
17. Wilson, P. D., et al. An objective assessment of physiotherapy for female genuine stress incontinence. *Br. J. Obstet. Gynecol.* 94:575, 1987.
    Successful treatment with pelvic floor exercises with or without faradic stimulation is more likely in younger patients and in those with lesser degrees of SUI.
18. Bhatia, N. N., Bergman, A., and Karram, M. M. Effects of estrogen on urethral function in women with urinary incontinence. *Am. J. Obstet. Gynecol.* 160:176, 1989.
    Improvement in half the cases was associated with increased urethral closure pressure and improved abdominal pressure transmission to the proximal urethra.
19. Eriksen, B. C., Bergmann, S., and Mjolnerod, O. K. Effect of anal electrostimulation with the 'Incontan' device in women with urinary incontinence. *Br. J. Obstet. Gynecol.* 94:147, 1987.
    Intraanal electrostimulation may provide an alternative treatment to surgical therapy.
20. Stanton, S. L. Stress incontinence. Why and how operations work. *Urol. Clin. North Am.* 12:279, 1985.
    Discusses the mechanisms producing continence accomplished with various procedures. Also provides a good review of the causes of and treatment for failed operations.
21. McGuire, E.J. Abdominal procedures for stress incontinence. *Urol. Clin. North Am.* 12:285, 1985.
    The author prefers the Burch colposuspension to the classic Marshall-Marchetti procedure, because the latter is more likely to cause urethral compression. A rectus fascia sling is used for the nonfunctioning urethral sphincter mechanism resulting from multiple failed operations, scarring, and some types of neurologic disease.
22. Hadley, H. R., et al. Transvaginal needle bladder neck suspension. *Urol. Clin. North Am.* 12:291, 1985.
    This is the most popular type of operation done for the treatment of SUI today. Cystoscopic examination during placement of suspending sutures allows accurate placement at the bladder neck and prevents bladder perforation by the sutures.
23. Beckingham, I. J., Wemyss-Holden, G., and Lawrence, W. T. Long-term follow-up of women treated with periurethral Teflon injections for stress incontinence. *Surg. Gynecol. Obstet.* 175:173, 1992.
    Symptoms abated in 80 percent immediately after operation. Only 27 percent remained improved 3 years later.
24. Blaivas, J. G., and Jacobs, B. Z. Pubovaginal fascial sling for the treatment of complicated stress urinary incontinence. *J. Urol.* 145:1214, 1991.
    A fascial sling was used in the treatment for complicated UBI. Eighty-two percent of the patients were continent afterward. Three percent had permanent urinary retention requiring intermittent self-catheterization.
25. Raz, S., et al. The Raz bladder neck suspension: Results in 206 patients. *J. Urol.* 148:845, 1992.
    Successful results were achieved in 90.3 percent.
26. Webster, G. D., et al. Management of type III stress urinary incontinence using artificial urinary sphincter. *Urology* 39:499, 1992.

The artificial sphincter is an excellent first option for treating type III stress incontinence due to intrinsic urethral weakness resulting from various causes.

27. Juma, S., Little, N. A., and Raz, S. Vaginal wall sling: four years later. *Urology* 39:424, 1992.

The vaginal wall was used to fashion a sling. After operation, 94.4 percent of the patients were continent. Long-term intermittent self-catheterization for urinary retention was needed in 5.5 percent.

28. Eckford, S. D., and Abrams, P. Para-urethral collagen implantation for female stress incontinence. *Br. J. Urol.* 68:586, 1991.

Transurethral injection of collagen appears to produce the best results in patients whose previous operations for the treatment of incontinence have failed.

29. Meschia, M., et al. Recurrent incontinence after retropubic surgery. *J. Gynecol.* 9:25, 1993.

The most important risk factors for failed surgical treatment are age, parity, work conditions, menopause, and a low urethral closure pressure.

30. Bump, R. C. Racial comparisons and contrasts in urinary incontinence and pelvic organ prolapse. *Obstet. Gynecol.* 81:421, 1993.

Black women have a different set of symptoms, different conditions causing their incontinence, and different risk profiles than do white women.

50. DYSMENORRHEA AND PELVIC PAIN
Michel E. Rivlin

Dysmenorrhea, the occurrence of painful uterine cramps during menstruation, may be either *primary* and due to no discernible organic cause, or *secondary*, and due to a demonstrable pelvic lesion. It is estimated that more than 50 percent of menstruating women experience dysmenorrhea, and, in about 10 percent, the symptoms are incapacitating for several days each month. Absenteeism among the women with severe cramps has been estimated to account for approximately 600 million lost working hours, which costs employers 2 billion dollars annually. Primary dysmenorrhea usually begins at menarche or shortly thereafter. The pain appears either several hours before or immediately after the start of menses and is most severe on the first and second days. The pain is spasmodic, occurs over the lower abdomen, and may radiate to the back and thighs. Systemic symptoms, such as nausea, vomiting, and diarrhea, may accompany the pain. The relationship between premenstrual syndrome (PMS) and dysmenorrhea is obscured by the traditional definitions, as PMS is regarded as a constellation of variable symptoms and dysmenorrhea is restricted to pain. However, PMS has been shown to more commonly afflict women with dysmenorrhea, and menstrual pain may precede the onset of bleeding. Furthermore, PMS symptoms may persist into the menstrual period and dysmenorrhea sufferers often have symptoms like those in PMS (e.g., nausea, breast discomfort, and depression). It is therefore an artificial distinction to separate the premenstrual stage from the menstrual period, and appropriate management must be based on this perspective.

Primary dysmenorrhea and its frequently associated symptoms appear to be related to the increased production and release of endometrial prostaglandins ($PGE_{2\alpha}$ and PGE_2) during menstruation, which triggers increased and abnormal uterine activity. The condition is limited to the ovulatory cycles because the estrogen-primed endometrium requires luteal-phase progesterone levels to enhance the production and concentration of prostaglandins. The abolition of ovulation by oral contraceptives is therefore highly effective in relieving dysmenorrhea.

The myometrial contractions brought about by the particularly high prostaglandin levels reduce uterine blood flow, resulting in uterine ischemia and hypersensitization of pelvic nerve terminals to prostaglandins and endoperoxides, thereby reducing the threshold for the physical and chemical stimuli of pain. Nonsteroidal antiinflammatory drugs (NSAIDs) inhibit prostaglandin production and thus represent another means of managing dysmenorrhea. They are successful in relieving the dysmenorrhea in about 80 percent of sufferers. Arachidonic acid is metabolized by two important enzyme systems: cyclooxygenase, leading to prostaglandin formation, and 5-lipoxygenase, leading to leukotriene production. The NSAIDs readily suppress menstrual prostaglandin release by inhibiting cyclooxygenase. It is possible that nonresponse to NSAIDs may be related to the continued production of leukotrienes, which also stimulate uterine contractions. Lipoxygenase inhibitor therapy may therefore prove useful in this event.

The causes of *secondary dysmenorrhea* include endometriosis, intrauterine devices (IUDs), pelvic inflammatory disease, adenomyosis, congenital müllerian system malfusions, cervical stenosis, ovarian cysts, and, arguably, pelvic congestion and Allen-Master's syndrome. The diagnosis is based on the patient's history, physical examination findings, and response to NSAIDs. These drugs are usually ineffective in relieving secondary dysmenorrhea, so that a failure of response may help identify those patients who need to undergo diagnostic laparoscopy. NSAIDs can effectively suppress IUD-induced prostaglandin production to normal levels and, as a result, significantly reduce IUD-induced dysmenorrhea and menorrhagia.

The treatment of primary dysmenorrhea depends on the patient's choice of contraception, if any. If oral contraception is not requested, NSAIDs are prescribed for patients not suffering from a gastric ulcer or NSAID hypersensitivity. If patients do not respond to this treatment after 3 to 4 months, an alternative NSAID is prescribed or oral contraception is added. If there is still no response, laparoscopy is performed, and, if an organic cause is found, further therapy is directed at the underlying disease. Prostaglandin induces uterine contractions by causing the formation of free calcium within the myometrial cell. It does so by acting at the adenylate cyclase level and by preventing binding of calcium to the sarcoplasm. A possible therapeutic approach might therefore be to block calcium entry into the cell with a calcium channel blocker; however, the side effects from these drugs are significant. Surgical interruption of the uterine nerves is occasionally performed for the treatment of severe intractable cases.

Chronic pelvic pain (which, by definition, persists for more than 6 months) is one of the most common complaints of gynecologic patients. Even after a thorough evaluation, including diagnostic laparoscopy, the cause may remain obscure. Furthermore, the relationship between certain types of pathologic conditions and the pain response may be inconsistent and often inexplicable. For instance, the incidence and severity of pain that occur in endometriosis do not correlate with the amount of disease present, nor does the site, density, or amount of adhesions (postinfective or postoperative) in those with a complaint of pelvic pain differ from those in patients without pain. Many of these women are presumed to suffer from chronic pelvic inflammatory disease and are given repeated courses of antibiotics, which may result in chronic vaginal candidiasis. Many others undergo a variety of surgical procedures, including dilatation and curettage, cyst aspiration, lysis of adhesions, hysterectomy, and oophorectomy. Some sufferers see physicians 20 times a year. Thus, the outcome of traditional management has often led to loss of hormonal and reproductive function, continued pain, and frustration for both the patient and physician.

Nerves carrying pain impulses from the pelvic organs are numerous, and knowledge in this area is incomplete. Sympathetic fibers from T10 to L1, which are contained within the inferior hypogastric nerve, course along the vena cava and sacrum to enter the uterus through the uterosacral ligaments. Parasympathetic fibers from S1 to S4 travel within the nervi erigentes, emerging in the lateral pelvis and forming ganglia lateral to the cervix (Frankenhäuser's ganglion). Autonomic nerves from the outer two thirds of the tubes and from the ovaries enter the cord at the T9-T10 level and are carried via the aortic and mesenteric ganglia and plexuses. Somatic pain is readily perceived and well localized, whereas visceral pain is poorly localized and the patient's description is usually vague. The most effective triggers of visceral pain are stretch, inflammation, and ischemia.

Characteristically, women who suffer from chronic pelvic pain are aged 25 to 35 and also complain of dysmenorrhea and dyspareunia. The pain is continuous and poorly localized to the lower abdomen. There is an insistent belief that the pain has an organic cause, and there is a desire for surgical therapy. There is a history of menorrhagia, but the hematocrit is generally normal. Careful questioning often reveals a history of sexual or physical abuse (36%) in these women with an attendant lack of self-esteem and a negative attitude toward sex. The patient usually has a poor relationship with her partner and family. Previous pelvic procedures, especially tubal ligation, are common. Invariably these patients resent suggestions that their problem has a psychiatric or psychosomatic basis.

The initial evaluation, once the history is taken, includes a physical and pelvic examination. A pelvic ultrasound examination may be helpful in confirming the normalcy of the pelvic structures. Other causes of pelvic pain may be ruled out with further studies, including barium enema, proctoscopy, and pyelography. Consultation with a gastroenterologist, urologist, orthopedist, or neurologist may be indicated. The patient should then be asked to keep a diary describing the pain for about 2 months, rating the pain on a scale of 1 to 10 and noting when any stressful events occur and their relationship to the pain. Laparoscopy is the major tool for guiding diagnosis and management in these women. About a third each will be found to have endometriosis, adhesions, or a normal pelvis. The finding of minor pelvic pathology may prove difficult to interpret; however, endometriosis should, of course, be treated with standard therapy. The role of pelvic adhesions in causing pain is controversial, and although adhesiolysis has been found to relieve pain in some patients, surgical measures to achieve lysis might produce more adhesions, and patients should be made aware of this fact. When pelvic findings are normal, such patients may be helped by understanding the emotional origins of their problem. Referral to a pain clinic for management, together with psychologic or psychiatric treatment, is frequently necessary, as these patients need to understand the connection between stress and pain. Psychologic evaluation provides information about the patient's treatment responses and prognosis. Women accept this when they are reassured that it is a routine measure and not performed to ascertain whether the pain is psychogenic. Psychologic treatment may include behavior therapy and either marital or sexual therapy, or both, plus psychotherapy, as necessary. At the outset, the patient must understand not to expect a "cure." Instead, she will be seen regularly by interested therapists, with the goal to achieve a reduction in the level of pain sufficient to permit her return to normal activities.

Pelvic congestion has been proposed as an entity causing pelvic pain. Congestion of the uterus and broad ligament has been noted on radiographic studies and at laparoscopy. A constellation of findings, including secondary dysmenorrhea, low back pain, dysuria, menorrhagia, dyspareunia, and, frequently, retroflexion of the uterus, are thought to stem from this syndrome. Various approaches to therapy, including psychiatric consultation, vasoconstrictor drugs, and hysterectomy, have been tried, with differing results. Traumatic laceration of uterine supporting tissues, the *Allen-Master's syndrome*, has also been explored as a cause of pelvic pain. Similar complaints and findings have been associated with repair of the lacerations or hysterectomy.

In patients with recalcitrant pain who still wish to have children, especially those with associated dysmenorrhea, a presacral neurectomy may be performed. The presacral nerve (superior hypogastric plexus) fibers may also be interrupted in the uterosacral ligaments via the laparoscope. Resection does not interfere with bladder or bowel function, as the innervation of these organs is predominantly parasympathetic. The procedure is commonly performed in association with conservative surgical treatment for endometriosis, with results that are better than those when surgical treatment is performed for the chronic midline pelvic pain alone. Patients who respond to uterosacral block appear to be suitable candidates for the procedure. In the worst cases, the patient undergoes extremes of treatment, including castration with hysterectomy, in futile efforts to relieve her pain. An operation may bring tremendous relief and even euphoria. However, this elation lasts only until suspicion falls on another body part. Unconscious feelings of guilt or unworthiness return, and the patient repeats the process.

Experience with the multidisciplinary management of pelvic pain at specialized pain clinics suggests that many of these patients have coexisting problems, which are both somatic and nonsomatic in nature. Conditions such as the irritable bowel syndrome, urethral syndrome, interstitial cystitis, and myofascial syndrome are important somatic disorders, which must be kept in mind in such patients; concurrent psychopathology includes the somatoform pain disorder, somatization, posttraumatic stress disorder, and depression. Advocates of a multidisciplinary approach, including both organic and psychologic interventions, suggest that the frequency with which hysterectomy is performed for this disorder can be markedly reduced.

Dysmenorrhea

1. Dawood, M. Y. Dysmenorrhea. *Clin. Obstet. Gynecol.* 33:168, 1990.

   It is postulated that a decline in the progesterone output gives rise to lysosomal labilization, releasing phospholipase A_2, which hydrolyzes phospholipids, thus generating arachidonic acid. Cellular trauma that occurs with menses stimulates the arachidonic cascade, producing prostaglandins.

2. Creatsas, G., et al. Prostaglandins: $PGF_{2\alpha}$, PGE_2, 6-keto-$PGF_{1\alpha}$ and TXB_2 serum levels in dysmenorrheic adolescents before, during and after treatment with oral contraceptives. *Eur. J. Obstet. Gynecol. Reprod. Biol.* 36:292, 1990.

   The role of prostacyclin in relation to other prostanoids such as thromboxane, $PGF_{2\alpha}$, and PGE_2 needs to be considered. Some patients have reduced prostacyclin (prostacyclin relaxes the uterus, induces vasodilatation, and is platelet antiaggregatory) levels as the source of their dysmenorrhea. NSAIDs block production of all these prostanoids.

3. Rees, M. C. P., et al. Leukotriene release by endometrium and myometrium throughout the menstrual cycle in dysmenorrhoea and menorrhagia. *J. Endocrinol.* 113:291, 1987.

   The pattern of leukotriene release is similar to that of the prostaglandins: the endometrial concentrations varied throughout the menstrual cycle and were always higher than the myometrial values.

4. Pulkkinen, M., Monti, T., and Macciocchi, A. Analysis of uterine contractility after administration of the nonsteroidal anti-inflammatory drug nimesulide. *Acta Obstet. Gynecol. Scand.* 71:181, 1992.

   Uterine activity in dysmenorrheic patients is characterized by high resting pressure, high frequency, and high active pressure.

5. Ekström, P., et al. Stimulation of vasopressin release in women with primary dysmenorrhoea and after oral contraceptive treatment—effect on uterine contractility. *Br. J. Obstet. Gynaecol.* 99:680, 1992.

   Oral contraceptives reduce the sensitivity of the uterus to $PGF_{2\alpha}$ and vasopressin.

6. Sundell, G., Milsom, I., and Andersch, B. Factors influencing the prevalence and severity of dysmenorrhoea in young women. *Br. J. Obstet Gynaecol.* 97:588, 1990.

   A beneficial effect of childbirth may be related to uterine neuronal degeneration and a decrease in the uterine noradrenaline level that has been demonstrated in the third trimester of pregnancy.

7. Åkerlund, M. Modern treatment of dysmenorrhea. *Acta Obstet. Gynecol. Scand.* 69:563, 1990.

   An oxytocin analogue that competitively inhibits the effects of vasopressin and oxytocin has been developed and is effective, but no oral preparation of this agent is available.

8. Tilyard, M. W., and Dovey, S. M. A comparison of tiaprofenic acid, mefenamic acid and placebo in the treatment of dysmenorrhoea in general practice. *Aust. N.Z. J. Obstet. Gynaecol.* 32:165, 1992.

   If NSAIDs are unsuccessful, additional analgesics should not be added because this may potentiate gastrointestinal and other side effects.

9. Dawood, M. Y., and Ramos, J. Transcutaneous electrical nerve stimulation

(TENS) for the treatment of primary dysmenorrhea: a randomized crossover comparison with placebo TENS and ibuprofen. *Obstet. Gynecol.* 75:656, 1990.
Transcutaneous electrical nerve stimulation is effective in the treatment of dysmenorrhea, possibly due to the "gate-control" mechanism postulated for stimulation-produced analgesia. This involves the bombardment of the thalamic receptors with impulses traveling on myelinated A fibers, which prevents slower-transmitting A-delta and C fibers from passing their information through the "gate" to the central nervous system pathways and receptors.

10. Gurgan, T., et al. Laparoscopic CO_2 laser uterine nerve ablation for treatment of drug resistant primary dysmenorrhea. *Fertil. Steril.* 58:422, 1992.
The menstrual pain in 20 women was assessed by a linear analog pain score, and this showed a 33 percent reduction after surgical treatment.

Pelvic Pain

11. Quan, M. Diagnosis of acute pelvic pain. *J. Fam. Pract.* 35:422, 1992.
The various causes of acute pelvic pain were found to be pegnancy-related, gynecologic, nonreproductive tract in origin, and not related to an organic abnormality.

12. Rapkin, A. J., et al. History of physical and sexual abuse in women with chronic pelvic pain. *Obstet. Gynecol.* 76:92, 1990.
Victims of abuse have been noted to exhibit an unusually high frequency of somatic complaints, including, but not limited to, chronic pelvic pain.

13. Stenchever, M. A. Symptomatic retrodisplacement, pelvic congestion, universal joint, and peritoneal defects: fact or fiction? *Clin. Obstet. Gynecol.* 33:161, 1990.
An objective appraisal of several time-honored but poorly documented diagnoses, including Allen-Masters syndrome (universal joint), retrodisplacement, and pelvic congestion, that have been implicated in the causation of pelvic pain.

14. Slocumb, J. C. Chronic somatic, myofascial, and neurogenic abdominal pelvic pain. *Clin. Obstet. Gynecol.* 33:145, 1990.
The author suggests that many patients suffer from abdominal wall or myofascial pain, or both, rather than from pelvic visceral pain. Hyperpathic "trigger points" can be identified and treated with local anesthetic blocks, followed by long-lasting improvement.

15. Pelvic congestion [editorial]. *Lancet* 337:398, 1991.
Pelvic pain secondary to congested pelvic veins responds to treatment with a vasoconstrictor such as dihydroergotamine or medroxyprogesterone acetate. This editorial suggests further investigation is warranted.

16. Bonney, R. C., et al. Endometrial phospholipases A_2, polycystic ovaries and pelvic pain. *Br. J. Obstet. Gynaecol.* 99:486, 1992.
These authors suggest that the frequency of pelvic pain in women with polycystic ovaries is increased, and is associated with pelvic venous congestion and increased endometrial prostaglandin formation.

17. Reiter, R. C., and Gambone, J. C. Nongynecologic somatic pathology in women with chronic pelvic pain and negative laparoscopy. *J. Reprod. Med.* 36:253, 1991.
It is critically important to rule out occult nongynecologic diagnoses such as myofascial syndrome, irritable bowel syndrome, urethral syndrome, interstitial cystitis, and psychogenic problems, including somatization, depression, stress disorders, and hypochondriacal or hysterical neuroses.

18. Baker, P. N., and Symonds, E. M. The resolution of chronic pelvic pain after normal laparoscopy findings. *Am. J. Obstet. Gynecol.* 166:835, 1992.
Six months after laparoscopy yielded negative findings, 58 percent of the patients were pain free. The authors suggest that treatment should be limited to patients whose symptoms persist 6 months after laparoscopy.

19. Peters, A. A., et al. A randomized clinical trial to compare two different approaches in women with chronic pelvic pain. *Obstet. Gynecol.* 77:740, 1991.
These authors maintain that equal attention to both organic and other causative factors from the outset is more likely to be successful than a standard approach; they believe that laparoscopy is seldom helpful.

20. Peters, A. A., et al. A randomized clinical trial on the benefit of adhesiolysis in

patients with intraperitoneal adhesions and chronic pelvic pain. *Br. J. Obstet. Gynaecol.* 99:59, 1992.
Adhesiolysis is not useful for alleviating moderate adhesions, but may be beneficial in patients with severe adhesions involving the intestinal tract.
21. Stovall, T. G., Ling F. W., and Crawford, D. A. Hysterectomy for chronic pelvic pain of presumed uterine etiology. *Obstet. Gynecol.* 75:676, 1990.
Nearly a fourth of the patients had persistent pelvic pain after the hysterectomy.
22. Steege, J. F., Stout, A. L., and Somkuti, S. G. Chronic pelvic pain in women: toward an integrative model. *Obstet. Gynecol. Surv.* 48:95, 1993.
The model proposed includes elements of the gate control theory, the cognitive-behavioral theory, and operant conditioning.
23. Heisterberg, L. Factors influencing spontaneous abortion, dyspareunia, dysmenorrhea, and pelvic pain. *Obstet. Gynecol.* 81:594, 1993.
Spontaneous abortion and postabortal pelvic inflammatory disease carry significantly elevated risks of dyspareunia and chronic pelvic pain.

51. ENDOMETRIOSIS
Eric R. Strasburg

Endometriosis is the condition in which endometrial tissue occurs aberrantly in various locations. It is not a neoplasm, although it can, on rare occasions, be the site for the development of a malignant growth. It assumes two forms: adenomyosis (sometimes called internal endometriosis), in which the endometrial glands and stroma extend diffusely through tissue spaces in the myometrium and are by convention located more than one high-power field from normal-surface endometrium on microscopic examination; and external endometriosis (usually abbreviated to endometriosis), in which the glands and stroma are located outside the uterus, usually on other pelvic or abdominal organs, although it can occur almost anywhere in the body.

Adenomyosis is thought to represent a downgrowth from the basal endometrium, but it may be due to venous or lymphatic embolization. Because it is composed of basal-type endometrium, which is normally insensitive to hormonal stimulus, secretory activity occurs in less than 30 percent of the cases. On gross examination, the lesion is not found to be encapsulated and exhibits a honeycomb appearance. Clinically, the condition is usually found in older multiparous women. Menorrhagia is the most common symptom, and the large uterus may also cause pelvic discomfort, bladder and bowel pressure, deep dyspareunia, and even a noticeable abdominal mass. It is, however, rare for the uterus to be larger than a 12 to 14 weeks' gestational size. The treatment for symptomatic adenomyosis is hysterectomy. Rarely, local excision with metroplasty may be attempted in the young woman still desirous of having children.

The etiology of endometriosis is not known, but there are three major theories. The first is retrograde endometrial spill with local implantation. This would also explain the endometriosis that occurs in abdominal incisions and on a traumatized cervix or vagina. To explain endometriosis in sites such as the ureter, urethra, or umbilicus, another theory suggests that the coelomic epithelium, which forms the müllerian ducts from which the endometrium arises, can, at any time in adult life, be restimulated by some unknown mechanism and transformed once again into endometrial tissue. Finally, endometriosis in pelvic lymph nodes or distant sites, such as the lung or limbs, can be explained by the theory of lymphatic or vascular embolization. More recently it has been suggested that changes in the immune system may play a role in the pathogenesis of endometriosis.

Endometriosis has been reported to affect from 7 to 50 percent of menstruating women, according to different studies, but the true incidence is unknown. Endometriosis may be found in adolescents and in older women after menopause. It affects most commonly upper middle income white women between the ages of 30 and 40 who have postponed marriage and childbearing. The incidence of infertility is approximately 30 to 40 percent in patients with the disease, and the remaining sufferers are usually of low parity.

Half of the patients with endometriosis are asymptomatic. For this reason, it must always be considered in infertile women. Other symptoms of endometriosis depend more on the site of involvement and its nerve supply than on the size of individual endometriomata or the extent of the involvement. The ovary is the most common site, and is affected in approximately 40 percent of the cases. Its involvement leads to menorrhagia, epimenorrhea, and epimenorrhagia. Involvement of the cul-de-sac and uterosacral ligaments, the next most common site, causes a fixed retroversion and is associated with deep dyspareunia. Progressively worsening dysmenorrhea is another common secondary symptom. Painful defecation due to bowel involvement and hematuria due to bladder involvement are more rarely encountered symptoms. The diagnosis must always be considered in cases of vague, chronic abdominal pain. Rupture of an endometriomatous cyst may cause acute abdominal pain accompanied by all the signs of an "acute abdomen." If the lesions are small and few, pelvic examination may yield completely negative findings. More extensive pathologic involvement produces tender, nodular swellings along the uterosacral ligaments, a tender, fixed retroverted uterus, and tender, fixed ovarian tumors with surrounding fibrosis. These patients are often incorrectly diagnosed as suffering from pelvic inflammatory disease.

The correct diagnosis of endometriosis depends on a thorough history, careful physical examination, and confirmation by laparoscopy. Early lesions appear as bluish purple or reddish brown "powder burn" lesions located on the peritoneal surface. However, protean black, yellow, white, or red lesions and adhesions may all represent sites of endometriosis. There is often an excessive amount of peritoneal fluid containing large amounts of prostaglandin. This has been postulated as the possible source of the associated infertility—perhaps by affecting tubal transport—in those patients with minimal lesions. Numerous other theories have also been postulated to explain how endometriosis may cause infertility. In severe cases, physical factors such as scarring and adhesions that interfere with tubal mobility, obstruct tubes, or interfere with ovulation and ovum transport are self-explanatory. In mild cases, these factors do not apply. Other explanations include luteinized unruptured follicle syndrome, luteal-phase defects, a cytotoxic effect of peritoneal fluid, peritoneal macrophages phagocytosing and degrading sperm, and many more. These are, however, all theories, and none has been conclusively shown to explain endometriosis-associated infertility.

The laparoscopic visualization of a classic lesion is considered sufficiently diagnostic to allow treatment to begin, even in the absence of a histologic diagnosis. Atypical lesions require biopsy. Histologic specimens may not always supply information that permits a pathologic diagnosis because there may have been so much pressure or scarring that the endometriomatous tissue, such as in the case of a "chocolate" or tarry cyst of the ovary, can no longer be seen. The best treatment for endometriosis depends on the age of the patient, the severity of the symptoms (e.g., pain), the patient's desire for pregnancy, and the stage of the disease, as determined by laparoscopy (e.g., an adnexal mass). Laparoscopy is considered mandatory before any form of medical therapy is instituted. If the patient is asymptomatic, she should be advised of the condition, checked by pelvic examination every 6 months, and advised to undertake pregnancy if she so desires. Although pregnancy may not cure endometriosis, it usually causes considerable involution of the lesions. Therapy based on the induction of pseudopregnancy with a combination oral contraceptive (or with medroxyprogesterone acetate) given continuously for 6 to 9 months was suggested by the observation of what occurred during pregnancy. This therapy is indicated in unmarried patients with maximal symptoms and minimal palpable findings and in patients with recurrent disease after a previous conservative operation. Short-term hormonal therapy for 6 to 8 weeks may also be used before conservative surgical treatment to make the identification and excision of lesions simpler and more complete. The pregnancy rates, after the hormonal treatment of endometriosis in appropriate cases, have varied from 20 to 90 percent. Hormonal treatment does not cure endometriosis and is only advised for those infertile patients who are found to have moderate degrees of surface ovarian endometriosis at laparoscopy.

Improved results, with a higher fertility rate, have been claimed for danazol, a synthetic derivative of testosterone that may act by causing suppression of gonadotropin-releasing hormone (GnRH) or gonadotropin secretion, or both. Side effects include menopausal symptoms, weight gain, edema, and mild virilization, when prescribed at high dosages. However, mild to moderate cases can be managed effectively with fewer side effects at lower dosage levels. These cases require nonhormonal contraception, however, because ovulation may occur with subsequent virilization of the female fetus. Danazol therapy may also be carried out for 6 to 8 weeks before conservative surgical treatment to make dissection of the lesions simpler and more complete. Five to 20 percent of the patients will experience a recurrence of their endometriosis each year. Either the adequacy of therapy or recurrence may be confirmed after the completion of medical therapy by second-look laparoscopy or by measuring the cell surface antigen CA-125 level, which has been noted to be elevated in patients with endometriosis and correlates with the amount of disease present. It should be remembered, however, that an elevation in the level is nonspecific and has been noted in many other conditions. More recently, the administration of GnRH analogues in the form of a nasal spray, nafarelin, daily injections of leuprolide acetate, or monthly injections of leuprolide acetate depot (3.75 mg intramuscularly) has been successful in the treatment of endometriosis, and the menopausal-like side effects are better tolerated than the androgenic side effects of danazol. GnRH analogues have become the most popular form of medical treatment for endometriosis.

In most patients whose major complaint is infertility, conservative surgical treatment produces the best results. The procedure may be completed at laparoscopy or laparotomy. Such operations involve excision rather than electrocoagulation of visible endometrial implants. Vaporization of such implants can also be achieved with the carbon dioxide or argon laser. Ovarian endometriomata are removed, and ventral suspension of the uterus and appendectomy may be performed. In the presence of severe dysmenorrhea, presacral neurectomy or transection of the uterosacral ligaments, which carry afferent pain fibers at their junction with the uterus, may be carried out. In older patients in whom pregnancy is not a consideration and relief of pain is the main objective, laparotomy with total hysterectomy and bilateral salpingo-oophorectomy with excision of any other visible endometriomatous lesions and lysis of adhesions is the treatment of choice. These women may be placed on maintenance estrogen therapy postoperatively because exacerbation of the endometriosis is uncommon.

Rarely, surgical intervention is indicated for relieving obstruction of the rectosigmoid colon at the level of the cul-de-sac due to an endometrioma, or for eliminating small bowel obstruction of the distal ileum or at the ileocecal junction. In the latter case, obstruction is most likely due to adhesions that have formed between loops of bowel with subsequent kinking. Surgical treatment may also be indicated for endometriomatous involvement of the ureter. Malignant change is rare, occurring in less than 1 percent of the patients; the lesion is an endometrioid adenocarcinoma. The prognosis for 5-year survival is good in these patients, averaging more than 70 percent. Stromal endometriosis is a rare myometrial tumor composed of endometrial stroma. It often spreads locally, but true malignant change with remote metastases owing to sarcomatous transformation is extremely uncommon.

Review
1. Barbieri, R. L. Endometriosis. A comprehensive review. *Curr. Prob. Obstet. Gynecol. Fertil.* 11:1, 1989.
   Staging each patient according to the American Fertility Association classification provides a baseline from which to measure disease regression, stability, or progression.
2. Olive, D. L., and Haney, A. F. Endometriosis-associated infertility; a critical review of therapeutic approaches. *Obstet. Gynecol. Surv.* 41:538, 1986.

Despite extensive literature on the treatment of endometriosis-associated infertility, there are very few answers that can be called definitive.

Etiology

3. Ridley, J. H. The histogenesis of endometriosis. *Obstet. Gynecol. Surv.* 23:1, 1968.
   None of the theories explain why all women do not get the disease.
4. Scott, R. B., TeLinde, R. W., and Wharton, L. R., Jr. Further studies on experimental endometriosis. *Am. J. Obstet. Gynecol.* 62:1082, 1953.
   Six of ten monkeys with experimentally induced retrograde menses developed endometriosis.
5. DiZerega, G. S., Barber, D. L., and Hodgen, G. D. Endometriosis, role of ovarian steroids in initiation, maintenance, and suppression. *Fertil. Steril.* 33:649, 1980.
   Estrogen is essential for the development of endometriosis and its continued activity.

Clinical Presentation

6. Simpson, J. L., et al. Heritable aspects of endometriosis: I. Genetic studies. *Am. J. Obstet Gynecol.* 137:327, 1980.
   An apparently unaffected patient with an affected first-degree relative has a 7 percent risk of suffering endometriosis. A polygenic, multifactorial form of inheritance seems most likely.
7. Metzger, D. A., et al. Association of endometriosis and spontaneous abortion: effect of control group selection. *Fertil. Steril.* 45:18, 1986.
   The results from this study suggest that the spontaneous abortion rate in patients with untreated endometriosis may not be as high as previously reported. The importance of well-defined control groups is also stressed.
8. Mostoufizadeh, M., and Scully, R. E. Malignant tumors arising in endometriosis. *Clin. Obstet. Gynecol.* 23:951, 1980.
   These tumors are rare, but their true incidence is not known. Endometrioid carcinoma, clear cell carcinoma, stromal sarcoma, and mixed mesodermal adenosarcoma have been described.
9. Wheeler, J. M. Epidemiology of endometriosis-associated infertility. *J. Reprod. Med.* 34:41, 1989.
   Population-based epidemiologic methods using accepted criteria for causality, when applied to the endometriosis literature, failed to demonstrate an association between endometriosis and infertility.

Diagnosis

10. Buttram, M. V., Jr. Evolution of the revised American Fertility Society classification of endometriosis. *Fertil. Steril.* 43:347, 1985.
    Endometriosis is classified into four stages, I through IV (mild, moderate, severe, and extreme), depending on the extent of the disease.
11. Martin, D. C., et al. Laparoscopic appearances of peritoneal endometriosis. *Fertil. Steril.* 51:63, 1989.
    An increase in the awareness and histologic confirmation of the protean presentation of endometriosis is associated with a significant increase in the diagnosis of endometriosis at laparoscopy.

Medical Management

12. Management of endometriosis. *ACOG Tech. Bull.* No. 85, March 1985.
    This communication emphasizes that the management should be strictly individualized.
13. Barbieri, R. L. CA-125 in patients with endometriosis. *Fertil. Steril.* 45:767, 1986.
    The development of the CA-125 antigen is reviewed. Its value in monitoring the course of treated endometriosis is discussed.

14. Buttram, V. C., Jr., Reiter, R. C., and Ward, S. Treatment of endometriosis with danazol: report of a 6-year prospective study. *Fertil. Steril.* 43:353, 1985.
    A summary of modern concepts and approaches to management.
15. Henzl, M. D., et al. Administration of nasal nafarelin as compared with oral danazol for endometriosis. *N. Engl. J. Med.* 318:485, 1988.
    Nafarelin is equally effective and is better tolerated than danazol.
16. Waller, K. G., and Shaw, R. W. Gonadotropin-releasing hormone analogues for the treatment of endometriosis: Long-term follow-up. *Fertil. Steril.* 59:511, 1993.
    The women in this study were found to be highly likely to suffer a recurrence, particularly if their disease was severe at the outset.
17. Taylor, P. J., and Kredenster, J. V. Nonsurgical management of minimal and moderate endometriosis to enhance fertility. *Int. J. Fertil.* 37:138, 1992.
    A rational clinical approach is described aimed at discouraging too rapid recourse to the apparent panacea of the highly technological new reproductive approaches.
18. Malinak, L. R. Surgical therapy and adjunct therapy of endometriosis. *Int. J. Gynecol. Obstet.* 40:S43, 1993.
    Combined surgical treatment and pre- or postoperative medical therapy is recommended for young noninfertile women and those with extensive or severe disease.

Surgical Management
19. Adamson, G. D., et al. Comparison of CO_2 laser laparoscopy with laparotomy for treatment of endometriomata. *Fertil. Steril.* 57:965, 1992.
    This is the first controlled study using prospectively tabulated data which confirms that carbon dioxide laser laparoscopy is safe and effective treatment for endometriomata.
20. Meyers, W. C., Kelvin, F. M., and Jones, R. S. Diagnosis and surgical treatment of colonic endometriosis. *Arch. Surg.* 114:169, 1979.
    The radiographic findings are nonspecific.
21. Moore, J. G., et al. Urinary tract endometriosis: enigmas in diagnosis and management. *Am. J. Obstet. Gynecol.* 134:162, 1979.
    If the ureter is involved, danger to renal function is great and castration is nearly always indicated, in addition to freeing the ureter.

52. PEDIATRIC GYNECOLOGY
Michel E. Rivlin

Most children are seen regularly by pediatricians and are referred to gynecologists only for specific problems. In obtaining the history and performing the physical examination, great care and sensitivity must be exercised, in view of the physical and emotional immaturity of the patient. Inspection of the external genitalia is part of the neonatal and well-child examination, while complete gynecologic examination is reserved for the child with symptoms or signs of a genital disorder. Specially designed equipment may be necessary (e.g., a vaginoscope and virginal speculum) or adapted (e.g., nasal speculum, otoscope, or laparoscope).

Newborn infants demonstrate the effects of maternal hormones, with breast budding, prominent external genitalia, and vaginal discharge. The ratio between the cervix and the corpus is 3:1, and the ovaries are abdominal organs. In early childhood (2 months to 7 years), an estrogen-poor phase, the uterus regresses and only regains the size present at birth by age 6. The breasts are undeveloped, and the diameter of the hymenal orifice is 0.5 cm. During late childhood (7 to 10 years), the onset of ovarian estrogen production results in the appearance of the breast bud, but external genital effects are not yet apparent. In the premenarche period (11 to 12 years), the hymenal orifice increases from 0.7 to 1.0 cm and the ratio of the cervix to the corpus alters from 1:1 toward the adult ratio. Puberty is the early stage of adolescence culminating in menarche. The changes and problems of puberty are discussed in Chapter 82.

Congenital anomalies of the genitalia may be related to intersex problems with sexual ambiguity in which the true gender cannot be immediately determined. These include genetic abnormalities and are discussed in the endocrinology section of this manual. A newborn with ambiguous genitalia requires immediate investigation, not only because of parental anxiety but because one of the causes, salt-losing congenital adrenal hyperplasia, may be rapidly fatal in the first week of life if the serum electrolyte levels are not closely monitored and corrected. Congenital anomalies of the genital tract in chromosomally normal females can result from agenesis or abnormalities of tissue fusion and canalization. Because the wolffian and müllerian ducts develop in close proximity, urinary tract anomalies are commonly associated, occurring in up to 20 percent of the cases. Persistence of the urogenital membrane results in an imperforate hymen, which may be found at birth as a mucocolpos. However, it may not be diagnosed until adolescence, when primary amenorrhea with recurrent pelvic pain leads to the discovery of a hematocolpos. A portion of the membrane should be removed for drainage.

The upper two thirds of the vagina are formed by the canalization of müllerian tissue, and the lower one third from the urogenital sinus. Varying degrees of failure of canalization may occur, including longitudinal and transverse vaginal septa and absence of the vagina. Asymptomatic longitudinal septa require no treatment, but transverse septa usually require excision, and vaginal agenesis requires the construction of an artificial vagina, generally when sexual maturity is achieved.

Uterine anomalies range from the minor arcuate deformity (subseptate uterus) to a double uterus (didelphia) with one (unicollis) or two (bicollis) cervices. These anomalies are seldom discovered until pregnancy occurs, with the exception of a rudimentary uterine horn that does not communicate with the other uterine cavity or the vagina, resulting in a hematometra or pyometra and necessitating surgical intervention. If pregnancy occurs in such a horn, it may result in rupture with hemoperitoneum. Ideally, a horn should be removed before pregnancy occurs.

Vulvar pruritus may be due to any of several vulvar or perineal dermatologic disorders. *Lichen sclerosus*, a hypotrophic disorder usually affecting postmenopausal women, is occasionally seen in young girls. Treatment is symptomatic and progesterone cream may also be helpful. The lesion may abate or resolve during puberty. A *labial adhesion* is quite common in prepubertal children, probably related to the thin skin covering the labia becoming denuded by local irritation and scratching, resulting in adherence at the midline. No therapy is required unless it becomes symptomatic with dysuria and recurrent vulvar and vaginal irritation. Treatment consists of twice daily local application of estrogen cream for 7 to 10 days and proper instruction with regard to perineal hygiene. Surgical separation is rarely required. Recurrence is quite common until puberty.

Vulvovaginitis is probably the most common gynecologic disorder in children because the estrogen-poor atrophic mucosa is susceptible to infection and because perineal hygiene is often inadequate, resulting in contamination by stool. Symptoms include a mucopurulent discharge, perineal pruritus, and dysuria. Nonspecific infections are usually polymicrobial. Specific infections include *Neisseria gonorrhoeae, Gardnerella vaginalis,* and *candidiasis*. Inoculation may occur secondary to upper respiratory or urinary tract infections. Allergic and chemical reactions are common, and careful inquiry into the kinds of soaps and detergents the patient is exposed to may suggest the cause. Panties made of synthetic material and tight clothing may aggravate the situation; loose cotton clothing should be recommended. If the predominant symptom is pruritus, a pinworm (*Enterobius vermicularis*) infestation is likely; diagnosis is based on identifying the eggs on a sticky tape placed on the perianal area overnight. A foreign body is suspected if the discharge is bloody and malodorous. In first infections, inspection of the external genitalia with microscopic examination and culture of the discharge is sufficient. Rectal examination should be performed to evaluate the pelvic organs. In the event of recurrence or nonresponse, vaginoscopy is necessary to rule out the presence of a foreign body or tumor. Therapy is directed toward the specific cause, and proper hygienic instructions are given to the mother and child. Recurrence with foreign bodies is quite common, and removal may require general anesthesia.

Injuries to the genitalia during childhood are usually accidental. Most are minor, but a few require major surgical treatment. It is important to determine how the injury was sustained, as the child will require protection if she is a victim of physical or sexual abuse. General anesthesia is frequently necessary in order to perform an adequate examination. Contusions and hematomas of the vulva may be relieved by ice packs and analgesics, but, if large or increasing in size, surgical incision and control of bleeding points or packing may be necessary. Vaginal wounds generally involve the lateral walls but may extend above the pelvic floor, and a retroperitoneal hematoma may develop or may involve the peritoneal cavity, necessitating laparotomy. Thus, if the hymen is torn, an intravaginal examination should be performed and the bladder and rectum checked for trauma.

Genital tumors, although rare, must be considered in girls with a chronic genital ulcer, nontraumatic genital swelling, fetid or bloody discharge, abdominal pain or enlargement, or premature sexual maturation. Almost every tumor of the adult has also been encountered in children, but about half of the genital tumors in the pediatric group are premalignant or malignant. Vulvar tumors are generally benign, and include hymenal cysts of the newborn, which usually disappear within a few weeks. Condyloma acuminatum, viral warts similar to those in the adult, teratomas, and hemangiomas also occur. Most benign vaginal tumors are cystic remnants of the mesonephric duct (Gartner's duct cyst) and require surgical excision or marsupialization if they become large enough to cause symptoms. Sarcoma botryoides is the most common neoplasm of the lower genital tract in girls younger than 16 years of age. The tumor usually involves the vagina, but the cervix may also be affected. In this condition, the vaginal mucosa bulges into a series of polypoid growths. Diagnosis is made on the basis of biopsy findings that usually indicate the presence of rhabdomyoblasts. Prognosis has improved with the advent of combination chemotherapy together with conservative surgical treatment, with or without irradiation. Clear cell adenocarcinoma of müllerian origin, often associated with antenatal exposure to synthetic estrogens, is now primarily seen in postmenarcheal females.

Ovarian tumors are the most frequent genital neoplasm encountered in children and adolescents. Nonneoplastic ovarian cysts occasionally occur in children or infants and are generally follicular or corpus luteal in origin. Unless acute complications occur, conservative management is preferable. The incidence of malignant degeneration of neoplasms is higher in children than in adolescents or adults, and ovarian neoplasms in children have a malignancy rate of 35 percent overall. The tumors in about 65 percent are of germ cell origin (e.g., teratoma, dysgerminoma, endodermal sinus tumor, gonadoblastoma, and choriocarcinoma); 12 percent are derived from specialized stroma (e.g., granulosa-theca cells or Sertoli-Leydig cells). The remaining tumors are chiefly epithelial in origin, as in the adult. The most common symptoms are abdominal pain and an abdominal mass. Stromal tumors and germ cell tumors may cause isosexual precocious puberty. At least a fourth of all childhood ovarian tumors are diagnosed only at the time of exploratory laparotomy. Conservative surgical treatment (unilateral adnexectomy) is justified for most premenarcheal patients with stage I cancer, once localization to the ovary has been established by surgical staging. If extension has occurred, a more radical operation (removal of the uterus with adnexa) is indicated. Adjunctive chemotherapy, with or without radiotherapy, may also be indicated, especially in the event of advanced disease or for those lesions with greater malignant potential, such as the papillary serous epithelial tumor.

General
1. Gardner, J. J. Descriptive study of genital variation in healthy, nonabused premenarcheal girls. *J. Pediatr.* 120:251, 1992.
   The colposcopic appearance of the genitals, widely used for evidence in court for alleged child sexual abuse, is complicated by the wide variations encountered in normal genital anatomy.
2. Cacciatore, B., et al. Ultrasonic characteristics of the uterus and ovaries in re-

lation to pubertal development and serum LH, FSH, and estradiol concentrations. *Adolesc. Pediatr. Gynecol.* 4:15, 1991.
The sonographic evaluation of the uterus and ovaries identifies the functional changes and appears useful for the assessment of gonadal development during puberty.
3. Blake, J. Gynecologic examination of the teenager and young child. *Obstet. Gynecol. Clin. North Am.* 19:27, 1992.
External genitalia are most easily examined with the child in a frog-legged position. Allowing the mother to hold the child on her lap may also be helpful.
4. Pokorny, S. F., et al. Acute genital injury in the prepubertal girl. *Am. J. Obstet. Gynecol.* 166:1461, 1992.
Straddle injuries, nonpenetrating injuries, penetrating injuries, and torque injuries are discussed.

Congenital Anomalies of the Genital Tract
5. The American Fertility Society classification of müllerian anomalies. *Fertil. Steril.* 49:944, 1988.
Class I, hypoplasia/agenesis; class II, unicornuate; class III, didelphus; class IV, bicornuate; class V, septate; class VI, arcuate; class VII, diethylstilbestrol related.
6. Doyle, M. B. Magnetic resonance imaging in müllerian fusion defects. *J. Reprod. Med.* 37:33, 1992.
Sonography, computed tomography, and magnetic resonance imaging have largely replaced purely diagnostic surgery.
7. Bergh P. A., Breen, J. L., and Gregori, C. A. Congenital absence of the vagina—the Mayer-Rokitansky-Kuster-Hauser syndrome. *Adolesc. Pediatr. Gynecol.* 2:73, 1989.
These patients have normal ovaries, XX chromosomes but an absent or rudimentary uterus, tubes, and the upper two thirds of the vagina (müllerian aplasia).
8. Kaufman, R. H., et al. Upper genital tract abnormalities and pregnancy outcome in diethylstilbestrol-exposed progeny. *Am. J. Obstet. Gynecol.* 148:97, 1984.
Upper genital tract abnormalities are revealed by hysterosalpingography in about half the exposed females. These include a T-shaped uterus and hypoplasia of the uterine cavity.

Vulvovaginitis
9. Gerstner, G. J., et al. Vaginal organisms in prepubertal children with and without vulvovaginitis. A vaginoscopic study. *Arch. Gynecol.* 213:247, 1982.
The frequency with which anaerobic bacteria and yeasts were isolated was increased when vulvovaginitis was present.
10. Pokorny, S. F. Prepubertal vulvovaginopathies. *Obstet. Gynecol. Clin. North Am.* 19:39, 1992.
Most (95–98%) prepubertal gynecologic problems involve the vulva or the vagina. These consist of bleeding problems, which are the most serious, abnormal appearance, which is the most worrisome, and pruritus/discharge, which is the most annoying.
11. Paradise, J. E., and Willis, E. D. Probability of vaginal foreign body in girls with genital complaints. *Am. J. Dis. Child.* 139:472, 1985.
Vaginal bleeding is the most reliable clue to a vaginal foreign object in premenarcheal girls.
12. Berkowitz, C. D., Elvik, S. L., and Logan, M. K. Labial fusion in prepubescent girls: a marker for sexual abuse? *Am. J. Obstet. Gynecol.* 156:16, 1987.
This article considers ten cases of labial fusion in 500 girls evaluated for sexual abuse. The patient's history or physical findings, or both, were consistent with abuse in six of the ten. It is suggested that the fusion may have resulted from trauma, particularly vulvar coitus.
13. Pacheco, B. P., et al. Vulvar infection caused by human papilloma virus in children and adolescents without sexual contact. *Adolesc. Pediatr. Gynecol.* 4:136, 1991.

Condyloma acuminatum can be nonsexually transmitted; however, the possibility of sexual abuse must also be addressed.

14. Velcek, F. T., et al. Surgical therapy of urethral prolapse in young girls. *Adolesc. Pediatr. Gynecol.* 2:230, 1989.
    Surgical treatment is seldom necessary because most patients respond to a short course of locally applied estrogen cream.

Tumors
15. Farghaly, S. A. Gynecologic cancer in the young female: clinical presentation and management. *Adolesc. Pediatr. Gynecol.* 5:163, 1992.
    Unfortunately, the rarity of these tumors and the nonspecificity of their symptomatology results in delays in diagnosis past the point of potential cure.
16. Muram, D., et al. Ovarian cancer in children and adolescents. *Adolesc. Pediatr. Gynecol.* 5:21, 1992.
    Ovarian tumors are the most common genital neoplasm in children and adolescents, accounting for 1 percent of all cancers in this age group.
17. Millar, D. M., et al. Prepubertal ovarian cyst formation: 5 years' experience. *Obstet. Gynecol.* 81:434, 1993.
    Cysts larger than 5 cm are at risk for torsion; ultrasound-guided aspiration has been suggested for the eradication of these larger cysts.
18. Shulman, L. P., et al. Marker chromosomes in gonadal dysgenesis: avoiding unnecessary surgery. *Adolesc. Pediatr. Gynecol.* 5:39, 1992.
    Gonadoblastoma, dysgerminoma, and other germ cell malignancies occur in 15 to 30 percent of females possessing Y chromosomal material in their karyotype. Accurate identification is essential because early bilateral gonadectomy is recommended.
19. Hicks, M. L., and Piver, M. S. Conservative surgery plus adjuvant therapy for vulvovaginal rhabdomyosarcoma, diethylstilbestrol clear cell adenocarcinoma of the vagina, and unilateral germ cell tumors of the ovary. *Obstet. Gynecol. Clin. North Am.* 19:219, 1992.
    Early stage disease (I or II) for these three groups of childhood cancers may be treated with high cure rates and retention of childbearing capacity.
20. Stillman, R. J., et al. Ovarian failure in long-term survivors of childhood malignancy. *Am. J. Obstet. Gynecol.* 139:62, 1981.
    In 12 percent of 182 cases, the only risk factor was the location of the ovaries in relation to radiation treatment fields.

53. LAPAROSCOPY AND HYSTEROSCOPY
Michel E. Rivlin

Inspection of the internal pelvic organs with an illuminated telescope through a small incision in the gas-distended abdominal cavity is termed *laparoscopy* (less commonly, *celioscopy* or *peritoneoscopy*). The major diagnostic application of the procedure is in the evaluation of female infertility, with particular regard to tubal patency and ovarian evidence of ovulation. The other major diagnostic application lies in the elucidation of the cause of pelvic pain. The presence of endometriosis, pelvic inflammatory disease, or ectopic pregnancy explains the symptoms, or the absence of organic pathology may provide reassurance to both the patient and physician. Diagnostic laparoscopy may also be helpful in the staging and follow-up of patients with pelvic cancer.

The most common indication for performing therapeutic laparoscopy is tubal sterilization, with the fallopian tubes either fulgurated with electrocautery or closed by clips or bands. Many other surgical procedures have been performed with the laparoscope, including the removal of intraabdominal foreign bodies (particularly, perforated intrauterine devices [IUDs]), ovarian biopsy in patients with endocrine disorders such as suspected ovarian failure, or the fulguration of endometriotic implants. Skilled laparoscopists can aspirate ovarian cysts, capture intact ova for in vitro fertilization, drain pelvic abscesses, remove ectopic pregnancies, ventrosuspend the uterus, lyse tubal adhesions, and perform fimbriolysis and salpingostomy. In recent years, advances in instrumentation have greatly increased the applications of this "minimally invasive" surgical approach, allowing the performance of myomectomy, appendectomy, adnexectomy, bladder suspension, lymphadenectomy, presacral neurectomy, and, most significantly, hysterectomy. The adaptation of the carbon dioxide laser to the operating laparoscope has introduced a new format for the performance of a variety of operative procedures, such as the fulguration of endometrial implants and the dissolution of pelvic adhesions. The distinction between diagnostic and therapeutic laparoscopy is no longer clear-cut, because it has become common practice to deal with abnormalities found at laparoscopy at the time of diagnosis, as many such problems can be managed through the laparoscope.

Laparoscopy is contraindicated in patients with severe cardiorespiratory disease, diffuse peritonitis, or ileus. The presence of hiatal herniation or an ostomy is also a contraindication. The procedure is relatively contraindicated, dependent to a large degree on the laparoscopist's skill or experience, in obese patients and in those with abdominal scars from previous operations.

Peritoneoscopy may be regarded as a minor surgical but a major anesthetic procedure. This is because general anesthesia with endotracheal intubation and muscle relaxation is the usual anesthesia used. Regional or local anesthesia is also satisfactory, however, particularly when the operation is performed on an outpatient basis.

Celioscopy is carried out with the patient supine, her legs supported by stirrups angled 15 degrees downward, and her buttocks protruding over the edge of the table. This position is essential because manipulative instruments are introduced through the uterine cervix to enhance visualization by moving the pelvic organs during the procedure. Furthermore, these instruments are canalized so that colored dyes (indigo carmine or methylene blue) may be injected for the assessment of tubal patency (chromopertubation).

The first step in the procedure is creating the pneumoperitoneum. The gas used is either carbon dioxide or nitrous oxide and it is introduced through a spring-loaded needle (Veress or Palmer), generally inserted subumbilically. Gas is insufflated at 1 L/min and the gas pressure should not exceed 20 mm Hg. The usual amount of gas required varies from 2 to 5 L. When liver dullness in response to percussion is lost, the patient is placed in the Trendelenburg position and the needle is withdrawn.

Next, the telescope is introduced. To do this, a 1-cm subumbilical incision is made through the skin and fascia. A trocar and valve sleeve are introduced at an angle of 45 degrees toward the pelvis. The trocar is removed, and the telescope is passed through the sheath. (Some surgeons prefer to introduce the trocar and valve sleeve directly and before the creation of the pneumoperitoneum.) The gas insufflator is attached on automatic flow to maintain the pneumoperitoneum. The fiberoptic light source is attached to the telescope, and viewing commences. Telescope diameters vary from 4 to 10 mm, and their objectives are usually angled 180 degrees forward. If a double-channeled operating laparoscope is used, this may obviate the need for placement of ancillary instruments through a further incision.

Additional instruments, if required, are passed through further incisions, generally placed in the iliac fossae through a smaller trocar and cannula. These incisions are made under direct laparoscopic vision. A wide variety of ancillary instruments are available. These include tubal clip or band applicators; ovarian biopsy forceps; apparatus for suction or aspiration; electrocautery or laser instruments capable of coagulation, vaporization, or cutting; forceps; graduated probes; scissors; loops; and needles for the placement of intraabdominal sutures. Either individual titanium clips can be applied or two lines of clips may be placed simultaneously with an inbuilt knife to cut the tissue between the lines of staples.

The mortality associated with diagnostic laparoscopy is 11 per 100,000, and the incidence of laparotomy performed for intraabdominal complications is 8.5 per 1000. Complications may occur owing to the anesthesia, improper gas insufflation, and perforation of viscera or vessels, as well as to the operative procedure itself, including hemorrhage or burns.

Anesthetic complications are related to increases in intraabdominal pressure over 20 mm Hg, particularly when carbon dioxide is the insufflating gas. Reduced pulmonary excursion and carbon dioxide absorption result in hypercapnia, causing cardiac arrhythmias and cardiac arrest (1 in 5000 procedures). Careful technique that includes close cardiac and abdominal pressure monitoring, as well as active ventilation, minimizes the incidence of this problem. The alternative use of nitrous oxide, which does not cause hypercapnia and is nonirritant, is not entirely without problems, as it is an ignitable gas and is only slowly absorbed. This must be kept in mind, particularly when electrocautery is used.

Almost every conceivable viscus or vessel has been injured by the Veress or other cannulas. Most of these injuries are minor and require no special attention other than close observation. Of course, immediate laparotomy is necessary to manage major bleeding or visceral injury.

When operative procedures are performed, bleeding is the most common complication encountered. Hemostasis can generally be achieved by electrocoagulation, although laparotomy may be required. The more serious complications are due to electrical burns. These result from accidentally touching adjacent tissues or from sparking of the current to these structures. Bowel burns are commonly involved and, if recognized and superficial, may be treated conservatively, as most resolve when managed in this way. In those cases in which unrecognized bowel burns become progressive, a clinical picture similar to that of pelvic inflammatory disease or appendicitis develops. Laparotomy with bowel resection, together with antibiotic therapy, is then necessary. The hazards of electrical burns are lessened by the use of bipolar rather than unipolar electrodes, while regular inspection and testing of equipment with particular attention to insulation is mandatory. Many surgeons prevent these problems by using clips or bands rather than electrosurgical techniques when performing tubal sterilization.

The introduction of minimally invasive surgical techniques into the practice of operative gynecology has had a revolutionary impact, such that, within a few years, the discipline may become almost exclusively endoscopic. The down side of the situation is that much expensive equipment is required and operating times may be prolonged ("foreveroscopy"). Extensive retraining and study are also required so that gynecologic endoscopic surgery, with its advantages of a shortened hospital stay and postoperative convalescent time, can be effective, safe, and free of unnecessary complications.

Hysteroscopy is the direct visualization of the endometrial cavity using an endoscope. It may be performed under local or general anesthesia. Women with recurrent abnormal bleeding, repetitive abortion, uterine synechiae, abnormal hysterosalpingograms, and infertility are all candidates for diagnostic hysteroscopy. Operative procedures that can be performed under hysteroscopic guidance with video monitoring include removal of IUDs, resection of submucous myomas, lysis of synechiae, incision of uterine septa, removal of endometrial polyps, electrosurgical or laser ablation of the endometrium, falloposcopy and balloon tuboplasty for obstructed fallopian tubes, and the placement of silicone plugs into the tubes for sterilization. The cavity of the uterus must be distended for the procedure, and the mediums used for this purpose include 32% dextran, 5% dextrose and water, 1.5% glycine, and carbon dioxide gas. Dextran is preferred by many for its good optic qualities and immiscibility with blood. However, it is antigenic, which may lead to anaphylaxis; instruments must also be cleaned shortly after the procedure because it is sticky. The flow of carbon dioxide must be limited to less than 100 ml/min, and the volume of 5% dextrose and water or 1.5% glycine must be carefully monitored to prevent fluid overload. A variant instrument, the contact hysteroscope, does not require a distending medium. The interpretation of findings is similar to that for colposcopy, relying on the color, contour, and vascular pattern. A microhysteroscope may be used to examine the endocervical canal after vital staining.

Contraindications to hysteroscopy include acute pelvic infection and pregnancy. Active bleeding and uterine cancer are relative contraindications. Complications occur in fewer than 2 percent of the procedures and include uterine perforation, pelvic infection, and hemorrhage. Complications due to the distending media include the potential for gas embolism with carbon dioxide.

Light amplification by the stimulated emission of radiation (*laser*) is a technique that is widely used in medicine. It involves the use of energized light to vaporize tissue. Lasers generate an intense narrow beam of light in waves that must all be of one wavelength (monochromatic), exactly in phase (coherent), and parallel (collimated), so that the peaks and valleys of the waves line up and amplify each other until they are absorbed by a target. In an atomic laser, the lasing medium emits only a single, predominant wavelength of light when its atoms have been excited and then allowed to return to the resting state. This wavelength is determined by the medium, which may be solid, liquid, or gas. Three types of lasers are commonly used in gynecology: the argon, Nd:YAG (neodymium: yttrium-aluminum-garnet), and carbon dioxide. Each of these lasers is used for specific purposes, as dictated by its wavelength and tissue-absorption qualities. The carbon dioxide laser has been evaluated most extensively for pelvic procedures and may be handheld or used through a laparoscope. It destroys tissue by instantaneously boiling intracellular water. Adjusting the spot size helps control the power density, which ranges from warming to incisional vaporization. The depth of laser action is precisely controlled by the power density, exposure time, and the use of energy-absorbing "backstop" probes or fluids. Nd:YAG lasers have been favored for use in hysteroscopy procedures because they can penetrate deep into tissue, producing an excellent coagulative effect. Protective goggles must be warn while this laser is in operation. As with electrocautery, great care must be taken to prevent injury to vessels and viscera.

Reviews

1. Nezhat, C., Nezhat, F., and Nezhat, C. Operative laparoscopy (minimally invasive surgery): state of the art. *J. Gynecol. Surg.* 8:111, 1992.
   The average postoperative stay is 0.5 to 2 days for operative laparoscopy versus 5 to 5.7 days for laparotomy. Women can return to full activity in 7 to 10 days.

2. Garry, R. Laparoscopic alternatives to laparotomy: A new approach to gynaecological surgery. *Br. J. Obstet. Gynaecol.* 99:629, 1992.
   Incorporating a laparoscopy-mounted videocamera, a videorecorder, and a videomonitor allows the surgeon to operate in an upright position directly from the videomonitor. Magnification of the pelvic organs by the monitor simplifies the procedure.

Technique

3. Philipsen, T., and Hansen, B. B. Comparative study of hysterosalpingography and laparoscopy in infertile patients. *Acta Obstet. Gynecol. Scand.* 60:149, 1981.
   For a conclusive evaluation of the tubal factor, hysterosalpingography should be replaced by laparoscopy, according to the findings in this series of 168 patients investigated by both techniques.

4. Penfield, A. J. How to prevent complications of open laparoscopy. *J. Reprod. Med.* 30:660, 1985.
   For the procedure of open laparoscopy, a special cannula is inserted through a small laparotomy incision; sutures ensure a gas-tight seal. This is an especially useful approach in the obese or when adhesions are suspected.

5. Shapiro, B. S., Diamond, M. P., and DeCherney, A. H. Salpingoscopy: an adjunctive technique for evaluation of the fallopian tube. *Fertil. Steril.* 49:1076, 1988.
   During laparoscopy, the fallopian tube is cannulated with an endoscope for examination of the endosalpinx. A discordance of 23 percent has been noted between the fimbrial appearance at operation and that revealed by the salpingoscopic examination. In patients with marked endosalpingeal damage, the prognosis for pregnancy with in vitro fertilization may be better than that with tuboplasty.

Anesthesia

6. Tan, P. L., Lee, T. L., and Tweed, W. A. Carbon dioxide absorption and gas exchange during pelvic laparoscopy. *Can. J. Anaesth.* 39:677, 1992.

A sharp rise in the arterial carbon dioxide tension and a fall in pH was noted with carbon dioxide, but there were no changes with nitrous oxide.

7. Versichelen, L., et al. Physiopathologic changes during anesthesia administration for gynecologic laparoscopy. *J. Reprod. Med.* 29:697, 1984.
   Large changes in total lung compliance and venous pressures yielded only marginal general effects, probably because of volume-controlled mechanical respiration and the limitation of insufflation pressures.

8. Peterson, H. B., et al. Local versus general anesthesia for laparoscopic sterilization: a randomized study. *Obstet. Gynecol.* 70:903, 1987.
   In properly selected patients (probably not the obese or those with a previous abdominal incision), local anesthesia may even be a preferable alternative. However, it appears to be used in only about 4 percent of cases nationwide.

9. Sengupta, P., and Plantevin, O.M. Nitrous oxide and day-case laparoscopy: effects on nausea, vomiting and return to normal activity. *Br. J. Anaesth.* 70:570, 1988.
   The use of nitrous oxide might contribute to the approximately 80 percent incidence rate of nausea and vomiting noted after outpatient laparoscopy. The authors conclude that the use of nitrous oxide may be readily avoided in these patients.

Applications

10. Paulson, J. D. The use of carbon dioxide laser laparoscopy in the treatment of tubal ectopic pregnancies. *Am. J. Obstet. Gynecol.* 167:382, 1992.
    In a surgically stable patient, especially with an unruptured accessible tube, both conservative and radical procedures are possible using electrocautery, endocoagulation, laser, or intraabdominal sutures.

11. Adamson, G.D., et al. Laparoscopic endometriosis treatment: Is it better? *Fertil. Steril.* 59:35, 1993.
    The author concluded that operative laparoscopy is the treatment of choice for infertile women with endometriosis unless they have severe tubal disease.

12. Hulka, J. F, et al. Management of ovarian masses. AAGL 1990 survey. *J. Reprod. Med.* 37:599, 1992.
    Seventy percent of the patients with adnexal masses were managed by laparoscopy alone. An overall incidence of 4 per 1000 cases of ovarian cancer was found.

13. Daniell, J. F., and Gurley, L. D. Laparoscopic treatment of clinically significant symptomatic uterine fibroids. *J. Gynecol. Surg.* 7:37, 1991.
    This describes an experience with laparoscopic myomectomy after shrinkage of the fibroids preoperatively using gonadotropin-releasing hormone analogs.

14. Livengood, C. H., III, Hill, G. B., and Addison, W. A. Pelvic inflammatory disease: findings during inpatient treatment of clinically severe, laparoscopy-documented disease. *Am. J. Obstet. Gynecol.* 166:519, 1992.
    The advantages of accurate diagnosis, possible identification of the organisms causing the infection, and the potential adjuvant role afforded by laparoscopic surgery are described.

15. Stovall, T. G., et al. Method failures of laparoscopic tubal sterilization in a residency training program. A comparison of the tubal ring and spring-loaded clips. *J. Reprod. Med.* 36:283, 1991.
    Electrical methods are preferable in women with adhesions and tubal pathology. Clips (Hulka and Filshie) and rings (Yoon) are preferable in women who may later request sterilization reversal.

16. Gürgan, T., et al. The effect of short-interval laparoscopic lysis of adhesions on pregnancy rates following Nd-YAG laser photocoagulation of polycystic ovaries. *Obstet. Gynecol.* 80:45, 1992.
    This represents an alternative to wedge resection for women in whom initial medical management fails.

17. Bryson, K. Laparoscopic appendectomy. *J. Gynecol. Surg.* 7:93, 1991.
    This is an effective alternative to open appendectomy for noninflamed and inflamed appendices.

18. Lavy, G., et al. Laparoscopic and transvaginal ova recovery: the effect of ova quality. *Fertil. Steril.* 49:1002, 1988.
    Transvaginal routes have largely replaced laparoscopic methods of ovum collec-

tion for in vitro fertilization and embryo transfer. However, laparoscopy is essential for gamete intrafallopian transfer procedures.

19. Tulandi, T. Reconstructive tubal surgery by laparoscopy. *Obstet. Gynecol. Surv.* 42:193, 1987.
   Laparoscopic salpingostomy, fimbrioplasty, and adhesiolysis may achieve results equivalent to those of surgical procedures performed through a laparotomy. However, for tubal anastomosis, the superior results of microsurgical procedures are unlikely to be accomplished by laparoscopic techniques.

20. Bahary, C. M., and Gorodeski, I. G. The diagnostic value of laparoscopy in women with chronic pelvic pain. *Am. Surg.* 53:672, 1987.
   Laparoscopy is necessary to establish the definitive diagnosis in women with chronic pelvic pain, to guide the proper treatment, and to prevent unnecessary laparotomies.

21. Liu, C. Y. Laparoscopic hysterectomy: a review of 72 cases. *J. Reprod. Med.* 37:351, 1992.
   In practice, it is unusual for a hysterectomy to be performed laparoscopically; generally, endoscopic procedures are performed to the point where a vaginal hysterectomy can be accomplished.

Complications

22. Franks, A. L., Kendrick, J. S., and Peterson, H. B. Unintended laparotomy associated with laparoscopic tubal sterilization. *Am. J. Obstet. Gynecol.* 157:1102, 1987.
   It is sometimes necessary to complete the sterilization or manage complications by laparotomy. Women who have undergone prior abdominal or pelvic operations are at greatest risk for requiring an unintended laparotomy.

23. Levy, B. S., Soderstrom, R. M., and Dail, D. H. Bowel injuries during laparoscopy. Gross anatomy and histology. *J. Reprod. Med.* 30:168, 1985.
   Bowel injuries ascribed to electrical damage may have in fact resulted from trauma. The authors suggest that unipolar techniques with appropriate low-voltage generators should be reconsidered in view of the increased failure rate associated with bipolar methods.

24. Peterson, H. B., et al. Deaths associated with laparoscopic sterilization in the United States, 1977–79. *J. Reprod. Med.* 27:345, 1982.
   This study reported nine deaths—five related to general anesthesia, three to bowel burns caused by unipolar electrocoagulation, and one to hemorrhage.

Hysteroscopy

25. March, C. M. Hysteroscopy. *J. Reprod. Med.* 37:293, 1992.
   There are three types of hysteroscopes: rigid panoramic, rigid contact, and flexible panoramic.

26. Itzkowic, D. Hysteroscopy. Its place in modern gynaecology. *Aust. Fam. Physician* 21:425, 1992.
   The infertility investigation includes hysterosalpingogram as a vital screening procedure; when an intrauterine abnormality is detected, hysteroscopic identification of the lesion is necessary.

27. Parasnis, H. B., and Parulekar, S. V. Significance of negative hysteroscopic view in abnormal uterine bleeding. *J. Postgrad. Med.* 38:62, 1992.
   Dilatation and curettage and hysteroscopy are similar in terms of specificity, but hysteroscopy is significantly more sensitive (98% versus 65%). In particular, dilatation and curettage may miss fibroids and polyps.

28. Choe, J. K., and Baggish, M. S. Hysteroscopic treatment of septate uterus with neodymium-YAG laser. *Fertil. Steril.* 57:81, 1992.
   Hysteroscopic metroplasty is superior to the transabdominal procedure in several respects, including the avoidance of pelvic adhesions and the need for cesarean section.

29. Daniell, J. F., Kurtz, B. R., and Ke, R. W. Hysteroscopic endometrial ablation using the rollerball electrode. *Obstet. Gynecol.* 80:329, 1992.
   The iatrogenic Asherman's syndrome may obviate the need for hysterectomy in

many women with uterine bleeding problems. This is particularly valuable in patients for whom a major surgical procedure is contraindicated. The most common technique is the use of a resectoscope with either a cutting loop or rollerball electrode.

30. Valle, R. F., and Sciarra, J. J. Intrauterine adhesions: hysteroscopic diagnosis, classification, treatment, and reproductive outcome. *Am. J. Obstet. Gynecol.* 158: 1459, 1988.

    An operative hysteroscopy for the treatment of Asherman's syndrome is often followed by the placement of an IUD and the institution of cyclic hormone therapy to prevent the reformation of adhesions and to encourage endometrial regeneration. However, the necessity for this adjunctive therapy has not been demonstrated.

31. Brooks, P. G. Complications of operative hysteroscopy: How safe is it? *Clin. Obstet. Gynecol.* 35:256, 1992.

    Bleeding, infection, and uterine perforation were attributed to the procedure. Allergic reactions and a symptom complex consisting of acute noncardiogenic pulmonary edema and disseminated intravascular coagulation, related to the distending medium, are the major, albeit rare, complications.

32. Mangar, D. Anaesthestic implications of 32% dextran-70 (Hyskon) during hysteroscopy: hysteroscopy syndrome. *Can. J. Anaesth.* 39:976, 1992.

    The author recommends limiting the total amount of Hyskon used to less than 500 ml and the frequent monitoring for signs of impending pulmonary edema. Monitoring the serum sodium content and osmolality may also be helpful.

33. Perino, A., et al. Role of leuprolide acetate depot in hysteroscopic surgery: a controlled study. *Fertil. Steril.* 59:507, 1993.

    Preoperative agonist therapy led to a significant reduction in operating time, blood loss, and the amount of distention medium required.

54. HYSTERECTOMY
Michel E. Rivlin

The uterus may be removed through an incision in the abdominal wall. A total abdominal hysterectomy is the removal of both the corpus and cervix. On rare occasions, the cervix may be left in situ; this is a subtotal hysterectomy. An alternative method, vaginal hysterectomy, consists of removal of the uterus through the vagina. At the time of hysterectomy, one or both tubes or ovaries may also be removed. For instance, in postmenopausal patients requiring hysterectomy, it is customary to remove the adnexa, a procedure termed a *bilateral salpingo-oophorectomy.*

Hysterectomy is the second-most common surgical procedure performed in the United States. Annually, over 650,000 women undergo the procedure at a cost of approximately $3 billion. Recent advances in operative techniques, the development of alternative therapies, the reevaluation of indications, and the reassessment of health-care expenditures and cost-benefit analysis are likely to lead to changes in the thinking regarding the procedure, as large differences in hysterectomy rates exist among different countries and even among different regions of the same country. For instance, rates in the Southern United States are one third higher than those in the Northeast. Hysterectomy in the treatment of cancer is discussed in relevant chapters in Section XVI, Gynecologic Oncology.

Leiomyomas, dysfunctional uterine bleeding, and pelvic relaxation account for more than half of the procedures performed. Other indications include adnexal diseases, such as endometriosis or pelvic inflammatory disease (PID), and, in this event, the uterus is removed together with the abnormal adnexa. Obstetric emergencies may necessitate the procedure, although in the absence of preexisting gynecologic abnormalities, hysterectomy during pregnancy should be discouraged because of the increased risk of hemorrhage and urinary tract injury. Hysterectomy for sterilization should generally be performed only when preexisting gynecologic disease or other circumstances warrant the increased risk over alternative procedures. Quality-of-life considerations, including menstrual problems, contraceptive difficulties, and cancer fears, may play an important role in a woman's decision to undergo the operation.

A preoperative workup to rule out the existence of preinvasive or invasive cancer is necessary, including colposcopy, curettage, or cone biopsy, if indicated by the results of Papanicolaou (Pap) smears or endometrial biopsy. In nonurgent cases, anemia and local infections should be treated preoperatively. Many surgeons require that an intravenous pyelogram and barium enema be obtained in patients before the operation. Adequate counseling, especially regarding menstrual, reproductive, and sexual function, is essential, as the procedure carries profound physical and psychologic implications.

The vaginal approach is used in 30 to 35 percent of the hysterectomies. The usual indication for this is pelvic relaxation, although the method is suitable for any hysterectomy in skilled hands, provided no contraindications exist. These contraindications include the presence of intraabdominal or pelvic abnormalities that necessitate abdominal exploration, a uterus too large to remove vaginally, or a narrow subpubic angle that would limit access. The vaginal route is associated with a shorter and more comfortable recovery but a higher incidence of febrile morbidity than the abdominal procedure.

Abdominal hysterectomy is performed through a transverse or vertical abdominal incision. No clear consensus exists regarding the age at which normal ovaries should be removed as prophylaxis against cancer. In view of the adverse effects of castration in terms of menopausal symptoms, osteoporosis, and vascular disease, many gynecologists remove these organs only in perimenopausal or postmenopausal patients. There is no similar controversy regarding the subtotal procedure. It should be reserved only for emergency situations in which operating time is a crucial factor or when technical difficulties render cervical removal hazardous, because the retained cervical stump may cause problems later, including vaginal discharge, infections, and cervical cancer. The safety of total hysterectomy is increased by the use of an intrafascial technique, although this is not suitable for patients with cervical precancer; in these women, an extrafascial approach is indicated.

In performing both vaginal and abdominal hysterectomy, it is important to support the vaginal vault (cuff) with the transverse cervical and uterosacral ligaments as prophylaxis against vault prolapse, an uncommon late complication of hysterectomy. Most gynecologists close the cuff routinely, although many leave it open to provide pelvic drainage if infection is present.

In recent years, a variety of hysterectomy procedures involving laparoscopy have been introduced. These range from diagnostic laparoscopy before vaginal hysterectomy, through laparoscopy-assisted vaginal hysterectomy, in which variable portions of the procedure are begun through the laparoscope with completion of the operation per vaginam, all the way to complete laparoscopic hysterectomy. It is not yet clear what place this new technology will hold in the future, and at present, the number of cases reported is too small to judge morbidity and mortality rates accurately.

Occasionally, postoperative bleeding may occur early or late and may be manifested by frank bleeding or a pelvic hematoma. Vaginal or abdominal resuturing is necessary in most instances, although late hemorrhage from the cuff usually responds to vaginal packing. Postoperative infections are not uncommon and may affect the urinary tract, abdominal or vaginal incisions, adnexa, or lungs. In severe cases, pelvic abscess, peritonitis, wound dehiscence, septicemia, and septic pelvic thrombophlebitis can occur. Febrile morbidity is most common in premenopausal patients undergoing vaginal hysterectomy. The administration of prophylactic antibiotics in high-risk patients has markedly lessened the incidence of all these infectious complications, although their routine use remains controversial. Thromboembolism is a major source of postoperative mortality. The use of low-dose prophylactic heparin may lessen the incidence, especially in patients at high risk, such as the markedly overweight.

Injuries to the bladder, ureters, or bowel are uncommon but, if not recognized and repaired at the time of operation, may lead to serious infections and the formation of urinary or fecal fistulas. Complications common to major abdominal or pelvic procedures, such as anesthetic and blood transfusion problems, drug reaction, and ileus and intestinal obstruction, may also arise.

The emotional and psychosexual sequelae of hysterectomy are of great significance. The incidence of depression after the procedure has been estimated to be two to three times that after other operations. Hormone replacement in premenopausal patients undergoing surgical castration and adequate preoperative and postoperative counseling and support are both important elements of care.

From this review of the complications, although the more serious are uncommon, it is clear that the added risks do not warrant hysterectomy purely for sterilization or as cancer prophylaxis. Nevertheless, it remains one of the safest major procedures, with a death-to-case ratio of 1 to 2 : 1000. The average patient may expect to be discharged from 4 to 5 days after the operation, and few procedures improve the quality of life more than an indicated hysterectomy in a well-informed patient.

Incidence

1. Vessey, M. P., et al. The epidemiology of hysterectomy: findings in a large cohort study. *Br. J. Obstet. Gynaecol.* 99:402, 1992.
   Almost 20 percent of the women in this study from England had had a hysterectomy by age 55.
2. Treloar, S. A., et al. Pathways to hysterectomy: Insights from longitudinal twin research. *Am. J. Obstet. Gynecol.* 167:82, 1992.
   Genetic influences were substantial but the important sources of genetic influence were not identified.
3. Bachmann, G. A. Hysterectomy. A critical review. *J. Reprod. Med.* 35:839, 1990.
   Possibly the most important unresolved aspect is whether removal of the cervix, uterus, or both, influences coital orgasm, lubrication, or satisfaction thereafter.
4. Stergachis, A., et al. Tubal sterilization and the long-term risk of hysterectomy. *J.A.M.A.* 264:2893, 1990.
   Women sterilized while 20 to 29 years old were three to four times more likely to undergo a subsequent hysterectomy. Married women sterilized at age 40 or older exhibit no higher risk. Results did not support a biologic basis for the relationship between tubal sterilization and hysterectomy.

Series

5. Browne, D. S., and Frazer, M. I. Hysterectomy revisited. *Aust. N.Z. J. Obstet. Gynaecol.* 31:148, 1991.
   More than 80 percent of the hysterectomies in this series were performed by the vaginal route. The indications for abdominal hysterectomy are the contraindications to the vaginal procedure.
6. Reiter, R. C., Gambone, J. C., and Lench, J. B. Appropriateness of hysterectomies performed for multiple preoperative indications. *Obstet. Gynecol.* 80:902, 1992.
   In this series, multiple indications were found to correlate with decreased diagnostic accuracy and decreased compliance with preoperative validation criteria.
7. Suchartwatnachai, C., Linasmita V., and Chaturachinda, K. Obstetric hysterectomy: Ramathibodi's experience 1969–1987. *Int. J. Gynaecol. Obstet.* 36:183, 1991.
   The indications for emergency obstetric hysterectomy generally include uterine rupture, placental disorders, and extension of the incision during cesarean section.
8. Summitt, R. L., Jr., et al. Randomized comparison of laparoscopy-assisted vaginal hysterectomy with standard vaginal hysterectomy in an outpatient setting. *Obstet. Gynecol.* 80:895, 1992.
   New surgical technology should be applied cautiously and prudently.

Management

9. Jaszczak, S. E., and Evans, T. N. Intrafascial abdominal and vaginal hysterectomy: a reappraisal. *Obstet. Gynecol.* 49:435, 1982.

Intrafascial dissection, clamping, and cuff closure lessens the risk of urinary tract and bowel injury.

10. Sack, R. A. The value of intravenous urography prior to abdominal hysterectomy for gynecologic disease. *Am. J. Obstet. Gynecol.* 134:208, 1979.
Benefits from intravenous urography include the demonstration of unsuspected pathology, defense against malpractice suits, and assistance in the prevention of urinary tract injury.

11. Williams, T. J., Johnson, T. R., and Pratt, J. H. Time interval between cervical conization and hysterectomy. *Am. J. Obstet. Gynecol.* 107:790, 1970.
Unless hysterectomy is done within 48 hours of conization, 6 weeks should elapse before proceeding, as an increase in morbidity is otherwise likely.

12. Pratt, J. H., and Jefferies, J. A. Retained cervical stump: a 25-year experience. *Obstet. Gynecol.* 48:711, 1976.
The indications for removal of the cervix after a subtotal hysterectomy appear to be similar to the indications for removal when the rest of the uterus is still present.

13. Kim, Y. B., DuBeshter, B., and Niloff, J. M. Continuous single-layer closure of midline abdominal incisions in high-risk gynecologic patients. *J. Gynecol. Surg.* 8:15, 1992.
The incidence of disruption of a suture line (dehiscence) ranges from 0.28 to 0.51 percent for abdominal hysterectomy. Obesity, anemia, vertical incision, and medical disorders (diabetes and renal) are all risk factors. Closure of a vertical incision should utilize the Smead-Jones technique with a nonabsorbable suture.

The Ovaries

14. Siddle, N., Sarrel, P., and Whitehead, M. The effect of hysterectomy on the age at ovarian failure: identification of a subgroup of women with premature loss of ovarian function and literature review. *Fertil. Steril.* 47:94, 1987.
The mean age of ovarian failure in the group undergoing hysterectomy was 45.4 years, which was significantly lower than the mean age of 49.5 years in the control group made up of women not undergoing hysterectomy.

15. Colditz, G. A., et al. Menopause and the risk of coronary heart disease in women. *N. Engl. J. Med.* 316:1105, 1987.
Women who underwent bilateral ovariectomy and women who never received estrogens had more than double the risk of coronary heart disease of the index group of premenopausal women. Women who went through a natural menopause without estrogen replacement or women who underwent ovariectomy with replacement estrogens did not exhibit an increased risk.

16. Centerwall, B. S. Premenopausal hysterectomy and cardiovascular disease. *Am. J. Obstet. Gynecol.* 139:58, 1981.
The incidence of cardiovascular disease when hysterectomy with ovarian conservation was performed was calculated to be 2.6 to 5 times that in control populations. There was a 4 percent chance of a myocardial infarction within 10 years of the procedure.

17. Bukovsky, L., et al. Ovarian residual syndrome. *Surg. Gynecol. Obstet.* 167:132, 1988.
In 1 to 3 percent of cases in which one or both ovaries are retained at the time of hysterectomy, subsequent symptoms of lower abdominal and back pain, deep dyspareunia, and urinary complaints may necessitate removal of the residual adnexa.

18. Pettit, P. D., and Lee, R. A. Ovarian remnant syndrome: Diagnostic dilemma and surgical challenge. *Obstet. Gynecol.* 71:580, 1988.
The patient who has pain after undergoing bilateral oophorectomy (usually for endometriosis) may harbor remnants of ovarian tissue, whether or not a mass is present. Surgical correction requires mobilization of the ureter throughout its entire pelvic course to facilitate resection of the mass.

19. Parazzini, F., et al. Hysterectomy, oophorectomy, and subsequent ovarian cancer risk. *Obstet. Gynecol.* 81:363, 1993.
Hysterectomy halves the risk of ovarian cancer, possibly because it permits the opportunity to examine the ovaries or because it leads to altered ovarian blood flow.

Infection
20. Hemsell, D. L., et al. Cefazolin for hysterectomy prophylaxis. *Obstet. Gynecol.* 76:603, 1990.
    Antimicrobial prophylaxis for vaginal hysterectomy is generally indicated, whereas for abdominal hysterectomy, it should be reserved for patients at high risk for infection. A single dose, given relatively soon before operation, of an antibiotic active against either aerobic or anaerobic flora is recommended. The pharmacokinetics and antimicrobial spectrum of an agent, although paramount in determining the efficacy for established infection, have little impact in terms of prophylactic efficacy.
21. Hemsell, D. L. Major Posthysterectomy Infections: Diagnosis and Management. In H. J. Buchsbaum and L. A. Walton (eds.), *Strategies in Gynecology Surgery.* New York: Springer-Verlag, 1988.
    Fever during the first 24 to 48 hours is usually pulmonary in origin, requiring treatment of atelectasis. A pelvic abscess or cuff abscess, on the other hand, causes fever at about 72 hours. Wound infections become evident at about the third day, with the exception of clostridial or streptococcal infections, which present earlier.

Complications
22. Perineau, M., Monrozies, X., and Reme, J. M. Complications of hysterectomy. *Rev. Fr. Gynecol. Obstet.* 87:120, 1992.
    A delayed complication of a subclinical hemorrhage is hematoma. Most are self-limiting and resolve. Drainage is unnecessary, unless there is infection or the location relative to the vaginal cuff allows easy access.
23. Bakri, Y. N., and Linjawi, T. Angiographic embolization for control of pelvic genital tract hemorrhage: report of 14 cases. *Acta Obstet. Gynecol. Scand.* 71:17, 1992.
    Approximately 30 percent of the blood volume is lost before a significant drop in blood pressure occurs. In the event of postoperative hypovolemic shock, an immediate return to the operating room is mandated. In less acute cases, restoration of the blood volume in conjunction with angiographic embolization of the bleeding vessel is possible.
24. Rosenzweig, B. A., et al. Urologic injury during vaginal hysterectomy: a case-control study. *J. Gynecol. Surg.* 6:27, 1990.
    Many vesicovaginal fistulas develop from an unsuspected bladder injury. It is recommended that, after a difficult dissection, the bladder should be distended with fluid or a dye solution to rule out such an injury.
25. Shaikh, N., Saveranamuthu, J., and Williams, G. Ureteric injury unrecognised during gynaecological operations. *J. Obstet. Gynecol.* 12:133, 1992.
    Bleeding is a common problem that attends pelvic procedures, and can lead to ureteral injury. Direct pressure can control most bleeding. The ureter and the bleeding point are positively identified before suturing or cauterizing, to ensure hemostasis without ureteral damage.
26. Farghaly, S. A., Hindmarsh, J. R., and Worth, P. H. L. Posthysterectomy urethral dysfunction: evaluation and management. *Br. J. Urol.* 58:299, 1986.
    Posthysterectomy urethral dysfunctions can occur secondary to injury to pelvic nerves, postoperative bladder changes, accidental lesions caused by inadequate postoperative bladder drainage, and urinary tract infections.
27. Clark-Pearson, D. L., et al. Variables associated with postoperative deep venous thrombosis: a prospective study of 411 gynecology patients and creation of a prognostic model. *Obstet. Gynecol.* 69:147, 1987.
    Patients at high risk for thrombosis benefit from low-dose prophylactic heparin (5000 units every 12 hours subcutaneously). This must be started 2 hours before operation, as thrombosis can occur intraoperatively.
28. Kvist-Poulsen, H., and Borel, J. Iatrogenic femoral neuropathy subsequent to abdominal hysterectomy: incidence and prevention. *Obstet. Gynecol.* 60:516, 1982.
    Femoral neuropathy with thigh numbness, paresthesia, and weakness may result from improper positioning in the stirrups with marked thigh flexing or nerve

stretching, or from retractor pressure on the psoas muscles through which the nerve runs. Perineal or sciatic nerve damage may occur in the lithotomy position resulting from compression along the leg or buttock.

29. Lalinec-Michaud, M., Englesmann, F., and Marino, J. Depression after hysterectomy: a comparative study. *Psychosomatics* 29:307, 1988.

In contrast to others, this study revealed a general decrease in the depression scores after operation, and hysterectomy patients did not differ from other groups of patients in terms of depression scores, quality of sexual life, postoperative adjustment, or relationship to partner.

30. Helström, L., et al. Sexuality after hysterectomy: a factor analysis of women's sexual lives before and after subtotal hysterectomy. *Obstet. Gynecol.* 81:357, 1993.

Some Swedish surgeons routinely perform subtotal hysterectomy for the treatment of nonmalignant disorders, believing that total hysterectomy adversely affects later sexual function.

31. Stuart, G. C. E., Allen, H. H., and Anderson, R. J. Squamous cell carcinoma of the vagina following hysterectomy. *Am. J. Obstet. Gynecol.* 139:311, 1981.

This analysis of 29 cases revealed the importance of follow-up, as vaginal cancer may follow hysterectomy for either cervical dysplasia or for an unrelated disease.

XI. INFECTIOUS AND VENEREAL DISEASES

55. GONORRHEA

Michel E. Rivlin

Neisseria gonorrhoeae is the causative agent of gonorrhea (GC), an infection that primarily involves the mucous membranes of the genitourinary tract, pharynx, and anus. The organism is a gram-negative diplococcus found in polymorphonuclear leukocytes. The virulence of the organism is associated with specific colony types. Only those that contain pili are capable of producing infection. Pili are proteinaceous surface appendages and are the primary mediators of attachment. Piliated gonococci have been shown to adhere to sperm and a variety of human epithelial cells. Colonies isolated from men with uncomplicated infection and from the endocervix in women are opaque, whereas colonies isolated in the setting of disseminated infection and the endocervix during menstruation are transparent. Gonococcal typing is essential for carrying out effective epidemiologic study. Auxotyping entails identifying the specific nutritional requirements of the organism; the most common is the wild type (requiring no additives). Auxotypes correlate well with patterns of infection and antibiotic sensitivity. Thus, arginine, hypoxanthine, and uracil–requiring (AHU) strains are associated with disseminated infection and are very sensitive to antibiotics. A less useful typing method is plasmid analysis. In 1976, strains of gonococci were found to contain an extrachromosomal deoxyribonucleic acid (DNA), a plasmid, which produces beta-lactamase, and this in turn inactivates penicillin. Similar strains of penicillinase-producing *N. gonorrhoeae* (PPNG) have since appeared worldwide. Another resistant strain that has appeared is beta-lactamase negative. Chromosomally mediated resistant *N. gonorrhoeae* (CMRNG) has intranuclear DNA that renders the cell membrane impermeable to penicillin. Both PPNG and CMRNG respond to therapy with either spectinomycin, quinolones or a third-generation cephalosporin. More recently, CMRNG strains resistant to tetracycline and spectinomycin have been recognized. Finally, serology is used to type the organism, often in conjunction with auxotyping, and this yields information on the auxotype/serovar classes.

The current epidemic of GC started in 1957, peaked in 1975, and is decreasing at approximately 1 percent per year, except in the young age group (15 to 19 years), in which the increase continues. The estimated annual incidence of infection in the United States is 1.3 to 2 million; the male to female ratio is 1.5:1. This ratio is reversed in young teenagers. Prevalence rates vary from 1 to 25 percent, depending on the population sampled. Risk factors include young age (15 to 24 years), an increased number of sex partners, and nonuse of barrier contraception. Transmission is almost entirely accomplished by sexual contact. A male has a 20 to 25 percent risk and a female has an 80 to 90 percent risk of transmission per single sexual contact. There is a short incubation time of 3 to 5 days, but this can range from 1 to 14 days. In adults, transmission can take place after fellatio and genital-rectal exposure, in addition to genital intercourse. In children, besides sexual exposure, nonsexual contact with the infectious discharge may lead to vaginal or ocular infection.

Uncomplicated urogenital or anal infection is frequently asymptomatic. There is a much higher prevalence of signs and symptoms in women who seek care, including dysuria, suprapubic discomfort, purulent cervical discharge, intermenstrual spotting and bleeding, or menorrhagia. The cervix or urethra, or both, may be red and edematous, and there may be a purulent discharge. Pharyngitis may be present with edema, erythema, and complaints of sore throat, or it may be asymptomatic. Proctitis may be associated with blood and pus in stools and diffuse erythema, or it may be asymptomatic. Ophthalmia neonatorum arises between 2 and 3 days after delivery and symptoms consist of bilateral conjunctivitis and a profuse purulent discharge. If left untreated, corneal ulceration and scarring occur. In 15 to 20 percent of women with uncomplicated anogenital GC, upper genital tract infection (pelvic inflammatory disease [PID]) occurs, usually at the end of or just after menstruation (see Chap. 63). Gonococcal vaginitis is rare, although it may be seen in prepubertal and postmenopausal females. Perihepatitis (Fitz-Hugh-Curtis syndrome) may be found in conjunction with PID, and results from either the direct or contiguous spread of the infection. Disseminated gonococcal infection (DGI) affects 1 to 3 percent of infected patients, but predominates in women, showing a female to male ratio of approximately 4:1. This usually appears during pregnancy, especially in the third trimester or within 7 days of the onset of menses. DGI manifests an early bacteremic stage consisting of chills, fever, and a dermatitis that includes a variety of skin lesions of gonococcal emboli that are asymmetrically distributed. These start as a macule, which becomes vesicular, pustular, and then purpuric, and are mostly seen on the hands, fingers, feet, and toes. Blood cultures are positive in half of the patients during this stage. Joint symptoms are frequently present and are then characteristic of the later septic arthritis stage, in which purulent synovial effusions occur commonly in the knees, ankles, and wrists. Tenosynovitis, involving the extensor and flexor tendons of the hands and feet, is also a common finding. Patients also experience erythema, swelling, tenderness, and pain on motion along the tendon sheath.

Culture of the organism is the gold standard for the diagnosis of GC. To obtain material for culture, a dry, sterile cotton-tipped swab is inserted into the endocervical canal; this is moved from side to side, and, after 15 to 30 seconds, organisms should be absorbed into the swab. (A single endocervical swab will miss approximately 10 percent of GC infections.) Ideally, the specimen is cultured directly onto selective medium (Thayer-Martin) and incubated immediately at 36°C in 5 to 7% carbon dioxide (a candle jar provides an adequate concentration of carbon dioxide). Fermentation reactions differentiate *N. gonorrhoeae* from *Neisseria meningitidis*. The former ferments glucose, the latter, maltose. Microscopic examination of a Gram's-stained specimen obtained from the infected site yields diagnostic findings of GC in only 40 to 50 percent of women, compared with 95 percent of men. The Gonozyme test is a solid-phase enzyme immunoassay (ELISA) for detecting gonococcal antigens and is more sensitive than Gram's staining (78–100%), but the specificity is variable (70–100%). The number of false-positive results that this would produce, particularly in low-prevalence populations, has consequently limited use of the test. Depending on the patient's history, samples may be taken from the urethra, pharynx, or rectum, in addition to the endocervical sample. Furthermore, blood testing for syphilis is indicated if GC is diagnosed. The differential diagnosis includes trichomoniasis, candidiasis, anaerobic vaginosis, herpes, and chlamydial cervicitis.

The Centers for Disease Control (CDC) has recommended regimens for the treatment of uncomplicated anogenital GC, and these include concomitant therapy for coexisting *Chlamydia* infection, as this organism is found in up to 45 percent of GC cases. A single-dose regimen is given for the treatment of GC and this is followed by doxycycline for the *Chlamydia* infection. Ceftriaxone (125 mg, intramuscularly) and, thereafter, doxycycline (100 mg twice daily for 7 days orally) are given. Alternatively, azithromycin may be given in a single 1-g dose for the chlamydial infection. If tetracyclines are either contraindicated (during pregnancy and in children) or not tolerated, erythromycin ethylsuccinate (800 mg four times daily) may be substituted. For patients who cannot take ceftriaxone, ciprofloxacin (500 mg, orally) or ofloxacin (400 mg, orally) or cefixime (400 mg, orally) is recommended. Other alternatives include spectinomycin (2 g, intramuscularly), cefoxitin (1 g, intramuscularly), cefotetan (1 g, intramuscularly), cefotaxime (500 mg), cefuroxime axetil (1 g, orally), enoxacin (400 mg, orally), or lomefloxacin (400 mg, orally). In the proven absence of penicillin resistance, a penicillin such as amoxicillin (500 mg four times daily) may be given. Pharyngeal infections should be treated with ceftriaxone; patients who cannot receive ceftriaxone should be treated with ciprofloxacin. Patients with incubating syphilis are likely to be cured by all the aforementioned regimens other than spectinomycin and the quinolones.

The disease is notifiable and contacts should be identified, examined, cultured, and treated presumptively. Follow-up culture ("test of cure") after combined ceftriaxone and doxycycline therapy is not essential, as failure is rare. Reculture 1 to 2 months later ("rescreening") can detect both failures and reinfections. Those patients with persistent symptoms or those treated with alternative regimens should have a culture performed 4 to 7 days after therapy. If GC persists after treatment, determination of antibiotic sensitivities is indicated, though reinfection is more commonly the problem than is resistance. Additional therapy with ceftriaxone and doxycycline should be carried out.

The endocervical GC culture should be done at the first visit in pregnant women and repeated in late pregnancy in high-risk cases. The treatment regimens in pregnant women are the same as those in nonpregnant women, except for quinolones and doxycycline, which are contraindicated in pregnancy. The therapy for PID is discussed in Chapter 63. Patients with DGI should be hospitalized for therapy, the details of which are beyond the scope of this chapter. Infants born to mothers with untreated GC should be treated, and those with GC ophthalmia require parenteral therapy. The dosage schedules for this are included in the CDC recommendations.

The major long-term complications of GC include PID and the sequelae of PID, such as ectopic pregnancy, infertility, and chronic pelvic pain (see Chap. 63). More recently, an association between maternal gonorrhea and DGI, and perinatal complications, such as premature ruptured membranes, chorioamnionitis, prematurity, intrauterine growth retardation, neonatal sepsis, and postpartum endometritis, has been recognized. The gonococcus is a highly adapted pathogen that has acquired or developed antibiotic resistance and possesses surface structures that can undergo phase and antigenic variation, ensuring the continuing high prevalence of the disease. The search for a vaccine continues; the ideal candidate would have conserved antigenic components common to all gonococci.

Review
1. Easmon, C. S. F., and Ison, C. A. *Neisseria gonorrhoeae*: A versatile pathogen. *J. Clin. Pathol.* 40:1088, 1987.
   Widespread use and abuse of beta-lactam–producing agents, together with increasing global travel, have facilitated the dissemination of antibiotic-resistant gonococci.
2. Sehgal, V. N., and Srivastava, G. Gonorrhea and the story of resistant *Neisseria gonorrhoeae*. *Int. J. Dermatol.* 26:206, 1987.
   Includes a discussion of tetracycline-resistant N. gonorrhoeae.

Epidemiology
3. Pencillinase-producing *Neisseria gonorrhoeae*—United States, 1986. *M.M.W.R.* 36:107, 1987.
   Beta-lactamase produced by the gonococcus hydrolyzes the beta-lactam ring of the antibiotic's molecule. The ability to produce the enzyme is transmitted in a plasmid, a small extranuclear DNA particle.
4. Schwarcz, S. K., et al. National surveillance of antimicrobial resistance in *Neisseria gonorrhoeae*. *J.A.M.A.* 264:1413, 1990.
   In 1991, the CDC reported that roughly 30 percent of gonococcal isolates in the United States were resistant to one or more antibiotics.
5. Schwarcz, S. K., et al. Crack cocaine and the exchange of sex for money or drugs. Risk factors for gonorrhea among black adolescents in San Francisco. *Sex. Transm. Dis.* 19:7, 1992.
   In addition to the classic sexually transmitted diseases, there are no fewer than twenty others.
6. Pereira, L. H., et al. Prevalence of human immunodeficiency virus in the patient population of a sexually transmitted disease clinic. *Sex. Transm. Dis.* 19:115, 1992.
   The likelihood of human immunodeficiency virus transmission is increased in the setting of sexually transmitted diseases.

Genital Gonorrhea
7. Louv, W. C., et al. Oral contraceptive use and the risk of chlamydial and gonococcal infections. *Am. J. Obstet. Gynecol.* 160:396, 1989.

Oral contraceptive led to an approximately 70 percent increase in the infection rates for both conditions.
8. Philpot, C. R., and Tapsall, J. W. Single-dose antibiotic therapy for the treatment of uncomplicated anogenital gonorrhoea. *Med. J. Aust.* 146:254, 1987.
Of females with GC, 44 percent had a positive anorectal culture; 10 percent had only a positive anorectal culture.
9. Niruthisard, S., Roddy, R. E., and Chutivongse, S. Use of nonoxynol-9 and reduction rate of gonococcal and chlamydial cervical infections. *Lancet* 339:1371, 1992.
Spermicides together with a diaphragm or condom can bring about an appreciable decrease in the risk of acquiring GC.

Extragenital Gonorrhea
10. Rompalo, A. M., et al. The acute arthritis-dermatitis syndrome. The changing importance of *Neisseria gonorrhoeae* and *Neisseria meningitidis*. *Arch. Intern. Med.* 147:281, 1987.
The early (septicemic) phase of migratory polyarthritis with fever is followed by a septic phase, consisting of inflammation and effusion in one joint. Blood culture is diagnostic in the early phase and joint culture in the later phase.
11. Suleiman, S. A., Grimes, E. M., and Jones, H. S. Disseminated gonococcal infections. *Obstet. Gynecol.* 61:48, 1983.
Disseminated disease is more common in the presence of asymptomatic than of symptomatic infection.
12. Laga, M., et al. Prophylaxis of gonococcal and chlamydial ophthalmia neonatorum. A comparison of silver nitrate and tetracycline. *N. Engl. J. Med.* 318:653, 1988.
Ophthalmic ointments or drops containing tetracycline or erythromycin should be instilled into the conjunctiva of all newborns to protect against gonococcal and chlamydial conjunctivitis.
13. Smith, L. G., Jr., et al. Gonococcal chorioamnionitis associated with sepsis: a case report. *Am. J. Obstet. Gynecol.* 160:573, 1989.
These authors present evidence suggestive of transplacental spread.

Diagnosis
14. Lieberman, R. W., and Wheelock, J. B. The diagnosis of gonorrhea in a low-prevalence female population: enzyme immunoassay versus culture. *Obstet. Gynecol.* 69:743, 1987.
In a high-incidence population, the predictive values of a positive and negative Gonozyme result are 96.4 and 97.1 percent, respectively; however, in a low-incidence population, the predictive value of a positive result was only 55.1 percent, mandating culture for confirmation.
15. Schink, J. C., and Keight, L. G. Problems in the culture diagnosis of gonorrhea. *J. Reprod. Med.* 30:244, 1985.
When culture specimens are transported elsewhere for testing, instead of tested on-site, 16 percent fewer infections are detected.

Treatment
16. Centers for Disease Control. 1993 Sexually transmitted diseases treatment guidelines. *M.M.W.R.* 42(RR-14): Sept. 24, 1993.
This contains recommendations for the treatment of uncomplicated, complicated, and disseminated disease as well as resistant organisms in adults, children, neonates, and pregnant women.
17. Plourde, P. J., et al. Single-dose cefixime versus single-dose ceftriaxone in the treatment of antimicrobial-resistant *Neisseria gonorrhoeae* infection. *J. Infect. Dis.* 166:919, 1992.
A single oral 400-mg dose of cefixime was an effective alternative to ceftriaxone in the treatment of uncomplicated gonococcal cervicitis.
18. Kaplowitz, L. G., et al. Norfloxacin in the treatment of uncomplicated gonococcal infections. *Am. J. Med.* 82:35, 1987.

Many antibiotics are effective against GC. These include the cephalosporins such as ceftazidime and cefoxitin; combinations of ampicillin or amoxicillin with beta-lactamase inhibitors such as clavulanic acid and sulbactam; aminoglycosides; and newer agents such as the monobactams and quinolones.

19. Yeung, K. H., and Dillon, J. R. Norfloxacin-resistant *Neisseria gonorrhoeae* in North America (letter). *Lancet* 336:759, 1990.
   Quinolones have a high tendency to induce resistance in N. gonorrhoeae organisms and are not considered safe for pregnant women or children.
20. Cavenee, M. R., et al. Treatment of gonorrhea in pregnancy. *Obstet. Gynecol.* 81:33, 1993.
   Repeat cultures during the third trimester are recommended for any patient treated for GC earlier in that pregnancy.
21. Handsfield, H. H., et al. Evaluation of new anti-infective agents for the treatment of uncomplicated gonorrhea in adults and adolescents. *Clin. Infect. Dis.* 15:5123, 1992.
   The lower limit of the 95 percent confidence interval for the efficacy of an antibiotic should not be less than 90 percent.

56. SYPHILIS
Michel E. Rivlin

Syphilis is a sexually transmitted disease caused by *Treponema pallidum*, a spirochete with a length of 6 to 15 mm and a width of only 0.15 mm, which is not easily grown in vitro. On dark-field microscopic examination, the organism is observed to exhibit a rotatory motion. Serologic studies provide the usual means of diagnosis. From 1985 to 1989, the incidence of syphilis in the United States increased by 61 percent to 18.4 cases per 100,000 population. This increase has primarily occurred among inner-city ethnic groups of low socioeconomic status. There was a 132 percent jump in the incidence among African-Americans, with a larger increase among women than men. This has led to a similar rise in the number of cases of congenital syphilis. This increase in the syphilis rates is associated with drug use, drug-related sexual behavior, prostitution, and the use of gonococcal therapies, such as spectinomycin and the quinolones, which, unlike penicillin, are not therapeutic for incubating syphilis. There is a suggestion that genital ulcer diseases, including syphilis, augment the likelihood of human immunodeficiency virus (HIV) acquisition or transmission. It is also possible, but not proved, that patients with HIV infection may be subject to more aggressive syphilitic infections and that the responses to therapy may be less successful in these patients.

The transmission of syphilis by sexual contact requires exposure to moist mucosal or cutaneous lesions. The incubation period before the primary lesion develops at the site of initial inoculation ranges from 10 to 90 days, with an average of 21 days. The chancre (the initial lesion of primary syphilis) is usually solitary, although multiple lesions can occur. It begins as a papule that erodes and ulcerates. It is usually painless, punched out, and clean with raised borders. The entire lesion is indurated, and draining lymph nodes are enlarged, hard, and nontender. The lesions are usually genital. Extragenital sites include the lips, tongue, tonsils, fingers, nipples, and anus. Diagnosis at this stage may be based on the findings from dark-field examination of a direct scraping from the lesion. The results of serologic tests are often negative initially. The differential diagnosis includes neoplasm, chancroid, lymphogranuloma venereum, granuloma inguinale, herpes, and fungal infection. Untreated, the chancre heals in a few weeks.

Within a few weeks or months, secondary syphilis may develop. This is a stage of spirochetemia that can involve any cutaneous or mucosal surface as well as any organ. Four major syndromes may be seen: rash, a generalized lymphadenopathy, a flulike illness, and visceral involvement. The skin lesions are usually dry and symmetrical and are most marked on the palms and soles. In warm, moist areas, such as the perineum, condylomata lata may form. Lesions may occur on mucosal surfaces and are called mucous patches; these are found in about 30 percent of the patients, generally in the mouth, palate, and pharynx. Organs that may be involved include the liver (10%) and long bones (rarely). The skin lesions must be differentiated from common skin eruptions, including drug reactions and acute exanthemata. Serology results are invariably positive and, like the chancre, the lesions are highly infective. In the latent stage that follows, there are no clinical signs, and the diagnosis is based on positive serology findings in the absence of concurrent disease that may produce a false-positive reaction. The early latent phase begins after the the first attack of secondary syphilis has passed and lasts for about 1 year. Late latent syphilis is rarely infectious, except that the pregnant woman may transmit infection to the fetus regardless of the duration of the illness. Tertiary syphilis is manifested by a diffuse vascular disease and the formation of lesions, termed gummas, that may occur throughout the body. It arises many years after the secondary stage of syphilis in about 30 percent of untreated patients. Most commonly, the cardiovascular and central nervous systems are involved. Serology is usually reactive. The clinical spectrum of syphilis acquired in utero includes stillbirth, neonatal death, neonatal illness in the first months of life, and development of the stigmata of congenital syphilis in later life.

Two blood tests are commonly performed for the detection of syphilis: a reagin test, such as the rapid plasma reagin (RPR) or the Venereal Disease Research Laboratory (VDRL) test, and a treponemal test, such as the fluorescent treponemal antibody–absorption (FTA-ABS) test. The preferred test for both screening and monitoring a patient's response to treatment is the VDRL test. The test result becomes positive 1 or 2 weeks after the appearance of the chancre. It is positive in about 66 percent of the primary cases, 99 percent of the secondary cases, and 70 percent of the tertiary cases. False-positive results may occur transiently in the setting of acute febrile illnesses, immunizations, and pregnancy. Repeated false-positive results may be caused by other chronic infections (e.g., chronic active hepatitis), autoimmune diseases (e.g., systemic lupus erythematosus), or narcotic addiction. The false-positive VDRL titer is usually low (no more than 1:8). The FTA-ABS test is used as a confirmatory test. Results are positive in 85 percent of the primary and 100 percent of the secondary cases, and it may be the only positive test result in patients with tertiary syphilis. False-positive results may occur in patients with diseases associated with hypergammaglobulinemia, although the VDRL result is usually negative in these diseases. Treponemal tests are expensive and not quantitative. Once results are positive, they do not reverse. They are not, therefore, used for either screening or evaluating the response to treatment. Mothers with treated syphilis may passively transfer immunoglobulin G (IgG) to the fetus, resulting in positive serology findings in the newborn. Because maternal immunoglobulin M (IgM) is not passively transferred, an IgM–FTA-ABS is used to diagnose congenital infection. Unfortunately, there is a 35 percent false-negative and 10 percent false-positive rate associated with the test. Many physicians therefore choose to treat all VDRL-positive neonates. Cerebrospinal fluid (CSF) examination, consisting of serology plus a search for cells and determination of the protein content, is essential in all syphilitics with unexplained neurologic abnormalities. The Centers for Disease Control (CDC) also recommends CSF examination for any patient with syphilis that has lasted for more than 1 year, or an undetermined duration, to rule out neurosyphilis.

Penicillin is the drug of choice for treating all stages of syphilis, and resistance of the organism to the antibiotic has never been described. The CDC recommendations for primary, secondary, or latent (<1 year) infection are to administer a depot form of the drug (benzathine penicillin G; 2.4 million units intramuscularly as a single dose). In penicillin-allergic patients, doxycycline (100 mg 2 times a day for 14 days) or, in those unable to tolerate that drug, erythromycin four times a day (500 mg for 14 days) is recommended. Ceftriaxone has also been recommended as an alternative therapy, but there is only limited experience with this regimen. For patients with late latent infection (>1 year), the penicillin regimen is extended to three injections administered at weekly intervals, and the duration of therapy with the alternative drugs is increased to 30 days. The therapy for neurosyphilis and congenital syphilis is beyond the scope of this manual. The therapy in pregnant women is the same, except that doxycycline is contraindicated; in addition, the fetal levels achieved with erythromycin are only 6 to 20 percent of the maternal levels. The CDC recommendations have therefore been modified for pregnancy, in that penicillin is deemed the only acceptable therapy. If allergy to penicillin is documented by skin testing, reactive patients should be desensitized in consultation with an expert, and penicillin given only where adequate emergency facilities are available.

After the initiation of antibiotic therapy, the Jarisch-Herxheimer reaction may occur. This is an acute flulike syndrome that peaks by 12 hours and resolves by 24 hours. Treatment is symptomatic and consists of antipyretics and fluids. Patients may resume sexual activity once the lesions have healed, and from 7 to 10 days after a complete course of therapy. Follow-up is accomplished by repeat quantitative nontreponemal tests performed at 3, 6, and 12 months after treatment. Repeat treatment is indicated if the VDRL titer increases fourfold or fails to decrease fourfold within a year. The retreatment schedules are the same as those for syphilis of more than 1 year's duration. Careful follow-up is particularly important in patients treated with antibiotics other than penicillin. In the setting of late syphilis, the titers may not decrease, and, if there are no other signs of disease activity, this is not an indication for retreatment. Cases of syphilis should be reported to the local or state health department within 48 hours of diagnosis, which can usually offer referral and follow-up services. Sexual partners of the patient are notified without identification of the index case.

Review
1. Buckley, H. B. Syphilis: a review and update of the 'new' infection of the '90s. *Nurse Pract.* 17:25, 1992.
   The stages of syphilis are used as a guide for therapy, as well as to indicate the duration of the disease and identify the infectious individual.
2. Farnes, S. W., and Setness, P. A. Serologic tests for syphilis. *Postgrad. Med.* 87:37, 1990.
   Acute false-positive results occur in 1 to 2 percent of the general population, and may reflect febrile or viral illness, the effects of immunizations, other spirochetal infections, or pregnancy.

Syphilis in Pregnancy
3. Wendel, G. D. Gestational and congenital syphilis. *Clin. Perinatol.* 15:287, 1988.
   Maternal follow-up should include a monthly nontreponemal serologic test for syphilis for the remainder of pregnancy. Retreatment is necessary for women who exhibit a fourfold rise in the test titer or who do not show a fourfold decrease in the titer within 3 months of treatment.
4. Hutchinson, C. M., and Hook, E. W. Syphilis in adults. *Med. Clin. North Am.* 74:1389, 1990.
   Premature labor or fetal distress may be precipitated by the Jarisch-Herxheimer reaction in the second half of pregnancy.
5. Barton, J. R., et al. Nonimmune hydrops fetalis associated with maternal infection with syphilis. *Am. J. Obstet. Gynecol.* 167:56, 1992.
   Fetuses with hydrops as a result of maternal syphilis survived the perinatal period after penicillin therapy and preterm delivery.
6. Wendel, G. D., Jr., et al. Identification of *Treponema pallidum* in amniotic fluid and fetal blood from pregnancies complicated by congenital syphilis. *Obstet. Gynecol.* 78:890, 1991.
   The first report of the diagnosis of fetal syphilis accomplished by funipuncture.
7. Stoll, B. J., et al. Clinical and serologic evaluation of neonates for congenital syphilis: a continuing diagnostic dilemma. *J. Infect. Dis.* 167:1093, 1993.
   A major problem is the inability to identify which asymptomatic but possibly infected neonate is really uninfected.

8. Chhabra, R. S. Comparison of maternal sera, cord blood, and neonatal sera for detecting presumptive congenital syphilis: relationship with maternal treatment. *Pediatrics* 91:88, 1993.
   Maternal treatment during pregnancy was not associated with a lower incidence of positive maternal serology findings nor with lower maternal titers at the time of delivery.

Epidemiology
9. Rolfs, R. T., and Nakashima, A. K. Epidemiology of primary and secondary syphilis in the United States, 1981 through 1989. *J.A.M.A.* 264:1432, 1990.
   In Philadelphia, from 1985 through 1989, the number of cases of early syphilis increased by 551 percent, from 696 to 4528 cases per year.
10. Andrews, J. K., et al. Partner notification: can it control epidemic syphilis? *Ann. Intern. Med.* 112:539, 1990.
    The trading of sex for drugs at crack houses encourages frequent sexual encounters with anonymous partners, rendering traditional methods of contact tracing much less effective.
11. Centers for Disease Control. Progress toward achieving the 1990 objectives for the nation for sexually transmitted diseases. *M.M.W.R.* 39:53, 1990.
    All sexually transmitted diseases are inextricably linked—behaviorally, epidemiologically, biologically, clinically, economically, organizationally, and historically. Health professionals should build on the similarities and draw on their common skills in the prevention of sexually transmitted diseases.

Diagnosis
12. Hira, S. K., et al. Clinical manifestations of secondary syphilis. *Int. J. Dermatol.* 26:103, 1987.
    Do not believe that lumbar puncture in the search for evidence of neurosyphilis is necessary in patients with secondary syphilis.
13. Feder, H. M., Jr., and Manthous, C. The asymptomatic patient with a positive VDRL test. *Am. Fam. Physician* 3:185, 1988.
    A patient with a low VDRL or RPR titer may have active disease. Lumbar puncture is indicated (1) for patients with possible congenital syphilis or with signs or symptoms of neurosyphilis; (2) before nonpenicillin treatment of latent or tertiary syphilis; and (3) in cases of syphilis treatment failure.
14. Shew, M. L., and Fortenberry, J. D. Syphilis screening in adolescents. *J. Adolesc. Health* 13:303, 1992.
    In areas where there is a high incidence of infection, screening should be carried out in high-risk groups (prostitutes, male homosexuals, intravenous drug users, and those with other sexually transmitted diseases).
15. Sanchez, P. J., et al. Molecular analysis of the fetal IgM response to *Treponema pallidum* antigens: implications for improved serodiagnosis of congenital syphilis. *J. Infect. Dis.* 159:508, 1989.
    IgG can be passively transferred from the mother, but IgM is not transferred. Fetal serum IgM reactivity can therefore be used as an important molecular marker for the diagnosis of congenital syphilis.

Treatment
16. Centers for Disease Control. 1993 Sexually transmitted diseases treatment guidelines. *M.M.W.R.* 42(RR-14): Sept. 24, 1993.
    This represents the CDC treatment recommendations for the spectrum of syphilitic diseases. Approximately 50 percent of those treated for primary syphilis will experience the Jarisch-Herxheimer reaction.
17. Schroeter, A. L., et al. Therapy for incubating syphilis: effectiveness of gonorrhea treatment. *J.A.M.A.* 218:711, 1971.
    Standard gonorrhea therapy is successful for clearing incubating syphilis, but it will not clear established infection. The routine use of spectinomycin (which does not appear to cure incubating syphilis) in geographic areas where a sizable proportion of gonorrhea infections are caused by beta-lactamase–producing organ-

isms may partially explain the increasing number of cases of infectious syphilis.

18. Guinan, M. E. Treatment of primary and secondary syphilis: defining failure at three- and six-month follow-up. *J.A.M.A.* 257:359, 1987.
    In patients treated successfully, there was an approximate fourfold and eightfold drop in the VDRL titers at 3 and 6 months, respectively. All patients should be followed until they are symptom free and seronegative or, if positive at 2 years, until a stable low titer is reached.

19. Shenep, J. L., Feldman, S., and Thornton, D. Evaluation for endotoxemia in patients receiving penicillin therapy for secondary syphilis. *J.A.M.A.* 256:388, 1986.
    The Jarisch-Herxheimer reaction was not found to be due to endotoxemia.

20. Rudolph, A. H., and Price, E. V. Penicillin reactions among patients in venereal disease clinics. A national survey. *J.A.M.A.* 223:499, 1973.
    Penicillin reactions occurred irrespective of a negative history of reaction or previous penicillin usage.

21. Hutchinson, C. M., et al. Characteristics of patients with syphilis attending Baltimore STD clinics. Multiple high-risk subgroups and interactions with human immunodeficiency virus infection. *Arch. Intern. Med.* 151:511, 1991.
    It is unresolved whether RPR titers respond to treatment in the same way in HIV-negative patients as in HIV-positive patients, and whether the response to therapy varies with the stage of HIV infection.

57. GENITAL HERPES
Michel E. Rivlin

Herpes simplex virus (HSV) belongs to a large group of deoxyribonucleic acid (DNA) viruses that includes varicella zoster, cytomegalovirus, and the Epstein-Barr virus. The virus is fairly large and complex, measuring 150 to 200 μm in diameter. The DNA core of HSV is surrounded by a glycoprotein envelope derived from the host cell. After the virus penetrates the cell wall, the nucleocapsid is released and the DNA enters the nucleus. There are two subtypes of HSV, but clinical differentiation is not necessary. Fifty percent of the DNA differs between HSV type 1 and type 2. Herpes infections that occur above the waist are generally caused by HSV type 1, and those below the waist are usually due to HSV type 2, although between 20 and 25 percent of genital cases are due to type 1. In both HSV types, the dorsal spinal ganglia are thought to harbor latent viral infection. When this latent virus is activated, it migrates down the axons and produces lesions in the skin supplied by the sensory neurons. Type 2 infections have a recurrence rate of about 95 percent, versus about 50 percent for type 1 infections. The prevalence of type 2 genital infections in the middle-class population of the United States ranges between 20 and 55 percent, but only about a third of these patients have a history of genital infections. The prevalence in lower socioeconomic groups is between 40 and 60 percent. An estimated 300,000 to 500,000 new cases occur annually in the United States.

Transmission is known to result from genital or oral-genital sexual contact. The attack rate (percentage of those who contract it after exposure) for susceptible individuals is thought to be 75 percent. If intercourse is avoided during symptomatic periods, transmission to the partner does not appear to be inevitable. The incubation period tends to range from 2 to 10 days, although it may vary from 1 to more than 30 days.

The clinical manifestations depend on the immune status of the individual. There are three distinct clinical syndromes. First-episode primary infection occurs in patients who do not have circulating antibodies to either herpes viral type. The second syndrome occurs in women who already have antibody to HSV, and this is termed a first-episode nonprimary genital infection. The third group comprises those patients with recurrent disease who have previously had primary genital herpes infection and now have activation of latent herpes, or recurrent disease. The most severe forms of disease are confined to patients with first-episode primary infection or those whose immune system is compromised (e.g., resulting from corticosteroid therapy, pregnancy, malignancy, or immunosuppression). Both humoral and cell-mediated immune responses are important. Antibodies appear about 7 days after the primary infection and peak in 2 to 3 weeks. There is little rise in the antibody titer during recurrent episodes. When the cell-mediated immune response is suppressed, life-threatening infections may occur. Generally the area of outbreak is more limited and the symptoms are less severe in patients with antibodies from previous type 1 infections.

The characteristic signs of the first-episode primary infection include systemic symptoms in association with pain, dysuria, and the presence of multiple, painful vesicular or ulcerative genital lesions. More than 40 percent of the patients complain of systemic symptoms such as fever and malaise, 85 percent have multiple bilateral lesions, and 80 percent suffer a tender lymphadenopathy. The mean duration of viral shedding is 11 days, and 87 percent of women shed virus from the cervix. Lesions first appear in the form of vesicles or pustules that ulcerate, crust, and finally heal in an average of 19 days. Local pain lasts for a mean of 12 days. Local and systemic symptoms have a mean duration of almost 3 weeks. Dysuria, which occurs in 83 percent of the women, may be due to urine passing over the genital lesions or to a true urethritis, as the organism is also one of the causes of the urethral syndrome. Viral shedding takes place when the lesions are in the vesicular, pustular, and wet ulcer form.

Extragenital infection occurs in about 26 percent of the women with primary genital herpes. These lesions usually appear in the second week and are most commonly a result of autoinoculation from infected genital sites. They are usually located on the buttocks and fingers. Pharyngitis is noted in 10 percent of the women with primary disease. Other complications, generally of the primary episode, include secondary urethral and bladder infections, urinary retention, and secondary bacterial invasion. Rectal herpes can cause significant pain and debilitation. Neurologic complications include inflammatory radiculomyelopathy, transverse myelitis, and aseptic meningitis. These are all uncommon but have been reported.

Recurrent infections exhibit a periodicity of 1 to 3 months. Fifty percent of affected women experience a protracted remission after 7 years, and the duration of recurrences is considerably briefer than the initial episode. Many patients believe emotional stress, coitus, insomnia, and menstrual distress play major roles in initiating recurrent disease. Unique to recurrent infection is the prodrome, which affects 50 percent of the women and lasts just over a day. It is characterized by a tingling or itching sensation in the area where the eruption will occur. Viral shedding lasts up to a week, and healing is usually complete by 2 weeks. Urethritis is unusual, and typically there are only a few lesions that tend to recur in the same site. Local symptoms of pain or itching, if present, are generally mild.

Most cases are diagnosed clinically based on the appearance of typical herpetic lesions and the patient's history. The usual diagnostic laboratory procedure is viral culture. To perform this, the lesions are swabbed after the vesicles or pustules are broken with a sterile needle and the exudate sample is transferred immediately for viral culture. Cytologic examination of a Tzanck preparation or Papanicolaou (Pap) smear may reveal multinucleated giant cells. These preparations can be made using scrapings obtained from the bases of the vesicles or the cervix. Unfortunately, cytologic analysis positively identifies only about 30 to 50 percent of the patients with herpes, whereas culture results are positive in 80 percent of the same patients. Herpes antigen detection methods include direct immunofluorescence and enzyme-linked immunosorbent assays. The diagnostic sensitivities of these tests are intermediate between those of cytologic studies and viral culture. HSV DNA detection by the polymerase chain reaction (PCR) is as effective as viral culture but is not yet widely available for clinical use.

The differential diagnosis of HSV includes ulcerative lesions of the genital tract. In Western countries, HSV accounts for 20 to 50 percent of such lesions. *Treponema pallidum* is another important etiologic agent. In developing countries, chancroid (*Haemophilus ducreyi* infection) is the most common cause. Lymphogranuloma venereum strains of *Chlamydia trachomatis* are also associated with genital ulcers, often in conjunction with a suppurative lymphadenopathy. Granuloma inguinale, or donovanosis, causes a chronic, slowly progressive genital ulceration that is spread by contiguity. The causative organism is *Calymmatobacterium granulomatis*. There is no adenopathy in this condition. In view of the multiple infectious causes of genital ulcers, clinical and laboratory confirmation of a diagnosis should be sought.

Noninfectious causes of genital ulcerations, such as the mucosal lesions associated with Behçet's syndrome or inflammatory bowel disorders (Crohn's disease), may also be confused with genital herpes. A history of inflammatory bowel disease symptoms in a patient with Crohn's disease and the finding of oral, ocular, and central nervous system involvement in a patient with Behçet's syndrome may help differentiate the conditions, although the differentiation between herpes and Behçet's syndrome may be difficult if there is not a long history of either.

The treatment of choice for primary herpetic episodes is the antiviral nucleoside acyclovir. The drug's specificity for HSV-infected cells depends on its phosphorylation to its active form, acyclovir triphosphate, which is carried out far more efficiently by HSV-specific thymidine kinase in infected cells than by cellular kinases in normal cells. The drug inhibits viral replication but does not eradicate latent infection. Therapy consisting of 200 mg orally five times daily for 7 to 10 days, initiated within 6 days of the onset of lesions, shortens the median duration of first-episode eruptions by 3 to 5 days and may reduce the number and intensity of systemic symptoms. Only about 2 percent of patients require hospitalization, and these may be treated intravenously. The topical application of acyclovir ointment confers only marginal benefit in decreasing viral shedding. Treatment for recurrent episodes should be limited to those patients who typically have severe symptoms and are able to begin therapy at the time of the prodrome or within 2 days of the onset of lesions. Acyclovir shortens the mean clinical course of recurrences by about 1 day. The safety of acyclovir in pregnancy and in neonates and children has not been established, and prophylactic administration to women with lesions at delivery or to their infants is not indicated.

The prevention of transmission depends on patient education. Patients should be advised to abstain from skin-to-skin contact when active oral or genital infections are present. The use of a condom may be helpful, although it is by no means always successful. Continuous oral acyclovir (200 mg orally two to five times daily) can reduce the frequency of recurrent episodes by at least 75 percent, but, when discontinued, the disease reverts to its natural course. Continuous treatment should be reserved for patients who suffer six or more recurrences annually, or those who either have severe symptoms or are immunocompromised. Most patients prefer suppressive to episodic treatment, and long-term therapy (up to 3 years) appears to be well tolerated. Acyclovir-resistant strains are associated with decreased or absent viral thymidine kinase enzyme activity. In immunocompromised patients, these strains may cause serious infections and other antiviral agents may be indicated.

Psychologic disability has been reported in up to 80 percent of the patients surveyed. Nearly half of those infected avoid interpersonal relationships or abstain from sexual activity for varying periods. In one survey, 25 percent of the patients reported that they had been rejected by partners because of the herpetic infection, and 18 percent felt that herpes contributed to the dissolution of a relationship. If the physician is not able to offer sufficient educational and psychologic support, these patients should be encouraged to seek out the services offered by national support groups and the assistance of trained psychologic or psychiatric personnel.

Besides the fear of infecting a sexual partner, women are frequently concerned about transmission of the infection during pregnancy; this problem is dealt with in Chapter 9. Furthermore, HSV infections have been associated with genital cancers. Women with HSV-2 antibodies exhibit a higher incidence of cervical dysplasia and cancer; however, when controlled for sexuality, these differences are not significant. In addition, HSV-2–specific DNA binding antigens have been found in the setting of cervical dysplasia and cancer. However, although an epidemiologic association exists, a causal link has not been established. Nevertheless, the epidemiologic associations do indicate that women with genital HSV infections should have a Pap smear at least once a year.

Reviews
1. Lycke, E. The pathogenesis of the genital herpes simplex virus infection. *Scand. J. Infect.* 78:71, 1991.
   The herpesviruses cause a primary, virus-productive infection followed by a latent phase, during which the viral genome is maintained inactive until reactivation occurs and the genome is again wholly expressed.
2. Baker, D. A. Herpes simplex virus infections. *Curr. Opin. Obstet. Gynecol.* 4: 6776, 1992.
   In immunocompromised patients, genital herpes infection may produce excessive lesions, both during primary and reactivated infections.
3. Arvin, A. M., and Prober, C. G. Herpes simplex virus infections: the genital tract and the newborn. *Pediatr. Rev.* 13:107, 1992.
   Infection may occur in utero, by means of transplacental or ascending infection, or through exposure to genital lesions during delivery, or it may be acquired postnatally from relatives or attendants.

Diagnosis
4. Nahass, G. T., et al. Comparison of Tzanck smear, viral culture, and DNA diagnostic methods in detection of herpes simplex and varicella-zoster infection. *J.A.M.A.* 268:2541, 1992.
   The polymerase chain reaction was equivalent to viral culture in its accuracy, but with fewer practical and technical limitations.
5. Cone, R. W., et al. Extended duration of herpes simplex virus DNA in genital lesions detected by the polymerase chain reaction. *J. Infect. Dis.* 164:757, 1991.
   Herpesvirus DNA was demonstrated by the polymerase chain reaction in lesions on 15 of 17 days, versus 3 of 17 days by viral isolation, suggesting that polymerase chain reaction techniques are more sensitive than viral culture.
6. Koutsky, L. A., et al. Underdiagnosis of genital herpes by current clinical and viral-isolation procedures. *N. Engl. J. Med.* 326:1533, 1992.
   Newly developed type-specific serologic methods can identify both recurrent and subclinical infections.

Clinical Features
7. Mertz, G. J., et al. Risk factors for the sexual transmission of genital herpes. *Ann. Intern. Med.* 116:197, 1992.
   The risk for acquisition was higher in females, but previous type 1 infection lessened the risk; in 70 percent, transmission occurred during periods of asymptomatic viral shedding.
8. Prober, C. G. Herpetic vaginitis in 1993. *Clin. Obstet. Gynecol.* 36:177, 1993.
   Virus can be isolated from approximately 90 percent of the vesicles or pustules, 70 percent of the ulcers, and only 25 percent of the crusted lesions.
9. Koelle, D. M., et al. Asymptomatic reactivation of herpes simplex virus in women after the first episode of genital herpes. *Ann. Intern. Med.* 116:433, 1992.
   Asymptomatic genital shedding occurs more often during the first 3 months after primary type 2 disease than during later periods.
10. Bryson, Y., et al. Risk of acquisition of genital herpes simplex virus type 2 in sex partners of persons with genital herpes: a prospective couple study. *J. Infect. Dis.* 167:942, 1993.
    The infection is commonly asymptomatic; the overall risk of transmission in couples is low (10/y), but may be significantly increased in women and in seronegative individuals.
11. Kulhanjian, J. A., et al. Identification of women at unsuspected risk of primary infection with herpes simplex virus type 2 during pregnancy. *N. Engl. J. Med.* 326:916, 1992.

Serologic testing of couples can identify women who are at risk for primary or reactivated HSV-2 infections during pregnancy.

12. Keller, M. L., Jadack, R. A., and Mims, L. F. Perceived stressors and coping responses in persons with recurrent genital herpes. *Res. Nurs. Health* 14:421, 1991.

    The distress associated with the initial diagnosis may be similar to that of a grief reaction, with initial shock, numbness, and early denial. Thereafter, insomnia, depression, and rage are common.

Therapy

13. Centers for Disease Control. 1993 Sexually transmitted diseases treatment guidelines. *M.M.W.R.* 42(RR-14): Sept. 24, 1993.

    Acyclovir is currently not recommended for the treatment of recurrent episodes in pregnancy nor as suppressive therapy near term.

14. Renkel, L. M., et al. Pharmacokinetics of acyclovir in the term human pregnancy and neonate. *Am. J. Obstet. Gynecol.* 164:569, 1991.

    Acyclovir was found to be concentrated in the amniotic fluid, with no accumulation in the fetus. The authors suggest safety and efficacy studies be performed with a view toward its clinical use for the suppression of recurrences in pregnant women near term.

15. Andrews, E. B., et al. Acyclovir in pregnancy registry: Six years' experience. *Obstet. Gynecol.* 79:7, 1992.

    At this time, no increase in risk has been found, but the sample size is still too small for interpretation. Use in pregnancy at present is recommended only in the presence of life-threatening maternal infection.

16. Kaplowitz, L. G., et al. Prolonged continuous acyclovir treatment of normal adults with frequently recurring genital herpes simplex virus infection. The Acyclovir Study Group. *J.A.M.A.* 265:747, 1991.

    It is recommended that patients interrupt therapy after 1 year to reassess the frequency of recurrences, as marked pattern changes may occur in up to 25 percent of the cases.

17. Shupack, J., et al. Topical alpha-interferon ointment with dimethyl sulfoxide in the treatment of recurrent genital herpes simplex. *Dermatology* 184:40, 1992.

    Acyclovir-resistant strains of HSV are occurring with increasing frequency, and alternative therapies may be necessary. In this study, patients treated with topical interferon exhibited a more rapid cessation of viral shedding when compared to a placebo group.

18. Safrin, S., et al. A controlled trial comparing foscarnet with vidarabine for acyclovir-resistant mucocutaneous herpes simplex in the acquired immunodeficiency syndrome. The AIDS Clinical Trials Group. *N. Engl. J. Med.* 325:551, 1991.

    Foscarnet was more effective and less toxic than vidarabine; however, there was a high frequency of relapse once treatment was stopped.

58. CHLAMYDIA
Michel E. Rivlin

Two species make up the genus *Chlamydia. C. psittaci* is the causative agent of psittacosis and *C. trachomatis* is a specifically human pathogen. There are three major groups of infections caused by the fifteen *C. trachomatis* serotypes that have been recognized. L1, L2, and L3 cause lymphogranuloma venereum and are more invasive with a broader tissue spectrum than the other strains. Serotypes A, B, and C are the agents responsible for endemic blinding trachoma. The remaining serotypes, D through K, are the sexually transmitted agents that cause urethritis, cervicitis, epididymitis, salpingitis, urethral syndrome, newborn conjunctivitis, and pneumonia.

The chlamydial organism has a unique growth cycle, existing in two forms. The infectious particle, the elementary body, is capable of entering uninfected cells where it reorganizes to produce an initial body. The initial body undergoes binary fission with coexisting initial and elementary bodies contained within an expanding lysosome, which appears as a rounded intracytoplasmic inclusion. Within 48 to 72 hours, the host cell bursts, releasing the highly infectious elementary bodies. In this manner, infection spreads from cell to cell along the epithelial surface. There is an affinity for columnar and pseudostratified epithelium. *C. trachomatis* is a bacterium containing DNA and RNA; it possesses a cell wall and is susceptible to antibiotics. However, it has similarities to viruses, in that it is an obligate intracellular parasite.

Genitourinary chlamydial infection is the most common sexually transmitted disease (STD) in the United States, with an estimated 3 million cases occurring annually—more than those of gonorrhea (GC), syphilis, and herpes combined! Infections are most prevalent in young, promiscuous, indigent, unmarried, inner-city women, especially those with a concomitant STD or a prior history of other STDs. For instance, if endocervical GC is present, there is a 25 to 50 percent likelihood of chlamydial infection. If a male partner has nongonococcal urethritis (NGU), there is a 29 to 68 percent chance of chlamydial infection. In the United States, the *Chlamydia* organisms reside in the cervix of approximately 4 to 5 percent of sexually active women, and this site appears to play a central role in transmission, with horizontal spread to male partners and vertical spread to neonates. The risk of transmission to an infant from an infected mother is 60 to 70 percent, with an attendant 10 to 20 percent risk of pneumonia and 25 to 55 percent risk of conjunctivitis. The likelihood of ascending infection to the endometrium, fallopian tubes, and pelvic peritoneum is not known, but it is estimated that *Chlamydia* is associated with 5 to 10 percent of the cases of acute pelvic inflammatory disease (PID) that occur in the United States.

Seventy percent of the women with genital chlamydial infections are asymptomatic. Mucopurulent cervicitis has been associated with 50 percent of the cases of chlamydial infection. Diagnosis of this disease is established by the finding of yellow or green endocervical secretions on a white swab, the presence of ten or more polymorphonuclear leukocytes per microscopic oil immersion field in a Gram's-stained smear of secretions, and the existence of cervical friability (bleeds to touch). When compared to women with gonococcal or mixed aerobic and anaerobic salpingitis, women with chlamydial salpingitis are often less clinically ill, with minimal or no leukocytosis. However, paradoxically, the sequelae may be even more severe in these women, possibly because of delayed or absent treatment, resulting in tubal infertility and an increased risk of ectopic pregnancy and chronic pelvic pain. The acute urethral syndrome is characterized by frequency of urination, dysuria, and pyuria with a negative urinary culture. Chlamydial infection has been found in the majority of these cases studied. Acute epididymitis complicates NGU in 5 percent of the males with the disease, and *Chlamydia* is the etiologic agent in the majority. Here again, the condition is clinically milder than the GC infection. *Chlamydia* has also been associated with proctitis and prostatitis. Its role in the development of endometritis and bartholinitis is unclear, but the organism has been found in both entities. Acute perihepatitis associated with salpingitis (Fitz-Hugh-Curtis syndrome) is probably usually chlamydial rather than gonococcal in origin. Chlamydial infection is the leading cause of conjunctivitis and afebrile interstitial pneumonia among infants younger than 6 months of age in the United States, and may also cause otitis media in this group. The impact of maternal chlamydial infection on pregnancy outcome and perinatal complications, such as preterm delivery, premature rupture of membranes, and postpartum endometritis, remains controversial.

The isolation of *C. trachomatis* on tissue cultures is the gold standard for definitive diagnosis. To perform this, cycloheximide-treated McCoy cells are first incubated and then stained with iodine or Giemsa, or both, and examined microscopically for the presence of inclusions. Culture, however, is difficult, expensive, and slow. There are two major rapid direct antigen tests that are commercially available. They are faster but require skilled personnel for interpretation. These tests react to chlamydial antigen in clinical specimens. They use either fluorescein-conjugated monoclonal antibodies to visualize the chlamydial elementary bodies in smears or enzyme immunoassay, which provides an objective colorimetric test. In addition, recently marketed DNA probe tests have proved to be approximately as efficient as the direct antigen methods and are less labor intensive for laboratory personnel. These tests are less expensive to perform than cultures and do not require the maintenance of a cold chain for preserving specimens en route to the laboratory. For all methods, good sampling is essential. The endocervical or urethral secretions should contain exfoliated (and presumptively infected) columnar cells. The sensitivity of either method using endocervical specimens ranges from 70 to 80 percent and the specificity varies from 94 to 96 percent, as compared to tissue culture. The rapid direct methods seem most useful for large-scale screening in high-risk, high-prevalence populations, because, in a low-prevalence population, there are a significant number of false-positive results. In addition, these methods miss up to 20 percent of the true positives. Serologic testing is of little clinical value, as neither seropositive nor seronegative results reliably correlate with either infection or absence of infection.

The diagnosis and treatment of chlamydial infections are frequently based on the nature of the clinical syndrome. Uncomplicated urethral, endocervical, or rectal infections are best treated with tetracycline (500 mg orally four times a day for 7 days) or doxycycline (100 mg orally twice a day for 7 days). Erythromycin is the treatment of choice for obstetric cases, and erythromycin ethylsuccinate (800 mg four times a day for 7 days) is preferred in this setting. As discussed in Chapter 63, an antichlamydial agent is part of a combination approach to the treatment of PID. Neonatal infections are best treated with systemic erythromycin. Additional drugs that have demonstrated activity against *Chlamydia* include ofloxacin, amoxicillin, sulfamethoxazole-trimethoprim, rifampin, and clindamycin. A single 1-g dose of azithromycin, an azalide antibiotic, is as effective as a standard course of doxycycline in the treatment of uncomplicated genital chlamydial infection. Sex partners should be treated and tests-of-cure performed, if available. Cure rates of 95 percent can be expected, and persistent positive test results suggest either noncompliance or reinfection.

Empiric treatment is effective in an individual patient but does not address the larger issues of epidemiologic control. Three general approaches can be utilized to this end. First, the reservoir can be reduced by routinely instituting antichlamydial therapy when treating patients with GC; by effectively treating NGU, including the sexual contact; and by managing mucopurulent cervicitis, as with NGU in men. Second, topical erythromycin should replace silver nitrate for ocular prophylaxis in the neonate. Third, the routine testing of pregnant women is probably cost-effective when the prevalence of the disease in a given population exceeds 6 to 12 percent.

Clinical Features
1. Freund, K. M. Chlamydial disease in women. *Hosp. Pract.* 27:175, 1992.
   The annual cost of treating the infection and its complications exceeds $1.4 billion.
2. Ruijs, G. J., et al. Further details on sequelae at the cervical and tubal level of *Chlamydia trachomatis* infection in infertile women. *Fertil. Steril.* 56:20, 1991.
   Association between antibodies to C. trachomatis and infertility due to tubal occlusion.
3. Brunham, R. C., et al. *Chlamydia trachomatis*–associated ectopic pregnancy: serologic and histologic correlates. *J. Infect. Dis.* 165:1076, 1992.
   C. trachomatis antibodies and tubal plasma cell infiltration were associated with ectopic pregnancy.
4. Phillips, R. S., et al. The effect of cigarette smoking, *Chlamydia trachomatis* infection, and vaginal douching on ectopic pregnancy. *Obstet. Gynecol.* 79:85, 1992.
   Cigarette smoking was associated with ectopic pregnancy; previous chlamydial infection and vaginal douching were not.

Diagnosis
5. Ferris, D. G., and Martin, W. A comparison of three rapid chlamydial tests in pregnant and nonpregnant women. *J. Fam. Pract.* 34:593, 1992.
The positive predictive value of these assays in a low-prevalence population can be surprisingly low, although their performance in a high-prevalence population is usually satisfactory.
6. Hosein, I. K., Kaunitz, A. M., and Craft, S. J. Detection of cervical *Chlamydia trachomatis* and *Neisseria gonorrhoeae* with deoxyribonucleic acid probe assays in obstetric patients. *Am. J. Obstet. Gynecol.* 167:488, 1992.
Detection of chlamydial nucleic acids by DNA hybridization techniques, including enzymatic amplification of the chlamydial target DNA (polymerase chain reaction).
7. Krettek, J. E., et al. *Chlamydia trachomatis* in patients who used oral contraceptives and had intermenstrual spotting. *Obstet. Gynecol.* 81:728, 1993.
Intermenstrual bleeding in women who were previously well regulated on oral contraceptive pills appears to be a marker for chlamydial infection.

Prevalence/Screening
8. Sellors, J. W., et al. Effectiveness and efficacy of selective vs universal screening for chlamydial infection in sexually active young women. *Arch. Intern. Med.* 152:1837, 1992.
Selective screening based on the identification of specific risk factors in the history and physical examination was found to be effective in a low-prevalence setting.
9. Brännström, M., et al. Prevalence of genital *Chlamydia trachomatis* infection among women in a Swedish primary health care area. *Scand. J. Infect. Dis.* 24:41, 1992.
No differences were found between Chlamydia-positive and -negative women with regard to any clinical or anamnestic factor.
10. Lloyd, F., et al. Screening for *Chlamydia trachomatis* in women referred for legal abortion. *J. Obstet. Gynaecol.* 11:224, 1991.
Doxycycline prophylaxis can prevent C. trachomatis infection after legal abortion. Infected women tended to be younger and unmarried; the prevalence of infection was 9.8 percent.
11. Blythe, M. J., et al. Recurrent genitourinary chlamydial infections in sexually active female adolescents. *J. Pediatr.* 121:487, 1992.
Frequent recurrences with the same serovar suggest reinfection or relapse. Female adolescents should be rescreened regularly.

Treatment
12. Sweet, R. L., et al. *Chlamydia trachomatis* infection and pregnancy outcome. *Am. J. Obstet. Gynecol.* 156:824, 1987.
Management of chlamydial infection consists of treatment in the late third trimester to prevent perinatal transmission to the vaginally delivered neonate.
13. Hammerschlag, M. R., et al. Efficacy of neonatal ocular prophylaxis for the prevention of chlamydial and gonococcal conjunctivitis. *N. Engl. J. Med.* 320:769, 1989.
Because neither silver nitrate nor antibiotics were effective in preventing neonatal chlamydial ophthalmia, the most effective control method may be the screening and treating of pregnant women.
14. Jones, R. B., et al. *Chlamydia trachomatis* in the pharynx and rectum of heterosexual patients at risk for genital infection. *Ann. Intern. Med.* 102:757, 1985.
Pharyngeal infection occurs in 3 to 5 percent of persons with genital Chlamydia infection who engage in orogenital sex. It is not clear whether C. trachomatis causes symptomatic pharyngitis.
15. Magat, A. H., et al. Double-blind randomized study comparing amoxicillin and erythromycin for the treatment of *Chlamydia trachomatis* in pregnancy. *Obstet. Gynecol.* 81:81, 1993.
Amoxicillin is a reasonable alternative for patients intolerant to erythromycin.
16. Faro, S., et al. Effectiveness of ofloxacin in the treatment of *Chlamydia tra-*

chomatis and *Neisseria gonorrhoeae* cervical infection. *Am. J. Obstet. Gynecol.* 164:1380, 1991.

Ofloxacin is effective against chlamydia *in a dose of 300 mg, taken twice daily for 7 days; it is contraindicated in pregnancy and pediatric patients.*

17. Martin, D. H., et al. A controlled trial of a single dose of azithromycin for the treatment of chlamydial urethritis and cervicitis. *N. Engl. J. Med.* 327:921, 1992.

The azolide antibiotics are related structurally to the macrolide, erythromycin. The long half-life and good bioavailability allow single-dose therapy. The therapeutic spectrum includes Ureaplasma urealyticum.

18. Centers for Disease Control. 1993 Sexually transmitted diseases treatment guidelines. *M.M.W.R.* 42(RR-14): Sept. 24, 1993.

This contains the treatment regimens and guidelines for the management of chlamydial infections from the Centers for Disease Control.

19. Mecsei, R., et al. Genital *Chlamydia trachomatis* infections in patients with abnormal cervical smears: effect of tetracycline treatment on cell changes. *Obstet. Gynecol.* 73:317, 1989.

Mild cellular atypia in patients with C. trachomatis *should initially be treated with tetracycline. More advanced atypia is unlikely to be caused by* Chlamydia.

59. HUMAN PAPILLOMAVIRUS
Michel E. Rivlin

The spectrum of disease resulting from infection with human papillomavirus (HPV) includes both the clinical (genital warts and condyloma acuminatum) and subclinical involvement of the cervix, vagina, vulva, perineal body, and anus. Furthermore, there is an association with intraepithelial neoplasia of these areas and the male genitalia. It has also been shown that HPV deoxyribonucleic acid (DNA) is present in most squamous cell cancers of the female and male genital tracts. Although HPV is probably not the primary etiologic agent responsible for these cancers, it is probably a strong co-carcinogen. Finally, juvenile laryngeal papillomatosis is an uncommon, but important, disorder caused by the virus.

The prevalence of HPV is linked to sexual activity, and HPV frequently coexists with other sexually transmitted diseases (STDs). Genital warts are the most common viral STD in the United States, and a minimum of 10 to 20 percent of sexually active adults are thought to be infected, with the predominant age, 15 to 30 years. Approximately 2 to 3 percent of unselected Papanicolaou (Pap) smears are positive for the virus and DNA testing indicates an additional 20 percent. Finding HPV in any area of the genital tract suggests that the virus is present in the remainder of the tract. HPV lesions are difficult to eradicate, with a very high recurrence rate that is possibly related to the existence of untreated lesions in sexual partners, but probably more often to persistent, latent virus in otherwise normal-appearing skin and squamous mucous membranes in other areas.

HPV is classified as a subgroup of the papovaviruses because of its icosahedral virion capsids (i.e., the protein shell of a virus that acts as an antigen) and circular double-stranded DNA. Attempts to cultivate the virus have been unsuccessful, but advances in molecular biology, in particular nucleic acid hybridization (i.e., the formation of a complex between two single-stranded nucleic acid molecules), have led to the definition of more than sixty distinct types of HPV. The types are based on the viral DNA sequence (genotype) rather than on the antigenic features (serotype). Twelve virus types have been found to be associated with anogenital tract lesions. HPV types 16, 18, 31, 33, and 35 tend to be found in the presence of high-grade lesions and invasive cancers, whereas types 6 and 11 are usually associated with condyloma acuminatum or low-grade lesions. However, cervical intraepithelial neoplasia (CIN) type I frequently contains types 16 and 18. In minor and early lesions, the DNA is circular and remains episomal (i.e., a foreign DNA molecule that is distinct from the host DNA and replicating autonomously). In more severe lesions, the virus is integrated into the host cell genome by opening its circular form, binding covalently to the host DNA, and then replicating with it (integrated DNA). In advanced lesions, abnormal host cell DNA replication results in a marked tendency toward aneuploidy, as demonstrated by flow cytometry. The lesions associated with HPV 6 and 11 usually have a diploid or polyploid DNA histogram.

The carcinogenic potential of HPVs was first recognized when squamous cell cancers arose from Shope HPV-induced warts of domestic rabbits. The rate of malignant conversion depended on the viral strain, host species, and individual rabbit response. The frequency and speed of conversion were strongly accentuated by concomitant exposure to chemical carcinogens. Furthermore, the viral genome persisted in the cancer cells in a high copy number and continuously expressed viral gene products. The potential role of HPV was first substantiated in the setting of squamous cell cancers arising in epidermodysplasia verruciformis (a disease characterized by multiple flat warts of nongenital skin in patients with congenitally impaired cellular immunity). The importance of host immunity is further demonstrated by the rapid enlargement and spread of condylomata associated with the natural immunosuppression of pregnancy and the abnormal immunosuppression observed for some drugs and diseases (e.g., renal transplantation). Humoral immunity appears to protect against infection and spread, but cell-mediated immunity probably determines whether lesions regress, persist, or progress to become premalignant and malignant disease. Molecular cloning techniques of HPV DNA types from benign and malignant tumors of the oral, laryngeal, epidermal, and anogenital areas have provided probes (known DNA- or ribonucleic acid [RNA]–labeled to detect a given target DNA or RNA, respectively; the label is a radioactive or biotinylated nucleotide that is incorporated into the probe) to establish the consistent relationship between the HPV types of various pathologic conditions. Molecular probe technologies screening for virus infection by hybridization analysis are more accurate than cytologic smears. These techniques include filter hybridization (dot blot or Southern blot) and in situ hybridization. The tests vary in their sensitivity, the type of specimen needed (swabs or fixed tissues), level of difficulty, time required, and cost. Some of the tests incorporate the use of restriction endonucleases (enzymes that cut DNA at unique sites). Polymerase chain reaction (PCR) technology has further expanded the ability to recognize specific viral DNA using extremely small samples. The clinical application of this technology is unclear, as the natural history of HPV infections is not known, so the use of routine HPV DNA typing may be indicated only in questionable situations.

Many HPV-infected women complain of fleshy warts on the external genitals, usually around the vulva, introitus, perineum, anus, or urethra. The cervix may also have fleshy fibroepithelial proliferations. The virus has a predilection for adolescents, probably because of their cervical biologic immaturity. Teenagers typically have larger areas of squamous cell metaplasia than do adults, and this affords the easy access to basal epithelium necessary for infection. Condylomata acuminatum cause symptoms of itching, burning, pain, and tenderness. Cervical or vaginal infections are usually asymptomatic. Up to 50 percent of the patients with perineal warts also have them in the anal canal. The latent period from the time of exposure to the development of lesions averages about 3 months, but can be much longer. Warts may be difficult to control in pregnant women, and may bleed or even necessitate abdominal delivery to prevent extensive vaginal damage. There is also a small, but potentially serious, risk of transmission to the infant, who may later manifest anogenital or laryngeal papillomata (HPV types 6 and 11). Possible modes of transmission include the transplacental and intrapartal route, as well as postnatal contact, and there is usually a latent period of years before the lesions become clinically significant. Because the mode of transmission is unknown and the risk unclear, there is no consensus regarding the need for cesarean versus vaginal delivery. To avoid this dilemma, many advocate eradication of the warts during pregnancy and have reported success with various modes of therapy.

HPV preferentially infects the basal cell layer, thereby inducing cellular proliferation. Exophytic warts are characterized by the marked proliferation of epithelial cells and upward papillomatous protrusion. Basal layers contain many mitoses; superficial layers exhibit marked koilocytosis, acanthosis, and parakeratosis. Flat warts, commonly seen on the cervix, display similar changes but are nonpapillomatous. Exfoliated cells exhibit koilocytosis (perinuclear cavitation), nuclear enlargement, and chromatin smudging. After the application of 5% acetic acid (vinegar), flat cervical warts were found to be blanched, white, flat, epithelial lesions on colposcopy. Blood vessels protruding through the epithelial surface may create an undulating or "spiked" appearance. CIN owing to HPV is similar but may also have an irregular vascular pattern with a punctate or mosaic appearance. Exophytic warts seldom require biopsy for diagnosis, although cervical flat warts usually do to rule out CIN. The differential diagnosis of anogenital warts includes molluscum contagiosum (poxvirus), verruca vulgaris (nongenital HPV infection), secondary syphilis (condylomata lata), hypertrophic vulvar dystrophies, and vulvar intraepithelial and invasive neoplasias. It is advised that the genitals and perianal area in the male partner also be inspected under magnification after the application of 5% acetic acid, as the reported rate of condyloma transmission is 64 percent, the virus frequently being of the same type in both men and women.

Visible lesions can be eradicated by means of any of a wide variety of treatment alternatives, but all are associated with a high rate of symptomatic clinical recurrence. Therefore, both the patient and her partner must be counseled about the unpredictable natural history of the disease and the possible increased risk of lower genital tract malignancy. A widely used treatment is topical podophyllin, a keratolytic agent that is then washed off thoroughly in 4 hours because it is toxic and otherwise absorbed. Recurrence is common, and, if there is no response after four weekly applications, other treatments are indicated. Topically applied trichloroacetic acid, another keratolytic, is more efficacious, but repeated treatments may be required. Topically administered 5-fluorouracil may be the treatment of choice for vaginal, perianal, and urethral warts, but severe reactions are common. Cryotherapy and electrocautery reportedly achieve cure rates of 63 and 90 percent, respectively, and may be performed under local anesthesia in an ambulatory setting. Carbon dioxide laser ablation using colposcopic guidance can be expanded to include all HPV-related diseases; however, the time, cost, and morbidity rates of laser vaporization must be taken into account. There is also a possibility, although no conclusive documentation exists, that the smoke from vaporized tissue may contain viral particles that could possibly induce respiratory tract lesions in treatment personnel. Alpha-interferon therapy is modestly effective, with complete remission observed in about 50 percent of cases. However, dose-related side effects and high costs have limited the use of this treatment to refractory cases.

The treatment of lesions in pregnant women is difficult, but good results have been reported for both cryotherapy and laser ablation. Trichloroacetic acid may be used, but podophyllin, 5-fluorouracil, and immunotherapy should be avoided during pregnancy. The male partner should be examined, and any visible lesions should be treated using the same therapeutic modalities as those used in the woman. There is no vaccine against HPV, nor is there any specific antiviral drug or protocol. The only currently effective means of minimizing the risk of transmission is barrier contraception. Frequent anxiety-provoking follow-up visits and repeated treatments over the course of many years may be required. This is often difficult and frustrating for both the patient and the physician.

Reviews
1. Richart, R. M., and Wright, T. C., Jr. Human papillomavirus. *Curr. Opin. Obstet. Gynecol.* 4:662, 1992.
   If the disease persists for 6 months despite therapy, it is referred to as resistant *and* persistent *HPV disease.*
2. Moscicki, A. B. Human papillomavirus infections. *Adv. Pediatr.* 39:257, 1992.
   Recurrences indicate failure of therapy, failure to treat all the involved areas, resistant virus, or reinfection; most occur within 3 to 6 months of treatment.

Virology
3. Bergeron, C., et al. Human papillomaviruses associated with cervical intraepithelial neoplasia. Great diversity and distinct distribution in low- and high-grade lesions. *Am. J. Surg. Pathol.* 16:641, 1992.
   The unpredictable clinical evolution of cervical dysplasia is linked to the diversity of genital types associated with the disease.
4. Hording, U., et al. Human papillomavirus types 16 and 18 in adenocarcinoma of the uterine cervix. *Gynecol. Oncol.* 46:313, 1992.
   Type 16 is more common in squamous cell carcinoma and type 18 in adenocarcinoma of the cervix. This may reflect different virus receptors, or specific infections may govern carcinogenesis.
5. Johnson, J. C., et al. High frequency of latent and clinical human papillomavirus cervical infections in immunocompromised human immunodeficiency virus–infected women. *Obstet. Gynecol.* 79:321, 1992.
   Impaired immune status, as reflected by the CD4 T-cell count, is an important factor in increasing the severity of HPV-induced cervical infections in this population.

HPV Infections
6. Reid, R., et al. Sexually transmitted papillomaviral infections. I. The anatomic distribution and pathologic grade of neoplastic lesions associated with different viral types. *Am. J. Obstet. Gynecol.* 156:212, 1987.
   Differing disease patterns arise partly from the predilection of specific viral types for certain sites and through variations in host response. Disease expression may represent the focal breakdown of host surveillance within a field of latent infection.
7. Rome, R. M., Chanen, W., and Pagano, R. The natural history of human papillomavirus (HPV) atypia of the cervix. *Aust. N.Z. J. Obstet. Gynaecol.* 27:287, 1987.
   Progression to CIN occurred in 15.8 percent, persistence occurred in 39.4 percent, and regression occurred in 44.8 percent of 259 untreated patients observed for a median of 18 months.
8. Sawchuk, W. S. Vulvar manifestations of human papillomavirus infection. *Dermatol. Clin.* 10:405, 1992.
   In contrast to the natural history of cervical lesions, the natural history of vulval, vaginal, and anal intraepithelial neoplasia is poorly understood.
9. Scholefield, J. H., et al. Anal intraepithelial neoplasia: part of a multifocal disease process. *Lancet* 340:1271, 1992.
   Nineteen percent of women with high-grade cervical lesions had anal intraepithelial neoplasia.
10. Panici, P. B., et al. Oral condyloma lesions in patients with extensive genital human papillomavirus infection. *Am. J. Obstet. Gynecol.* 167:451, 1992.
    There was a high incidence (85%) of oral HPV lesions in patients with genital condylomata. All patients were asymptomatic and 99 percent practiced orogenital sex.
11. Bergman, A., and Nalick, R. Prevalence of human papillomavirus infection in men. Comparison of the partners of infected and uninfected women. *J. Reprod. Med.* 37:710, 1992.
    There were HPV-associated lesions in 69 percent of the men with infected partners and in 2 percent of the men with uninfected partners.
12. Carlson, J. W., and Twiggs, L. B. Clinical applications of molecular biologic screening for human papillomavirus: diagnostic techniques. *Clin. Obstet. Gynecol.* 35:13, 1992.
    PCR techniques are highly efficient in detecting specific viral DNA.
13. De Villiers, E. M., et al. Human papillomavirus DNA in women without and with cytological abnormalities: results of a 5-year follow-up study. *Gynecol. Oncol.* 44:33, 1992.
    The progression of HPV-positive women from normal cytologic findings to dysplasia or cancer exhibited an annual frequency of 0.082 percent, with an assumed infected life span of 45 years and a lifetime risk of about 3.7 percent.
14. Koutsky, L. A., et al. A cohort study of the risk of cervical intraepithelial neopla-

sia grade 2 or 3 in relation to papillomavirus infection. *N. Engl. J. Med.* 327:1272, 1992.
Cervical dysplasia is a common and early manifestation of cervical HPV infection, particularly types 16 and 18.
15. Cox, J. T., et al. An evaluation of human papillomavirus testing as part of referral to colposcopy clinics. *Obstet. Gynecol.* 60:389, 1992.
Suggests that HPV testing and repeated cytologic screening provide a reliable method of triage for the purpose of limiting the use of colposcopic services, which are currently overburdened.

HPV and Pregnancy
16. Kemp, E. A., et al. Human papillomavirus prevalence in pregnancy. *Obstet. Gynecol.* 79:540, 1992.
There was no significant relationship between pregnancy and HPV prevalence.
17. Bennett, R. S., and Power, K. R. Human papillomaviruses: associations between laryngeal papillomas and genital warts. *Pediatr. Infect. Dis. J.* 6:229, 1987.
Laryngeal papillomas exhibit a bimodal age distribution, with the first peak in children aged 2 to 5 and the second peak in adults. The clinical course is commonly characterized by multiple recurrences after surgical excision. They may produce respiratory obstruction. In most juvenile patients, they regress, generally at about the time of puberty.
18. Shah, K., et al. Rarity of cesarean delivery in cases of juvenile-onset respiratory papillomatosis. *Obstet. Gynecol.* 68:795, 1986.
Whether adult-onset disease is due to latent virus or to later infection (e.g., by oral sex) is not known. Because genital infection is common and respiratory papillomatosis is rare (350 new cases in the United States annually), it is estimated that 80 cesarean deliveries would be needed to protect one baby at risk.

Treatment
19. Matsunaga, J., Bergman, A., and Bhatia, N. N. Genital condylomata acuminata in pregnancy: effectiveness, safety and pregnancy outcome following cryotherapy. *Br. J. Obstet. Gynaecol.* 94:168, 1987.
Affected women were treated as outpatients every 2 weeks until the warts resolved. Labor and delivery were unaffected, even by cervical cryotherapy.
20. Schwartz, D. B., et al. Genital condylomas in pregnancy: use of trichloroacetic acid and laser therapy. *Am. J. Obstet. Gynecol.* 158:1407, 1988.
This combination therapy was effective in controlling condylomata in 97 percent of the patients. The complication and recurrence rates were low.
21. Krebs, H., and Helmkamp, F. Chronic ulcerations following topical therapy with 5-fluorouracil for vaginal human papillomavirus-associated lesions. *Obstet. Gynecol.* 78:205, 1991.
A pyrimidine antimetabolite, 5-fluorouracil, causes sloughing of growing tissue. It is usually applied into the vagina and/or vestibule weekly for 12 weeks.
22. Hernandez, E., et al. Interferon as an adjunct to laser therapy in the treatment of recalcitrant vulvar condylomata acuminata: a pilot study. *Am. J. Gynecol. Health* 6:35, 1992.
The interferons, a family of glycoproteins with antiviral, antiprolific, and immunomodulatory properties, may be administered by either intralesional or intramuscular injection, alone or in combination with other therapies.

60. ACQUIRED IMMUNODEFICIENCY SYNDROME
Michel E. Rivlin

When the acquired immunodeficiency syndrome (AIDS) first came to the attention of the medical community in the United States in 1981, the affected groups seemed to comprise a sort of "4-H Club" of homosexual and bisexual men, heroin and other illicit intravenous drug users, hemophiliacs, and Haitians. Since then, it has become clear that the sexual partners of patients with the infection are at risk for developing AIDS (horizontal transmission) and that pregnant women can transmit the disease to their children (vertical transmission). The occurrence of a disease that is at least moderately predictive of a defect in cell-mediated immunity in an individual with no other known source of diminished resistance to that disease constitutes the core concept of AIDS. However, AIDS is just one facet of the many manifestations of infection with the human immunodeficiency virus (HIV), and represents the very small tip of the large iceberg of infection with HIV. Diseases that indicate immunocompromise include both opportunistic infections (e.g., *Pneumocystis carinii* pneumonia, cytomegalovirus infection, and toxoplasmosis) and neoplasias such as Kaposi's sarcoma and non-Hodgkin's lymphoma.

The HIV virion has a diameter of about 10 nm. It is classified as a retrovirus because its genetic material is ribonucleic acid (RNA), which directs production of deoxyribonucleic acid (DNA) (the *reverse* of the usual pattern), which then directs production of RNA, and this, in turn, directs production of viral proteins. The virus survives in the host in a latent state, during which viral genes are integrated into the DNA of host cells. Survival outside the host is limited, and the fragile organism is readily destroyed by simple disinfection. The virus most readily attacks cells with receptors for the T peptide, such as helper T4 lymphocytes (CD4-positive cells) and neural cells. Helper cells play a key role in coordinating a variety of immune functions, including B-lymphocyte activity and the induction of natural killer cells. When helper cells are inactivated, the immune system is effectively disabled. The system is further damaged by HIV infection of the monocytes/macrophages. The striking lymphopenia typically found is specifically due to a quantitative and qualitative defect in the T4-inducer or -helper subset of T lymphocytes, with a consequent reversal of the normal ratio to T8 suppressor-cytotoxic cells.

The effect of HIV on the nervous system is manifested by subacute encephalitis, vacuolar myelopathy, chronic meningitis, and peripheral neuropathy. Histologic studies reveal demyelination, focal necrosis, and the presence of multinucleated giant cells. The virus resides in the lymphocytes in semen and has also been isolated from cervical and vaginal secretions and breast milk. These fluids and blood have all been implicated in the transmission of the virus. Saliva, spinal fluid, urine, tears, and amniotic fluid also contain smaller amounts of virus but have not been implicated as a source of transmission. Thus, any sexual act that can injure the mucosa, thereby providing a portal of entry for the virus, involves a risk of transmission. Although oral intercourse and deep kissing pose theoretic risks, the exact probability of transmission is unknown. No evidence of casual transmission exists (e.g., by the sharing of utensils or shaking hands). Accidental transmission to health-care workers has been infrequent and has always been related to direct inoculation or exposure of the skin to infected blood.

The AIDS epidemic among women is increasing rapidly, having grown from constituting 6.6 percent of the total cases of AIDS in adults in 1985 to 12.8 percent in 1991. The findings from seroprevalence studies of HIV infection suggest that some 80,000 women aged 15 through 44 years may be infected. Latin American and African American women represent 14 percent of the population of the United States, but constitute approximately 72 percent of the women with AIDS. Although it appears that most patients with AIDS are residents of large urban areas, the proportion of rural and suburban cases is increasing. Two major reasons for women's greater susceptibility to HIV infection during heterosexual intercourse are that (1) more men than women in the United States are infected and (2) HIV appears to be more easily transmitted from men to women than the reverse.

The majority of women with AIDS are intravenous drug users; the second most commonly affected group are those who have heterosexual contact with a person at risk for AIDS. Most childhood cases occur as perinatal infections—in most cases, from mothers who abuse intravenous drugs or whose partners do. Since the screening of all blood and blood products for transfusions was implemented in 1985, the risk associated with transfusions has now become minimal. At this time, the three major risk groups are the sex partners of HIV-infected persons, infants born to infected mothers, and needle-sharing partners (or others with de facto parenteral contact) of those infected. Although the nature of transmission of HIV is similar to that of hepatitis B, HIV is less readily transmitted. In one report, the risk of transmission of hepatitis B from a needlestick-like exposure was cited to range from 6 to 30 percent; the risk associated with HIV was 0.49 percent. Factors associated with an increased risk of transmission include an increased number of sex partners, the presence of genital ulcers (e.g., syphilis or herpes), and anal receptive intercourse. An estimated 20 to 40 percent of the infants born to infected mothers acquire HIV.

Antibodies to HIV are detected weeks to months after initial infection; thus, the virus is present and transmissible before antibody is detectable. It is therefore postulated that the clinical course of HIV infection commences with an initial asymptomatic incubation period, followed by a mild, self-limited acute mononucleosis-like infection, probably occurring from 2 weeks to 3 months after exposure. This is followed by a period of asymptomatic seropositivity consisting in some patients of the development of generalized persistent lymphadenopathy and, in others, of severe systemic manifestations. Some patients manifest not AIDS but the AIDS-related complex. This is an imprecisely defined and less severe set of manifestations that include anorexia, weight loss, fever, night sweats, rashes, fatigue, diarrhea, susceptibility to infection, or lymphadenopathy, or a combination of these. When lymphocytes are stimulated by a secondary infection, the latent virus replicates and breaks out of the lymphocytes, resulting in a depletion of T4 cells and leaving the patient vulnerable to opportunistic infections. Each infected lymphocyte is capable of producing thousands of virus particles. Opportunistic infections often stem from the reactivation of childhood infections that were latent until the immunosuppression occurs, such as in the case of *P. carinii*. Protozoal infections also include cryptosporidiosis and toxoplasmosis. Viral diseases consist of cytomegalovirus and herpes. Bacterial infections comprise tuberculosis, nocardiosis, and atypical mycobacteria. Fungal infections include *Candida*, histoplasmosis, and cryptococcosis. The immunologic and hematologic abnormalities encountered include hemolytic anemia, thrombocytopenia, and lymphadenopathy. In addition to the central nervous system manifestations of opportunistic infections, many of the neurologic findings may reflect a direct effect of HIV infection.

Tests for the immunoglobulin G (IgG) antibody to HIV begin with a serologic test of high, but not 100 percent, sensitivity (i.e., the percentage of diseased patients with a positive test result). This is an enzyme-linked immunosorbent assay (ELISA) and is used as a screen. The results of these tests may be falsely positive, sometimes reflecting either autoimmune disease or the existence of cross-reacting antibodies resulting from transfusion or other viral infections. Tests are repeated if results are positive and, if results are again positive, usually a Western blot assay or a fluorescent method is used for confirmation. The blot assay involves the digestion of HIV virus with the electrophoretic separation of HIV proteins on material such as nitrocellulose paper. If the test specimen contains antibodies that bind to the specific HIV proteins, this represents a positive result. The Western blot is highly specific but is technically demanding to perform and requires subjective interpretation. Virus culture is available only in specialized laboratories and is not generally available for diagnostic purposes. Although these positive test results for HIV may indicate HIV infection, the diagnosis of AIDS requires the additional demonstration of an opportunistic disease and the exclusion of other causes of immunodeficiency. If testing programs are developed, consent for testing must be obtained and seropositive patients must be provided with counseling given by properly trained persons. Knowledge of test results must be confined to those directly involved in the patient's care, or as required by law, with assurance of confidentiality. Infected patients must be provided with needed optimal care. HIV is a chronic infection with a variable course; it takes about 10 years from the time of infection for AIDS to develop in 50 percent of infected persons.

Several laboratory and clinical markers predict the risk of progression from asymptomatic HIV infection to AIDS, and the most useful of these is the absolute CD4 lymphocyte count. Antiretroviral therapies interfere with the replication of

HIV. Three reverse transcriptase inhibitors (i.e., prevent translation of RNA to DNA), zidovudine (AZT), didanosine (DDI), and zalcitabine (DDC), are approved for use in the treatment of HIV infection and appear to slow the progression of HIV to AIDS. The major limiting toxicity of AZT is bone marrow suppression, and that of DDI is pancreatitis. The use of AZT in pregnancy is undergoing study, as is its use in persons after significant exposure to HIV. Both primary prophylaxis (prevention of illness before it occurs) and secondary prophylaxis (prevention of recurrence) for opportunistic infections are available and indicated for the suppression of several diseases, including pneumocystic pneumonia, candidiasis, herpes, tuberculosis, toxoplasmosis, cryptococcosis, cytomegalovirus, and the *Mycobacterium avium*-intracellulare complex. Patients should be screened for the existence of syphilis, hepatitis, cervical dysplasia, tuberculosis, and fungal disorders. Vaccine schedules should be updated, nutritional needs met, and mental health and substance abuse interventions supplied.

The available strategy for preventing the spread of HIV is to eliminate the vectors that are responsible for spreading the disease: Sex or needle-sharing with infected persons, births to infected persons, injections of HIV by means of transfusions or needlestick injuries, and unusual de facto parenteral transfer. The combined use of education, motivation, and skill building; serologic screening; and contact tracing and notification could substantially reduce the rate of transmission. The message that should be communicated is that any sexual intercourse (outside of mutually monogamous or HIV antibody–negative relationships) must be protected with a condom. Unsterile needles or syringes should not be shared, and all exposed women should be tested before pregnancy and, if positive, should avoid pregnancy. Because medical history and examination cannot reliably identify all infected patients, blood and body-fluid precautions should be consistently adopted for all patients (universal precautions). Barriers should be used to prevent skin and mucous membrane exposure when contact with blood or body fluids of any patient is anticipated. Gloves may protect the hands, masks and protective eyewear may protect the head, and gowns or aprons may protect against splashes. The hands or other skin areas should be washed immediately after contamination. Needles should not be recapped or manipulated by hand. After use, sharp instruments should be discarded in readily available puncture-proof containers. In order to avoid contact with body fluids during resuscitation, specially designed ventilation devices should be readily available, and wall suction devices should be employed for clearing the airway. Blood spills should be cleaned off with 0.5% sodium hypochlorite solution (diluted bleach). Isolation is required only if the patient's hygiene is poor. If a needlestick injury occurs, the health-care worker should be assessed and receive routine care for hepatitis B exposure. Antibody testing should be carried out and repeated at 6 weeks, 3 months, and 6 months; if this proves HIV seronegative, follow-up may be discontinued. The care of pregnant women infected with HIV and of their children is detailed in Chapter 9.

Any communicable disease that affects primarily young, previously healthy individuals and has a mortality rate in excess of 80 percent clearly requires an urgent remedy. Unfortunately, until effective treatment and control programs are developed, the incidence of AIDS will continue to increase and its impact on human health and health-care resources will be felt throughout the world.

Reviews
1. Priolo, L., and Minkoff, H. L. HIV infection in women. *Baillière's Clin. Obstet. Gynaecol.* 6:617, 1992.
   For all adults with HIV infection, routine immunization against influenza, Pneumococcus, Haemophilus influenza B, hepatitis B, tetanus, and diphtheria is indicated and advised.
2. Ziegler, J. B., et al. Pediatric HIV: Australian perspective. *J. Acquir. Immune Defic. Syndr.* 6:S20, 1993.
   Most babies born to HIV-infected mothers will test positive because of the passive transmission of maternal IgG antibodies. Testing for HIV-specific immunoglobulin A antibodies may be helpful in confirming HIV infection in young infants.

3. Centers for Disease Control. Revised classification system and expanded AIDS surveillance definition for adolescents and adults. *M.M.W.R.* 41:RR-17, 1992.
   The revised system emphasizes CD4 lymphocyte testing and is based on three ranges of CD4 counts and three clinical categories, giving a matrix of nine exclusive categories.

Epidemiology
4. Pertowski, C. A., and Rutherford, G. S. Epidemiology of human immunodeficiency virus infection and the acquired immunodeficiency syndrome. *Semin. Liver Dis.* 12:108, 1992.
   It is estimated that nearly 1.5 million Americans are infected with HIV-1. More than 195,000 cases of AIDS had been reported as of September 1991, and over half of the patients involved have died.
5. Kline, M. W., and Shearer, W. T. Impact of human immunodeficiency virus infection on women and infants. *Infect. Dis. Clin. North Am.* 6:1, 1992.
   As of September 1992, there were 25,947 women with AIDS in the United States; 50 percent occurring through injecting drug use, 36 percent through heterosexual contact, and 9 percent from exposure to blood products.
6. Centers for Disease Control. AIDS and HIV update: acquired immunodeficiency syndrome and human immunodeficiency virus infection among health-care workers. *J.A.M.A.* 259:2817, 1988.
   The occupational risk of acquiring HIV in health-care settings is low and is most often associated with the percutaneous inoculation of blood from an infected patient.

Diagnostic Testing
7. Centers for Disease Control. Update: serologic testing for antibody to human immunodeficiency virus. *J.A.M.A.* 259:653, 1988.
   The ELISA is exquisitely sensitive (percentage of diseased patients with a positive test result) but is less than 100 percent specific (percentage of nondiseased patients with a negative test result). This feature means that the test has a relatively poor positive predictive value for populations with a low percentage of HIV infections.
8. Consortium for Retrovirus Serology Standardization. Serological diagnosis of human immunodeficiency virus infection by Western blot testing. *J.A.M.A.* 260:674, 1988.
   Unfortunately, the current "gold standard" for confirmation of HIV serology suffers from a lack of standardization in terms of reagents, methods, and interpretation.
9. Fehrs, L. J., et al. Trial of anonymous versus confidential human immunodeficiency virus testing. *Lancet* 2:379, 1988.
   A flexible HIV testing program should consider offering both confidential and anonymous HIV testing.
10. Burke, D. S., et al. Measurement of the false positive rate in a screening program for human immunodeficiency virus infections. *N. Engl. J. Med.* 319:961, 1988.
    In a program for screening applicants to the U.S. military, the rate of false-positive diagnosis was 1 in 135,187 persons tested. The overall prevalence of HIV in this population was 1.4 per 1000.

Therapy and Prevention
11. Jewett, J. F., and Hecht, F. M. Prevention health care for adults with HIV infection. *J.A.M.A.* 269:1144, 1993.
    This article describes different stage-specific health maintenance needs that form an important part of comprehensive care.
12. Centers for Disease Control. Guidelines for the performance of CD4+T-cell determinations in persons with human immunodeficiency virus infection. *M.M.W.R.* 1:1, 1992.
    Guidelines are given for initiating antiretroviral treatment and pneumocystic pneumonia prophylaxis based on CD4 counts, generally less than 500/μl for zi-

dovudine and less than 200 μl for trimethoprim-sulfamethoxazole. The T-cell levels decline slowly, such that 3- to 6-monthly testing intervals are generally acceptable.

13. Meng, T.-C., et al. Combination therapy with zidovudine and dideoxycytidine in patients with advanced human immunodeficiency virus infection. *Ann. Intern. Med.* 116:13, 1992.
Side effects of zidovudine include granulocytopenia and anemia (dose-limiting toxicities), headaches, nausea, vomiting, muscle weakness, and fatigue. Didanosine and dideoxycytidine, also nucleoside analogue reverse transcriptase inhibitors, can serve as alternative therapy if the zidovudine proves too toxic or when drug resistant strains emerge during therapy.

14. Hudson, C. N. Nosocomial infection and infection control procedure. *Baillieres Clin. Obstet. Gynaecol.* 6:137, 1992.
Details "universal precautions"; the greatest risk to health-care workers is posed by needlestick injuries, with a risk of 1 in 250.

15. Potts, D. M., and Smith, J. B. Contraception and safer sex. *Baillieres Clin. Obstet. Gynaecol.* 6:199, 1992.
These authors recommend use of a latex condom with nonoxynol-9 lubricant and a reservoir tip during vaginal, oral, or rectal sex. Users should also have condoms available at all times, know that HIV can penetrate animal skin condoms, and that oil-based lubricants damage condoms.

16. Dolin, R., et al. The safety and immunogenicity of a human immunodeficiency virus type 1 (HIV-1) recombinant gp160 candidate vaccine in humans. *Ann. Intern. Med.* 114:119, 1991.
Multiple strategies for inducing HIV immunity are being tested, including the administration of inactivated virus, recombinant viral proteins, or recombinant live vaccines that express viral antigens.

General

17. Lindsay, M. K., et al. Crack cocaine: a risk factor for human immunodeficiency virus infection type 1 among inner-city parturients. *Obstet. Gynecol.* 80:981, 1992.
Drug use in shooting galleries, sharing of equipment, and either the trading of sex for money to buy the drug and for the drug all increase the risk of acquiring HIV.

18. Tichy, A. M., and Talashek, M. L. Older women. Sexually transmitted diseases and acquired immunodeficiency syndrome. *Nurs. Clin. North Am.* 27:937, 1992.
Expresses the sentiment that a full life requires balancing moderate and extreme risks because life itself can be considered a universally lethal sexually transmitted disease.

19. Schafer, A., et al. The increased frequency of cervical dysplasia-neoplasia in women infected with the human immunodeficiency virus is related to the degree of immunosuppression. *Am. J. Obstet. Gynecol.* 164:593, 1991.
The frequency and severity of dysplasia appear to increase with diminishing numbers of CD4-positive helper/inducer T lymphocytes.

20. Herbert, W. N. P., Owen, H. G., and Collins, M. L. Autologous blood storage in obstetrics. *Obstet. Gynecol.* 72:166, 1988.
The old "hemoglobin of 10/hematocrit of 30" rule, below which transfusion was considered necessary, is increasingly being challenged because of the perceived risk of getting AIDS by many patients. Autologous blood transfusion provides a safe and satisfactory alternative.

21. Jaffe, L. R., et al. Anal intercourse and knowledge of acquired immunodeficiency syndrome among minority-group female adolescents. *J. Pediatr.* 112:1005, 1988.
This discusses common sexual practices among a population of heterosexually active inner-city black and Hispanic female adolescents. Condoms are even less likely to be used during anal than during vaginal intercourse.

22. Sunderland, A., et al. The impact of human immunodeficiency virus serostatus on reproductive decisions of women. *Obstet. Gynecol.* 79:1027, 1992.
Seropositive women often become pregnant again, even when they receive optimal social and medical support services and education.

23. Perry, S., et al. Effectiveness of psychoeducational interventions in reducing emotional distress after human immunodeficiency virus antibody testing. *Arch. Gen. Psychiatry* 48:143, 1991.
This article considers the value of supportive and cognitive counseling, the treatment of severe anxiety and depression, stress management techniques, and the merits of support groups and assistance that meet practical stage-specific needs at different points in the course of HIV infection.

61. VAGINITIS
Abraham Rubin

Vaginal discharge is the most common gynecologic complaint, but it is important to distinguish between leukorrhea and an infected vaginal discharge. Leukorrhea may be mucinous, owing to reactive hypersecretion resulting from the presence of cervical polyps or "erosions"; hyperestrogenic (postovulatory or resulting from the use of birth control pills); or caused by hyperdesquamation stemming from an exaggerated response of the vaginal mucosa to normal or abnormal hormonal stimulation. Hyperdesquamation is classically associated with a nonadherent, abundant, whitish discharge. There may be an associated itch in 30 percent of such patients. Therapy may be confined to reassuring the patient and confirming the noninfective nature of the condition.

A nonspecific vaginal discharge in adult women may be related to the presence of foreign materials, such as forgotten diaphragms, cotton balls, sponges, tampons, or even condoms. There is also an increased discharge associated with use of an intrauterine device (IUD). Tight underwear or nylon may cause chafing, thus producing itching, vulvitis, and vaginitis with an excessive discharge. Allergies to various types of clothing fabrics, feminine deodorant sprays, detergents, soaps, and douches may produce a profuse leukorrhea. These conditions frequently become secondarily infected stemming from damage to the epithelium caused by chemicals or after scratching in response to the intense pruritus.

Atrophic vaginitis results from the loss of natural estrogens. It is seen in women after radiation therapy or oophorectomy and in menopausal women. The mucosa is easily fractured in these settings, and, initially, there is a nonspecific, often blood-stained discharge. Invasion by pathogenic organisms may follow.

The three most common vaginal infections in women of reproductive age are *Trichomonas vaginalis, Candida albicans,* and bacterial vaginosis (previously called *Gardnerella vaginitis*). *T. vaginalis* is transmitted sexually, usually in the immediate postmenstrual phase. The discharge involved is characteristically malodorous, frothy, and yellow and has a pH of 5.0 to 5.5. The infection may produce vulvovaginal erythema and edema. In its most severe form, petechiae with swollen vaginal papillae (strawberry vagina) may be seen. It must be stressed, however, that many infections can cause reddened vaginas in conjunction with malodorous discharges, and *T. vaginalis* infection should therefore not be assumed based solely on these findings. Specimens for examination should be obtained from fairly high up on the posterior vaginal wall. The swab is placed in a saline tube and rotated several times, then applied to a slide and a coverslip placed over the area of application. Motile trichomonads can be seen without the use of a specific stain. Trichomonads can also be seen on routine Papanicolaou (Pap) smears. Either metronidazole or analogues (500 mg taken twice daily for 7 days, or 2 g as a single dose) can cure 90 percent of the cases. It is important that the male partner also be treated. Metronidazole should not be used in the first trimester of pregnancy, but it may be used thereafter if symptoms are severe. If metronidazole is contraindicated, *T. vaginalis* infection can be treated with local applications of povidone-iodine at night for a week at a time. If alcohol is consumed, metronidazole can produce side effects such as nausea and dizziness. In pregnant women, 15 percent of *T. vaginalis* infections are combined with candidiasis.

C. albicans is the most important of the specific agents causing vaginitis in pregnant or diabetic women; it can, however, be present in the vagina as a commensal organism, inciting neither reactions nor symptoms. In the past two decades, there has been a worldwide increase in the incidence of fungal diseases. This is ascribed to the increased use of antibiotics, corticosteroids, cytotoxic agents, and oral contraceptives. Candidiasis occurs in 6 to 28 percent of women, but its incidence doubles in pregnant women. Typical complaints include leukorrhea, pruritus, and dyspareunia. Examination usually reveals the classic features of a red, edematous vulva and vagina with a thick, creamy discharge that adheres in patches to the vaginal wall. Removal of these patches may leave petechiae. The malodor is usually due to associated *G. vaginalis* infection or trichomoniasis. Diagnosis is based on the microscopic examination of the discharge, which is mixed with 10% potassium hydroxide. Distinct translucent spores and hyphae (filaments) are seen after the potassium hydroxide destroys the cellular elements. Confirmatory cultures can be made by plating the discharge on Nickerson's medium. Nightly insertions of miconazole cream or equivalent agents placed high up into the vagina for a week are usually quite efficacious, though a repeat course is sometimes necessary. Oral plus vaginal medication with nystatin may produce better results if repeated infection occurs.

Recurrent *C. albicans* infections are associated with cell-mediated immunization responses, and there is a 50 percent decrease in the luteal phase. Maintenance low-dose oral ketoconazole for 6 months can effectively prevent recurrences, though relapses may occur when therapy is stopped. Long-term treatment with ketoconazole may be hepatotoxic. The microwave sterilization of underwear at a high setting kills all the organisms in 5 minutes, thereby reducing the risks of reinfection. Depo-Provera (medroxyprogesterone) injections substantially reduce the number of recurrences. Topical flucytosine can be used for strains that are resistant to common preparations. Refractory infections may be treated by painting the whole vagina with 1% gentian violet.

Bacterial vaginosis is probably a sexually transmitted disease but recently there have been many reports of nonsexually transmitted infections. It occurs when the pH in the vagina is low (i.e., hyperestrogenic states), between 5.0 to 5.5. Concomitant treatment of the male partner has not been shown to be beneficial. There is a significant association between bacterial vaginosis in pregnancy and both low-mean-birth-weight infants and premature rupture of membranes. If the leukorrhea is heavy, this usually indicates a mixed infection. Many patients are asymptomatic, whereas others have mild pruritus and burning. The discharge is malodorous, grayish, and homogeneous. The symptoms and the odor are probably related to the effects of the commonly associated anaerobes, and *G. vaginalis* may be only a "marker" organism. Because it is a surface infection, inflammation is rare. A wet mount shows clumps of dark, stippled epithelium ("clue cells," but at least 20% must be present to establish diagnosis) exhibiting the *Gardnerella* rods. There are few pus cells and often no lactobacilli. Gram's staining confirms the presence of small gram-negative rods. Two species of motile, curved gram-negative anaerobic rods (*Mobiluncus mulieris* and *curtisii*) with gram-positive cell walls have been isolated from patients with bacterial vaginosis. Recent evidence indicates that vaginitis emphysematosa (bullous vaginitis) is associated with *Trichomonas* and *G. vaginalis* infection in immunocompromised patients. Metronidazole is very effective in its treatment at a dosage of 500 mg twice daily for a week. Vaginal metronidazole gel is only 2 percent absorbed, thus reducing the side effects and making it suitable for use in pregnancy. Twice daily application for 5 days is very effective. An alternative regimen is clindamycin (300 mg twice daily for 7 days or intravaginally as a cream).

Atrophic vaginitis is characterized by a pale, thin, diffuse redness. The mucosa is smooth with ecchymoses and petechiae and loss of the normal rugae. The discharge is variable, ranging from blood-stained, thick, or watery to purulent. The pH is only slightly acidic. Cultures reveal mixed, nonspecific bacterial flora. Vaginal cytologic examination reveals the presence of abundant parabasal or basal epithelial cells. Rapid relief of the burning, itching, and dyspareunia is obtained with the local application of estrogen cream. In severe cases in which there are other symptoms of menopause, orally administered estrogens may also be used. Secondary infection, like any nonspecific infection, can be treated with local sulfonamide preparations.

Allergic and chemical vulvovaginitis may be treated with local corticosteroid preparations. The prolonged use of antibiotics may allow fungal overgrowth to take place, and therapy should be combined with an antifungal cream in such cases. Intercourse should be avoided during any treatment for vaginitis.

Reviews
1. Sparks, J. M. Vaginitis. *J. Reprod. Med.* 36:745, 1991.
   An excellent review article.
2. Martius, J., et al. The role of bacterial vaginosis as a cause of amniotic fluid infection, chorioamnionitis and prematurity—a review article. *Arch. Gynecol. Obstet.* 247:1, 1990.
   Detailed review article on the role of bacterial vaginosis and prematurity.
3. Ross, C. A. Postmenopausal vaginitis. *J. Med. Microbiol.* 11:209, 1975.
   A survey of infected and noninfected cases of postmenopausal vaginitis is discussed.
4. Moi, H., et al. *Mobiluncus* species in bacterial vaginosis: aspects of pathogenesis. *A.P.M.I.S.* 99:1049, 1991.
   Mobiluncus is a newly designated genus of bacilli that is highly associated with the presence of bacterial vaginosis, although the role of these organisms in this entity is unclear.
5. Fong, I. W., et al. Cellular immunity of patients with recurrent or refractory vulvo-vaginal moniliasis. *Am. J. Obstet. Gynecol.* 166:887, 1992.
   There is normal cellular immunity in most women with recurrent moniliasis.
6. Josey, W. E., et al. Vaginitis emphysematosa. A report of 4 cases. *J. Reprod. Med.* 35:974, 1990.
   The association between vaginitis emphysematosa and infectious vaginitis is well demonstrated. It may be a feature of these infections in the immunosuppressed patient.

Epidemiology
7. Holst, E. Reservoir of four organisms associated with bacterial vaginosis suggests lack of sexual transmission. *J. Clin. Microbiol.* 28:2035, 1990.
   The infection is frequently unrelated to sexual activity.
8. Spinillo, A., et al. Epidemiologic characteristics of women with idiopathic recurrent vulvovaginal candidiasis. *Obstet. Gynecol.* 81:721, 1993.
   Appropriate counseling about contraception, sexual activity, and personal hygiene habits could be an important preventive measure in these women.
9. De Oliveira, J. M., et al. Prevalence of *Candida albicans* in vaginal fluid of asymptomatic Portuguese women. *J. Reprod. Med.* 38:41, 1993.
   The overall prevalence of infection was 10.4 percent, and rates were lower in women taking birth control pills (6.8%).
10. Kent, H. L. Epidemiology of vaginitis. *Am. J. Obstet. Gynecol.* 165:1168, 1991.
    This article reviews the epidemiology of three major causes of vaginitis in the United States and Scandinavia. There has been an increase in non-albicans monilia and a decrease in Trichomonas.

Diagnosis
11. Wolner-Hanssen, P., et al. Clinical manifestations of vaginal trichomoniasis. *J.A.M.A.* 261:571, 1989.
    The sensitivity of symptoms and signs was relatively low.
12. Hay, P. E., et al. Diagnosis of bacterial vaginosis in a gynecology clinic. *Br. J. Obstet. Gynaecol.* 99:63, 1992.
    Defines and describes the diagnosis very well.
13. Schoomaker, J. N., et al. A new proline aminopeptide assay for diagnosis of bacterial vaginosis. *Am. J. Obstet. Gynecol.* 165:737, 1991.

Refinement of the "whiff test" (the amine odor released when the discharge is mixed with 10% potassium hydroxide).

14. Platz-Christensen, J., et al. Detection of bacterial vaginosis in Papanicolaou smears. *Am. J. Obstet. Gynecol.* 160:132, 1989.
    The demonstration of clue cells in Pap smears is a useful method for identifying women with probable bacterial vaginosis.

Risk Factors

15. Soper, D. E., et al. Bacterial vaginosis and *Trichomonas* vaginitis are risk factors for cuff cellulitis after abdominal hysterectomy. *Am. J. Obstet. Gynecol.* 163:1016, 1990.
    Patients with bacterial vaginosis were found to have a dramatic increase in the total anaerobic bacteria. Advise pH and wet mount evaluation prior to hysterectomy.
16. Barbone, F., et al. A follow-up study of method of contraception, sexual activity and rates of trichomoniasis, candidiasis and bacterial vaginosis. *Am. J. Obstet. Gynecol.* 163:510, 1990.
    There was a 40 percent lower incidence of T. vaginalis infection in association with oral contraceptive use than with the use of IUD or tubal ligation. There was a reduced incidence (15–20%) of trichomoniasis and bacterial vaginosis associated with spermicidal use.

Treatment

17. Sobel, J. D., Schmitt, C., and Meriwether, C. Clotrimazole treatment of recurrent and chronic *Candida* vulvovaginitis. *Obstet. Gynecol.* 73:330, 1989.
    There was initial clinical remission in 90 percent of the cases; however, only a modest long-term protective effect was observed for intermittent prophylaxis.
18. Nystatin Multicenter Group Study. Therapy of candidal vaginitis. The effect of eliminating intestinal candidiasis. *Am. J. Obstet. Gynecol.* 155:651, 1986.
    Some benefit was realized when oral and vaginal treatment was used, compared to vaginal treatment with nystatin only.
19. Sobel, J. D. Recurrent vulvovaginal candidiasis. A prospective study of the efficacy of maintenance ketoconazole therapy. *N. Engl. J. Med.* 315:1455, 1986.
    This discusses the topic of elective treatment in preventing recurrences. Relapses commence when treatment is stopped. Long-term therapy may be hepatotoxic.
20. Gordon, W. E., et al. Treatment of atrophic vaginitis in postmenopausal women with micronized estradiol cream. *J. Ky. Med. Assoc.* 77:377, 1979.
    There are distinct advantages if the estrogen cream is micronized.
21. Livengoode, C. H., et al. Bacterial vaginosis: treatment with topical intravaginal clindamycin phosphate. *Obstet. Gynecol.* 76:118, 1990.
    Topical clindamycin cured 93.5 percent of the infections with 5-day treatment. There was virtually no absorption and no side effects.
22. Ison, C. A., et al. Local treatment for bacterial vaginosis. *Br. Med. J.* 295:866, 1987.
    Vaginal chlorhexidine is as effective as oral metronidazole in the cure of bacterial vaginosis.
23. Dennerstein, G. J. Depo-Provera in the treatment of recurrent vulvovaginal candidiasis. *J. Reprod. Med.* 31:801, 1986.
    Long-acting injectable progestogen (evaluated in a pilot study) appeared to substantially reduce women's susceptibility and recurrence.

62. TOXIC SHOCK SYNDROME
Michel E. Rivlin

Toxic shock syndrome (TSS) gained great notoriety in 1980 when the connection between menses, tampon use, and disease was recognized, resulting in the withdrawal of certain high-absorbency tampons from the market. It soon became clear that the syndrome was also associated with a wide variety of surgical conditions unrelated to menses, and, in recent years, almost one case in three has been nonmenstrual and caused by *Staphylococcus aureus* infections at other sites. For the epidemiologic and clinical identification of TSS, a case definition was formulated by the Centers for Disease Control (CDC). According to it, a patient must have the following four major signs: fever (>38.9°C), rash (diffuse macular erythroderma), hypotension (<90 mm Hg), and desquamation (1–2 weeks from the onset, particularly affecting the palms and soles). In addition, at least three organ systems must be involved with characteristic abnormalities: gastrointestinal (nausea, vomiting, or diarrhea at the onset of illness), mucous membranes (vaginal, oropharyngeal, or conjunctival hyperemia), muscular (severe myalgia or creatine kinase level at least twice normal), renal (creatinine level at least twice normal or pyuria without infection), hepatic (bilirubin, serum glutamic-oxaloacetic transaminase, or serum glutamic-pyruvic transaminase levels at least twice normal), hematologic (thrombocytopenia or leukocytosis with left shift), or nervous system (disorientation or altered consciousness). In addition, specific diagnostic tests for other possible causes must yield negative results. These include blood, throat, or cerebrospinal fluid cultures (blood culture may be positive for *S. aureus*). Such tests also include a search for rising antibody titers for Rocky Mountain spotted fever, leptospirosis, or rubeola, or the presence of any bacteria other than *S. aureus,* such as group A streptococci. Use of this strict case definition probably eliminates a large number of milder cases of the disease, but it is important to diagnose these mild cases in order to prevent recurrence.

The syndrome is caused by infection with strains of *S. aureus* possessing a unique phenotype, high levels of proteolytic activity, and the production of an exoprotein called toxic shock syndrome toxin-1 (TSST-1), either alone or in combination with one or more enterotoxins. Whereas colonization with, and antibody formation to, these organisms is common, TSS is relatively uncommon. Women who suffer TSS have absent or low levels of serum antibody to TSST-1. The formation of antibodies after a bout with TSS is variable, and those patients who do not form them are prone to relapse. The syndrome is associated with a potential focus of infection (e.g., abscess or menses with a tampon in use), and focal growth conditions may play a major role; for instance, some tampon fibers that have a high absorbency for water also absorb ions, particularly magnesium. Low concentrations of magnesium promote greater production of TSST-1 by *S. aureus*, perhaps explaining the increased risk of TSS associated with high-absorbency tampons. It therefore appears that TSS reflects a multifactorial pathogenic process that includes exposure to a toxin-producing organism, absence of preexisting immunity, and growth under optimal conditions for toxin production. The toxins cause direct cell membrane damage and activate vasodilators, resulting in increased permeability and decreased vasomotor tone with subsequent tissue hypoxia, metabolic acidosis, and ischemia. The gastrointestinal, epidermal, and mucous membrane manifestations are caused by direct toxin damage. The toxins also exert a direct effect on the myocardium, resulting in impaired contractility. The ischemia can lead to renal shutdown and central nervous system dysfunction.

The incidence of TSS declined from 890 cases in 1980 to 61 cases in 1990. The percentage of menstrual cases has leveled off at about two thirds of all cases in women. At highest risk are women in the 15- to 34-year-old group. The mortality, previously in the range of 5.6 to 8.3 percent, is currently 2.7 to 3.3 percent and is twice as high (8%) in men for reasons that are not clear. Nonmenstrual TSS can be associated with a wide variety of infections caused by *S. aureus,* including skin, bone, and soft tissue infections. Postpartum and postoperative obstetric cases have occurred, and rare cases of TSS complicating contraceptive diaphragm and sponge use have been described. Oral contraceptives may be protective for reasons that are not known, but this is possibly related to changes they effect in the vaginal environment, as staphylococci are part of the normal vaginal flora in 10 percent of women.

Typically the onset of TSS occurs during menses, and a vaginal tampon may be found in place in such women. It may also appear 1 or 2 days after menses. The clinical presentation of menstrual and nonmenstrual TSS is essentially the same, but the patient characteristics and onset of disease differ. The most common presentation consists of fever, myalgias, headache, dizziness, diarrhea, and vomiting. Physical examination reveals fever, hypotension, or orthostasis, and the existence of a diffuse sunburnlike erythroderma that blanches with pressure. Scleral or conjunctival infection is also common, and diffuse abdominal tenderness without rebound may be present. Thereafter, changes in the patient's sensorium and profound shock may develop. The characteristic desquamation begins at about day 7 and progresses to become a castlike desquamation, with cleavage at the basal layer, particularly of the fingers, palms, toes, and soles, between days 10 and 14.

The multisystem organ involvement caused both directly by the toxin and indirectly by the hypotension may lead to many laboratory-detected abnormalities that are reflected in the blood count, liver and renal functions, and serum electrolyte levels. In arriving at the diagnosis, the critical finding is diffuse erythroderma, which is not found in other compatible diseases. If the erythroderma, which may be evanescent, is not seen, any bacteremic disease is possible and must be considered. Finding a site of S. aureus infection in nonmenstrual cases is strong evidence for a presumptive diagnosis of TSS in cases that may be otherwise somewhat atypical. Unfortunately, there are as yet no simple laboratory tests to confirm the diagnosis. Several complications have been reported that are related to disease severity and a delay in therapy. These include adult respiratory distress syndrome (ARDS), reversible acute oliguric and nonoliguric renal failure, myoglobinuria, myocardial dysfunction, disseminated intravascular coagulopathy (DIC), tetany with hypocalcemia, arthritis, and vasculitis. Survivors generally begin to recover within 7 to 10 days. The three major causes of death are ARDS, intractable hypotension, and DIC.

Patients must undergo aggressive fluid resuscitation in an intensive care area. A Swan-Ganz catheter should be inserted, and fluid challenges should be given until the wedge pressure is elevated to 15 to 20 mm Hg. Urine output should be kept above 20 ml/hr. Positive-pressure ventilation may be needed to prevent respiratory failure and ARDS. If adequate blood pressure cannot be maintained, vasopressor drugs may be required. The administration of corticosteroids may decrease the severity of illness, if given early, but their efficacy has not been proved. Once the patient's condition is stabilized and the source of infection has been identified, the source of the toxin must be eliminated through the drainage of infected wounds, debridement, or removal of an infected nidus such as surgical packings. Vaginal examination, with removal of tampons, diaphragms, and other contraceptive devices, is essential. Cultures of blood, mucous membranes, discharges, and foreign devices must be performed. There are few data to suggest that antibiotics affect the course of TSS. However, their use does lead to a decrease in the recurrence rate and can benefit those rare patients with S. aureus bacteremia. A penicillinase-resistant semisynthetic penicillin (nafcillin or oxacillin), given in a dosage of 1 or 2 g administered intravenously every 4 hours for 10 to 14 days, is recommended. A first-generation cephalosporin or, in penicillin-allergic patients, vancomycin may be used. Patients with sequestered infections, such as osteomyelitis, may require more prolonged therapy.

TSS may recur within the first 2 to 3 months after the initial episode in 25 to 30 percent of patients. The cornerstone of prevention is education of the patient, in conjunction with effective antimicrobial therapy of the initial infection and avoidance of tampon use. Women who choose to use tampons should be advised to use them intermittently throughout menses, and for the shortest period consistent with personal comfort, perhaps alternating with pads or napkins. Tampons with the lowest absorbency compatible with hygienic protection should be used. Women who use tampons should be made aware of the syndrome and should be reassured that it is an uncommon disease. They should be familiar with the early symptoms and signs and know to remove the tampon and seek medical care if an illness associated with fever, dizziness, rash, or diarrhea develops. Women with a history of TSS should be urged not to resume tampon use at all. If they insist on using them, S. aureus should first be eliminated from the lower genital tract and, if necessary, from the sexual partner. Nonmenstrual TSS may be largely prevented by the prompt institution of medical and surgical treatment of localized suppurative staphylococcal infection.

In recent years, there have been numerous descriptions of a similar constellation of findings associated with group A streptococci. This syndrome, termed the *toxic streptococcal syndrome* or *toxic shock-like syndrome,* may stem from a general re-emergence of invasive streptococcal infections. Factors associated with the syndrome include the serotype, especially M-types 1 and 3, pyrogenic exotoxins, and protein-ases. Immunologic factors, such as preexisting M-type–specific antibody, and other host characteristics may also be important. Surveillance for the syndrome has been hindered by the lack of an accepted case definition, and currently the diagnosis and management are similar to those applied in the setting of staphylococcal TSS.

Reviews
1. Helms, C., and Wintermeyer, L. Menstrually-related toxic shock syndrome. *Iowa Med.* 81:17, 1991.
   The many similarities between TSS and gram-negative septic shock suggest that endotoxin may play a role in the disease.
2. Jones, J., and MacRae, D. L. Toxic shock syndrome. *J. Otolaryngol.* 19:211, 1990.
   Additional staphylococcal toxins may cause TSS, including enterotoxins. Thus, TSST-1 production may not be essential to the pathogenesis of TSS.

Etiology
3. Todd, J., et al. Toxic-shock syndrome associated with phage-group 1 staphylo-cocci. *Lancet* 2:1116, 1978.
   This is the original report describing TSS. Phage-group 1, types 29 and 52, was originally implicated, but, since then, many phage groups have been involved and may represent a regional distribution rather than a genetic association of the dis-ease with a specific phage.
4. Kass, E. H., and Parsonnet, J. On the pathogenesis of toxic shock syndrome. *Rev. Infect. Dis.* 9:S482, 1987.
   An endogenous endotoxin contributes to rabbit susceptibility to TSST-1 and may play a role in human TSS.
5. Crass, B. A., and Bergdoll, M. S. Toxin involvement in toxic shock syndrome. *J. Infect. Dis.* 153:918, 1986.
   TSS patients may have an immunodeficiency that inhibits the production, main-tenance, or both, of antibodies to the staphylococcal enterotoxins and TSST-1.
6. Fast, D. J., Schlievert, P. M., and Nelson, R. D. Toxic shock syndrome–associated staphylococcal and streptococcal pyrogenic toxins are potent inducers of tumor necrosis factor production. *Infect. Immunol.* 57:291, 1989.
   Streptococcal pyrogenic exotoxins A through C are similar to TSST-1 and staphy-lococcal enterotoxins A through E in their ability to stimulate cytokine release.

Menstrual TSS
7. Reduced incidence of menstrual toxic-shock syndrome—United States, 1980–1990. *M.M.W.R.* 39:421, 1990.
   TSS may not be an important public health problem at this time, probably due to the removal of polyacrylate rayon tampons from the market and accompanying reductions in tampon absorbency.
8. Chesney, P. J. Clinical aspects and spectrum of illness of toxic shock syndrome: overview. *Rev. Infect. Dis.* 2:S1, 1989.
   In arriving at the diagnosis, there should be reasonable evidence for the absence of other bacterial, viral, or rickettsial infections, drug reactions, or autoimmune disorders.
9. Crews, J. R., et al. Stunned myocardium in the toxic shock syndrome. *Ann. In-tern. Med.* 117:912, 1992.
   The left ventricular dysfunction that occurs in TSS is reversible, similar to the

behavior of postischemic myocardial dysfunction, a process termed stunned myocardium.

Nonmenstrual TSS

10. Petitti, D., D'Agostino, R. B., and Oldman, M. J. Nonmenstrual toxic shock syndrome. Methodologic problems in estimating incidence and delineating risk factors. *J. Reprod. Med.* 32:10, 1987.
    Reliable estimates of the incidence of nonmenstrual TSS are largely unavailable, and systematic studies of risk factors have not been done.
11. Remington, K. M., Buller, R. S., and Kelly, J. R. Effect of the Today contraceptive sponge on growth and toxic shock syndrome toxin-1 production by *Staphylococcus aureus. Obstet. Gynecol.* 69:563, 1987.
    Five to 10 menstrual cases of TSS are expected per 100,000 regular tampon users per year. Eighteen definite instances of TSS associated with diaphragm use and 13 cases associated with contraceptive sponge use were reported to the CDC up to 1984.
12. Hughes, D., and Stapleton, J. Postoperative toxic shock syndrome. *Iowa Med.* 81:55, 1991.
    Nonmenstrual TSS begins a median of 2 days after operation in patients with surgical wound infections; from 1 day to 8 weeks in patients with nonsurgical, skin, subcutaneous, or soft tissue infections; and in postpartum and postabortion cases.
13. Cone, L. A., et al. A recalcitrant, erythematous, desquamating disorder associated with toxin-producing staphylococci in patients with AIDS. *J. Infect. Dis.* 165:638, 1992.
    This article adds immunoincompetence to the equation.
14. Erstad, B. L., et al. Toxic shock–like syndrome. *Pharmacotherapy* 12:23, 1992.
    Broad-spectrum antibiotics are advisable for treatment because beta-lactam antibiotics may be less effective than antibiotic combinations that suppress protein synthesis. Surgical debridement and aggressive supportive care are essential.

Streptococcal TSS

15. The Working Group on Severe Streptococcal Infections. Defining the group A streptococcal toxic shock syndrome. Rationale and consensus definition. *J.A.M.A.* 269:390, 1993.
    The occurrence of shock and multiorgan failure early in the course of the infection helps differentiate streptococcal TSS from other types of streptococcal infection.
16. Hoge, C. W., et al. The changing epidemiology of invasive group A streptococcal infections and the emergence of streptococcal toxic shock–like syndrome. A retrospective population-based study. *J.A.M.A.* 269:384, 1993.
    Both the rate and severity of invasive group A streptococcal infections have increased since the mid-1980s.
17. Barry, W., et al. Intravenous immunoglobulin therapy for toxic shock syndrome. *J.A.M.A.* 267:3315, 1992.
    Dramatic improvement was observed within hours of intravenous immunoglobulin administration in a patient with streptococcal TSS whose condition was deteriorating while on standard therapy.

63. PELVIC INFLAMMATORY DISEASE
Michel E. Rivlin

Pelvic inflammatory disease (PID) is defined as the acute clinical syndrome attributed to the ascending spread of microorganisms from the vagina and endocervix to the endometrium, fallopian tubes, one or both ovaries, and the pelvic and perhaps abdominal peritoneum. The suprahepatic space may also be involved. In most cases, it is a community-acquired bacterial infection presumed to be initiated by sexual activity. Infections related to pregnancy or surgical procedure are usually not included in the definition and are regarded as separate entities. There are an estimated 1 million cases per year in the United States. Late sequelae develop in one fourth of the women with acute PID, including involuntary infertility, which occurs in 15 to 20 percent. Other sequelae include chronic pelvic pain, dyspareunia, and inflammatory masses, which require surgical intervention in 15 to 20 percent of the cases. In addition, the incidence of ectopic pregnancy is increased several-fold to about 8 percent in women who have had PID.

Several risk factors for PID can be identified. Previous PID damages endothelial resistance and predisposes to recurrence. Women with multiple sex partners have a relative risk factor of 4.6. The microbiologic causes of PID vary greatly. In general, *Neisseria gonorrhoeae* has been estimated to account for 10 to 66 percent of the cases, whereas, at least in the United States, *Chlamydia trachomatis* is causally linked to approximately 20 percent of the cases. Infection with *N. gonorrhoeae* or *Chlamydia* is associated with an approximate 10 to 20 percent risk of developing clinically recognizable PID. Oral contraceptive users have an increased risk of chlamydial cervicitis but a lesser risk of overt PID. Pill use does not affect the risk of tubal infertility. The use of an intrauterine device (IUD) increases the risk of PID by seven- to ninefold, chiefly in young nulliparous women, whereas the risk is much lower in older women who are multiparous and have only one partner. On the other hand, barrier contraceptives combined with spermicides reduce the risk of PID.

PID frequently has a polymicrobial etiology, no matter what organisms are cultured from the cervix. The traditional role of *N. gonorrhoeae* as the initiator of infection that paves the way for a subsequent invasion by gram-positive and -negative aerobic and anaerobic vaginal or enteric organisms has become less tenable, as it now seems probable that all the organisms enter the upper tracts at the same time. Many studies have demonstrated a poor correlation between the bacteria obtained by cervical culture and those grown from cul-de-sac or laparoscopic samples, taken at the same time. In addition, genital mycoplasmas (e.g., *Mycoplasma hominis* and *Ureaplasma urealyticum*) may play a role in some cases of PID. Although the traditional division of PID into gonococcal and nongonococcal forms is therefore no longer widely alluded to, there is a difference between *N. gonorrhoeae* and chlamydial infections, in that *Chlamydia* infection appears to be associated with a more indolent, less acute, and less severe clinical picture, with more potential for permanent tubal damage and its sequel, tubal infertility. Both *N. gonorrhoeae* and *Chlamydia* spread along the endocervix to the endometrium and then to the tubal mucosa. Characteristically (66–77%), gonococcal PID presents in the first postmenstrual week. There is also some evidence that bacteria may attach to sperm and reach the upper tract by means of bacteriospermia. The mechanism of spread appears to differ from that seen for IUD use. Here, the string may act as a wick (especially the multifilament string of the Dalkon Shield), and the chronic local endometritis generated by the device may breach host defenses, leading to a lymphatic spread into the parametrium similar to that seen for postabortal or postpartum infections.

For the purposes of clinical management, PID may be subdivided into two major types: uncomplicated, which is not associated with an adnexal mass or inflammatory complex; and complicated, which is associated with an adnexal complex or more advanced condition. The presence of abdominal, adnexal, and cervical motion tenderness in a patient with a history of abdominal pain, together with at least one objective indication of infection or inflammation, such as fever (>38.3°C; 100.4°F), leukocytosis (>10,500), or an elevated erythrocyte sedimentation rate (>20), constitute the clinical criteria recommended for establishing the diagnosis of PID. Further objective evidence supporting the diagnosis includes the presence of gram-negative intracellular diplococci on an endocervical smear, purulent material obtained from the peritoneal cavity by culdocentesis or laparoscopy, and an adnexal mass found during bimanual or sonographic examination. Endocervical tests for *Chlamydia* and the estimation of C-reactive protein levels provide further important diagnostic information. Endometrial biopsy samples are obtained by some clinicians, with findings of plasma cell endometritis reported for almost all patients with proven PID. The clinical diagnosis of PID is incorrect in up to 35 percent of women, and the differential diagnosis is broad and includes ectopic pregnancy, appendicitis, ovarian cyst accidents, endometriosis, and, not infrequently, a normal pelvis. As a consequence, laparoscopy is increasingly used in doubtful cases, because it exhibits a near 100 percent sensitivity and affords access to the tubes for culture. However, economic factors and logistic difficulties have, until now, prevented the routine use of laparoscopy diagnosis in all suspected PID cases in the United States. If laparoscopy is used, PID is deemed mild if the tubes are edematous, erythematous, and freely mobile; and as moderate if spontaneous gross purulence is seen with tubes that may not be mobile and stomata that may not be patent. In severe disease, there is an inflammatory complex or abscess (pyosalpinx or tuboovarian abscess) that may be leaking.

The goals of therapy are to cure the present illness and to prevent infertility and other chronic sequelae. Women with mild disease receive ambulatory therapy. The criteria for hospital admission include a suspected pelvic abscess, uncertain diagnosis, severe illness, and failure to respond to outpatient care within 48 hours; those patients who are unable to follow or tolerate the regimen or to be seen for follow-up within 48 to 72 hours should also be hospitalized. In many areas, the hospitalization criteria are more liberal, especially with regard to nulliparous women with first infections. Because no single antibiotic is active against all possible pathogens, the Centers for Disease Control (CDC) recommend several possible combination regimens that are directed against *N. gonorrhoeae,* including penicillinase-producing strains and *Chlamydia.* Cefoxitin, or an equally effective cephalosporin, plus doxycycline or tetracycline, is an example of a regimen that provides this activity. Therapy is maintained for 7 to 10 days. An alternative outpatient regimen also recommended by the CDC includes ofloxacin and either clindamycin or metronidazole for 14 days. Bed rest, sexual abstinence, analgesics, referral of sexual partners for examination and possible treatment, removal of an IUD if present, and contraceptive counseling are further important measures. If specific pathogens are cultured, the cultures should be repeated after therapy is completed. The CDC recommends two regimens for inpatient therapy: (1) cefoxitin or cefotetan plus doxycycline or (2) clindamycin plus gentamicin, followed by doxycycline. It is recommended that intravenous therapy be maintained for at least 4 days and for at least 48 hours after clinical improvement takes place.

Unfortunately, the clinical efficacy and even the efficacy of ambulatory versus inpatient therapy are not well established. In practice, those patients requiring hospitalization but who do not have an adnexal mass are often treated with single-agent regimens, with results equal to those observed for the CDC recommendations, but with lower costs and side effects. The drugs include the newer broad-spectrum cephalosporins and the expanded-spectrum penicillins. Accumulating data indicate that the penicillins, cephalosporins, and clindamycin may have antichlamydial activity. Adnexal inflammatory masses are usually treated with combinations of agents, including an aminoglycoside or aztreonam and an agent with specific antianaerobic activity (clindamycin, chloramphenicol, or metronidazole). In using these drugs, the possibility of nephrotoxicity and pseudomembranous enterocolitis must be kept in mind. Existing data do not establish the need for lengthy parenteral therapy, and many clinicians discontinue intravenous therapy when patients have become afebrile and asymptomatic. In general, fever is a poor prognosticator of response, unless it is elevated or rising. Instead, reduced abdominal pain and degree of peritonism and decreased cervical motion tenderness are better guides. About 15 percent of the patients fail to respond to the initial medication, requiring a change of agents. Surgical treatment is not indicated for acute PID, other than to rule out possible surgical emergencies or in the event of pelvic abscess formation in certain circumstances. The surgical management of PID is reviewed in Chapter 64.

The relationship of infertility to the number of episodes is linear, with 11 percent of the patients infertile after one attack, 23 percent after two attacks, and 54 percent after three or more attacks. It is also related to the severity of disease, with 6 percent infertile after mild changes, 13 percent after moderately severe inflammation, and 30 percent after severe disease. PID recurs in 25 percent of the patients. In women who suffer one episode of salpingitis, the risk of ectopic pregnancy increases to 5 percent of live births (normally 1–2%); in those with multiple previous episodes, the risk may be as high as 20 percent. Good results of therapy depend on early diagnosis and rational antibiotic selection and administration, together with the prevention of reinfection by means of patient education and the treatment of sexual partners. At issue is the reproductive capacity of an unfortunately ever-increasing group of young women.

Review

1. Morgan, R. J. Clinical aspects of pelvic inflammatory disease. *Am. Fam. Physician* 43:1725, 1991.
   The existence of chronic tubal infection is often only diagnosed in conjunction with ectopic pregnancy or during an infertility investigation.
2. Pelvic inflammatory disease: guidelines for prevention and management. *M.M.W.R.* 40:1, 1991.
   Differentiating lower from upper genital tract infections is often difficult.

Etiology

3. Soper, D. E., Brockwell, M. J., and Dalton, H. P. Microbial etiology of urban emergency department acute salpingitis: treatment with ofloxacin. *Am. J. Obstet. Gynecol.* 167:653, 1992.
   Gonorrhea was found in 69 percent of the patients, Chlamydia infection in 17 percent, and the source was polymicrobial in one patient only. All responded to ofloxacin treatment.
4. Beck, E. Intrauterine devices and pelvic inflammatory disease—a reanalysis of the literature. *West. J. Med.* 154:328, 1991.
   The rates of PID were lower in association with the current types of IUDs than with the older types.
5. Scholes, D., et al. Vaginal douching as a risk factor for acute pelvic inflammatory disease. *Obstet. Gynecol.* 81:601, 1993.
   It appears that vaginal douching can predispose a woman to PID.
6. Cates, W., Jr., Rolfs, R. T., Jr., and Aral, S. D. Sexually transmitted diseases, pelvic inflammatory disease, and infertility: an epidemiologic update. *Epidemiol. Rev.* 12:199, 1990.
   Tubal infertility may follow symptomatic or asymptomatic PID.
7. Clark, K., and Baranyai, J. Pelvic infection and the pathogenesis of tubal ectopic pregnancy. *Aust. N.Z. J. Obstet. Gynaecol.* 27:57, 1987.
   The increase in the incidence of ectopic pregnancies is strongly associated with an increase in the prevalence of PID.
8. Kahn, J. G., et al. Diagnosing pelvic inflammatory disease: a comprehensive analysis and considerations for developing a new model. *J.A.M.A.* 266:2594, 1991.
   In the long term, a false diagnosis of PID can be a heavy emotional burden.
9. Cacciatore, B., et al. Transvaginal sonographic findings in ambulatory patients with suspected pelvic inflammatory disease. *Obstet. Gynecol.* 80:912, 1992.
   Thickened fluid-filled tubes were found in 11 of 13 patients with plasma cell endometritis and in none of those without. In this study, the finding of plasma cell endometritis was considered diagnostic of PID.
10. Livengood, C. H., III, et al. Pelvic inflammatory disease: findings during inpatient treatment of clinically severe, laparoscopy-documented disease. *Am. J. Obstet. Gynecol.* 166:519, 1992.
    The laparoscopic grading of severity is much more accurate than clinical diagnosis and grading. Laparoscopic grading can also be useful in predicting the duration of hospital stay and the future of tubal factor infertility.

Clinical Features

11. Hager, W. D., et al. Criteria for diagnosis and grading of salpingitis. *Obstet. Gynecol.* 61:113, 1983.
    The article tabulates the clinical criteria required for diagnosis and the grading

of severity based on the findings from clinical and laparoscopic examination, as recommended by the Infectious Disease Society for Obstetrics and Gynecology.

12. Morcos, R., et al. Laparoscopic versus clinical diangosis of acute pelvic inflammatory disease. *J. Reprod. Med.* 38:53, 1993.
    PID was established laparoscopically in 76.1 percent of 176 women admitted with a clinical diagnosis of PID.

13. Rolfs, R. T., Galaid, E. I., and Zaidi, A. A. Pelvic inflammatory disease: trends in hospitalizations and office visits, 1979 through 1988. *Am. J. Obstet. Gynecol.* 166:983, 1992.
    Hospitalization rates decreased by 36 percent while office visit rates remained unchanged. Surgery was performed in 42 percent of the patients with acute PID and 90 percent of those with chronic PID who were hospitalized.

14. Omens, S., et al. Laparoscopic treatment of painful perihepatic adhesions in Fitz-Hugh-Curtis syndrome. *Obstet. Gynecol.* 78:542, 1991.
    This paper describes a form of PID associated with perihepatitis and on occasion, perisplenitis and perinephritis. Chlamydia and N. gonorrhoeae have been implicated as etiologic agents.

15. Safrin, S., et al. Long-term sequelae of acute pelvic inflammatory disease: a retrospective cohort study. *Am. J. Obstet. Gynecol.* 166:1300, 1992.
    Subsequent PID occurred in 43 percent of the patients, 24 percent experienced pelvic pain for 6 months or more, and 40 percent were involuntarily infertile after hospitalization for acute PID.

16. Green, M. M., et al. Acute pelvic inflammatory disease after surgical sterilization. *Ann. Emerg. Med.* 20:344, 1991.
    Salpingitis can occur after tubal ligation.

17. Blanchard, A. C., Pastorek, J. G., II, and Weeks, T. Pelvic inflammatory disease during pregnancy. *South. Med. J.* 880:1363, 1987.
    This is a rare complication that is generally amenable to antibiotic therapy, although the diagnosis may only be made at exploratory laparotomy.

18. Hoegsberg, B., et al. Sexually transmitted diseases and human immunodeficiency virus infection among women with pelvic inflammatory disease. *Am. J. Obstet. Gynecol.* 16:1135, 1990.
    Human immunodeficiency virus–infected patients with PID were more likely to have abscesses and to require surgical intervention. Early hospitalization is therefore recommended.

Treatment

19. Centers for Disease Control. 1993 Sexually transmitted diseases treatment guidelines. *M.M.W.R.* 42(RR-14): Sept. 24, 1993.
    Cephalosporins that are equivalent in efficacy to cefoxitin include cefotetan, ceftizoxime, cefotaxime, and ceftriaxone.

20. Peterson, H. B., et al. Pelvic inflammatory disease: key treatment issues and options. *J.A.M.A.* 266:2605, 1991.
    No single agent that provides sufficient coverage is currently available. Hospitalization, where feasible, is called for, particularly if further childbearing is desired.

21. Landers, V., et al. Combination antimicrobial therapy in the treatment of acute pelvic inflammatory disease. *Am. J. Obstet. Gynecol.* 164:849, 1991.
    The response rate was 98.5 percent in uncomplicated cases of PID and 81 percent in cases complicated by tuboovarian abscess. Surgical treatment during the initial hospitalization was required in 5 of 148 patients.

22. Carey, M., and Brown, S. Infertility surgery for pelvic inflammatory disease: success rates after salpingolysis and salpingostomy. *Am. J. Obstet. Gynecol.* 156:296, 1987.
    Adhesiolysis led to an intrauterine gestation in 41 percent and an ectopic pregnancy in 23 percent. Adhesiolysis in combination with terminal salpingostomy resulted in an intrauterine gestation in 18 percent and an ectopic pregnancy in 9 percent.

23. Washington, A. E., Cates, W., Jr., and Wasserheit, J. N. Preventing pelvic inflammatory disease. *J.A.M.A.* 266:2574, 1991.

The best strategies for preventing PID are: (1) prevention of Chlamydia infection and gonorrhea in both sexes, and (2) when this fails, early detection and treatment of lower-tract infection.

24. Washington, E., and Katz, P. Cost of and payment source for pelvic inflammatory disease: trends and projections, 1983 through 2000. *J.A.M.A.* 266:2565, 1991.
    For 1990, the cost was $4 billion; for 2000, the cost will be $9 billion.

64. PELVIC ABSCESS
Michel E. Rivlin

Most pelvic abscesses are a sequela of infection in the upper genital tract originating as pelvic inflammatory disease (PID). Abscesses usually form as a result of inadequate treatment or patient delay in seeking care, and are more commonly seen in women who have had multiple episodes of PID. Less frequently, pelvic abscesses are a complication of appendicitis, diverticulitis, or gynecologic or obstetric surgical procedures. The abscess may be largely confined to the uterine tube (pyosalpinx), but more commonly involves a tuboovarian complex. In some instances, purulent material extends into the posterior pelvis and becomes walled off by multiple structures, including the tube, ovaries, broad ligaments, small bowel, and omentum. Whereas the PID is almost always a bilateral process, the abscess may be unilateral in up to 71 percent of the cases, especially if an intrauterine device (IUD) is present. Adnexal masses in the presence of pelvic infections are not necessarily abscesses, but frequently represent conglutination of the tubes and ovaries to the adjacent pelvic and abdominal structures as a reaction to the purulent exudate from the inflamed tube. This condition is better described as a tuboovarian complex rather than an abscess, for it lacks the classic abscess wall. The appropriate use of broad-spectrum antibiotics has led to a marked decrease in the incidence of tuboovarian abscess. An intraovarian abscess, contained within the parenchyma of the ovary, may arise through inoculation of an open wound, such as that produced by ovulation or by surgical procedures. This variety of pelvic abscess is relatively uncommon. Rupture into the general peritoneal cavity, with subsequent diffuse peritonitis, is the major complication of a pelvic abscess. The rupture may either be spontaneous or precipitated by trauma, such as that produced by a pelvic examination or barium enema, a fall, or abdominal blow. If not diagnosed and correctly treated within 24 to 48 hours, septicemia and septic shock ensue, with a resultant high mortality. Pelvic thrombophlebitis and ovarian vein thrombosis are other late complications of major pelvic infections that may be associated with significant morbidity and mortality.

The bacteria responsible are those normally found in the lower genital tract, including aerobes such as *Streptococcus* and *Escherichia coli;* anaerobes such as *Peptococcus, Peptostreptococcus*, and *Bacteroides;* and, rarely, *Clostridia* or *Actinomyces.* The infection is virtually always polymicrobial, with three or more organisms commonly recovered. The sexually transmitted organisms such as *Neisseria gonorrhoeae* and *Chlamydia* are usually not present in the abscess but may be recovered from the cervix in approximately one third of the cases. The onset of symptoms is usually insidious, with the most common complaint pelvic pain and tenderness. Patients frequently experience fever and tachycardia, and some may complain of abnormal vaginal bleeding, vaginal discharge, nausea, anorexia, or diarrhea. On examination, lower abdominal and pelvic tenderness with or without evidence of peritonism, may be noted. An abnormal mass may not be found by clinical means, depending on its location, the woman's weight, and the degree of tenderness. Some patients may be afebrile and the white blood cell count may be normal. Ultrasonography can usually show a complex adnexal mass, although a purely cystic lesion may be seen. Sonography will usually demonstrate the mass, and computed tomography (CT), which is probably the most accurate technique for localizing intraabdominal abscesses, can be reserved for those cases in which other diagnostic procedures have failed to confirm the diagnosis. The clinician must determine whether the abscess is confined to the pelvis and lower abdomen, or whether there is evidence of leakage or rupture. For the former to be the case, evidence of peritoneal irritation should be limited to the pelvis or lower abdomen; peritoneal signs above the umbilicus suggest leakage or rupture, which constitutes a surgical emergency. The differential diagnosis includes appendicitis, diverticulitis, ectopic pregnancy, a twisted ovarian cyst, and septic abortion. In this respect, serum pregnancy tests are most helpful in identifying these problems associated with pregnancy. The physical findings of endometriosis may be very similar to those of chronic adnexal sepsis, but, in the acute phase, the systemic evidence of infection provides the diagnostic clue.

The initial approach to treatment in the patient with an unruptured abscess should usually be medical, consisting of antibiotics effective against anaerobes and aerobes, including *E. coli*. A commonly used regimen comprises an aminoglycoside in combination with clindamycin or metronidazole. The monocyclic beta-lactam aztreonam may be used in place of the aminoglycoside, which thus avoids potential nephrotoxicity. Fluid and electrolyte balance are maintained with intravenous fluids and nasogastric suction. Such conservative management may be successful in 33 to 74 percent of the cases. Surgical management is urgently indicated for patients with a ruptured abscess and in those whose condition deteriorates rapidly while they are being treated, with evidence of increasing peritonitis. Abscesses that are situated in the cul-de-sac and dissect down the rectovaginal septum should be drained via a colpotomy. Surgical intervention is also indicated for patients who do not respond to medical therapy, as evidenced by persistent fever and leukocytosis, pain, enlarging masses (based on the findings from examination, ultrasound, or CT), and persistent ileus. Many clinicians set a time limit and proceed to surgical intervention if there has not been a good response within 48 to 72 hours. Surgical treatment is also indicated for those patients who, after discharge, continue to have pain and a persistent tender mass. Removal of the uterus and both adnexa may confer the least risk of postoperative morbidity and the least risk of the need for reoperation for an unresolved infection, but this results in castration, often at a young age. An operation that preserves the uterus and some ovarian tissue offers at least a possibility of childbearing, but the likelihood of recurrent or persistent infection is greater. Consultation with the woman and her family with an explanation of the risks and benefits involved are important factors in choosing the best operation for the particular patient. Novel approaches in the management of pelvic abscesses that may be more widely used in the future include laparoscopic drainage as well as sonographically or CT-directed percutaneous aspiration or catheter drainage.

The clinical picture exhibited by a woman with a ruptured abscess is highly variable. In some, the rupture is heralded by a severe and sudden exacerbation of pain, tachycardia that is out of proportion to the temperature, and signs of peritonitis and shock. Operative intervention is imperative as soon as the patient's condition has been stabilized through the admininstration of intravenous fluids. The placement of a central line or Swan-Ganz catheter may be helpful for this purpose. Conservative surgical treatment may be indicated under selected circumstances when preservation of reproductive function is a high priority and the patient is willing to accept the possibility of reoperation. In most instances, the patient is best served by a complete hysterectomy with bilateral adnexectomy. If the abscess is unilateral, an adnexectomy of the involved side may be sufficient. Careful exploration of the whole abdomen and examination of the entire bowel is necessary for achieving complete drainage, followed by copious irrigation and the liberal use of suction drains or drainage via the vaginal cuff. Mass closure of the abdominal incision with nonabsorbable suture material and delayed closure of the subcutaneous tissue and skin are advisable. Postoperative ileus is to be expected, requiring continued nasogastric drainage and possible total parenteral nutrition.

The pregnancy rates in patients treated for pelvic abscesses after all methods of treatment appear to range from about 10 to 20 percent. It is becoming apparent that the most appropriate approach to management is individual therapy that takes into account the age, clinical status, and desires of the properly informed patient.

Reviews

1. Burnett, L. S. Gynecologic causes of the acute abdomen. *Surg. Clin. North Am.* 68:385, 1988.
   The complex environment of an abscess frequently limits the effectiveness of antibiotics, so that surgical intervention often becomes necessary.
2. Osborne, N. G. Tubo-ovarian abscess: Pathogenesis and management. *J. Natl. Med. Assoc.* 78:937, 1986.
   Whether a true abscess will respond to conservative treatment remains undocumented. The size of the abscess may play a major role in responsiveness to therapy.
3. Wiesenfeld, H. C., and Sweet, R. L. Progress in the management of tuboovarian abscesses. *Clin. Obstet. Gynecol.* 36:433, 1993.
   Ultrasound-guided transvaginal drainage of pelvic abscesses and fluid collections has been reported to lead to a successful outcome in 86 to 100 percent of the cases.

Etiology/Diagnosis

4. Edelman, D. A., and Berger, G. S. Contraceptive practice and tuboovarian abscess. *Am. J. Obstet. Gynecol.* 138:541, 1980.
   The proportions of women with unilateral and bilateral abscesses were similar regardless of the contraceptive method.
5. Pearlman, M., et al. Abdominal wall *Actinomyces* abscess associated with an intrauterine device. A case report. *J. Reprod. Med.* 36:398, 1991.
   Female genital tract actinomyces infection may result in a wide variety of sequelae, including asymptomatic colonization, salpingitis, pelvic masses, and tuboovarian abscess.
6. Livengood, C. H., III, and Addison, W. A. Adnexal abscess as a delayed complication of vaginal hysterectomy. *Am. J. Obstet. Gynecol.* 143:596, 1982.
   The prolonged latency periods before the clinical manifestation of these postoperative adnexal abscesses were ascribed to the use of prophylactic antibiotics.
7. McCausland, V. M., et al. Tuboovarian abscesses after operative hysteroscopy. *J. Reprod. Med.* 38:198, 1993.
   The authors suggest the use of prophylactic doxycycline at the onset of hysteroscopy in patients with a history of PID.
8. Hoffman, M., et al. Tuboovarian abscess in postmenopausal women. *J. Reprod. Med.* 35:525, 1990.
   No age is exempt, although the condition is rare in the very young and in the old. Older patients, who have failed medical therapy should usually undergo definitive surgical intervention, if there are no major contraindications to this approach.
9. Dobrin, P. B., et al. Radiologic diagnosis of an intraabdominal abscess. Do multiple tests help? *Arch. Surg.* 121:41, 1986.
   CT was superior to ultrasound and ultrasound was superior to gallium-enhanced scanning in terms of the sensitivity, specificity, accuracy, and positive and negative predictive values.
10. Hoogewoud, H. M., et al. The role of computerized tomography in fever, septicemia and multiple system organ failure after laparotomy. *Surg. Gynecol. Obstet.* 162:539, 1986.
    As soon as sepsis is suspected, an abdominal and pelvic CT study should be performed so that therapeutic procedures may be carried out at a stage when no organ is yet failing—that is, in a period when the risk of mortality is lowest.

Series

11. Landers, B. V., and Sweet, R. L. Current trends in the diagnosis and treatment of tuboovarian abscess. *Am. J. Obstet. Gynecol.* 151:1098, 1985.
    The failure to respond to adequate medical therapy may be the most reliable way of distinguishing those patients with true adnexal abscess from those with an adnexal inflammatory complex or salpingitis alone.
12. Kaplan, A. L., Jacobs, W. M., and Ehresman, J. B. Aggressive management of pelvic abscess. *Am. J. Obstet. Gynecol.* 98:482, 1967.

The authors advocate routine hysterectomy with adnexectomy (often referred to as "pelvic clean-out," "pelvic sweep," "pelvic clearance") to prevent long-term complications.

Therapy

13. Reed, S. D., Landers, D. V., and Sweet, R. L. Antibiotic treatment of tuboovarian abscess: comparison of broad-spectrum beta-lactam agents versus clindamycin-containing regimens. *Am. J. Obstet. Gynecol.* 164:1556, 1991.
Extended-spectrum antibiotic coverage exhibited an efficacy equivalent to that of clindamycin-containing regimens.
14. Rivlin, M. E. Conservative surgery for adnexal abscess. *J. Reprod. Med.* 30:726, 1985.
Reviews the reoperation and pregnancy rates after conservative surgical treatment.
15. Rivlin, M. E. Clinical outcome following vaginal drainage of pelvic abscess. *Obstet. Gynecol.* 61:169, 1983.
The likelihood of pregnancy after colpotomy drainage when the uterus is left in place is quoted to be about 10 percent.
16. Reich, H., and McGlynn, F. Laparoscopic treatment of tuboovarian and pelvic abscess. *J. Reprod. Med.* 32:747, 1987.
The authors claim that laparoscopy provides the opportunity to accurately diagnose tuboovarian abscess in terms of the degree of involvement, while at the same time affording definitive treatment.
17. Worthen, M. N., and Gunning, J. E. Percutaneous drainage of pelvic abscesses: management of the tubo-ovarian abscess. *J. Ultrasound Med.* 5:551, 1986.
Of 35 cases, the success rate for aspiration drainage was 94 percent, and that for catheter drainage was 77 percent. There was one abscess rupture and one bowel perforation.
18. Hajj, S. N., Merce, L. J., and Ismail, M. A. Surgical approaches to pelvic infections in women. *J. Reprod. Med.* 33:159, 1988.
Pelvic thrombophlebitis is of late onset in the course of the disease. It presents like a resistant infection with tachycardia, fever, and dull, low abdominal pain. The clinical response to a therapeutic trial of heparin provides the presumptive diagnosis.
19. Stubblefield, P. G. Intraovarian abscess treated with laparoscopic aspiration and povidone-iodine lavage. A case report. *J. Reprod. Med.* 36:407, 1991.
Ovarian abscesses are primary infections involving the substance of the ovary. An association with IUD use has been noted, and some cases have occurred as complications of hysterectomy.
20. VanDerKolk, H. L. Small, deep pelvic abscesses: Definition and drainage guided with an endovaginal probe. *Radiology* 181:283, 1991.
CT scanning, fluoroscopy, and transabdominal or transvaginal ultrasound have all been successfully used for guidance in draining pelvic abscesses per vaginam or per rectum.
21. Mecke, H., et al. Pelvic abscesses: pelviscopy or laparotomy. *Gynecol. Obstet. Invest.* 31:231, 1991.
The results of small studies that compare laparoscopic and percutaneous drainage are encouraging, but studies that compare antibiotic therapy alone versus therapy with antibiotics and drainage procedures, or that compare different drainage techniques, have not yet been attempted.
22. Sterghos, S. N., Jr., and Hoffman, M. S. Primary wound closure after laparotomy for tuboovarian abscess. *J. Gynecol. Surg.* 8:73, 1992.
There was no increased risk of wound infection associated with immediate skin closure after laparotomy for a tuboovarian abscess.

Ruptured Tuboovarian Abscess

23. Vermeeren, J., and Te Linde, R. W. Intra-abdominal rupture of pelvic abscesses. *Am. J. Obstet. Gynecol.* 68:402, 1954.

This is the classic paper on the topic; mortality was reduced from 90 to 12 percent.
24. Pedowitz, P., and Bloomfield, R. D. Ruptured adnexal abscess (tuboovarian) with generalized peritonitis. *Am. J. Obstet. Gynecol.* 88:721, 1964.
    This reports the best results ever published; a survival rate of 96.9 percent was obtained.
25. Rivlin, M. E., and Hunt, J. A. Ruptured tuboovarian abscess. Is hysterectomy necessary? *Obstet. Gynecol.* 50:518, 1977.
    Conservative procedures directed at the preservation of reproductive potential are possible, even in the most severe forms of PID.

65. GENITAL TUBERCULOSIS
Michel E. Rivlin

Infection of the genital tract with *Mycobacterium tuberculosis* is almost always secondary to a primary lesion elsewhere, usually in the lungs. Although rare in developed countries, the possibility of pelvic tuberculosis (TB) must be kept in mind, especially in foreign-born patients or in those living in conditions of poverty, overcrowding, and poor health care.

The incidence of pelvic TB varies widely, depending on the source of the estimation. For instance, in patients with problems of infertility living in India, the incidence is 5 to 10 percent; in a similar group in the United States, the incidence is under 0.5 percent. Ten to 50 percent of the patients with genital TB either have a history of pulmonary TB or x-ray evidence of the disease. The age range for patients with the disease is between 20 and 40 years in 80 to 90 percent of cases, although it may occur in the young and in women after menopause.

The decline in TB in the United States ceased in 1984, and, since then, has increased 18 percent, with 26,283 cases reported in 1991. This increase is largely due to the activation of latent disease in immunosuppressed persons and the rapid development of newly acquired infections in this group. The disease disproportionately affects young black and Hispanic people, many of them human immunodeficiency–virus (HIV)–positive, intravenous drug and alcohol abusers. TB is included in the list of acquired immunodeficiency syndrome (AIDS)–defining diseases and, in some 30 percent of the new TB cases, the patients also have AIDS. The chance of an HIV-positive, TB-infected person suffering active disease is about 10 percent each year. Poor compliance with treatment has also resulted in multidrug-resistant TB, which is now found in up to 20 percent of the patients with active disease. Although pulmonary disease accounts for most of these infections, as many as 25 percent of the patients have extrapulmonary disease.

The fallopian tubes usually bear the brunt of the hematogenous spread from the primary lesion. Less commonly, there may be direct or lymphatic spread from adjacent viscera or peritoneal surfaces. The earliest tubal lesions are generally mucosal and bilateral, and may spread to the uterus and ovaries by direct extension. The endometrium is thus repeatedly reinfected from the tubes. The reported rates of infection for the various pelvic organs are: tubes, 90–100 percent; uterus, 50 percent; ovaries, 30 percent; cervix, 5–15 percent; and vagina/vulva, 1 percent.

The appearance of tubes affected by tuberculous salpingitis varies. In severe infections, they are distended with caseous material; in milder cases, they are not enlarged, but small tubercles may be seen on the serosal surface. The microscopic findings in the tubes and endometrium are similar, and characterized by tuberculous granulomas consisting of epithelioid cells surrounded by a zone of lymphocytes and plasma cells, together with the presence of giant cells and areas of caseating necrosis. The fimbrial end of the tube often remains patent and the fimbria is everted, producing the so-called tobacco pouch appearance.

There is a family history of TB in about 20 percent of the patients; 50 percent have had pleurisy, peritonitis, erythema nodosum, or renal, osseous, or pulmonary TB. Up to 85 percent of the patients have never been pregnant, and half of the remaining 15 percent manifest symptoms within a year of their last delivery.

The most common complaint is infertility; the most common symptom is pelvic pain. The pain is seldom severe, unless there is secondary infection. The pain may be worsened by coitus, exercise, and menses. Menstrual disorders, which often occur, include menorrhagia and metrorrhagia; amenorrhea is most frequent in the setting of advanced endometrial disease. In 2 percent of the cases, postmenopausal bleeding occurs. Frequently, there is a history of poor health that includes weight loss, fatigue, and malaise. A diagnosis of pelvic inflammatory disease (PID) nonresponsive to antibiotics is characteristic.

There may be no abnormalities encountered during physical examination. If abdominal involvement is present, there may be ascites with a "doughy" abdomen and irregular masses. The pelvic findings may be difficult to distinguish from those of nontuberculous PID. The bilateral masses, however, may be less tender and have a less uniform consistency. The finding of bilateral inflammatory tuboovarian masses in a virgin constitutes strong presumptive evidence of genital TB.

The diagnosis depends on either the demonstration of the organism or the characteristic tubercles, usually on endometrial curetted specimens. The optimal time to perform biopsy or culture is during the late secretory phase. Direct microscopy and culture performed on selective media are especially valuable, not only to establish the diagnosis but also to ascertain the antibiotic sensitivities of the organism. It may take from 6 to 8 weeks for the bacteriologic results to become available, so therapy is usually begun based on the histologic findings. It must also be kept in mind that other conditions cause granulomas with giant cells. These include sarcoidosis, foreign body reactions, and actinomycosis. Furthermore, because there will be no endometrial involvement in 50 percent of the cases, curettage findings will not establish the diagnosis in at least half the cases. Other diagnostic methods include culturing menstrual blood, hysterosalpingography, and laparoscopy. Unfortunately, many cases are diagnosed only at the time of laparotomy performed to evaluate suspected PID or of tuboplasty to treat suspected blocked tubes. If the diagnosis is not then appreciated, the surgical procedure is associated with a high complication rate, including recrudescence of the infection and fistula formation.

The workup in the patient with suspected genital TB should include a chest x-ray film, but the original lesion may have healed by the time the genital lesion appears, so negative findings should not be interpreted to rule out TB. A tuberculin skin test should also be performed, and it is rare for a patient to have TB without a positive skin reaction. Active extragenital disease should be sought in proved cases, and this includes bacteriologic examination of sputum and urine.

The therapy for genital TB, with or without extragenital lesions, primarily consists of continuous, long-term, combined drug therapy lasting 1 to 2 years. The drugs available for treatment include isoniazid, ethambutol, rifampin, pyrazinamide, and streptomycin. Because of the problem of drug resistance, it is currently recommended that therapy start with isoniazid, rifampin, pyrazinamide, and either ethambutol or streptomycin, and the four drugs should be continued until the complete results of drug-susceptibility tests are available. General therapeutic measures, including adequate diet and rest, should not be neglected. It is essential to include an experienced chest physician on the therapeutic team. Most patients may be treated on an outpatient basis. Response to therapy is monitored by endometrial biopsy or curettage findings, obtained at 6 and 12 months, as well as by clinical observation, including pelvic examination. Long-term follow-up is essential, as late recurrence is not uncommon.

Surgical intervention is indicated if endometrial TB persists or recurs after a year of therapy or if pelvic symptoms do not abate with long-term treatment. Further indications for surgical treatment include persistent adnexal masses or masses that enlarge during therapy. Less commonly, surgical measures may be indicated for patients who do not comply with medical therapy or for those with persistent fistulas. If genital TB is encountered unexpectedly at operation, only biopsy should be performed, as procedures performed after 3 to 4 months of antimicrobial therapy are technically much easier and hence less prone to complication. For the same reason, operation should be delayed until chemotherapy has been carried out for 3 to 4 months, whenever possible.

If surgical intervention is necessary, patients older than 40 years should undergo a total hysterectomy with bilateral salpingo-oophorectomy. In younger patients, if menstrual function is desired, the uterus and one or both of the ovaries may be conserved, provided they are free of TB. Drug therapy must be resumed after operation. Only in exceptional cases should there be an attempt to preserve reproductive function or should tuboplasty be attempted, as the prognosis for further pregnancy is extremely poor. As of 1976, only 31 cases of well-documented, successful pregnancy out of 7000 cases of genital TB had been reported in the literature. Thus, although the prognosis for cure is good, the prospects for pregnancy are negligible.

Reviews
1. Saracoglu, O. F., Mungan, T., and Tanzer, F. Pelvic tuberculosis. *Int. J. Gynaecol. Obstet.* 37:115, 1992.
   In the United States, an estimated 1 out of every 5,000 gynecologic hospital admissions will be for pelvic tuberculosis, most gynecologists will never see a single case.
2. Margolis, K., et al. Genital tuberculosis at Tygerberg Hospital—prevalence, clinical presentation and diagnosis. *S. Afr. Med. J.* 4:81, 1992.
   Menstrual fluid collection and culture was the most reliable diagnostic procedure. Radiology and laparoscopy proved to be of little help in establishing the diagnosis.
3. Sutherland, A. M. Gynaecological tuberculosis: analysis of a personal series of 710 cases. *Aust. N.Z. J. Obstet. Gynaecol.* 25:203, 1985.
   A high level of suspicion is necessary to achieving a high detection rate of genital TB.

Diagnosis
4. Seigler, A. M., and Kontopoulos, V. Female genital tuberculosis and the role of hysterosalpingography. *Semin. Roentgenol.* 14:295, 1979.
   A hysterosalpingogram is useful, although not diagnostic. Pelvic calcification or irregular filling defects along the tube should arouse suspicion. Endometrial adhesions and deformity may be found.
5. Marana, R., et al. Incidence of genital tuberculosis in infertile patients submitted to diagnostic laparoscopy: Recent experience in an Italian university hospital. *Int. J. Fertil.* 36:104, 1991.
   Many clinicians try to avoid performing laparoscopy in the diagnosis of genital TB because of the risk of bowel injury related to adhesions.
6. Slutsker, L., et al. Epidemiology of extrapulmonary tuberculosis among persons with AIDS in the United States. *Clin. Infect. Dis.* 16:513, 1993.
   As of December 1991, 2.3 percent of the AIDS patients reported were also found to have extrapulmonary tuberculosis.
7. Pallen, M. J. Death knell for guinea pig test. *Lancet* 12:337, 1991.
   Animal inoculation to test for TB does not add to the diagnostic information and should no longer be employed.
8. Gürgan, T., et al. Pelvic-peritoneal tuberculosis with elevated serum and peritoneal fluid CA-125 levels. *Gynecol. Obstet. Invest.* 53:60, 1993.
   Serum levels of CA-125 returned to normal limits after antituberculous drug treatment in the two cases described in this report.

Therapy
9. Arora, R., et al. Prospective analysis of short course chemotherapy in female genital tuberculosis. *Int. J. Gynaecol. Obstet.* 38:311, 1992.
   Limited data on short-course chemotherapy in genitourinary tuberculosis are available; however, it appears likely that both 6- and 9-month regimens provide satisfactory results.
10. Gostin, L. O. Controlling the resurgent tuberculosis epidemic. *J.A.M.A.* 269:255, 1993.

Problems of compliance contribute to treatment failure and drug resistance. Directly observed therapy, in which a designated person actually observes the patient ingest the prescribed drugs, is recommended.

11. Skolinick, J. L., et al. Rifampicin, oral contraceptives, and pregnancy. *J. Am. Med. Assoc.* 236:1382, 1976.
   Rifampicin inhibits the effectiveness of oral contraceptives and several other drugs by accelerating their hepatic degradation.
12. Daley, C. L., et al. An outbreak of tuberculosis with accelerated progression among persons infected with the human immunodeficiency virus: an analysis using restriction-fragment-length polymorphisms. *N. Engl. J. Med.* 326:231, 1992.
   There are many reports of the transmission of multidrug resistant strains to patients and staff within hospitals, AIDS facilities, drug abuse treatment facilities, and prison systems.
13. Selwyn, P. A., et al. High risk of active tuberculosis in HIV-infected drug users with cutaneous anergy. *J.A.M.A.* 268:504, 1992.
   The finding of cutaneous anergy on delayed-type hypersensitivity testing, common in HIV-positive drug users, may render a negative tuberculin test result uninterpretable. Isoniazid prophylaxis may be indicated for these patients.
14. Jordan, T. J., et al. Isoniazid as preventive therapy in HIV-infected intravenous drug abusers: a decision analysis. *J.A.M.A.* 265:2987, 1991.
   Liver function monitoring is important in these patients because of a high prevalence of alcoholism and hepatitis. Isoniazid should be withheld or discontinued if there is evidence of significant biochemical dysfunction.
15. Sutherland, A. M. Surgical treatment of tuberculosis of the female genital tract. *Br. J. Obstet. Gynaecol.* 87:610, 1980.
   The place of tubal reconstructive surgery is not well established. Certainly it should not be undertaken before adequate chemotherapy has been carried out.

Less Common Forms
16. Sutherland, A. M. Gynaecological tuberculosis after the age of 40. *J. Obstet. Gynaecol.* 11:445, 1991.
   Eighty-one of the 711 cases occurred in women older than 40 years, 55 were premenopausal and 26 were postmenopausal. Fifty-seven percent of the patients had irregular bleeding and 20 percent had pelvic pain.
17. Tang, L. C. H. Postmenopausal tuberculous cervicitis. *Acta Obstet. Gynecol. Scand.* 65:279, 1986.
   This represents an unusual age and situation for the infection.
18. Ghattacharya, P. Hypertrophic tuberculosis of the vulva. *Obstet. Gynecol.* 51:21S, 1978.
   In a woman with an ascending infection, the possibility that the husband has an active genital lesion should not be overlooked.

Pregnancy
19. Nogales-Ortiz, F., Tarancon, I., and Nogales, F. F. The pathology of female genital tuberculosis. A 31-year study of 1436 cases. *Obstet. Gynecol.* 53:422, 1979.
   Four cases of active female genital TB were found that coexisted with intrauterine or ectopic pregnancies.
20. Frydman, R., et al. In vitro fertilization in tuberculous infertility. *J. In Vitro Fertil. Embryo Transfer* 2:184, 1985.
   Of 22 women, managed by invitrofertilization (IVF) in 49 attempts, six conceived and bore babies. Results suggest that IVF probably offers a better chance of pregnancy in such women.
21. Bate, T. W. P., Sinclair, R. E., and Robinson, M. J. Neonatal tuberculosis. *Arch. Dis. Child.* 61:512, 1986.
   The diagnosis of congenital or neonatal TB is difficult; the purified protein skin test derivative result is usually negative initially, and only becomes positive some 6 weeks to 4 months later.

XII. CONTRACEPTION

66. HORMONAL CONTRACEPTION
Michel E. Rivlin

Combination oral contraceptives are the most widely used form of reversible contraception in the United States. The major mechanism of action of oral contraceptives consists of an alteration in the gonadotropin sequence, resulting in the suppression of ovulation. Other mechanisms include an atrophic effect on the endometrium and endocervical mucus that renders them "hostile" to sperm. The pregnancy failure rate is about 0.5 to 2 percent, and this usually stems from compliance problems rather than from method failure, or results from interactions with other medications that lessen the contraceptive effect. These medications include anticonvulsants, nonsteroidal antiinflammatory agents, and antibiotics, particularly rifampicin. By comparison, pregnancy failure rates associated with condom contraception range from 2 to 10 percent and, with no method, up to 90 percent.

The modern combination pill contains estrogen in the form of ethinyl estradiol or mestranol, both of which appear to have virtually identical pharmacologic activity; the dose in each pill is 30 to 50 μg. The progestin component is provided by one of five synthetic progestins, all derivatives of 19-nortestosterone. They are norethindrone, ethynodiol diacetate, norethindrone acetate, norethynodrel, and norgestrel. Three recently developed progestins that are claimed to have lesser androgenic properties, norgestimate, desogestrel, and gestodene, are now also available. Whether they represent a clinical improvement over the older formulations is as yet uncertain. Monophasic pills contain constant doses of the two components, and multiphasic or varying-dose pills combine a steady or slightly varied dose of estrogen with varying doses of progestins in an effort to lower the total steroid dose. Lower doses of estrogen and progestins are associated with more breakthrough bleeding and amenorrhea; higher doses, especially of estrogens, are associated with the more serious complications.

Common minor side effects include nausea and vomiting (in approximately 10% of users in the first cycle), breakthrough bleeding and spotting, amenorrhea, mastalgia, weight gain and edema, and depression. These cause more discomfort than real harm, but account for much of the discontinuation of the method (about 35% in the first year). Most symptoms usually subside after 3 months. More serious side effects include a worsening of migraine headaches; a worsening of asthma or epilepsy; growth of preexisting fibroids; or a worsening of kidney or heart disease. These side effects necessitate medical evaluation of the individual patient. Oral contraceptives decrease carbohydrate tolerance; therefore, diabetic and prediabetic patients must be carefully monitored. There is also an increase in the levels of triglycerides and total phospholipids of unknown clinical significance, but with important implications in terms of possible atherogenic effects. There may be an increased risk of gallbladder disease after only 6 to 12 months of use, possibly with cholelithiasis. Ocular lesions, including optic neuritis or retinal thrombosis, may be associated with use of the pill.

The complications that have received the most attention are cardiovascular disease and cancer, though the data are often conflicting. Most of the mortality statistics offer little evidence for a relationship between the pill and cardiovascular events. Multiple variables, such as age, smoking, and differences in the pills, have not been allowed for in these studies; nevertheless, the risk must be considered when counseling individual patients.

Hypertension develops in an estimated 1 to 5 percent of pill users, and usually resolves when use is discontinued. The risk of venous thromboembolism may be increased by from three to eleven times; however, heavy smoking may be the major factor here. Estrogen is thought to be the cause, and the effect disappears 4 to 6 weeks after discontinuation, as the levels of coagulation factors, increased by estrogens, return to normal. It is therefore recommended that pill use cease at least 2 weeks before a woman undergoes a major surgical procedure or during prolonged immobilization. The risk of thrombotic stroke appears to be approximately doubled in users, and, as with the other circulatory diseases, the risk of myocardial infarction (MI) is

317

largely confined to those women older than 35 years who smoke. In younger women, the mortality risk of MI is less than that of pregnancy; however, longer duration of use increases the risk of MI, and this risk persists after the discontinuance of pill use, particularly in older women who have taken the pill for more than 5 years and those who are heavy smokers. The atherosclerotic change responsible for MI and stroke appears to be related to the progestin component, as progestins decrease the level of HDL (high-density lipoprotein) cholesterol and increase the level of LDL (low-density lipoprotein) cholesterol, an effect that promotes the development of heart disease. Estrogens have the opposite effect. There is no clinical evidence as yet regarding the relationship between these lipid changes and vascular diseases; however, the strong relationship between vascular disease and lipoprotein concentrations cannot be ignored. Furthermore, the risk associated with low HDL cholesterol levels is exaggerated when combined with other risks such as hypertension and elevated LDL cholesterol levels.

The data on the role of the pill and cancer are fairly clear. There is little evidence that oral contraceptives adversely affect the risk of breast cancer. Although there is some evidence of a higher incidence of cervical neoplasia, the influence of sexual activity could not be eliminated and the relationship to pill use is unclear. Pill use for 12 months or longer is protective against all three major subtypes of endometrial cancer, an effect persisting for at least 15 years after the discontinuation of pill use. There is also a protective effect against ovarian cancer. There does appear to be an increased incidence of rare liver tumors associated with pill use, including benign hepatic adenomas and hepatocellular cancers, and an increasing duration of pill use increases the risk, though the incidence is still very low. Pill use does not appear to have any bearing on the incidence of pituitary adenoma or malignant melanoma. The inadvertent use of contraceptive steroids during early pregnancy does not appear to lead to fetal anomalies. Beneficial side effects of pill use include a significantly decreased incidence of benign breast disorders, functional ovarian cysts, gonococcal pelvic inflammatory disease, iron-deficiency anemia, dysmenorrhea, and ectopic pregnancy.

Absolute contraindications to pill use include the existence of thrombophlebitis or thromboembolism or a history of these disorders; cerebral, vascular, or coronary artery disease; known or suspected breast or endometrial cancer; undiagnosed abnormal genital bleeding; pregnancy; and the presence of a benign or malignant liver tumor. The pill is virtually contraindicated in women older than 35 years who smoke or who have other high-risk factors such as hypertension or abnormal carbohydrate or lipid laboratory values, or both. Current recommendations are to use a multiphasic or low-dose monophasic pill in the 85 percent of women who are acceptable candidates for pill use. Women taking the high-dose pills should be stepped down to low-dose preparations. Blood pressure together with glucose and lipid levels should be monitored in women with risk factors who nevertheless wish to use the pill. One suggestion is that pills should not be prescribed if the total cholesterol level is over 300 mg/dl, the LDL cholesterol concentration is over 190 mg/dl, the HDL cholesterol level is less than 35 mg/dl, or the triglyceride content exceeds 500 mg/dl. Among the few reasons for considering use of a 50-μg pill are persistent breakthrough bleeding or amenorrhea (alternatives include switching from a low-dose monophasic to a multiphasic pill, or vice versa, or the intermittent use of estrogen); use of anticonvulsants; and long-term antibiotics, as used in acne therapy. Counseling is the key to the successful use and selection of oral contraceptives. Considering that fewer than 23 percent of women are well educated about health matters and that the average reading level in the United States is sixth grade, ensuring comprehension is a serious issue. For most women who meet the medical criteria, the benefits of the pill outweigh the risks, particularly the risks associated with pregnancy.

The pill may be started on the first day of menses or the "first Sunday" after the period commences. Seven days of continuous use are sufficient for full protection. Active pills are taken for 21 days, with either no pill or a placebo taken during days 22 to 28. Withdrawal bleeding, usually light and painless, generally occurs between courses. If a patient has had an abortion, the pill should be started a week later; with a viable gestation, a 2-week interval is allowed after delivery. The pill is excreted in breast milk and also decreases milk volume, so it should not be used by breast-feeding mothers. If a patient misses a pill for 2 days in a row, she should add barrier contraception for 7 days. If three or more pills are missed, or two pills are missed in the third week of the cycle, the next pill pack should be started directly. If a patient misses two consecutive periods, pregnancy must be ruled out. A pill with greater estrogen content may then be required.

About 65 percent of women conceive within 3 months of stopping the pill; however, about 1 percent have amenorrhea that persists for 6 to 12 months afterward. About 15 percent of these have associated galactorrhea. These patients require evaluation to rule out pituitary microadenoma. With therapy (e.g., clomiphene or gonadotropins), about 42 percent conceive.

Many clinicians advise delaying fertilization after pill discontinuation, because, in those patients who become pregnant within 1 to 2 months of stopping the pill, the risk of congenital anomalies may be slightly increased, although this finding is controversial. There is also a possible association between congenital abnormalities and use of the pill in the first trimester. Therefore, progestin-estrogen withdrawal bleeding should not be used as a pregnancy test.

The "minipill" (progestin alone) is taken daily in low doses. It is generally used for patients in whom estrogen is a risk factor (e.g., those with fibroids, hypertension, diabetes, or epilepsy). Because it does not suppress lactation, it may be given to lactating mothers. Unfortunately, irregular bleeding occurs in 70 percent of the patients and the pregnancy rate is 3 per 100 users per year, with an increased incidence of ectopic gestation.

Progestin-only contraception may also be given either by intermittent intramuscular injection using depot medroxyprogesterone acetate (150 mg every 3 months) or by the subdermal placement of levonorgestrel-releasing implants (Norplant), which provide protection for 5 years. Circulating levels of progestin are adequate to block ovulation and the failure rate is below 1 percent. Side effects include menstrual irregularity, amenorrhea, weight gain, headache, breast tenderness, and psychologic complaints such as depression, nervousness, fatigue, and loss of libido. Progestin-only methods are generally reserved for patients who refuse combination oral contraception or in whom estrogen is contraindicated.

The postcoital or "morning-after" pill may be taken within 72 hours of unprotected intercourse to prevent normal implantation. Generally, diethylstilbestrol (25 mg), or an equivalent estrogen, is taken twice daily for 4 days. An alternative that does not cause the nausea associated with a high estrogen dosage is to administer ethinyl estradiol (0.2 mg) and norgestrel (2.0 mg) in two doses over 24 hours. The antiprogestational agent mifepristone (RU 486) is also highly effective, but is not available for use in the United States at this time. Although postcoital pills are very effective, their drawback is that, if pregnancy occurs, the fetus has been exposed to exogenous hormones and termination may have to be considered.

Reviews
1. Masterson, B. J. Oral contraceptive agents: current status. *Am. J. Surg.* 155: 619, 1988.
   Although the reports on oral contraceptives are frequently contradictory and confusing in the data they provide, recall what Voltaire said several centuries ago: "Doubt is an uncomfortable condition, but certainty is a ridiculous one."
2. Grimes, D. A. The safety of oral contraceptives; epidemiologic insights from the first 30 years. *Am. J. Obstet. Gynecol.* 166:1950, 1992.
   The newer formulations no longer appear to be associated with an increased risk of fostering MI or stroke.

Metabolic Changes
3. Thomson, J. M., et al. A multicentre study of coagulation and haemostatic variables during oral contraception: variations with four formulations. *Br. J. Obstet. Gynaecol.* 98:1117, 1991.
   The adverse effects on coagulation are affected by the type and dose of estrogen.
4. Godsland, I. F., et al. Insulin resistance, secretion, and metabolism in users of oral contraceptives. *J. Clin. Endocrinol. Metab.* 74:64, 1992.
   The general metabolic effects of the pill are similar to those found in pregnancy,

although to a lesser degree. Carbohydrate metabolism is affected, with a resultant decrease in glucose tolerance, increased insulin resistance, and increased pancreatic insulin secretion.

5. Godsland, I. F., et al. The effects of different formulations of oral contraceptive agents on lipid and carbohydrate metabolism. *N. Engl. J. Med.* 323:1375, 1990.
   Increased levels of triglycerides and LDL cholesterol, and decreased levels of HDL cholesterol are all changes linked with atherogenesis and associated with pill use; however, the newer formulations appear to minimize these changes.

6. Fotherby, K. Interactions with oral contraceptives. *Am. J. Obstet. Gynecol.* 163: 2153, 1990.
   The incidence of serious interactions is low and unaffected by use of lower-dose preparations, probably because of the large intersubject variability in terms of the pharmacokinetics of oral contraceptives.

Adverse Reactions

7. Gram, I. T., Macaluso, M., and Stalsberg, H. Oral contraceptive use and the incidence of cervical intraepithelial neoplasia. *Am. J. Obstet. Gynecol.* 167:40, 1992.
   There is probably no increased risk of invasive cancer but a possible increased risk of precursor lesions in pill users. Women on oral contraceptives require annual Papanicolaou smears.

8. Wigo, P. A., et al. Age-specific differences in the relationship between oral contraceptive use and breast cancer. *Obstet. Gynecol.* 78:161, 1991.
   The subgroups of women who might be at increased risk for premenopausal breast cancer associated with pill use have consistently been difficult to target.

9. Wynn, V. Oral contraceptives and coronary heart disease. *J. Reprod. Med.* 36: 219, 1991.
   The newer progestins, possessing little or no androgenic activity, appear to have less effect on lipid and lipoprotein metabolism than the older, more androgenic progestins.

10. Lammer, E. J., and Cordero, J. F. Exogenous sex hormone exposure and the risk for major malformations. *J.A.M.A.* 255:3128, 1986.
    Exposure to oral contraceptives during pregnancy does not appear to increase the risk of birth defects in the offspring.

11. Vessey, M. P., et al. Oral contraceptives and venous thromboembolism: findings in a large prospective study. *Br. Med. J.* 252:526, 1986.
    The incidence of deep vein thrombosis after operation in young women taking the pill was not statistically different from that in patients not taking the pill.

12. Radberg, T., et al. Oral contraception in diabetic women: diabetes control, serum and high density lipoprotein lipids during low-dose progestogen, combined oestrogen/progestogen and non-hormonal contraception. *Acta Endocrinol.* 98:246, 1981.
    Contraception in the diabetic represents a difficult choice, and the risks versus benefits must be weighed for the individual.

13. Kay, C. R. The Royal College of General Practitioner's Oral Contraception Study: some recent observations. *Clin. Obstet. Gynecol.* 11:759, 1984.
    The mortality rates for various groups of women aged 40 to 44 were as follows: 6.6/100,000, nonsmoking pill users; 58.4/100,000, smoking and pill users; and 71.4/100,000, associated with pregnancy and childbirth. (These figures are based on the use of older pill formulations.)

14. Branham, J. Oral contraceptives and depression. *Br. Med. J.* 1:237, 1970.
    An underlying cause of this depression may be a disturbance in tryptophan metabolism precipitated by a pill-related pyridoxine deficiency. Therapy with vitamin B_6 may be useful to counteract these effects.

15. Luciano, A. A., et al. Hyperprolactinemia and contraception: a prospective study. *Obstet. Gynecol.* 65:506, 1985.
    The incidence of hyperprolactinemia in oral contraceptive users was higher than that in control subjects (12% versus 5%).

16. Scott, L. D., et al. Oral contraceptives, pregnancy, and focal nodular hyperplasia of the liver. *J.A.M.A.* 251:1461, 1984.

Rarely, hyperplasia or hepatoma may occur. The major danger is rupture with intraabdominal bleeding.

Benefits

17. Hankinson, S. E., et al. A quantitative assessment of oral contraceptive use and risk of ovarian cancer. *Obstet. Gynecol.* 80:708, 1992.
An estimated 1700 cases of ovarian cancer are averted in the United States annually by the use of oral contraceptives.

18. Williams, J. K. Oral contraceptives and reproductive system cancer. Benefits and risks. *J. Reprod. Med.* 36:247, 1991.
An estimated 2000 cases of endometrial cancer are averted in the United States every year by the use of oral contraceptives.

19. Lanes, S. F., et al. Oral contraceptive type and functional ovarian cysts. *Am. J. Obstet. Gynecol.* 166:956, 1992.
The protective effect of high-dose monophasic pills against functional cysts may be attenuated by newer pills with a lower hormonal potency.

Other Hormonal Contraceptives

20. Graham, S., and Fraser, I. S. The progestogen-only minipill. *Contraception* 26:373, 1982.
Findings indicate that the method is reasonably efficacious and the side effects are minor. The authors suggest use in diabetics, cardiac patients, breast-feeding patients, and older patients, as well as in those who suffer the depression and loss of libido associated with combination drugs.

21. Chi, I.-C. The safety and efficacy issues of progestin-only oral contraceptives—an epidemiologic perspective. *Contraception* 47:1, 1993.
This agent is particularly helpful for use as contraceptive in lactating women.

22. Van Santen, M. R., and Haspels, A. A. A comparison of high-dose ethinylestradiol and norgestrel combination in postcoital interception: a study in 493 women. *Fertil. Steril.* 43:206, 1985.
The efficacy of both methods of postcoital contraception was confirmed. The combination is preferable because treatment is limited to 1 day, and the incidence of nausea and vomiting is considerably lower.

23. Cundy, T., et al. Bone density in women receiving depot medroxyprogesterone acetate for contraception. *Br. Med. J.* 303:13, 1991.
The degree of estrogen deficiency induced by depot medroxyprogesterone acetate may adversely affect bone density. Women using the drug exhibit bone density values intermediate between normal premenopausal and postmenopausal controls.

24. Segal, S. J., et al. Norplant implants: the mechanism of contraceptive action. *Fertil. Steril.* 56:273, 1991.
Flexible Silastic capsules placed subcutaneously in the inner surface of the upper arm release 30 µg of levonorgestrel daily.

25. Shoupe, D., et al. The significance of bleeding patterns in Norplant implant users. *Obstet. Gynecol.* 77:256, 1991.
Bleeding patterns improve after the first year; those with regular cycles are at greatest risk of failure.

26. Ledipo, O. A. Norplant use by women with sickle cell disease. *Int. J. Gynecol. Obstet.* 41:85, 1993.
Appears to be safe for women with mild to moderate Hb SS disease.

67. INTRAUTERINE DEVICES
Michel E. Rivlin

Product liability and medical malpractice issues in the United States have resulted in a marked decline in the use of the intrauterine device (IUD). At this time, the only

IUDs available in the United States are the Progestasert and the Copper T 380A (ParaGard). The manufacturers of these devices have developed extremely detailed informed consent forms, which must be read and completed by the patient with guidance from her physician. These forms also have the effect of defining those patients at least risk for complications and those in whom the device is contraindicated. Partly as a result, there have been few if any medicolegal problems associated with the Progestasert or the ParaGard device.

Intrauterine contraception is very popular outside the United States, and is used by more than 50 million women worldwide. The IUD is convenient, effective, and relatively safe, with failure rates only slightly higher than those for oral contraceptives. Approximately 80 percent of the women continue use through the first year and about 60 percent use it through the second year.

The IUD is a foreign body that is placed in the uterus to prevent pregnancy. Devices may be either nonmedicated or medicated. Medicated devices contain progesterone (Progestasert) or copper (T 380A). A mild inflammatory reaction occurs around the IUD. However, the mechanism of action is uncertain, but appears to stem from the interference with fertilization rather than from implantation. Progestaserts are reinserted annually, and the copper devices are reinserted after 8 years when medication is exhausted. Inert devices can be left in for longer periods if there are no complications. Contraindications to IUD use include pregnancy; uterine abnormalities that distort the cavity; uterine malignancy; abnormal bleeding; acute cervicitis; and a history of pelvic inflammatory disease (PID), sexually transmitted disease (STD), ectopic pregnancy, postpartum endometritis, or infected abortion. Relative contraindications include hypermenorrhea, severe dysmenorrhea, multiple sexual partners, congenital or valvular heart disease, and nulliparity. Approximately 20 percent of the women require removal of the device during the first year because of side effects, such as heavy bleeding, cramping, and pain. Approximately 5 to 12 percent spontaneously expel the device.

Insertion is usually carried out during menses, so as not to disturb a pregnancy. Use of a careful aseptic technique performed by experienced personnel, prior sounding of the uterine cavity (it should be more than 6 cm and less than 9 cm in length), and atraumatic fundal placement in the correct plane are all measures that minimize complications. The IUD tail string is cut approximately 3 cm from the external os, and the patient is instructed in the technique of checking for the string. She should be informed of minor side effects, including cramping, intermenstrual bleeding, increased menstrual flow, and increased vaginal secretions. Women should be reexamined after their next menses, and thereafter at least annually.

If at follow-up the IUD string cannot be felt or seen, it must be determined whether pregnancy, expulsion, or perforation has taken place. Once pregnancy is ruled out, the device may be palpated with a sound or localized by ultrasound or x-ray, with the cavity indicated by placement of an instrument or dye. Hysteroscopy or laparoscopy may be required for this in some instances. Uterine perforation occurs in 1 per 1000 insertions. Because all devices are capable of eliciting peritonitis, adhesions, and organ penetration, the IUD must be removed by means of laparoscopy, hysteroscopy, or laparotomy when perforation is diagnosed. Expulsion occurs in from 3 to 12 per 100 women per year, usually in the first few months after insertion.

There is an increased risk of PID associated with the use of IUDs, though the risk is much lower if the Dalkon Shield figures are removed from the overall statistics. The risk of infection is highest in the first 4 months after insertion. The women at greatest risk are those at risk for STDs—that is, those who have more than one sexual partner or whose partner has multiple consorts. IUD use is not recommended in such women. If symptoms of PID do occur, antibiotics should be administered and the IUD should be removed. *Actinomyces*, an anaerobic gram-positive bacterium, is occasionally detected in IUD users by the appearance of the characteristic "Gupta bodies" on Papanicolaou (Pap) smears. In the absence of PID, penicillin therapy should be instituted and the IUD left in place. If PID is present, or the *Actinomyces* infection does not respond to penicillin, the IUD should be removed. Actual *Actinomyces* infection of the pelvic organs is rare; however, the risk of pelvic *Actinomyces* infection increases with the duration of IUD use.

The pregnancy rate for users of the IUD varies from 1.8 to 2.8 per 100 women per year. Women who become pregnant with an IUD in place must be advised of the increased risk of spontaneous abortion, together with an increased risk of septic abortion, septicemia, septic shock, and death. If the woman decides on pregnancy termination, the IUD can be removed at that time. If she decides to proceed with the pregnancy, the IUD should be removed if the strings are visible. She must be warned that abortion may follow removal. If any signs of infection or impending abortion appear, vigorous treatment with intravenous broad-spectrum antibiotics must be mounted. If the IUD is removed in the first trimester, the risk of a second- or third-trimester fetal loss is not increased. If the IUD remains in place, there is an increased risk of both first-trimester abortion and septic abortion, especially in the second trimester, and of premature birth in the third trimester. There does not appear to be an association between IUD use and an increased risk of congenital abnormalities in the offspring. Although most IUDs do not promote ectopic pregnancy, they do not offer protection against an ectopic gestation. In the case of the Progestasert, the likelihood of ectopic pregnancy appears to be increased, and users should be warned of this enhanced risk. In patients with IUDs who do become pregnant, there is a 1:20 ratio of ectopic to intrauterine gestation (1:200 in the general population) as a result of the contraceptive effect of the devices. These women must therefore be evaluated for this complication. The pregnancy rates in women after removal of IUDs appear to be similar to those in women who discontinue the use of other types of contraceptives. Unrecognized PID may, however, partially or completely interfere with the restoration of fertility among former IUD users, as it does among non-IUD users. The outcome of pregnancies conceived after the removal of an IUD appears to be no different than that in women discontinuing use of other contraceptive methods.

Reviews
1. The intrauterine device. *ACOG Tech. Bull.* No. 164, February 1992.
   The Food and Drug Administration, the United States Agency for International Development, and the World Health Organization still consider the IUD to be safe and effective.
2. Edelman, D. A., and van Os, W. A. A. Safety of intrauterine contraception. *Adv. Contracept.* 6:207, 1990.
   The IUD does not appear to impair subsequent fertility or affect the outcome of future pregnancies.
3. Richardson, A., and Paul, D. A national study to monitor the safety of IUCD use. *Contraception* 47:359, 1993.
   Twenty-seven percent of the insertions were in women who had a relative contraindication; 0.9 percent had an absolute contraindication.

Complications
4. Sivin, I. IUDs as contraceptives, not abortifacients: a comment on research and belief. *Stud. Fam. Plann.* 20:355, 1989.
   Studies do not show the presence of human chorionic gonadotropin in IUD users, and implantation does not occur; as such, the IUD is not an abortifacient.
5. Sivin, I., et al. Long-term contraception with the levonorgestrel 20 mcg/day (LNg 20) and the Copper T 380Ag intrauterine devices: a five-year randomized study. *Contraception* 42:361, 1990.
   The steroid-releasing IUD is associated with significantly higher termination rates for expulsion and amenorrhea, significantly lower termination rates for other menstrual problems and pain, and a lower continuation rate.
6. Zhou, S. W., and Chi, I. C. Immediate postpartum IUD insertions in a Chinese hospital—a two year follow-up. *Int. J. Gynecol. Obstet.* 35:157, 1991.
   Insertions performed at the time of cesarean section were associated with lower expulsion rates than were vaginal insertions. No perforations occurred.
7. Najarian, K. E., and Kurtz, A. B. New observations in the sonographic evaluation of intrauterine contraceptive devices. *J. Ultrasound Med.* 5:205, 1986.
   The authors claim that ultrasound is an accurate tool for determining whether an IUD is present within the uterus.

8. McKenna, P. J., and Mylotte, M. J. Laparoscopic removal of translocated intra-uterine contraceptive devices. *Br. J. Obstet. Gynaecol.* 89:163, 1982.
   There is an increased risk of perforation after pregnancy. Laparoscopic removal was successful in 77 percent overall and in 44 percent for copper IUDs.

Pregnancy

9. Herbertsson, G., Magnusson, S. S., and Benediktsdottir, K. Ovarian pregnancy and IUCD use in a defined complete population. *Acta Obstet. Gynecol. Scand.* 66:607, 1987.
   Women who have an ectopic pregnancy while using an IUD appear to be at significantly higher risk of having an ovarian implantation.
10. Anteby, E., et al. Intrauterine device failure: relation to its location within the uterine cavity. *Obstet. Gynecol.* 81:112, 1993.
    Sonographic follow-up and reinsertion for displaced devices is recommended to prevent pregnancy related to malpositioned devices.
11. Sivin, I., et al. Rates and outcomes of planned pregnancy after use of Norplant capsules, Norplant II rods, or levonorgestrel-releasing or copper TCu 380Ag intrauterine contraceptive devices. *Am. J. Obstet. Gynecol.* 166:1208, 1992.
    Normal fertility and pregnancy outcomes were unrelated to the method and duration of use.
12. Farr, G., and Rivera, R. Interactions between intrauterine contraceptive device use and breast-feeding status at time of intrauterine contraceptive device insertion: analysis of TCu-380A acceptors in developing countries. *Am. J. Obstet. Gynecol.* 167:144, 1992.
    This represents a viable option for lactating women; no uterine perforations were reported.
13. Biggerstaff, E. D., et al. Maternal midtrimester sepsis in association with the intrauterine contraceptive device: early histopathologic findings. *Am. J. Obstet. Gynecol.* 124:207, 1976.
    The insidious onset of a flulike syndrome, with a rapidly developing fulminant infection and an absence of pelvic findings, culminated in severe sepsis, septic shock, and maternal death within 72 hours.
14. Foreman, H., Stadel, B. V., and Schlesselman, S. Intrauterine device usage and fetal loss. *Obstet. Gynecol.* 58:669, 1981.
    Pregnancy with an IUD in place at the beginning of the second trimester carries a 10-fold increased risk of fetal loss. Third-trimester risk of fetal loss is also increased, but the magnitude is uncertain.

Pelvic Inflammatory Disease

15. Buchan, H., et al. Epidemiology of pelvic inflammatory disease in parous women with special reference to intrauterine device use. *Br. J. Obstet. Gynaecol.* 97:780, 1990.
    The relative risk of PID in users of medicated devices was 1.8, half that associated with the nonmedicated device. There was little risk elevation in ex-users of the IUD.
16. Kronmal, R. A., Whitney, C. S., and Mumford, S. D. The intrauterine device and pelvic inflammatory disease: the Women's Health Study reanalyzed. *J. Clin. Epidemiol.* 44:109, 1991.
    This is the richest source of information on infection risk. The risk was not increased for women in stable, monogamous relationships.
17. Sinei, S. K. A., et al. Preventing IUCD-related pelvic infection: the efficacy of prophylactic doxycycline at insertion. *Br. J. Obstet. Gynaecol.* 97:412, 1990.
    Doxycycline (200 mg) or erythromycin (500 mg orally 1 hour before insertion and repeated 6 hours later) has been suggested, but the results are inconclusive.
18. Toivonen, J., Luukkainen, T., and Allonen, H. Protective effect of intrauterine release of levonorgestrel on pelvic infection: three years comparative experience of levonorgestrel- and copper-releasing intrauterine devices. *Obstet. Gynecol.* 77:261, 1991.

The progesterone-containing IUD significantly protected against the development of PID, as compared to the copper device.

19. Yoonessi, M., et al. Association of *Actinomyces* and intrauterine contraceptive devices. *J. Reprod. Med.* 30:48, 1985.

Four to 8 percent of IUD users may have Actinomyces-*like organisms on a Pap smear, but this finding has not been equated with pelvic actinomycosis, nor has the risk of subsequent pelvic infection been quantified.*

68. BARRIER AND CHEMICAL CONTRACEPTIVES
Marc Vatin

Barrier methods of contraception aim to prevent conception by interposing a mechanical, chemical, or combination barrier between the spermatic ejaculate and the cervical os. Barrier methods are nonsystemic, have distinct advantages, such as their safety in lactating mothers, and can be quite effective, if used properly.

One must, however, distinguish between the theoretic effectiveness of a birth-control method and its use effectiveness. The theoretic effectiveness is the antifertility action of a contraceptive if it is used under ideal conditions without human error or negligence. Its use effectiveness is the antifertility action achieved in real-life circumstances. Effectiveness is measured in terms of failure rates by either the pregnancy rate (PR) or the Pearl index. The Pearl index is defined as the number of failures per 100 woman-years of exposure. The index is calculated by the number of pregnancies multiplied by 1200, divided by the number of women observed, multiplied by the months of exposure. In a population that does not use any contraceptive method, the PR is 80 pregnancies per 100 woman-years. The theoretic effectiveness of barrier methods is very high, with a PR ranging from 1 to 7 pregnancies per 100 woman-years; but the use effectiveness varies widely depending on motivation and education. The PR can reach 30 per 100 woman-years.

Modern mechanical barriers include the condom, the diaphragm, the cervical cap, the contraceptive sponge, and, the most recent development, the "female condom." Chemical barriers are the topical spermicides.

The condom is a disposable sheath used to cover the erect penis during intercourse and to collect the ejaculate. Condoms are made of latex in various colors, textures, and thicknesses, and can be perfumed. It is the most widely used and available contraceptive in the world. Its theoretic effectiveness is very high, at about 1 pregnancy per 100 woman-years; its use effectiveness ranges from 6 to 18 pregnancies per 100 woman-years. Method failure occurs when the condom breaks, but this is rare. Most failures are due to "user failure." Condoms should be stored in a cool, dry place and checked for tears before use. The condom must be applied before there is any contact between the penis and the vagina, with a space left at the tip as a reservoir for the ejaculate. The penis must be withdrawn before detumescence, with the rim of the condom held manually to prevent the spillage of semen. Petroleum or oil-based products should not be used for lubrication as they weaken the latex. There are rare side effects of local irritation. In addition to its contraceptive role, the condom has recently received tremendous publicity because of its protective role in sexually transmitted diseases (STD), including the acquired immunodeficiency syndrome (AIDS), and in cervical neoplasia. Laboratory studies have shown that latex condoms can block the passage of *Chlamydia* and *Neisseria* organisms, the human immunodeficiency virus (HIV), herpes simplex virus, cytomegalovirus, and hepatitis B virus. Proper use of latex condoms can reduce, although not eliminate, the risk of transmission of STDs. The use of spermicide-containing condoms may provide additional protection.

The diaphragm is a soft rubber cup with a metal-reinforced rim that is inserted into the vagina before intercourse to cover the cervix and thus prevent penetration of sperm into the uterus. It is also a receptacle for spermicidal cream or jelly. Diaphragms range in size from 50 to 105 mm in diameter. Most women can be fitted with a 70- to 80-mm diaphragm. The most commonly used types of diaphragms are the coil spring and flat spring ones for the woman with good pelvic support, and the arcing spring one for the woman with poor vaginal muscle tone or a cystocele. It is essential that a diaphragm be fitted properly. After a pelvic examination, the diagonal length of the vaginal canal, from the posterior aspect of the symphysis pubis to the posterior vaginal fornix, is assessed by digital examination and the correct size of diaphragm chosen. Alternately, several sizes of fitting rings can be inserted and tried for determination of the correct size. The largest diaphragm that can be tolerated comfortably should be chosen. It should fit snugly between the symphysis pubis and the cul-de-sac, covering the cervix and a great part of the anterior vaginal wall. A postpartum woman should not be fitted until 6 weeks after delivery. After the fitting, the user must be taught how to insert and remove the diaphragm and how to check the placement by feeling for the cervix.

The diaphragm can be inserted up to 8 hours before intercourse, but additional spermicide should be used if more than 2 hours elapse before coitus. Adding more spermicide prior to each coital act is also recommended. The diaphragm must be left in place for at least 8 hours after intercourse, but leaving it in for more than 24 hours may result in infection. Douching must be delayed for 8 hours after intercourse, as otherwise this can dilute the spermicide.

The theoretic effectiveness of the diaphragm used with spermicidal agents is high, with a PR of 3 pregnancies per 100 woman-years. The use effectiveness varies, however, ranging from 6 to 25 pregnancies per 100 woman-years. Method failures occur when the diaphragm is displaced in certain coital positions or when it is defective.

The diaphragm is contraindicated in certain clinical conditions, such as complete uterine prolapse, severe cystocele, or rectocele. Minor side effects consist of local irritation or allergic reactions. Diaphragm users may have more frequent urinary tract infections (UTIs) but do not appear to be at increased risk for toxic shock syndrome (TSS). A beneficial side effect conferred by diaphragm use may be a degree of protection against cervical cancer, pelvic infections, and STDs.

The cervical cap is a reusable, thimble-shaped rubber cup that blocks only the cervix and is held in place by suction. It is available in several sizes and should be initially fitted by a physician. Spermicidal cream or jelly should be placed inside the cap before each insertion. It can remain in place for 48 hours, during which the reapplication of spermicide is not necessary. However, it can be displaced during coitus. The cap is comparable to the diaphragm in effectiveness. It can be used by women with poor muscle tone or prolapse, but not when there is a cervical malformation, cervicitis, or an abnormal Papanicolaou (Pap) smear. There is an increased rate of conversion to an abnormal Pap test during the first 3 months of cervical cap usage; therefore, a follow-up Pap test should be performed after the first 3 months and, if the result is abnormal, use of the cap should be discontinued. The Pap test must be repeated annually thereafter. The cap cannot be used during menstrual periods or during postpartum and postabortal periods. There may be a slight increase in the risk of TSS associated with its use.

The disposable contraceptive sponge, made of polyurethane impregnated with spermicide, is shaped like a mushroom cap and fits in the upper vagina with a concave side covering the cervix. It is left in place to provide continuous protection for 24 hours, then discarded. It is about as effective as topical spermicides but less effective than the diaphragm plus spermicide. Side effects consist of allergic-type reactions and vaginal irritation; there may also be an increased risk of TSS. Sponges have a tendency to tear and can be difficult to remove from the vagina.

The recently approved "female condom" combines the features of male condoms and diaphragms. Also called a vaginal pouch, it is a lubricated polyurethane pouch that is designed to line the vagina and is inserted like a tampon. There is a flexible ring at the closed end of the pouch that covers the cervix, like a diaphragm. Another ring at the open end remains outside the body and helps keep the pouch in place during intercourse. This device gives the woman more control, as she can easily insert it in advance and is not dependent on the male's willingness to use a condom. Because the external genitalia are also covered, it should also afford increased protection against STDs. During clinical trials, it was found to be very acceptable to both men and women, although there were some complaints that the device was cumbersome and unaesthetic. On the positive side, it does not seem to increase the risk of UTIs. And one size fits all!

Vaginal chemical contraceptives or spermicides are packaged in four basic forms: foams (including aerosol and tablets), creams and jellies, suppositories, and soluble films. The spermicide is inserted high into the vagina before intercourse, allowing time for the spermicidal agent to disperse and block the cervix. Another application is required before each coital act and if more than 1 hour elapses before coitus. No douching is permitted for 6 hours after the last coital act. Occasionally, there are side effects of local irritation. Spermicides tend to have high failure rates (PR up to 30 pregnancies per 100 woman-years) but are readily available and easy to use. The most commonly used spermicidal agents are surfactants that destroy sperm cell membranes. There has been some concern about the potential teratogenicity of spermicides, but most epidemiologic studies addressing this problem have revealed no evidence of an association between spermicides and congenital malformations or spontaneous abortion. On the positive side, spermicides have been shown to provide some protection against STDs, including AIDS. Public health experts suggest the use of spermicides along with condoms to reduce the risk of transmitting STDs.

A "Must Read"
1. Trussell, J., et al. A guide to interpreting contraceptive efficacy studies. *Obstet. Gynecol.* 76:558, 1990.
   The authors discuss how to read reports of studies with a critical eye; misleading data and numerous fallacies render valid comparisons among the methods and products virtually impossible.

Reviews
2. Connell, E. Barrier contraceptives—their time has returned. *The Female Patient* 14:66, 1989.
   This article is quick and easy to read, with a discussion of the advantages (safety, efficacy, low cost, and good for occasional coitus), disadvantages (motivation, consistent use, and cultural acceptability), indications (mainly for safety or for short-term use), and contraindications (poor motivation).
3. Greydanus, D., et al. Contraception in the adolescent. Preparation for the 1990s. *Med. Clin. North. Am.* 74:1205, 1990.
   An overview of all the contraceptive methods, with an emphasis on oral contraceptives, but also a good review of the barrier methods.
4. Kulig, J. Adolescent contraception: nonhormonal methods. *Pediatr. Clin. North Am.* 38:717, 1989.
   Another good review with a comparison of the advantages, disadvantages, and costs of each method.

The Cervical Cap
5. Richwald, G., et al. Effectiveness of the cavity-rim cervical cap: results of a large clinical study. *Obstet. Gynecol.* 74:143, 1989.
   The article presents data from a clinical trial involving 3433 women that spanned from 1981 to 1988. The estimated first-year pregnancy risk was 11.3 percent, with risks of 8.3 and 3.8 percent for user and method failures, respectively. "Near-perfect" users had half the first-year pregnancy risk of others (6.1% versus 11.9%). There were no serious medical or gynecologic complications.
6. Brokaw, A., et al. Fitting the cervical cap. *Nurse Pract.* 13:49, 1988.
   A "how-to" article.

Beneficial Effects
7. Celentano, D., et al. The role of contraceptive use in cervical cancer: The Maryland Cervical Cancer Case-Control Study. *Am. J. Epidemiol.* 126:592, 1987.
   This article considers the importance of STDs in the etiology of cervical cancer. Overall, the lifetime use of contraceptives seems to protect against cervical cancer.

The effectiveness of vaginal spermicides in this prevention may be due to their antiviral action.

8. Cramer, D., et al. The relationship of tubal infertility to barrier method and oral contraceptive use. *J.A.M.A.* 257:2446, 1987.
In general, there is no association between the past use of oral contraceptives and tubal infertility. On the other hand, women who use both a mechanical and chemical barrier (such as a diaphragm plus spermicide) exhibit a significantly decreased risk of tubal infertility.

9. Li, D., et al. Prior condom use and the risk of tubal pregnancy. *Am. J. Public Health* 80:964, 1990.
In this case-control study made up of 227 women who had had a tubal pregnancy, it was found that a history of condom use for more than 1 year was associated with a decreased risk of subsequent tubal pregnancy. This is probably due to the protection that condoms offer against STDs, which are likely to be causally related to tubal pregnancy.

10. Centers for Disease Control. Condoms for prevention of sexually transmitted diseases. *M.M.W.R.* 37;133, 1988.
Recommends the use of condoms and spermicides to reduce the transmission of STDs.

11. Rosenberg, M., et al. Barrier contraceptives and sexually transmitted diseases in women: a comparison of female-dependent methods and condoms. *Am. J. Public Health* 82:669, 1992.
As compared with women using no contraceptives or those who had undergone tubal ligations, women using the sponge or diaphragm showed at least 65 percent lower rates of infection with Neisseria gonorrhoeae *and* Trichomonas vaginalis; *the rates were lower by 34 percent and 30 percent, respectively, for condom users. For* Chlamydia trachomatis *infection, the reduction was 13 percent for sponge users, 72 percent for diaphragm users, and 3 percent for condom users. Vaginal candidiasis was more common in diaphragm users, but the rates of bacterial vaginosis were similar among all groups. The conclusion is that women using female-dependent methods experience greater protection from STDs than those relying on condoms.*

12. Shervington, D. O. The acceptability of the female condom among low-income African-American women. *J. Natl. Med. Assoc.* 85:341, 1993.
Cultural norms of female submission and passivity in sexual negotiation is a major barrier to taking preventive actions among African-American women.

13. Kreiss, J., et al. Efficacy of nonoxynol 9 contraceptive sponge use in preventing heterosexual acquisition of HIV in Nairobi prostitutes. *J.A.M.A.* 268:520, 1992.
In this study, the authors were unable to demonstrate that the nonoxynol-9 sponge was effective in reducing the risk of HIV infection in an admittedly very highly exposed population.

69. FEMALE STERILIZATION
Marc Vatin

Sterilization is the voluntary destruction of the reproductive function. It can apply either to the male or female partner, but, in practice, female sterilization is performed more frequently than male sterilization.

The most frequent indication is multiparity. The woman typically has completed having her family and wants a permanent method of contraception. Another obvious indication is the presence of any disease process in which pregnancy would endanger the patient's life, such as cardiac disease. Generally, an adult woman (regardless of parity or marital status) can request sterilization, but the laws governing sterilization vary from state to state, and the physician should be familiar with them. Alternatives to sterilization, failure rates, complications, and possible long-term effects of sterilization should all be discussed with the patient. In the past 15 years, approximately half a million female sterilizations were performed annually in the United States. It is estimated that 1 percent of these women will seek reversal of the procedure within the subsequent 5 years; the usual reason given for this is a change in partner. Regret at undergoing sterilization is thus a public health problem.

A great variety of techniques have been used to prevent the union of the sperm and the ovum, generally by interrupting the fallopian tube. Unless there is a concomitant pelvic disorder, hysterectomy is not usually considered an acceptable method of sterilization owing to its potential risks and morbidity. Tubal "ligation" is actually a misnomer. In fact, it is a partial salpingectomy, performed through a standard laparotomy incision, consisting of either a small, 2.5- to 3.0-cm, suprapubic incision (minilaparotomy) or a 3- to 5-cm incision made through the posterior cul-de-sac (colpotomy). Both colpotomy and minilaparotomy can be done under local anesthesia. The colpotomy technique has been found to be associated with a significantly higher infectious morbidity than the abdominal approach.

The postpartum period is a very convenient time for performing sterilization, as the fundus is near the umbilicus and the fallopian tubes are easily accessible through a mini-infraumbilical incision; the failure rates are higher than those for interval procedures, however. In the interval procedure (sterilization done in the absence of pregnancy), the key to success is the elevation of the uterine fundus against the anterior abdominal wall. The most popular partial salpingectomy method is the Pomeroy, because of its simplicity and effectiveness (0.0–0.4% failure rate). To perform it, a 2.5-cm midportion loop of tube is picked up and ligated at its base with absorbable suture, after which the loop is excised. The stumps are left tied together, but absorption of the ligature causes them to separate after a few weeks. Many other techniques have been described: the Madlener, Irving, and Uchida, to name a few.

The most popular approach to interval sterilization in the United States uses laparoscopy. It is rapid, it allows visualization of the pelvic cavity, and it can be done under local anesthesia on an outpatient basis. First, the abdomen is insufflated with 2 to 4 liters of gas administered through a Veress needle inserted into the subumbilical area. A sharp trocar is then placed to allow introduction of the laparoscope. Alternately, the trocar can be inserted first and the pneumoperitoneum created through the trocar. Both methods are acceptable. Disposable shielded trocars can now be used to ensure sharpness and reduce the risk of injury. The fallopian tube is then identified, and its midportion is grasped with the forceps and either destroyed by fulguration or occluded by mechanical devices.

Complications include injury to major vessels or bowels during the blind insertion of the needle or trocar, bleeding from mesosalpingeal tears during manipulation of the tubes, and bowel burns resulting from electrical methods. Burns often go undetected at the time of laparoscopy. Only compatible electrosurgical units should be used, and the manufacturer's recommendations followed. Failures and complications have been traced to the unauthorized "mixing" of bipolar forceps and generators. The risk of burn is now greatly reduced through the use of bipolar forceps. With another method, endo- or thermocoagulation, no current enters the body. The coagulation instrument is merely heated to effect coagulation, though the failure rates associated with use of this method are higher than those observed for bipolar current. Transection or resection of a segment of tube, in addition to electrical coagulation, does not improve the effectiveness of the procedure and increases the risk of hemorrhage. Coagulation alone is very effective, if a minimum 3-cm length of tube is destroyed by creating multiple coagulation points.

For the nonelectrical or mechanical methods of laparoscopic sterilization, a special applicator is used to occlude the fallopian tube with a mechanical device. The Yoon band, or Falope ring, is a small Silastic ring that is slipped onto the base of a loop of the fallopian tube. If a tube is inadvertently transected, the ring can be applied to each stump or the stumps can be electrocoagulated. The clips (the spring-loaded clip of Hulka and the titanium-silicone rubber clip of Filshie) destroy the least amount of tissue (0.5 cm) and preserve the continuity of the uteroovarian vascular anastomosis. Compared with the otherwise very efficient Falope ring and Hulka clip, the Filshie clip can accommodate thick tubes with less trauma. Because of the minimal tissue destruction involved, the reversibility potential is better for clips. This should be an important consideration, given the number of such requests.

Among the widely used sterilization methods, there is little difference in effectiveness. Comparisons are made difficult, however, by the lack of standardization in data collection. If luteal pregnancies and the misidentification of pelvic structures are ruled out, the failure rate of the laparoscopic techniques varies from 0.9 to 6.0 per 1000 sterilizations. The most serious complication of laparoscopic sterilization failure is ectopic pregnancy. It has been suggested that electrocoagulation techniques lead to a higher rate of ectopic pregnancies, but, overall, laparoscopic sterilization is a safe procedure that is attended by very low morbidity and mortality. In the United States, a morbidity of 0.27 percent and mortality rate of 4 per 100,000 have been cited.

Many experimental methods of sterilization are now being tested. In the technique of hysteroscopic coagulation, a small endoscope is inserted via the cervix into the endometrial cavity, which is then distended by gas or liquid to afford proper visualization of the internal ostia. An electrode or a thermoprobe is then passed into the tubal orifices, which are fulgurated at the uterotubal junction. It is a procedure fraught with technical difficulties and potentially life-threatening complications (e.g., uterine perforations and burns, and interstitial or cornual pregnancies following failures), as well as a high failure rate (11–35%).

In another method, which uses a transcervical route and is performed through a hysteroscope, various chemicals are instilled into the fallopian tubes. These chemicals act either by destroying the inner lining of the tube, with subsequent fibrosis (sclerosing agents), or by forming solid occluding plugs. If improved, these methods could have a future as a quick, inexpensive outpatient procedure. For the present, however, their failure rate is still high.

Another promising avenue for research is immunization of the woman against sperm. Animal studies have shown that the local cervical secretion of antisperm antibodies can be induced. Each coital act then serves as a booster to keep the antibody titer high.

The long-term effects of sterilization are difficult to evaluate because the data published to date lack adequate controls. A poststerilization syndrome has been described that is characterized by menorrhagia, pelvic discomfort, and ovarian cyst formation. A very high (25–50%) rate of menstrual disturbance associated with electrocautery has been reported for some uncontrolled studies. This problem may stem from the fact that the blood flow to the ovaries undergoes cyclic changes and correlates with the systemic progesterone level. The mechanisms that underlie such changes in the blood flow are unknown. Surgical sterilization seems to interfere with the vascular supply of the ovaries, especially if coagulation involves the mesosalpinx.

Psychologic or sexual dysfunctions, or both, develop in some patients after sterilization, and are often related to a patient's ambivalence regarding the procedure. Furthermore, fertility is so intimately associated with femininity in the view of many women that they cannot easily relate to the loss of the reproductive function. Careful preoperative counseling is essential if these problems are to be prevented.

Reviews and Methods
1. Liskin, L., et al. Female sterilization. Minilaparotomy and laparoscopy: safe, effective, and widely used. *Popul. Rep.* [C] 9:125, 1985.
   An exhaustive review with a description of the methods, effectiveness, complications, long-term side effects, and research on new methods.
2. Khandwala, S. D. Laparoscopic sterilization: a comparison of current techniques. *J. Reprod. Med.* 33:463, 1988.
   Compares current techniques based on a large pool of international data. With electro- and endocoagulation, there are few technical failures and fewer surgical complications, but the complications are more serious and ectopic pregnancy is a greater problem. There are greater technical difficulties and complications associated with clips and rings in cases of tuboperitoneal abnormalities. The reversal rates are highest for clips.

3. Hulka, J., et al. American Association of Gynecologic Laparoscopists' 1988 membership survey on laparoscopic sterilization. *J. Reprod. Med.* 35:584, 1990.
   The membership continued to perform fewer sterilizations. The incidence of complications from diagnostic laparoscopies was consistently higher than that after sterilizations. Two deaths (4.8 per 100,000 procedures) were reported to have occurred after diagnostic laparoscopy; no deaths were reported after sterilization. The relative likelihood of ectopic pregnancy was substantially greater after a coagulation procedure than after a mechanical one. There was a relative increase in the performance of newer diagnostic and therapeutic endoscopic procedures.

4. Lipscomb, G., et al. Comparison of Silastic rings and electrocoagulation for laparoscopic tubal ligation under local anesthesia. *Obstet. Gynecol.* 880:645, 1992.
   Silastic rings appear preferable to bipolar coagulation when long-acting agents are used for tubal anesthesia.

5. Byron, J., et al. Evaluation of the direct trocar insertion technique at laparoscopy. *Obstet. Gynecol.* 74:423, 1989.
   Nine hundred thirty-seven laparoscopic procedures were performed using this technique. There were no major complications. With increased experience, the frequency of minor complications decreased from 5.3 to 1.3 percent. Obesity was a risk factor; a history of abdominal surgery was not.

6. Børdahl, P. E., et al. Laparoscopic sterilization under local or general anesthesia? A randomized study. *Obstet. Gynecol.* 81:137, 1993.
   A shorter operative time, quicker recovery time, less abdominal pain and sore throat, and substantial cost savings were realized with the use of local anesthesia.

7. Jarrett, J. Laparoscopy: direct trocar insertion without pneumoperitoneum. *Obstet. Gynecol.* 75:725, 1990.
   The technique is carefully described. It was used in 1002 patients. The disposable trocar with a shield enhanced the safety of this technique. The operating time was reduced. One complication occurred: a small self-limiting omental hematoma. In any patient suspected of having significant anterior peritoneal adhesions, open laparoscopy was performed.

8. Mehta, P. A total of 250,136 laparoscopic sterilizations by a single operator. *Br. J. Obstet. Gynaecol.* 96:1024, 1989.
   The patients were placed in a steep Trendelenburg position. Falope rings were applied by the laparocator under local anesthesia, with premedication but without vaginal manipulation. The number of women sterilized was generally 40 to 50 per hour!

Reversal

9. Spivak, M. M., et al. Microsurgical reversal of sterilization: a six-year study. *Am. J. Obstet. Gynecol.* 154:355, 1986.
   In this series of 113 patients, 50 percent of the women achieved intrauterine pregnancies and 5 percent had an ectopic pregnancy. Positive factors affecting the pregnancy rate were the length of the tube affected (>6 cm), the type of sterilization performed (rings or clips), the anastomotic site (isthmic-isthmic), and the availability of both tubes for reconstruction.

10. Pei, X., Fa, Y. Microsurgical reversal of female sterilization: long-term follow-up of 117 cases. *J. Reprod. Med.* 34:451, 1989.
    The term delivery, intrauterine pregnancy, spontaneous abortion, and ectopic pregnancy rates were 81.2, 83.8, 1.7, and 1.7 percent, respectively. The time interval between sterilization and reversal and the method of sterilization both influenced the pregnancy outcome. The success rate associated with intervals of less than 5 years was much higher than that with intervals of more than 5 years.

Complications

11. Rochat, R. W., et al. Mortality associated with sterilization: preliminary results of an international collaborative observations study. *Int. J. Gynaecol. Obstet.* 24:275, 1986.
    Data were collected from 28 countries. Of 41,834 sterilizations, 23 resulted in

death. The adjusted attributable case-fatality rates were 13.5 per 100,000 for interval procedures, 53.3 per 100,000 for postabortion procedures, and 43.4 per 100,000 after vaginal delivery.

12. DiGiovanni, M., et al. Laparoscopic tubal sterilization. The potential for thermal bowel injury. *J. Reprod. Med.* 35:951, 1990.
    Bowel burns often go undetected at the time of laparoscopy. There is controversy over whether they are caused directly by operator error or result indirectly from a hot oviduct or a hot recently used forceps. The study results indicate that only direct electrocoagulation of the bowel appears to cause injury.

13. Weisman, C. S., Teitelbaum, M. A., and Morlock, L. L. Malpractice claims experience associated with fertility-control services among young obstetrician-gynecologists. *Med. Care* 26:298, 1988.
    The types of services most frequently named as the basis for threatened lawsuits are sterilization and abortion procedures. The type of practice arrangement, physician gender, and attitudes toward physician-patient communication did not appear to affect the risk of litigation.

14. Kjersgaard, A. G., et al. Male or female sterilization: a comparative study. *Fertil. Steril.* 51:439, 1989.
    Vasectomies were less expensive, more easily performed as outpatient procedures, and associated with less postoperative symptoms. The failure rate associated with them was also lower than that for laparoscopic tubal ligation.

New Developments

15. Shuber, J. Transcervical sterilization with the use of methyl 2-cyanoacrylate and a newer delivery system (the FEMCEPT device). *Am. J. Obstet. Gynecol.* 160:887, 1989.
    Hysterosalpingography performed 4 months after the procedure showed bilateral tubal occlusion in 88.2 percent of the study participants. There were no complications. The technique appears to be safe and simple, but the failure rate remains a problem.

16. Eubanks, S., Newman, L., and Lucas, G. Reduction of HIV transmission during laparoscopic procedures. *Surg. Laparosc. Endosco.* 3:2, 1993.
    Evacuation of the pneumoperitoneum into a closed system diminishes exposure of the surgical team to aerosolized HIV-infected blood and peritoneal fluid.

XIII. INFERTILITY

70. EVALUATION OF THE INFERTILE COUPLE
John D. Isaacs

Infertility is defined as the inability of a couple to conceive after 1 year of unprotected intercourse. Approximately 10 to 15 percent of couples in the United States are affected (3–5 million). The major causes of infertility include ovulatory dysfunction (30%), fallopian tube compromise (30–35%), and defects of sperm function or delivery (30%). The initial infertility evaluation is designed to address these major causes as efficiently as possible, and can reveal the condition, or conditions, responsible in most couples (85%). With careful planning, the infertility evaluation can be completed in 2 to 3 months.

During the initial visit, a directed history should be obtained from both partners. Specifically, the woman should be asked about pelvic infection, the use of an intra-uterine device, previous surgical procedures, or recent changes in her body weight. Physical examination may reveal evidence of genetic defects, genital malformations, galactorrhea, androgen excess, or other factors contributing to female infertility. Information to be elicited from the man includes previous fathered pregnancies, urogenital operations, impotence, diabetes, or mumps orchitis. The gynecologist or urologist should evaluate the man for evidence of varicocele, testicular atrophy, or other urogenital malformations.

Confirmation of ovulation relies on the detection of progesterone, which is secreted by the corpus luteum. Menstrual cycles occurring at regular intervals of 28 to 38 days and preceded by moliminal symptoms (e.g., breast tenderness) due to elevated progesterone levels reliably predict ovulation (98%). A serum progesterone level greater than 15 ng/ml during the midluteal portion of the menstrual cycle or an endometrial biopsy specimen taken premenstrually, which shows less than 2 days' discrepancy between the histologic dating and the actual cycle day, provide confirmation of ovulation.

Progesterone is a thermogenic hormone; therefore, its secretion by the corpus luteum produces an elevation in the basal body temperature. Basal body temperature records that document an increase of 0.36°F (0.2°C) for 12 to 15 days provide retrospective evidence of ovulation and normal duration of the luteal phase of the cycle. Common causes of ovulatory dysfunction include hyperprolactinemia, androgen excess, polycystic ovarian disease, and thyroid dysfunction. Investigation of these causes may be warranted in patients with ovulation defects.

The uterine cavity and fallopian tubes may be evaluated by hysterosalpingography, usually performed during the follicular portion of the cycle. To perform it, contrast medium is injected into the uterus and tubes under fluoroscopic visualization, thereby allowing assessment of tubal patency and intrauterine contour. With the use of laparoscopy and hysteroscopy, it is possible to directly visualize the endometrial cavity, fallopian tubes, and pelvic peritoneum, and they also permit therapeutic interventions to be carried out, as needed.

A semen sample is obtained from the male partner for the microscopic analysis of ejaculate volume (2–5 ml), sperm density (20 million/ml), motility (50%), and morphology (50%), as well as evidence of infection (assessed by the white blood cell count). Abnormal findings should be confirmed with a second test 90 days later.

Postcoital testing provides information about the sperm–cervical mucus interaction and indicates whether sperm are reaching the upper reproductive tract. Two to 3 days before the expected date of ovulation, a sample of cervical mucus is obtained several hours after coitus and examined microscopically for evidence of at least 5 motile sperm per high-powered field. The cervical mucus is also assessed for evidence of excessive thickness. Abnormal cervical mucus may be improved by supplemental estrogen therapy. Oligospermia or immobilized sperm, when the semen analysis findings are otherwise normal, is an indication for intrauterine insemination.

Once abnormalities are identified, directed therapy can be instituted. Ovulatory dysfunction may be treated with clomiphene citrate or human menopausal gonadotropins. Intrauterine insemination may improve fertility in cases of male factor infertility, and may be done with semen obtained from either the husband or a donor. Pelvic adhesions, endometriosis, and other tuboperitoneal factors are usually treated surgically.

Approximately 5 to 10 percent of couples will remain without an explanation for their infertility after completion of this basic evaluation. Adjunctive studies are available for the evaluation of this group of patients.

General
1. Bronson, R., Cooper, G., and Rosenfeld, D. Sperm antibodies: their role in infertility. *Fertil. Steril.* 42:171, 1984.
   Sperm antibodies have been linked to infertility; this article reviews the diagnostic modalities available.
2. Barnea, E. R., Holford, T. R., and McInnes, D. R. A. Long-term prognosis of infertile couples with normal basic investigations: a life-table analysis. *Obstet. Gynecol.* 66:24, 1985.
   The natural history of untreated childless couples with normal results revealed by a basic infertility investigation reveals that 87 percent will be pregnant within 5 years.
3. Lobo, R. A. Unexplained infertility. *J. Reprod. Med.* 38:241, 1993.
   A nebulous diagnosis is justified only after a thorough investigation of both partners. Spontaneous pregnancies occur at a reported rate of 60 percent after 3 years.

Male Factor
4. Grunfeld, L. Workup for male infertility. *J. Reprod. Med.* 34:143, 1989.
   An excellent introduction to the evaluation of male infertility. Provides an overview of the most commonly used testing modalities and a classification of the causes of male infertility.
5. Dunphy, B. C., Neal, L. M., and Cooke, I. D. The clinical value of conventional semen analysis. *Fertil. Steril.* 51:324, 1989.
   Relates aspects of the semen analysis to conception in infertile couples.
6. Fisch, H., and Lipshultz, L. I. Diagnosing male factors of infertility. *Arch. Pathol. Lab. Med.* 116:398, 1992.
   An in-depth review of all aspects of the male infertility investigation, the history and physical examination, laboratory tests, and invasive diagnostic modalities.
7. Collins, J. A., et al. The postcoital test as a predictor of pregnancy among 355 infertile couples. *Fertil. Steril.* 41:703, 1984.
   A critical look at the role of postcoital testing in modern infertility practice.
8. Doody, M. C., and Good, M. C. The postcoital test: a quantitative method. *J. Androl.* 14:149, 1993.
   The postcoital test is performed to assess the ability of sperm to penetrate and survive in cervical mucus.

Tubal Factor
9. Rajah, R., McHugo, J. M., and Obhrai, M. The role of hysterosalpingography in modern gynaecological practice. *Br. J. Radiol.* 65:849, 1992.
   The authors provide evidence validating the continued use of hysterosalpingography by correlating findings obtained at laparoscopy with those obtained at hysterosalpingography.
10. Rice, J. P., London, S. N., and Olive, D. L. Reevaluation of hysterosalpingography in infertility investigation. *Obstet. Gynecol.* 67:718, 1986.
    Accurate diagnosis of tuboperitoneal abnormalities is more possible with laparoscopy than with hysterosalpingography.

Ovulation Factor
11. Moghissi, K. S. Ovulation detection. *Endocrinol. Metab. Clin. North Am.* 21:39, 1992.
    An excellent overview of the most widely used methods for detection of ovulation.

12. McNeely, M. J., and Soules, M. R. The diagnosis of luteal phase deficiency: a critical review. *Fertil. Steril.* 50:1, 1988.
Extensive review of the methods available for the diagnosis of luteal phase deficiency.

71. TREATMENT OF MALE-ASSOCIATED INFERTILITY
Michael D. Fox

Infertility affects 10 to 15 percent of couples attempting to conceive in the United States. Often the emphasis of diagnosis and treatment is on the female partner. However, at least one third of the infertility causes can be attributed to the male partner alone, and another 15 to 25 percent are a combination of male and female factors. In general, compared to female infertility, less is known about male infertility and the treatment outcomes have been poorer. A precise definition of male infertility is difficult because, as long as motile sperm can be found in the ejaculate, pregnancies have occurred. Additionally, the criteria for judging the findings from semen analysis as "normal" or acceptable have become less strict with time. This makes it difficult to interpret comparisons among scientific efforts aimed at investigating male infertility treatments.

In terms of gametogenesis, sperm undergo considerably more developmental steps than the ovum, any one of which can be interrupted by external influences. For normal spermatogenesis to take place, the male must possess end-organs (testes) capable of responding to an endocrine stimulus. A functioning epididymis is also required for sperm maturation to occur. Furthermore, a ductal and accessory gland system capable of depositing semen into the proximal urethra and an intact neural pathway which can produce erection and external ejaculation are necessary. To achieve pregnancy, the male must deposit an adequate number of functioning sperm into the woman's vagina. The sperm must then traverse the cervical mucus and travel into the upper genital tract, where, through capacitation (a 6- to 12-hour process that takes place in the female genital tract and results in hyperactive motility) and the acrosome reaction (release of proteolytic enzymes necessary to penetrate the oocyte), fertilization occurs. Thus, male reproductive physiology is a complex process possessing numerous vulnerable aspects.

The testicle is both an exocrine organ (seminiferous tubules) and an endocrine organ (Leydig's cells); both components must be functioning normally for adequate spermatogenesis to occur. The hypothalamus produces gonadotrophin-releasing hormone in a pulsatile fashion, causing the pituitary to release follicle-stimulating hormone (FSH; stimulatory to seminiferous tubules with resultant spermatogenesis) and luteinizing hormone (LH; causing testosterone production in the Leydig's cells). Both LH and FSH are initially required for normal spermatogenesis to take place. Negative feedback in this system is mediated by inhibin and testosterone for FSH and LH, respectively. Normal spermatogenesis occurs over a 72-day period, such that the initial semen analysis reflects events which may have occurred several months in the past.

The evaluation of male infertility requires a history, physical examination, and semen analysis, at a minimum. The history is important (see Chapter 70) and may reveal a history of toxic insults to spermatogenesis. The identification of such insults often merely gives the patient and physician a diagnosis, as treatment is rarely available unless the offending agent can be eliminated before the seminiferous tubules are completely destroyed. Antineoplastic agents, cimetidine, sulfasalazine, nitrofurantoin, alcohol, marijuana, androgenic steroids, radiation, insecticides, and a host of industrial chemicals are known spermatogenic toxins. A history of testicular trauma is only a significant factor as an explanation for infertility if resultant edema occurred or hospitalization was necessary. Sexual history should include lubricant use (many are spermicidal), coital frequency and timing in the menstrual cycle, and impotence. Men should be reassured that the use of boxer shorts, as opposed to tight briefs, and the frequency of hot baths have never been conclusively implicated as factors in infertility. The existence of galactorrhea, anosmia, or visual disturbances point to more unusual disorders of the hypothalamic pituitary axis. The presence of severe chronic or metabolic diseases such as uremia, cirrhosis, or sickle cell disease should be sought, as they can also cause impairment of fertility.

Blood pressure, pulse, body habitus, hair and fat distribution, breast examination for gynecomastia, evaluation of smell, and visual fields are components of the physical examination useful for identifying endocrine causes of infertility, such as hyperthyroidism, Kallmann's syndrome, and pituitary disorders. The presence of inguinal herniorrhaphy scars may bring to light damage to components of the spermatic cord. Careful genital examination should include evaluation for the presence of hypospadias, bilateral vas deferentia, and varicocele, as well as assessment of the size and consistency of the testicles. The normal testicular volume ranges from 15 to 25 ml (best determined by comparison to sized plastic models), and the length should be greater than 4.5 cm with moderately firm consistency. Small soft testicles are associated with loss of normal seminiferous tubules, while small, extremely firm testicles are found in the setting of Klinefelter's syndrome. Rectal examination to evaluate the prostate is important. If a urethral secretion is noted after examination, it should be viewed microscopically and cultured when necessary.

The cornerstone of laboratory evaluation for male infertility is semen analysis. The normal values quoted in published reports vary widely and have been progressively lowered with time. Interestingly, the average semen parameters are significantly lower among fertile males today than those cited in older reports. Generally accepted normal values are as follows: sperm volume more than 1 ml of total volume, 15 to 20 million sperm per milliliter, 30 percent motility after 2 hours, 60 percent normal morphology, and liquefaction within 60 minutes. Morphology and velocity (linear and curvilinear) are most closely correlated with pregnancy outcome. Samples should be collected within 2 hours of reading and prior abstinence is recommended for a minimum of 2 to 3 days. Because even a normal man exhibits significant variation in his semen parameters over time, samples should be collected and analysis repeated twice in the event of abnormal findings, but no closer than monthly. Some advocate computer-assisted semen analysis to assure more objective assessments as well as quantitative measures of velocity and linearity, but this is not routinely necessary.

Testosterone, FSH, and LH levels should be determined in all patients with oligospermia (<20 million sperm/ml) or azoospermia (absence of sperm in semen). Others also have the prolactin levels measured in these patients. Thyroid function studies and other hormonal evaluation are done when the findings from the history or physical examination indicate their need. Evaluation for antisperm antibodies is indicated for those patients with gross sperm agglutination, abnormal postcoital test results, or a history of previous vasectomy reversal, cryptorchidism, or significant trauma. A testicular biopsy specimen is obtained to differentiate between gonadal failure and ductal obstruction or agenesis in patients with azoospermia (total absence of sperm) and a normal FSH level. Aside from in vitro fertilization, the hamster egg penetration test is the only measure of fertilizing capacity. In this test, the zona pellucida is digested from hamster ova and mixed with the patient's sperm, with more than 20 percent penetrations considered normal. After this evaluation, patients can be assigned to one or more of the following diagnostic categories: genetic, anatomic, inflammatory, immunologic, exogenous (as previously discussed), ejaculatory dysfunction, endocrine, and idiopathic. The following discussion focuses on the discovery and treatment of these disorders.

Klinefelter's syndrome is the most common genetic abnormality associated with male infertility. It consists of decreased androgenicity, eunuchoid habitus, gynecomastia, azoospermia, and small firm testes, which are less than 3.5 cm long. The FSH level is elevated and the testosterone level is typically low, but can be normal. This syndrome is associated with an XXY karyotype and there is no specific therapy for it. Other genetic causes of male infertility, such as mosaicism and translocations, are extremely rare.

Bilateral anorchia (vanishing testes) is a rare disorder that may result from torsion, trauma, or vascular abnormality in the fetus. These patients present with primary testicular failure and also have a eunuchoid habitus. Subtle steroidogenic enzyme defects, with or without associated adrenal steroid abnormalities; partial androgen insensitivity syndromes; and congenital absence of germ cells (Sertoli cell only syndrome) are other unusual causes of male reproductive failure.

Varicoceles, discovered on scrotal examination and exhibiting the feel of a "bag of worms," are simply varicosities of the spermatic venous system. The examination is performed with the patient in both the supine and standing positions. The Valsalva maneuver can produce venous pulsations that aid in the diagnosis of subtle lesions. Ninety percent of the varicoceles are on the left side, and presumably due to the increased hydrostatic pressure associated with the higher insertion of the left testicular vein into the left renal vein. It has been proposed that male infertility results from increased temperature of the testicle, decreased testosterone production, or reflux of adrenal byproducts into the testes via the testicular vein. Varicoceles are found in 41 percent of infertile males, but they are also found in 15 percent of fertile men, which has raised questions concerning their true role in infertility. Some studies have shown that semen parameters improve the testosterone level increases by 50 percent, and pregnancy rates are better after repair. Others have failed to show improvement after surgical repair, but, because the procedure is minimally invasive, many consider repair is warranted when other measures have failed.

Several anatomic causes of infertility should be sought during the infertility evaluation. Elevated temperature and antisperm antibody production are the proposed causes of infertility associated with cryptorchidism. To ensure an optimal reproductive outcome, this condition should be addressed surgically before 1 year of age, and certainly before adolescence. Other anatomic abnormalities include hypospadias and epispadias, which interfere with the deposition of semen in the proximity of cervical mucus. These may be corrected surgically, or the problem may be circumvented by carrying out artificial insemination using the husband's sperm. A congenital absence of the vas deferens or seminal vesicles is suspected when azoospermia and lack of seminal fructose are discovered. Artificial spermatoceles have been surgically created, thereby allowing intermittent needle aspirations of sperm, but the pregnancy results associated with use of this technique have been disappointing. Infection and trauma can result in obstruction anywhere along the ductal system. Some of these abnormalities are amenable to surgical correction employing vasoepididymostomy, but successful outcome is seen in only 10 to 15 percent of the cases.

The most common reversible anatomic defect is that due to male sterilization (vasectomy). Using current microsurgical techniques, pregnancy rates of 45 to 60 percent can be expected. Prognostic factors for success include proximity to sterilization (<10 years is optimal), finding sperm in the proximal segment at operation, and the absence of antisperm antibodies. Nearly all men develop some level of antisperm antibodies after sterilization, and the level increases over time.

Epididymal infections with tuberculosis, gonococcus, or *Chlamydia* can result in obstruction at any point along the efferent duct system. Epididymal obstruction is a common sequela, with resultant azoospermia. Examination of testicular biopsy specimens and determination of the seminal fructose level are indicated to rule out additional defects, but results are normal in the setting of isolated obstructions. Vasoepididymostomy is an option for these patients, and pregnancy rates of 10 to 15 percent have been reported in association with its use.

Mumps orchitis is a complication in 10 to 25 percent of the cases of acute mumps infection. This complication is more likely to occur in cases of adolescent and adult infection. Fortunately, only one third of these patients have subsequent significant infertility. Male genital *Mycoplasma hominis* and *Ureaplasma urealyticum* infections have been associated with infertility; however, their significance and the value of their eradication are questioned.

Antisperm antibodies have been detected in the male and found to decrease motility and interfere with zona pellucida penetration. They are present most commonly after sterilization reversal. The recent widespread use of immunobead antibody identification techniques has allowed the detection of antibodies on the sperm surface itself, and hence differentiation between immunoglobulin A and G. This technique also allows for the indirect localization of antibody to serum, prostatic fluid, and seminal vesical fluid. As many as 50 percent of patients who were judged to have serum antisperm antibodies on the basis of older detection methods have been found not to have sperm surface antibodies based on the findings from the immunobead method. Fourteen percent of male infertility patients will be found to have antisperm antibodies in the setting of the following indications for antibody testing: gross agglutination of sperm, as revealed by semen analysis; an abnormal postcoital test despite a normal semen analysis; restricted sperm motility ("vibrating") in the cervical mucus; and unexplained infertility. Treatments include high-dose corticosteroid regimens, which are associated with significant side effects, such as aseptic necrosis of the femoral head, and ejaculation directly into a buffer solution to reduce the antibody binding originating from seminal vesicle or prostatic secretions. Neither of these regimens has consistently been associated with improved pregnancy rates when compared to the outcome after no therapy.

Neurologic integrity of the male genital system is required for normal erection and external ejaculation to occur. In brief, the parasympathetic system governs erection and the sympathetic system regulates ejaculatory contractions. Any neurologic condition, such as diabetes or spinal cord injury resulting in disruption of this system, can lead to retrograde ejaculation, impotence, or ejaculatory failure. Retrograde ejaculation has been effectively circumvented by the intrauterine insemination of sperm that has been separated from postejaculatory urine. In the absence of confounding infertility variables, this technique has enjoyed excellent results. Ejaculatory failure has been treated by electroejaculation, in which a transrectal probe is applied to electrically stimulate the ejaculatory sequence. In this situation, if the semen parameters are poor, its use in combination with in vitro fertilization (IVF), with or without micromanipulation (zona pellucida dissection and subzonal insertion of sperm), has led to improved pregnancy outcomes.

Less than 5 percent of infertile men are found to have an endocrinopathy responsible for their inability to impregnate. Men with oligospermia or azoospermia can be divided into hypergonadotropic (testicular failure) and hypogonadotropic (hypothalamic or pituitary failure) groups, based on their levels of testosterone, LH, and FSH. Patients with hypergonadotropic hypogonadism (low testosterone level, and elevated FSH and LH levels) generally have irreversible testicular damage stemming from the previously mentioned genetic factors, congenital absence of germ cells, or exogenous toxic insults to the testes, including chronic diseases, all of which carry an extremely poor prognosis. In contrast, hypogonadotropic hypogonadism (low testosterone level with normal FSH and LH levels) is generally associated with an excellent treatment prognosis. Causes of this disorder include Kallmann's syndrome (hypogonadism, anosmia, and midline somatic defects), isolated gonadotropin deficiency, pituitary failure (caused by tumors, infarctions, or infiltrative disease), excessive hormones (caused by body-building anabolic steroids, Cushing's syndrome, or congenital adrenal hyperplasia), thyroid disease, and hyperprolactinemia. Before any therapy is instituted, radiologic imaging of the pituitary and hypothalamus (computed tomography or magnetic resonance imaging) is an absolute necessity to rule out the presence of a tumor. For specific disorders, treatment alone usually results in the restoration of normal spermatogenesis. If spermatogenesis fails to resume or the cause is idiopathic, then gonadotropic replacement is indicated. An accepted regimen begins with human chorionic gonadotropin, which mimics LH (2500–5000 IU three times weekly for 8 to 12 months) to stimulate testosterone production. Generally, in men with postpubertal onset of hypogonadism, this is the only treatment required to normalize the semen analysis. If this fails or if the onset of hypogonadism occurred in the prepubertal period, then human menopausal gonadotropins (hMG; containing FSH and LH in equal proportions) are added at a dose of 75 units given three times weekly for 4 months, followed by 150 units three times weekly for 4 months. Although this treatment is expensive, the results of therapy are excellent, but may take 6 to 12 months to be realized.

Unfortunately, after a thorough evaluation, as described herein, most patients are given the diagnosis of idiopathic infertility. Empiric therapies such as intrauterine insemination, either alone or in combination with clomiphene citrate (a weak estrogen compound that increases LH and FSH release), hMG, or assisted reproductive technologies, including IVF, gamete intrafallopian transfer, and zygote intrafallopian transfer (ZIFT) have all been used as fertilization methods in this situation. The literature is mixed with regard to the efficacy of these treatments; some report improvement while others report no improvement in pregnancy rates. Many studies fail to include control groups. Without treatment, couples with an isolated male factor have a 9 to 18 percent chance of pregnancy over at least a 24-month follow-up period. Despite the disparity in overall pregnancy rates observed among investigators, most believe these treatments shorten the time to pregnancy. To some couples this may in fact be the most pressing goal in their pursuit of infertility treatment.

Both IVF and ZIFT involve in vitro techniques, and allow physicians to visualize fertilization before replacing zygotes into the female partner. Thus, these procedures provide the most accurate method of testing the fertilizing capacity of sperm. Using these techniques, pregnancy rates as high as 10 to 20 percent per cycle have been achieved. Often, however, the sperm from men with oligospermia fail to fertilize in vitro. In these cases, new and as yet not fully evaluated micromanipulation techniques may be tried before the couple resort to the use of donor sperm or adoption. Micromanipulation utilizes microinstruments to make it easier for sperm to penetrate the oocyte. Currently this is accomplished in one of three ways: (1) partial zona dissection (opening a hole in the zona pellucida); (2) subzonal insertion (injecting several sperm under the zona, thus placing them in direct contact with the oolemma); and (3) microinjection of sperm directly into the oocyte cytoplasm (the least-studied technique). These procedures, although achieving limited success at the present time, undoubtedly will be improved in the future. Using this technique to remove individual blastomeres from the zygote could facilitate genetic screening, and the injection of single-sex sperm (when separation is more precise) into the oocyte may revolutionize sex preselection.

The question of sex preselection is common among couples trying to achieve pregnancies. Currently a Sephadex column filtration technique is used to select X-bearing sperm and albumin separation has been used to isolate Y-bearing sperm. These techniques result in a 70 to 80 percent delivery rate of the desired sex. Undoubtedly in the future, techniques will be developed that can virtually assure the ability to choose the sex of children. In most centers performing separations, the ratio of male-to-female requests has been nearly equal, making initial fears of shifting population demographics unfounded.

Last, and most importantly, the practitioner must know when to recommend the cessation of therapy and counsel patients about adoption or donor insemination. Adoption laws are different in every state, but invariably there are several different options available to couples choosing this avenue. Artificial insemination using donor sperm is indicated in cases of failed treatment as well as cases involving a genetic disorder in the male genome, or when there is no desire to undergo vasectomy reversal. After a normal semen analysis, donors undergo history and physical examination, plus tests for human immunodeficiency virus (HIV), hepatitis B, and cytomegalovirus, as well as routine screening tests. Donated specimens are frozen and stored until a second HIV test is negative 6 months later. Donors are then screened on a 6-month basis. In the absence of female infertility factors, monthly fecundity rates are 8 to 10 percent. The timing of insemination is accomplished through the use of basal body temperature charting or urinary LH ovulation predictor kits administered at home by the couple.

Etiology and *Pathophysiology*
1. Sogor, L. Pathophysiology of male infertility. *Semin. Reprod. Endocrinol.* 6:309, 1988.
    This consists of a series of articles by different authors addressing the evaluation of infertile men and the causes and treatment of male infertility.
2. Liu, D. Y., et al. Tests of human sperm function and fertilization in vitro. *Fertil. Steril.* 58:465, 1992.
    A comprehensive review of semen analysis parameters and sperm function testing,

with special emphasis on which parameters correlated most closely with fertilization rates.

3. Adeghe, J.-H. A. Male subfertility due to sperm antibodies: a clinical overview. *Obstet. Gynecol. Surv.* 48:1, 1993.
   The inhibition of sperm transport within the female tract seems to be the main antifertility mechanism of sperm antibodies.

Treatment

4. American Fertility Society. New guidelines for the use of semen donor insemination. *Fertil. Steril.* 53:1S, 1990.
   Unfortunately, the pregnancy rates achieved with frozen sperm are much lower than those obtained with fresh semen.
5. Quagliarello, J. R. Artificial insemination. *Semin. Reprod. Endocrinol.* 5:1, 1987.
   This is a collection of works addressing pertinent issues concerning the use of artificial insemination techniques in the setting of male infertility.
6. Zarutskie, P. W., et al. The clinical relevance of sex selection techniques. *Fertil. Steril.* 52:891, 1989.
   A comprehensive review of current sex selection techniques.
7. Glover, T. D., et al. *Human Male Fertility and Semen Analysis.* London: Harcourt Brace Jovanovich, 1990.
   A refreshing, concise, and updated view of male fertility.
8. Horvath, P. M., et al. A prospective study on the lack of development of antisperm antibodies in women undergoing intrauterine insemination. *Am. J. Obstet. Gynecol.* 160:631, 1989.
   Women undergoing intrauterine insemination failed to develop antisperm antibodies compared to controls over time.
9. Friedman, A. J., et al. Life table analysis of intrauterine insemination pregnancy rates for couples with cervical factor, male factor, and idiopathic infertility. *Fertil. Steril.* 55:1005, 1989.
   Of 64 intrauterine insemination pregnancies for the above indications, all but one occurred in the first four cycles, and it occurred in the fifth.
10. Aboulghar, M. A., et al. Cryopreservation of the occasionally improved semen samples for intrauterine insemination: a new approach in the treatment of idiopathic male infertility. *Fertil. Steril.* 56:1151, 1991.
    Pregnancy rates were improved two- to threefold in oligospermic patients when occasionally improved semen was cryopreserved and later inseminated.
11. Gorelick, J. I., and Goldstein, M. Loss of fertility in men with varicocele. *Fertil. Steril.* 59:613, 1993.
    Men with a varicocele may benefit from early evaluation and prophylactic surgery to prevent future infertility.

72. TREATMENT OF FEMALE INFERTILITY
Michael D. Fox

Counseling patients about the treatment options for infertility is difficult owing to confusion in the literature regarding efficacy. Because term pregnancy rates are the only true indicators of success, the findings from many studies that have end points such as fertilization, ovulation, or chemical pregnancy do not necessarily support the efficacy of a particular therapy. Additionally, very few studies contain adequate numbers of patients. The background (treatment-independent) pregnancy rate is high for infertility patients, and therefore large numbers are required to demonstrate differences. For example, in those patients who have no cause identified after routine evaluation, as many as 60 to 80 percent will achieve a pregnancy after 3 years, even without treatment.

Tuboperitoneal factors are responsible for 30 to 40 percent of the cases of female infertility, and are correlated with the poorest outcome in response to primary therapy. These factors include pelvic adhesive disease resulting from endometriosis or previous infection, hydrosalpinx, proximal tubal obstruction, and obstruction due to previous sterilization. Laparoscopic surgical approaches for the correction of these defects have begun to replace traditional laparotomy microsurgical procedures, except for tubal anastomosis to reverse sterilization and the treatment of proximal tubal occlusion. The reported success rates have been similar for both methods. Results have been best in women who have undergone simple adhesiolysis and ablation of endometriosis, in whom pregnancy rates of 40 to 60 percent have been obtained, depending on the severity of disease. A less than 25 percent pregnancy rate is achieved when hydrosalpinges are treated surgically by neosalpingostomy. Proximal tubal obstruction is seen in up to 20 percent of hysterosalpingograms. Traditionally, the treatment approach for these lesions, if confirmed by chromotubation at laparoscopy, consisted of partial resection and microsurgical anastomosis. Recent transcervical tubal cannulation techniques have been developed, which are less invasive. These include fluoroscopic and ultrasound-guided cannulation and, most recently, falloposcopy. The pregnancy rates observed for these newer procedures are 25 to 30 percent, which are comparable to those seen for microsurgery. In women with severe tubal or peritoneal disease, surgical treatment has accomplished limited success and in vitro fertilization with embryo transfer is the preferred mode of therapy.

Endometriosis is a common finding in infertility patients. In those who undergo laparoscopy as part of the evaluation, 50 percent will be found to have endometriosis. The mechanisms proposed for endometriosis-associated infertility include adhesions with disrupted oocyte pickup, alterations in the composition of peritoneal fluid (increase in prostaglandin F and protein content), and an increase in the number of peritoneal macrophages and their activation. Medical and surgical treatments, alone or in combination, and observation have all been used in the treatment of endometriosis-associated infertility. Medical treatments for endometriosis include progestational agents (medroxyprogesterone), danazol, and gonadotropin-releasing hormone agonists (GnRHa). Each of these therapies has been shown to be effective in reducing the stage of disease, as confirmed by second-look laparoscopy, as well the severity of pain, and results in similar pregnancy rates of 30 to 60 percent. Restoration of normal anatomy is the primary goal of surgical management. The carbon dioxide laser, electrocautery, and electrofulguration have all been used to destroy peritoneal implants, with equivalent success. The pregnancy rates observed for these surgical treatments are similar to those of the medical therapies. Combined medical and surgical therapy offers no advantage over the use of either treatment alone. Some investigators question whether any of these therapies is superior to simple observation in painfree patients without adhesions. Others, however, believe that treatment, as opposed to observation, can prevent the pelvic pain and progression of disease in some of these patients. Moreover, most patients undergo a diagnostic laparoscopy during the evaluation, at which time surgical therapy can generally be easily performed. Due to the variety of acceptable treatment options, it is important to individualize therapy in this group of patients.

The therapy for ovulatory dysfunction, present in some 20 percent of couples seeking infertility treatment, has the best prognosis. The patient's history, basal body temperature (BBT) charting, urinary luteinizing hormone (LH) monitoring, and serum progesterone determinations are all measures utilized to confirm the diagnosis. BBT charting is helpful by demonstrating the 0.36° to 1.0°F (0.2° to 0.6°C) temperature rise seen in the luteal phase of ovulatory cycles. A history of irregular menses is highly predictive of anovulation. Usually more than a very basic evaluation can be deferred until three to four ovulatory cycles have been achieved with therapy. First-line treatment consists of clomiphene citrate (50 mg daily for 5 days) taken during the early follicular phase of the cycle, beginning 3 to 5 days after spontaneous or progesterone-induced menses. BBT charting, urinary LH monitoring, or serum progesterone determinations can be used to follow patients, and the dose increased by 50 mg per cycle, up to 150 to 200 mg, before abandoning clomiphene citrate therapy. Patients with amenorrhea must be evaluated for the presence of hyperprolactinemia, thyroid disorders, and hypogonadotropic hypogonadism before the institution of therapy.

Clomiphene citrate is a nonsteroidal molecule with weak estrogenic activity that acts at the level of the hypothalamus by interrupting the negative-feedback mechanism of estrogen. As a result, the hypothalamus amplifies its signal to the pituitary, resulting in increased LH and follicle-stimulating hormone (FSH) release, which promotes improved follicular development. Clomiphene therapy induces ovulation in 85 percent of patients and results in pregnancy in 50 percent. Side effects, such as vasomotor symptoms, abdominal discomfort, and abnormal ovarian enlargement, are unusual. Pelvic examination at the conclusion of each cycle can identify persistent ovarian enlargement, which commonly responds to the withholding of therapy until the next cycle. More than 75 percent of the pregnancies that occur do so in the first four ovulatory cycles. Beyond six cycles, pregnancies are rare, and therefore alternative therapies are recommended at this time. The multiple-gestation rate is less than 10 percent and the vast majority are twins. No increase in the congenital anomaly, abortion, or neonatal death rates has been observed for clomiphene therapy. A marginal improvement in outcome has been observed when cycles are monitored using ultrasound in conjunction with the administration of 5000 IU of human chorionic gonadotropin (hCG; used to mimic the midcycle LH surge and induce ovulation) when the largest follicle is greater than 15 to 17 mm, followed by intrauterine insemination; however, this method has not been studied in controlled trials. Last, clomiphene acts as an antiestrogen in the cervix, resulting in abnormal postcoital test results in 10 to 15 percent of patients. Intrauterine insemination may be used to overcome this abnormality.

For patients with hyperprolactinemia-induced anovulation, bromocriptine is effective in inducing ovulation 80 percent of the time. Elevated prolactin levels cause anovulation by decreasing the gonadotropin-releasing hormone amplitude and pulse frequency. Bromocriptine acts on the pituitary by inhibiting prolactin release. In addition to bringing about a restoration of cyclic menses, bromocriptine therapy can also effectively reduce the size of prolactin-secreting pituitary macroadenomas (greater than 1.0 cm in diameter) and ameliorate their associated symptoms of headache and visual disturbance. Like clomiphene, bromocriptine does not cause an increase in congenital anomalies, even when used during pregnancy for the treatment of recurrent symptoms. If bromocriptine fails to achieve ovulation, clomiphene or human menopausal gonadotropin (hMG) has been used for this purpose, with excellent results.

hMG is the next therapeutic step in cases of clomiphene resistance and hypogonadotropic hypogonadism, and as empiric therapy for unexplained infertility. Because of its high cost and the potential for severe and even life-threatening side effects, this therapy should not be undertaken until a complete diagnostic evaluation is performed and other less complex methods have been attempted. hMG is a urinary extract of FSH and LH (1:1) obtained from postmenopausal women. Several formulations (ratios) are available, including a nearly pure FSH preparation, and all appear to have similar efficacy. A multitude of protocols exist for the administration of gonadotropins. In general, hMG is administered early in the follicular phase at a beginning dosage of 150 units IM daily. Estrogen determinations and ultrasound examinations are performed every 3 days to monitor follicular development. The frequency of monitoring and the dose are adjusted according to the patient's response. When the dominant follicle reaches 16 mm or greater and the estrogen level is acceptable (200–300 pg per follicle >14 mm), 5000 IU of hCG is given, followed by natural or intrauterine insemination. Luteal support is provided either by hCG or supplemental progesterone. The pregnancy rates achieved by this therapy after six cycles range from 65 percent for anovulatory or hypogonadotropic patients to 25 percent in women with unexplained infertility. Side effects include multiple gestation (10%, with twins accounting for 75%) and ovarian hyperstimulation syndrome. Multiple gestation is more likely if more than four dominant follicles are present.

Ovarian hyperstimulation syndrome is the most significant side effect of hMG treatment. It occurs in a spectrum that ranges from mild ovarian enlargement and discomfort to a life-threatening derangement of water and electrolyte balance. The mild form occurs in 5 percent of the patients and is rarely a significant factor. The severe form occurs in less than 1 percent of the cycles and is characterized by massive ovarian enlargement (>12 cm), hypovolemia, hemoconcentration, weight gain, ascites, and pleural fluid. The underlying mechanism is a massive third spacing of fluid into the abdominal cavity. Thromboembolism and adult respiratory distress syndrome are responsible for the rare deaths associated with this disorder. Treatment is supportive and includes hospitalization and fluid replacement to correct hypovolemia and maintain urine output. Intercourse, pelvic examination, ultrasound examination, excessive activity, and diuretics should be strictly avoided in these patients. Surgical intervention is indicated only in the event of ovarian torsion, rupture, or hemorrhage. Risk factors for development of the syndrome include a peak estradiol level greater than 2000 pg/ml and the formation of more than ten nondominant (<14 mm) follicles at the time of hCG injection. The occurrence of the syndrome is dependent on ovulation, and, in high-risk cases, withholding hCG injection prevents its development. In the absence of pregnancy, symptoms abate in 5 to 7 days, whereas with pregnancy they may persist for up to 3 weeks due to continued hCG stimulation.

Chlamydia, gonorrhea, *Mycoplasma,* and tuberculosis are all infections that have been implicated in the etiology of infertility. In most cases, severe infection results in substantial residual adhesive disease, in addition to subtle abnormalities of tubal function. Electron microscopic studies have shown an extensive deciliation, flattening of the mucosal folds, and general cellular damage to the epithelial lining in such patients. These abnormalities are difficult to overcome with present methods. Assisted reproductive technology (see later discussion) is often the only option to offer these patients when conventional treatment fails.

A great deal of controversy surrounds the diagnosis and treatment of luteal-phase deficiency (LPD). It is likely that all women have an occasional LPD. Presence of the disorder is confirmed either if there is a sustained temperature rise in the luteal phase lasting less than 10 days or if late luteal phase biopsy specimens on two occasions are histologically out of phase by more than 2 days. Proposed treatment includes clomiphene citrate or supplemental progesterone (25 mg bid). However, there is little evidence in the literature supporting the efficacy of this treatment.

Another controversial area of the infertility evaluation is the postcoital test to assess cervical mucus and sperm competence. Proponents of postcoital testing hold that abnormal results can identify couples with coital abnormalities or abnormal cervical mucus, as well as those with either male- or female-derived immunologic infertility. The test is performed in the periovulatory period, which is best timed with BBT charting. Examination of the cervical mucus is best done 2 to 12 hours after coitus. The amount, clarity, stretchability, cellularity, and sperm presence in the endocervical mucus are recorded. When findings are abnormal, the tests should be repeated, as the most common source of the "abnormality" is poor timing. If the mucus is turbid, yellow, scant, and cellular, cultures should be done to exclude cervical or vaginal infection. Much debate over "normal" sperm numbers exists. Generally, more than 20 per high-powered field correlates with a normal sperm count and pregnancy outcome; less than 5 indicates a poor prognosis. The finding of either immobile sperm or "vibrating" sperm on examination of the mucus is indicative of the existence of male or female antisperm antibodies. If immobilization occurs within 2 hours of intercourse, cervical mucous abnormalities are usually the cause, but, if this is found after 4 or more hours, complement-mediated antibody immobilization is the likely cause. Crossed cervical mucus penetration tests can be performed to differentiate the two situations. In these, the female partner's mucus is incubated with the male donor and partner's sperm. If the donor sperm but not the partner's sperm penetrates the mucus, a diagnosis of male-derived antibody is likely. If both men's sperm penetrate, mucous abnormalities, such as infection or female-derived antibodies, could be the cause. The treatment of male antisperm antibody is described in Chapter 71. Treatment of the infection may reverse abnormal mucus qualities. Female-derived antisperm antibody is best managed by washed intrauterine insemination. Some have advocated hMG therapy to improve the cervical production of mucus. Additionally, assisted reproductive technologies (ARTs; see later discussion) have been used in patients with cervical factor infertility.

ART is the final common pathway for infertility patients with a variety of diagnoses. Despite its expense, it offers the only hope for patients who otherwise would have little chance for pregnancy. Tubal occlusion, severe pelvic adhesions unlikely to respond to surgical treatment, male factor abnormalities, failure of conventional treatment for any of the conditions mentioned, and unexplained infertility are all indications for the use of ART.

In vitro fertilization with embryo transfer (IVF-ET), gamete intrafallopian transfer (GIFT), and zygote intrafallopian transfer (ZIFT) are the most commonly used ART methods. All use a stimulation protocol similar to that described for hMG therapy. In general, the administration of hMG or purified FSH is begun early in the follicular phase at a daily dosage of 225 to 300 units per day. Some groups add short-acting GnRHa to the regimen in the luteal phase of the preceding cycle to prevent a premature LH midcycle surge. As with the hMG ovulation induction protocols, patients' conditions are monitored by frequent ultrasound scanning and estradiol measurements. With ART, estrogen levels can be stimulated to much higher levels than is possible with hMG protocols, as oocyte recovery disrupts the residual follicles and thereby decreases the risk of hyperstimulation. When follicular maturity is attained, an hCG injection is given and oocyte recovery is performed before 36 hours have elapsed to prevent ovulation. At this point, the three procedures mentioned diverge. For IVF-ET, the oocytes are recovered transvaginally in an outpatient setting under ultrasound-guided needle aspiration of the follicles and the gametes are cultured together in supportive media. Fertilization is easily documented by the presence of two pronuclei at 16 to 20 hours. In most programs, embryos are transferred after 48 hours when they are in the 2- to 8-cell stage; however, pregnancies have been achieved when embryos were transferred as late as the blastocyst stage. Transfer is accomplished by the careful injection of embryos into the uterine cavity via a thin plastic catheter. ZIFT and GIFT are only useful in patients with normal tubal architecture. These procedures offer the advantage of allowing fertilization, for GIFT, and early embryo development, for ZIFT, to occur in the tube, which is thought to be advantageous due to the presence of an unknown secretory factor. ZIFT differs from IVF-ET only in the location of the transfer. In ZIFT, embryos are transferred into the tube either by laparoscopy or by a transcervical route under ultrasound guidance. In the case of GIFT, the patient must undergo a laparoscopic procedure to harvest the oocytes, at which time the gametes are mixed, loaded into a flexible catheter, and replaced into the distal tube.

The success of the ART procedures is variable, depending on the cause of the infertility and the procedure used. For IVF-ET, the best prognosis is seen in patients with endometriosis or unexplained infertility; the worst prognosis is seen in the setting of male factor infertility. Overall success rates of 15 to 20 percent term pregnancy per transfer procedure have been noted. The pregnancy rate increases with the number of embryos transferred; with the transfer of more than four embryos, the multiple-pregnancy rates rise without an improvement in the pregnancy rate. The multiple-gestation rate has been 20 to 25 percent, of which 25 percent are triplets or higher. Patients with more than two gestations can undergo selective reduction to triplets or twins. Five to 7 percent of the pregnancies are ectopic. The results reported for GIFT and ZIFT have been somewhat better than those reported for IVF-ET; however, these procedures are relatively new and are still undergoing evaluation.

A simple extension of ART is oocyte donation, which is occasionally used in women with ovarian failure. In this situation, the donor undergoes hMG stimulation and oocyte retrieval, while the recipient is given exogenous estradiol and progesterone to mimic a normal cycle in synchrony with the donor's cycle. Term pregnancy rates with oocyte donation have approached 50 percent. This obvious improvement is thought to be due to the lower levels of estrogen stimulation in the recipient's endometrium.

Because large numbers of embryos are often produced with ART procedures, methods for cryopreserving oocytes and embryos have been developed. The social and ethical issues associated with cryopreserved embryos are currently being addressed. Today, the survival rate for thawed embryos is low, but likely to improve in the future.

General
1. Hull, M. G. R., et al. Population study of causes, treatment, and outcome of infertility. *Br. Med. J.* 291:1693, 1985.
   An often-quoted article elucidating the treatment outcomes for common infertility diagnoses.

Tubal Factors
2. Gomel, V. Operative laparoscopy: time for acceptance. *Fertil. Steril.* 52:1, 1989.
   Review of the operative laparoscopic techniques for assessing and treating infertility.
3. Kerin, J. F., et al. Tubal surgery from the inside out: falloposcopy and balloon tuboplasty. *Clin. Obstet. Gynecol.* 35:299, 1992.
   A comprehensive review of the latest techniques for the evaluation and treatment of intratubal disease.
4. Jansen, R. P. Early laparoscopy after pelvic operations to prevent adhesions: safety and efficacy. *Fertil. Steril.* 49:26, 1988.
   Adhesions were noted in 50 percent of the patients after surgery performed by laparotomy, and were significantly improved by laparoscopic lysis carried out between 8 and 21 days after the initial procedure.
5. Boer-Meisel, M. E., et al. Predicting the pregnancy outcome in patients treated for hydrosalpinx: a prospective study. *Fertil. Steril.* 45:23, 1986.
   Of five different factors, many adhesions, thick adhesions, and a thick tubal wall were the worst prognostic factors. The authors developed a useful scoring system to predict outcomes.

Endometriosis/Fibroids
6. Cook, A. S., and Rock, J. A. The role of laparoscopy in the treatment of endometriosis. *Fertil. Steril.* 55:663, 1991.
   A complete review of the laparoscopic treatment of endometriosis.
7. Corfman, R. S., et al. Endometriosis associated infertility, treatment options. *J. Reprod. Med.* 34:137, 1989.
   Overview of the pathophysiologic basis for the current treatment of infertility.
8. Gehlbach, D. L., et al. Abdominal myomectomy in the treatment of infertility. *Int. J. Gynecol. Obstet.* 40:45, 1993.
   The majority of women were able to conceive, but rates of adhesion formation and myoma recurrence were high.

Ovulation Induction
9. Dodson, W. C., and Haney, A. F. Controlled ovarian hyperstimulation and intrauterine insemination for the treatment of infertility. *Fertil. Steril.* 55:457, 1991.
   The authors advocate the use of hyperstimulation and intrauterine insemination in lieu of the more expensive ART methods; however, there are no controlled trials proving the efficacy of this approach.
10. Gysler, M., et al. A decade's experience with an individualized clomiphene treatment regimen including its effect on the postcoital test. *Fertil. Steril.* 37:161, 1982.
    Useful data are provided concerning the use of clomiphene.

Luteal Phase Defect
11. Karamardian, K. N., and Grimes, D. A. Luteal phase deficiency: effect of treatment on pregnancy rates. *Am. J. Obstet. Gynecol.* 167:1391, 1992.
    This review of the literature casts doubt on the efficacy of treatment for luteal phase deficiency.

Cervical, Immunologic, and Infectious Factors
12. Bronson, R. A., et al. Factors affecting the population of the female reproductive tract by spermatozoa. Their diagnosis and treatment. *Semin. Reprod. Endocrinol.* 4:371, 1986.

A thorough discussion of the cervical causes for infertility and their treatment.

13. Carson, S. A., et al. Antibody binding patterns in infertile males and females as detected by immunobead test, gel-agglutination test, and sperm immobilization test. *Fertil. Steril.* 49:487, 1988.
    This study supports the immunobead technique as the most useful screening test for antisperm antibodies in the male and female.
14. Patton, D. L., et al. A comparison of the fallopian tube's response to overt and silent salpingitis. *Obstet. Gynecol.* 73:622, 1989.
    This group examined tubal biopsy specimens obtained from patients with and without a history of pelvic inflammatory disease and tubal disease in comparison to normal tubes and found that the histologic features of both disease groups were similar and showed a correlation in those patients with positive Chlamydia *titers, when compared to the normal group.*

Assisted Reproductive Technologies
15. Paulson, R. J. Human in vitro fertilization and related assisted reproductive techniques. In D. R. Mishell, et al. (eds.), *Infertility, Contraception and Reproductive Endocrinology.* Boston: Blackwell, 1991.
    A thorough assessment of the current status of assisted reproduction.
16. Halman, L. J., Abbey, A., and Andrews, F. M. Why are couples satisfied with infertility treatment? *Fertil. Steril.* 59:1046, 1993.
    The most frequently mentioned reasons for satisfaction with infertility treatment were the technical skills and emotional support of infertility specialists.

73. ANOVULATORY INFERTILITY

Bryan D. Cowan

Repeated ovulation failure is manifested clinically as amenorrhea, menstrual irregularity, or infertility. An inability to conceive owing to failed ovulation accounts for 10 to 15 percent of the women who complain of infertility. The integrated function of the hypothalamic-pituitary-ovarian (HPO)–endometrial axis can be disrupted either by endogenous means (within the HPO axis) or by a perturbation of peripheral endocrine dysfunctions. In general, dysfunctions of the hypothalamic-pituitary system occur as a consequence of psychogenic causes, or develop as a result of structural defects or lesions within the central nervous system; on the other hand, peripheral endocrine disorders that induce ovulatory dysfunction do so by attenuating the proper cyclic sex steroids that signal the responding elements of the HPO axis.

Control of the self-regulated ovarian menstrual cycle is entrained in the "ovarian clock" conceptualized by Yen. In this model, nonlinear feedback of incremental estradiol (E^2) is generated over a well-defined time course. The two principal sources of circulating estrogen are gonadal (ovary) and extragonadal (adipose tissue). In the ovary, gonadotropin-dependent cyclic estrogen production is mediated by granulosa cell responses to follicle-stimulating hormone (FSH), in which androgens (androstenedione and testosterone) are converted to estrogens (estrone and estradiol). The extraglandular gonadotropin-independent conversion of androgens to estrogens provides a second and steady-state mechanism for estrogen production. The predominant estrogen produced by the peripheral conversion of androgens is estrone (E^1). The E^1/E^2 ratio is often used to compare the relative contributions of extraglandular (E^1) and ovarian (E^2) estrogen to the circulation. High E^1/E^2 ratios (>1) are associated with the excess extraglandular conversion of androgens and anovulation.

In addition to estrogens, androgens substantially affect the ability of the HPO axis to respond properly to feedback signals. In women, there are two sources of circulating androgens. The first, gonadotropin-stimulated ovarian stroma, primarily produces androstenedione and testosterone, whereas the second, corticotropin (ACTH)–stimulated adrenal zona reticularis, produces androstenedione, testosterone, dehydroepiandrosterone (DHEA), and DHEA-sulfate (DHEA-s). The most biologically important androgen produced by these two organs is testosterone. The ovary produces 25 percent of the circulating testosterone; 25 percent more is contributed by the adrenal glands; and a final 50 percent is derived from the peripheral metabolism of testosterone precursors. The principal testosterone precursor is androstenedione, which is transformed to testosterone at several sites.

Although estradiol and testosterone are important mediators of HPO responses, it is the hormone-binding globulins that unquestionably modulate the peripheral hormonal effects of these steroids. In general, specific binding globulins exist for all biologically potent hormones, and the bulk of steroid hormones that circulate in the plasma are bound by such proteins. Sex hormone–binding globulin (SHBG), also named testosterone-estradiol–binding globulin, has a high affinity for testosterone, estradiol, and 5-alpha dihydrotestosterone. Besides the specific steroid-binding hormone SHBG, albumin plays an additional major role in the binding of sex steroids. Approximately 60 percent of the circulating hormone is bound to albumin, 40 percent is bound to SHBG, and only 2 percent of estradiol is free in the circulation. SHBG-bound steroids are generally not available for binding and action in the target tissue.

Polycystic ovarian syndrome (PCOS) is the most common cause of chronic anovulation. The term *polycystic ovarian disease*, or PCOS, emphasizes the heterogenicity of this entity, as ovulatory failure, infertility, hirsutism, obesity, and bilateral polycystic ovaries are not unique to PCOS. Although hyperandrogenism is a well-established feature of PCOS, the issue of its source (adrenal versus ovarian) has been the subject of several studies. The findings yielded by direct adrenal or ovarian vein catheterization studies suggest that the androgen excess in PCOS patients has a combined adrenal and ovarian origin. Furthermore, selective "medical ovariectomy" using the gonadotropin-releasing hormone (GnRH) agonist has been used as a probe to determine the respective contributions of ovarian and adrenal androgens to this syndrome. After the suppression of ovarian function with the GnRH agonist, the subsequent measurements of peripheral androgens reveal that ovarian hormones (androstenedione, testosterone, and 17-hydroxyprogesterone) are reduced to castrate levels, whereas the concentrations of the adrenal hormones (DHEA and DHEA-s) are unaffected. Thus, the biglandular excess production of both ovarian and adrenal androgens contributes to the overall androgen excess present in patients with PCOS.

The secretion of excessive amounts of androgen, with subsequent conversion to estrogen, constitutes the basis for the chronic anovulation observed in PCOS. Relatively constant levels of estrogen are reflected mainly by chronically elevated levels of estrone (rather than estradiol), which is derived from the extraglandular conversion of androstenedione. This tonically elevated estrogen environment perpetuates acyclic feedback and the inappropriate secretion of luteinizing hormone (LH) and FSH by the hypothalamic-pituitary system. Patients with PCOS typically exhibit elevated blood LH concentrations together with relatively constant or low FSH levels, and the LH-FSH ratio is usually greater than 3. The disparity between LH and FSH secretion in patients with PCOS can be explained by the following: (1) the negative feedback inhibition of both estradiol and estrone has greater impact on FSH than on LH; (2) FSH release is relatively insensitive to GnRH stimulation; and (3) a multicystic ovary in PCOS patients may secrete large amounts of follicular inhibin (an inhibitor of FSH release), which further inhibits the release of FSH.

In addition to abnormal androgen and estrogen metabolism, PCOS is associated with a peripheral resistance to insulin and glucose intolerance. Both obese and non-obese women with PCOS demonstrate a positive correlation between hyperinsulinemia and hyperandrogenism, implying that androgen excess may somehow mediate peripheral insulin resistance.

The genesis of PCOS is not related to an inherent defect in the HPO axis, but rather it is initiated and then sustained by elevated circulating androgen levels arising from any source. Increased androgen production then leads to increased acyclic peripheral estrogen formation. Peripheral estrogen preferentially inhibits pituitary FSH secretion and causes a high LH-FSH ratio to be established that sustains the acyclic nonincremental estrogen feedback on the HPO axis. LH stimulation of the ovarian stroma cells in conjunction with an associated excess secretion of ovarian androgens then ensues. The excess production of adrenal and ovarian androgens causes SHBG production to diminish, and this alteration further augments the biologic activity of the circulating androgens. In addition, the increased availability of circulating androgens for end-organ action makes them more available for peripheral conversion to estrogen. Thus, elevated androgen concentrations induce an acyclic steady-state of estrogen production (predominantly E^1), which perpetuates chronic anovulation. Ovarian changes, such as inadequate follicular maturation and increased follicular atresia, are secondary events that stem from both inadequate FSH and excess LH stimulation of the follicle.

The association between amenorrhea and galactorrhea has long been known, and its relationship with prolactin excess is well established. Prolactin is secreted by the lactotrophs of the anterior pituitary, mainly under the control of the prolactin-inhibiting factor, dopamine. The mechanism by which hyperprolactinemia is associated with hypogonadism is not yet well established. Dopamine agonists such as levodopa and the ergot alkaloids (e.g., bromocriptine and pergolide) decrease the serum prolactin level, whereas antagonists increase it. Many pharmacologic agents induce hyperprolactinemia, including estrogens, neuroleptics, antiemetics, antihypertensives, hallucinogens, and anesthetic agents. Eliminating or replacing these drugs is frequently sufficient therapy to restore ovulation. Pituitary prolactinomas are generally small (microadenomas) and are commonly treated with bromocriptine, with good fertility outcomes. Side effects from therapy are common and include postural hypotension and gastrointestinal symptoms. The cessation of therapy is usually followed by return of the prolactin excess. Larger tumors (macroadenomas) may require surgical removal. However, medical therapy alone or in combination with surgical treatment has been used successfully for the management of some macroadenomas. The diagnosis and follow-up of patients with pituitary tumors are best conducted using computed tomographic (CT) scanning of the pituitary fossa, magnetic resonance imaging, and a visual field test to rule out pressure effects on the optic chiasma.

Central neuroendocrine failure (hypothalamic-pituitary system) results in hypogonadotropic hypogonadism. In this setting, the gonadotropin concentrations are depressed and estrogen activity is absent. Ovarian failure is manifested by hypergonadotropic hypogonadism, in which the gonadotropin levels are elevated and estrogen activity is insufficient. Asynchronous gonadotropin and estrogen production results in anovulation and manifests varying clinical features. The estrogen, LH, and FSH levels are usually normal, but the menstrual cycles are disrupted. Depending on the degree of impairment, the clinical spectrum of anovulation therefore encompasses amenorrhea, dysfunctional uterine bleeding, and infertility.

The treatment of PCOS or chronic anovulation depends on the clinical diagnosis rendered and the wishes of the patient. If pregnancy is not desired, therapy is directed at protecting the endometrium from unopposed estrogen stimulation, which either could produce endometrial hyperplasia or adenocarcinoma or result in dramatic dysfunctional bleeding. Therapy usually consists of cyclic endometrial shedding, which can be initiated with medroxyprogesterone (10-mg tablet taken orally for 10 to 13 days every 1 to 2 months) or with oral contraceptive pills. If androgen excess is also present, ovarian suppression through the use of oral contraceptive pills is usually the treatment of choice.

Women with chronic anovulation who wish to get pregnant require ovulation induction. Clomiphene citrate has been shown to be effective for this purpose in such women. However, before initiating therapy for ovulation induction, the clinician must be certain that serious disease states have been excluded. Pituitary tumors, anorexia nervosa, gonadal dysgenesis, masculinizing tumors, and adrenal and thyroid disease are all possible causes of chronic anovulation.

Clomiphene citrate is a novel synthetic preparation that acts as both a strong antiestrogen as well as a weak estrogen. It predominantly affects hypothalamic-pituitary receptors for estrogen and promotes an increase in pituitary gonadotropin release, which stimulates follicular development and maturation. We initiate therapy with the administration of 50 mg of clomiphene citrate on days 5 through 9 of the cycle, after a progestin withdrawal. Because approximately 75 percent of clomiphene-induced pregnancies occur during the first 3 months of treatment, a full infertility workup need not be pursued until the woman fails to conceive after several ovulatory cycles. Efficacy (ovulation) can be monitored with basal body temperature charts, luteal-phase progesterone measurements, or endometrial histologie studies. If ovulation does not occur at the 50-mg dose, the dose should be increased by 50 mg after each anovulatory cycle to a maximum of 150 mg. Side effects from clomiphene therapy include ovarian enlargement (13%), vasomotor flushes (10%), and abdominal discomfort (5%). The incidence of multiple gestation ranges from 5 to 10 percent. In patients with ovarian enlargement, therapy should be withheld until the ovaries are a normal size. Occasionally, mild adrenal androgen suppression is also desirable in such patients. Our choice for this has been to administer 2.5 to 5.0 mg of prednisone at 10 to 11 P.M. and to monitor the clinical responses with DHEA-s measurements. Prednisone is a potent glucocorticoid with a short duration of action. As such, the risks of adrenal insufficiency resulting from lengthy exposure to low doses of this preparation are small, but efficacy at low doses can be achieved only if the prednisone is given at night a few hours before the endogenous nocturnal ACTH rise.

Patients who fail to respond to clomiphene are candidates for gonadotropin therapy. This medication is expensive and its effects are difficult to monitor; in addition, treatment requires daily injections and carries a substantial complication rate. For these reasons, patients must undergo a complete infertility workup before gonadotropin therapy is begun. In particular, the uterotubal and male factors must be investigated and ovarian failure excluded. Patient counseling and instruction are essential.

Gonadotropin therapy requires only an ovary with responsive oocytes; about 90 percent of the patients ovulate with therapy. Women with hypogonadotropic hypogonadism have a 70 to 90 percent chance of conception after three to four successful inductions. Unfortunately, patients with PCOS have only a 30 to 40 percent chance during the same time interval. Multiple gestation is the major complication of the method, with an incidence of 20 to 35 percent. Three or more fetuses per pregnancy may be conceived in 5 percent of the women. Superovulation can be kept to a minimum by withholding human chorionic gonadotropin if the estrogen levels are excessive. The second major drawback of gonadotropin treatment is the ovarian hyperstimulation syndrome. The severe form is rare, consisting of large theca lutein cysts, ascites, hypovolemia, hypercoagulability, and even death. Ovarian rupture or hemorrhage may occur, necessitating laparotomy. A mild ovarian enlargement of 5 to 10 cm occurs in 30 percent of the ovulatory cycles.

GnRH, a hypothalamic decapeptide, is the neurohormone responsible for gonadotropin release. This decapeptide has been synthesized and its analogues used for ovulation induction. Physiologic GnRH secretion is pulsatile in nature, and thus its clinical use requires that the GnRH be administered by long-term pulsatile infusion. The early results of this method have proved promising in selected patients, generally women with hypothalamic amenorrhea.

General

1. Cowan, B. D. Anovulation. In R. L. Collins (ed.), *Clinical Perspectives in Obstetrics and Gynecology: Ovulation Induction.* New York: Springer-Verlag, 1990.
   Current review of the etiology and evaluation of anovulation.

2. Yen, S. S. C. Chronic Anovulation Caused by Peripheral Endocrine Disorders. In S. S. C. Yen and R. B. Jaffe (eds.), *Reproductive Endocrinology, Physiology, Pathophysiology, and Clinical Management.* Philadelphia: Saunders, 1986.
   Exceptionally thorough treatise on anovulation.

3. Hillier, S. G., Reichert, L. E., Jr., and Van Hall, E. V. Control of preovulatory follicular estrogen biosynthesis in the human ovary. *J. Clin. Invest.* 57:1320, 1976.
   Experimental observations of human theca and granulosa cell responses to gonadotropin stimulation.

4. Rebar, R., Judd, H. L., and Yen, S. S. C. Characterization of the inappropriate gonadotropin secretion in polycystic ovary syndrome. *J. Clin. Invest.* 45:301, 1966.
   The LH level is elevated in women with PCOS.

5. Horton, R., and Tait, J. F. Androstenedione production and interconversion rates

measured in peripheral blood and studies on the possible site of its conversion to testosterone. *J. Clin. Invest.* 45:301, 1966.
Peripheral conversion of androgens in women.

6. Bardin, C. S., and Lipsett, M. B. Testosterone and androstenedione blood production rates in normal women with idiopathic hirsutism or polycystic ovaries. *J. Clin. Invest.* 46:891, 1967.
Discusses androgen production in women with nonpathologic androgen excess conditions.

7. Rosenfeld, R. L., and Moll, G. W., Jr. The Role of Proteins in the Distribution of Plasma Androgens and Estradiol. In C. G. Molinatti, L. Martini, and G. H. T. James (eds.), *Androgenization in Women.* New York: Raven, 1983.
SHBG and albumin bind 98 percent of the testosterone and estradiol.

Polycystic Ovarian Syndrome

8. Goldzieher, J. W., and Green, J. A. The polycystic ovary. I. Clinical and histologic features. *J. Clin. Endocrinol. Metab.* 22:325, 1962.
A classic article that summarizes the clinical expressions of PCOS.

9. Kirschner, M. A., and Jacobs, J. B. Combined ovarian and adrenal vein catheterization to determine the site(s) of androgen overproduction in hirsute women. *J. Clin. Endocrinol. Metab.* 33:199, 1971.
In general, the ovary is the major source of androgens in women with PCOS or idiopathic hirsutism.

10. Chang, R. J., et al. Steroid secretion in polycystic ovarian disease after ovarian suppression by a long-acting gonadotropin-releasing hormone agonist. *J. Clin. Endocrinol. Metab.* 56:897, 1983.
Suppression of pituitary LH and FSH secretion reduces ovarian but not adrenal androgen secretion.

11. Chang, R., et al. Insulin resistance in nonobese patients with polycystic ovarian disease. *J. Clin. Endocrinol. Metab.* 57:356, 1983.
Women with androgen excess demonstrate a peripheral resistance to insulin.

12. Takai, T., et al. Three types of polycystic ovarian syndrome in relation to androgenic function. *Fertil. Steril.* 56:856, 1991.
Possible subsets of PCOS based on the extent of hirsutism and androgen excess.

Treatment

13. Blacker, C. M. Ovulation stimulation and induction. *Endocrinol. Metab. Clin. North Am.* 21:57, 1992.
Protocols for follicular stimulation.

14. Hoffman, D., and Lobo, R. A. Serum dehydroepiandrosterone sulfate and the use of clomiphene citrate in anovulatory women. *Fertil. Steril.* 43:196, 1985.
Suppression of adrenal androgen production may improve ovulatory responses in some women.

15. Garcia-Flores, R. F., and Vasquez-Mendez, J. Progressive dosages of clomiphene citrate in hypothalamic anovulation. *Fertil. Steril.* 42:543, 1984.
Extended therapy with clomiphene citrate may induce ovulation when standard therapy fails.

16. Adashi, E. Y. Clomiphene citrate: mechanism(s) and site(s) of action—a hypothesis revisited. *Fertil. Steril.* 42:331, 1984.
A well-written review describing the history of the development of clomiphene citrate therapy and its mechanism(s) of action.

17. Suginami, H., et al. A clomiphene citrate and tamoxifen citrate combination therapy: a novel therapy for ovulation induction. *Fertil. Steril.* 59:976, 1993.
The combination of clomiphene citrate and tamoxifen citrate was more effective than clomiphene alone.

18. Lunenfeld, B., Mashiach, S., and Blakenstein, J. Induction of Ovulation with Gonadotropins. In R. P. Shearman (ed.), *Clinical Reproductive Endocrinology.* New York: Churchill Livingstone, 1985.
This article considers the topic of human menopausal gonadotropin treatment and

monitoring protocols. Discusses the efficacy of treatment, the complications, and the therapeutic considerations.

19. Randall, S., Liang, I., and Chapman, A. J. Pregnancies in women with hyperprolactinemia: obstetric and endocrinological management of 50 pregnancies in 37 women. *Br. J. Obstet. Gynaecol.* 89:20, 1982.
    This article details the use of bromocriptine for the induction of ovulation and the establishment of pregnancy in women with hyperprolactinemic anovulation.

20. Vance, M. L., Evans, W. S., and Thamer, M. O. Bromocriptine. *Ann. Intern. Med.* 100:78, 1984.
    A review on the topic of bromocriptine.

21. Nakamura, Y., et al. Clinical experience in the induction of ovulation and pregnancy with pulsatile subcutaneous administration of human menopausal gonadotropin: a low incidence of multiple pregnancy. *Fertil. Steril.* 51:423, 1989.
    Discusses the administration of gonadotropins in a pulsatile mode by means of a portable peristaltic pump via a subcutaneous catheter inserted in the lower abdominal wall.

22. Society for Assisted Reproductive Technology, The American Fertility Society. Assisted reproductive technology in the United States and Canada: 1991 results from the Society for Assisted Reproductive Technology generated from The American Fertility Society Registry. *Fertil. Steril.* 59:956, 1993.
    Increases have been seen in the numbers of programs being reported on and the numbers of procedures performed. The overall success rates are slightly higher than those for 1990.

XIV. HUMAN SEXUALITY

74. ADOLESCENT SEXUALITY
Michel E. Rivlin

Along with the body and the mind, sexuality is one of the three elements most basic to being human. Fetal sexuality begins when an X or Y chromosome directs the development of either testicles or ovaries. Starting in the eighth week of gestation, the gonads elaborate hormones governing sex differentiation and function. In the male, ultrasound imaging has shown that erections occur in the same 90-minute cycle in the 17-week fetus as in adult men. By the end of the first year of life, the infant has experienced and exhibited the full range of the most basic emotions. The positive emotions include pleasure, joy, interest, and surprise; the negative emotions include fear, sadness, anger, disgust, and distress. Fear and sadness are both elements of anxiety, apathy, and depression. Between 18 months and 3 years, most children begin to add shame to the fear, probably already associated with the genital organs. Girls receive much more touching than do boys, despite the equal need for it. Sexually, the preschool age is the period of "playing doctor" and "comparing genitals." Between 4 and 5 years of age, intellectual and physical skills are added. Often, children learn to silence their own sexual feelings and activities, with a resulting breakdown in family communications. The prime time for formal education, between the ages of 6 and 11, the preadolescent book-learning years, is when basic facts and academic skills must be acquired in as many areas as possible to provide a solid basis for successful living.

The changes of adolescence occur along a continuum, which is divided arbitrarily into three stages, although the ages and events quoted here vary widely among individuals. Each stage is associated with certain behavioral characteristics and tasks. The early stage, ages 11 to 14, is characterized by a concern over body changes, egocentricity, and an ambivalence about family relationships. The tasks of this period involve separation from the family and the development of individual identity and independence. In the middle stage, ages 14 to 17, there is concern about peer group approval, conflict with the parents, and feelings of invincibility. The tasks of this period include a continued struggle for identity and independence and the development of adult social relationships with peers. In the late stage, ages 17 to 22, youths become concerned about life-planning issues and acquire an increasing ability to consider the consequences of their own behavior. Common tasks of this period are the development of a moral and ethical value system, career planning, and maturation toward autonomous decision-making.

Adolescence is regarded as a time of turmoil, with a significant disruption in psychologic equilibrium leading to a fluctuation in mood, confused thought, rebellion against parents, and unpredictable behavior. In fact, however, the percentage of disturbances among adolescents is similar to that found among adults—namely, 20 percent. This means that 80 percent cope well with the teenage years. They are not in constant turmoil. At age 16, a third of the adolescents have attained the highest level of cognitive development (formal operations)—the same percentage as is found in adults. The decision-making ability is the same in both, and is based less on rationality than on training and habit. Thus, when it comes to choices made regarding drugs, sex, smoking, and drinking, social acceptance by peers and parental example is more important than is logical information provided by education. When the information is intrinsically conflictive, adolescents, like adults, accept only the message they believe will make them acceptable in their social environment.

Much of adolescent behavior consists of experimenting with a variety of activities, many potentially perilous, including sex, substance abuse, and violence. The adolescent group is the only age group exhibiting an increasing mortality rate in America, with accidents, suicides, and homicides responsible for more than 75 percent of teenage mortality. Substance abuse contributes to this phenomenon. Sexual experimentation results in millions of cases of sexually transmitted diseases and unwanted pregnancies each year, as adolescents show little insight into the consequences of their actions. Youngsters younger than age 16 think in present terms and find it

357

difficult to consider the future or to truly comprehend their behavior in terms of cause and effect. Many of these risk-taking behaviors are interconnected with their origins in childhood experiences, parenting, peer pressure, timing of puberty, self-esteem, ethical and religious training, and education. It is important for adults to understand that thought processes continue to develop and change during adolescence.

National survey data indicate that age 16 is now the average age of first intercourse. Rates of sexual activity continue to climb among the youngest adolescents at a rate faster than that of older adolescents. Sexual activity among adolescents is as common in Canada, England, and France as it is in the United States, but the United States teen pregnancy rate is twice as high (see Chap. 16). The critical difference is a lack of contraceptive knowledge and use. Compliance with contraception is difficult to assess; however, only the birth control pill has been shown to achieve high contraceptive efficacy in teenagers. The number of 15- to 19-year-old women who use oral contraceptives (about 1.5 million) is more than twice the number who rely on condoms, the next most popular method.

Because adolescence represents a time of sexual experimentation, the 15- to 19-year age interval appears to be the highest risk interval for multiple sex partners, and the earlier sexual activity begins, the greater the likelihood for multiple sex partners. Four factors are especially linked to the early onset of coitus: the less the mother's education, the weaker the religious affiliation, the younger the age at menarche, and the less stable the family at age 14 years, the earlier the age at first intercourse.

Denial is a particular characteristic of adolescence and risk taking is a natural behavioral sequela; this adds to the likelihood of acquiring and transmitting sexually transmitted diseases. Some 18 to 30 percent of sexually active adolescents are infected with the human papillomavirus and some 5 to 30 percent with chlamydial cervicitis. Forty percent of the cases of gonorrhea occur in adolescents, as do 47 percent of the reported cases of genital herpes. Adolescents account for 1 percent of the cases of the acquired immunodeficiency syndrome (AIDS), and the incidence is increasing. Age-specific rates of pelvic inflammatory disease are highest for adolescent females and the risk of it in the sexually active 15-year-old girl is estimated to be 1 in 8.

The data for substance abuse are equally discouraging. About 71 percent of Americans aged 12 to 17 years have used cigarettes (21% are daily smokers), 93 percent have consumed alcohol (5.5% are daily drinkers), 57 percent have smoked marijuana (5.5% are daily smokers), 35 percent have used stimulants, and 16 percent have used cocaine.

Fortunately, not all teenagers are the alcoholic, sex-crazed, reefer-pulling aliens that many adults think they are. The important sources of the data show inevitable flaws, such as those related to self-reporting. Furthermore, there is a steady increase in the use of contraception by teenagers, although, unfortunately, adverse media publicity has led to a move from reliance on the birth control pill to less reliable methods, even though there has *never* been a single pill-related death involving a teenager reported in the medical literature. Nearly half of the sexually active girls have had only a single partner, and nearly 85 percent of the remaining half have had no more than three partners. Up to 25 percent have had intercourse only once or twice; 39 percent of sexually experienced teens think that premarital sex is wrong; and 83 percent cite a best age for intercourse older than the age at which they experienced it. The same conventional view is found with regard to substance abuse, in that teenage drug use may be a time-limited pattern of behavior that for many will be abandoned or lessened in young adulthood.

The physician has an important role in encouraging adolescents to be responsible for their own health care. Confidentiality is essential, so that the teen can speak freely and openly. Because most adolescents learn about sexual matters from their peers, peer group values are usually the dominant force in their lives. The physician and parents should attempt to keep their own values as adolescents out of the picture. A nonjudgmental and supportive parental attitude can spare the teenager enormous emotional stress and pain, and the physician, provided that confidentiality is not breached, can provide valuable support to both the parents and the child.

More effective than sermons about the dangers of sex is a relationship in which the young person believes her physician is concerned, and that concern is manifested by the sharing of accurate information. Conversations may address concerns about obesity, acne, and other body image issues, as sexual intercourse is often sought as a means of gaining reassurance about appearance. Adolescents of all ages, regardless of sexual activity, often need to be reassured that they are normal. Discussions of ways to handle peer pressure may also be helpful at all stages of adolescence. Questions or concerns about sexual orientation require the provision of accurate information and the opportunity to deal with these feelings and fears. If the physician is uncomfortable dealing with these issues, timely referral to a knowledgeable professional is essential.

Generally, the clinician functions best in a climate of parental knowledge, but, if confidentiality is requested, treatment need not be withheld. The "mature minor" rule allows the physician to supply full medical care if the minor is considered capable of understanding the nature, extent, and consequences of the invasion of her body. Full documentation of this is essential, however.

Reviews
1. Fisher, M. Adolescent sexuality: overview and implications for the pediatrician. *Pediatr. Ann.* 20:285, 1991.
   Television, rock videos, and fashion magazines bombard teenagers with the attractiveness of sex, without providing any counterbalancing prevention messages.
2. Bidwell, R. J. and Delsher, R. W. Adolescent sexuality: current issues. *Pediatr. Ann.* 201:293, 1991.
   Without an adequate knowledge base, teenagers are unequipped to deal with prevention decisions. Without negotiating skills to resist peer pressures, adequate knowledge cannot be translated into safer behaviors.
3. Alexander, B., McGrew, M. C., and Shore, W. Adolescent sexuality issues in office practice. *Am. Fam. Physician* 44:1273, 1991.
   A nonjudgmental manner, an emphasis on confidentiality, and an honest appraisal of the implications of early sexual activity can enhance discussions about sexual issues with adolescents.

Biology
4. Tanner, J. M. *Growth of Adolescence* (2nd ed.). Oxford: Blackwell, 1962.
   The staging of secondary sex characteristics allows the prediction of future events based on present developmental status.
5. Piaget, J. Intellectual evolution from adolescence to adulthood. *Hum. Dev.* 15:1, 1972.
   This discusses the development of the ability to plan and consider alternatives and their possible results before embarking on any action. This development is affected by genetics, environment, stimulation, education, and economics.

Statistical Sources
6. Centers for Disease Control. Premarital sexual experience among adolescent women, United States, 1970–1988. *M.M.W.R.* 39:929, 1990.
   By 1988, over one quarter of both black and white 15-year-old females had experienced coitus; by age 19 years, over four fifths of both races were sexually experienced.
7. Tyden, T., Bjorkelund, C., and Olsson, S.-E. Sexual behavior and sexually transmitted diseases among Swedish university students. *Acta Obstet. Gynecol. Scand.* 70:219, 1991.
   Ninety-four percent of the students surveyed were sexually active, with a mean number of sexual partners of 6.6 ± 7.7. These findings were compatible with those from similar surveys conducted in the United States.

Contraception
8. Adler, N., et al. Adolescent contraceptive behavior: an assessment of decision processes. *J. Pediatr.* 116:463, 1990.

One study of metropolitan area teenagers revealed that there was a mean delay between first intercourse and first use of a prescription method of contraception of 11 months for clinic patients and 13 months for private patients.

9. Makkonen, K., and Hemminki, E. Different contraceptive practices: use of contraceptives in Finland and other Nordic countries in the 1970s and 1980s. *Scand. J. Soc. Med.* 19:32, 1991.
   Lower rates of teenage pregnancy in other Western countries may be attributable to the teaching of thorough sex education starting in the elementary school.

10. Moore, S. M., and Rosenthal, D. A. Condoms and coitus: Adolescents attitudes to AIDS and safe sex behavior. *J. Adolesc.* 14:211, 1991.
    If teenagers are concerned about becoming infected with the human immunodeficiency virus (HIV), if they believe condoms are protective, if they are not embarrassed to discuss the issue with the partner, if they have discussed the use of condoms with a physician, and if they carry them, then they are more likely to use them consistently.

Problems

11. Cates, W., Jr. Gallagher lecture. Teenagers and sexual risk taking: the best of times and the worst of times. *J. Adolesc. Health* 121:84, 1991.
    Teenagers are at higher risk of acquiring sexually transmitted infections than are other age groups for a variety of behavioral, biologic, and psychosocial reasons.

12. Sugar, M. Adolescent pregnancy in the USA: Problems and prospects. *Adolesc. Pediatr. Gynecol.* 4:171, 1991.
    One million teenage pregnancies occur each year, 400,000 of which end with induced abortion; 85 percent of teens are already sexually active when they first request contraception.

13. Comerci, G. D., and Macdonald, D. I. Prevention of substance abuse in children and adolescents. *Adolesc. Med.* 1:127, 1990.
    Sexual practices as well as drug use are biologically based and complex behaviors. Sexual activity can be spontaneous and unplanned and can take place when judgment is impaired by the effects of alcohol or other drugs.

14. Rosenthal, S. L., and Biro, F. M. A preliminary investigation of the psychological impact of sexually transmitted diseases in adolescent females. *Adolesc. Pediatr. Gynecol.* 4:198, 1991.
    Adolescent females were grouped according to whether they had cervical dysplasia or gonorrhea/Chlamydia infection. Rates of psychopathologic conditions and the impact of the diagnosis were compared. Overall, the patients were more likely to have avoidant rather than intrusive thoughts.

15. Rotheram-Borus, M. J., et al. Reducing HIV sexual risk behaviors among runaway adolescents. *J.A.M.A.* 266:1237, 1991.
    The demonstrated effectiveness of the intensive HIV/AIDS program highlights the importance of enlarging the scope of most current HIV/AIDS prevention programs.

16. Moscicki, A. B., et al. The association between human papillomavirus deoxyribonucleic acid status and the results of cytologic rescreening tests in young, sexually active women. *Am. J. Obstet. Gynecol.* 165:67, 1991.
    In early puberty, columnar epithelium extends into the vagina. Infection with human papillomavirus involving the transformation zone at an early age apparently results in cervical cytologic changes during the teenage years.

17. Remafedi, G. Adolescent homosexuality: psychosocial and medical implications. *Pediatrics* 79:331, 1987.
    The majority of the adolescents in this study had experienced school problems related to sexuality, substance abuse, and emotional difficulties. Nearly half gave a history of having sexually transmitted diseases, running away from home, or conflicts with the law.

18. Rousso, H. Affirming adolescent women's sexuality. *West. J. Med.* 154:629, 1991.
    Although many disabled teenaged women have less satisfying social lives than do their nondisabled counterparts, this is not the inevitable consequence of disability.

Physicians can actively encourage these young women to become involved in the social scene.

19. Chamberlain, A., et al. Issues in fertility control for mentally retarded female adolescents: I. Sexual activity, sexual abuse, and contraception. *Pediatrics* 73:445, 1984.

The proportion of retarded female adolescents who had had intercourse was comparable to that seen in the general adolescent population. The currently available contraception methods did not appear to be adequate.

Education

20. Forrest, J. D., and Silverman, J. What public school teachers teach about preventing pregnancy, AIDS and sexually transmitted diseases. *Fam. Plann. Perspect.* 22:65, 1989.

Because the teacher's information is often inaccurate, what is taught varies greatly.

21. Graves, C. E., Budge, M. D., and Nyhuis, A. W. Residents' perception of their skill levels in the clinical management of adolescent health problems. *J. Adolesc. Health Care* 8:413, 1987.

The residents surveyed felt unskilled about dealing with sexuality, handicaps, family planning, psychosocial concerns, homosexuality, and sexual assault.

22. Schwartz, I. M. Affective reactions of American and Swedish women to their first premarital coitus: a cross-cultural comparison. *J. Sex Res.* 30:18, 1993.

Young women in a culture where premarital intercourse is deemed socially unacceptable are severely limited in their access to important information on which to base responsible sexual decisions.

23. Wielandt, H. B. Have the AIDS campaigns changed the pattern of contraceptive usage among adolescents? *Acta Obstet. Gynecol. Scand.* 72:111, 1993.

Campaigns in Denmark have led to an increase in condom usage, such that, in 1989, 37 percent of females and 52 percent of males had used condoms at their most recent sexual encounter.

75. ALTERATIONS IN SEXUALITY WITH AGING, DRUGS, AND DISEASE
Michel E. Rivlin

The aging process affects the entire body, with sexuality being among the last functions to decline. These involutional changes occur gradually and at different rates for different people. At menopause, reproduction ceases in women, whereas men may retain fertility throughout their lives. There appears to be no physiologic male menopause. Men reach their sexual peak in late adolescence, and this is followed by a gradual decline. Female peaks are reached in the late thirties and the subsequent decline is less than that in the male. Postmenopausal changes in the vagina include epithelial atrophy, disappearance of the rugae, elevation in pH, decrease in lubrication, reduced elasticity, vascular fragility, and narrowing of the outlet. There is also an increased susceptibility to vaginitis and dyspareunia. All these changes may be prevented or reversed to a major extent by estrogen replacement. In the male, the ejaculatory demand decreases as, too, do the expulsive force, seminal volume, erectile rigidity, and maintenance. However, although erection is slower and physical stimulation may be necessary, erection may be maintained for extended periods. The decline in the frequency of intercourse associated with aging is related primarily to male sexual dysfunction.

These alterations in sexuality with aging involve all three phases of sexual response. Men show a much greater decline in the sex drive (desire) than do women. Thus, at age 17, the average of four to ten ejaculations a week falls to about 1 at age 60. The sex drive in the male is very sensitive to stress and depression, and declining levels of testosterone may also be a factor. In contrast, many women have an increase in libido at menopause, perhaps associated with the unopposed action of adrenal testosterone when the ovarian supply of estrogen declines. Older men generally require both psychic and tactile stimuli to produce erection in the excitement phase. In the female, lubrication and swelling may diminish, but frequent intercourse, hormone replacement, and the use of lubricants readily restore adequate function. The phase of orgasm is shorter in older women, and, in older males, the refractory period usually increases substantially. The combination of declining physical capacity and a maintained psychologic need for sex in the male leads to his becoming more vulnerable sexually and more dependent on his partner.

A great number of aged people have an active sexual life. There is a large range of sexual behavior, including erotic fantasy, masturbation, coitus, and nongenital erotic pleasuring, that remains as satisfactory in later years as it does for the young. Social and economic factors have an important influence on the sexual life of the elderly, so that, for instance, married women and wealthy men (single or married) maintain a higher frequency of sexual activity. A relatively high level of sexual activity over the years sets the pattern in old age also.

Primary care physicians can promote sexual health in older women by always taking a sexual history. A wide variety of physical, emotional, and pharmaceutically induced disorders may influence sexuality. Physicians can reassure patients that sexual dysfunction is not inevitable with advancing age. If problems are identified, management is directed at reducing specific contributory organic, hormonal, psychologic, and social stresses. Because a lack of suitable male partners is common for older women, acceptable alternatives of sexual expression must be sought. If possible, older women should be encouraged to discard unnecessary strictures against masturbation. The staff of long-term care facilities should be nonjudgmental, understanding, and supportive. Privacy and the opportunity to express sexual desires should be provided. Most elderly people cease engaging in sexual activity because of psychologic and societal misconceptions, not because of aging processes or disease. The longer it has been since sexuality has ceased, the more difficult it is to resume; therefore, therapy should be prompt and vigorous.

The physiologic mechanisms involved in the normal sexual response include psychogenic, vascular, neurogenic, and hormonal factors, which are coordinated by centers in the hypothalamus, limbic system, and cerebral cortex. Many commonly used drugs can interfere with sexual function in either sex, causing a loss of libido, interfering with erection or ejaculation in men, and delaying or preventing orgasm in women. The pharmacologic mechanisms proposed to explain these adverse effects include anticholinergic activity, alterations in adrenergic tone, and changes in central serotonin and catecholamine levels, in addition to endocrine and sedative effects. Drug-related changes may be difficult to distinguish from sexual dysfunction stemming from the disease state per se; for instance, untreated hypertensive and depressed patients exhibit a higher incidence of sexual difficulties than does the general population. Patients experiencing drug-related sexual dysfunction may be able to discontinue the therapy responsible, and it is vital to inform them about this possibility and to reassure them that the changes are reversible. If possible, symptoms may be alleviated by either switching agents or lowering the dosage without loss of the desired therapeutic effect. Most reports concern male patients, and it is not known whether women's sexual functioning is less vulnerable to drug changes or whether information on these alterations has not been volunteered as freely.

Antihypertensive agents are probably the most frequent offenders. Thiazides, drugs with peripheral sympatholytic action, and centrally acting sympatholytics can all cause impotence and ejaculatory failure. Beta-adrenergic–blocking agents can produce loss of libido and impotence. Drugs less likely to cause sexual dysfunction include the angiotensin-converting enzyme inhibitors, calcium channel blockers, and the arteriolar dilator hydralazine. Cimetidine, a histamine H_2-receptor antagonist, increases the prolactin level and acts as an antiandrogen, causing loss of libido and impotence. Ranitidine and famotidine may have fewer adverse sexual side effects. The antipsychotic drugs, tricyclic antidepressants, and especially monoamine oxidase inhibitors may impair sexual function in both men and women, causing anorgasmy. Many of these medications also cause hyperprolactinemia. Central nervous system depressants, including sedatives, marijuana, alcohol, methadone, and heroin, can diminish desire, impair erection, and interfere with ejaculation. Antineoplastic drugs can cause gonadal damage and progressive loss of libido in both sexes.

If noncompliance or drug misuse to promote an aphrodisiac effect (alcohol, marijuana, benzodiazepines, or yohimbine) is suspected, sexual function should be assessed. Furthermore, a baseline sexual history should be obtained before high-risk agents are prescribed. If an organic basis for sexual dysfunction is identified, agents known to aggravate the problem should be avoided. A high index of suspicion is particularly important in the elderly, because inappropriate drug use in this group is not uncommon. In this way, many serious problems that result from active or passive underuse, misuse, or excessive use of either prescribed or over-the-counter drugs may be avoided.

The range of physical and mental illness and disability that may affect sexual function is enormous. In some instances, there is organic sexual dysfunction; in others, psychosocial factors induce the dysfunction; and, in yet a third group, sexual activity is modified as a result of physical illness. Here again, these changes have been studied mainly in men.

Adequate sexual function requires intact vascular, neurologic, and endocrine function. Neurologic disorders, including spinal cord injury and multiple sclerosis, severely impair function. Diabetes is a common cause of sexual dysfunction, probably as a result of a peripheral autonomic neuropathy. Vascular disease, particularly affecting the pelvic arteries and veins, may compromise engorgement enough to cause impotence. Endocrine disorders can influence sexuality; commonly, pituitary, adrenal, and ovarian disorders affect sexuality adversely because of the hormonal imbalance involved.

Either illness or a surgical procedure that involves the genitalia also causes sexual problems. These include urologic and gynecologic disorders, pelvic cancer, congenital and acquired anatomic defects, as well as sexually transmitted diseases. Procedures commonly implicated include hysterectomy, prostatectomy, mastectomy, sterilization, castration, and radiotherapy.

Many chronic illnesses require marked sexual adjustments. These include painful conditions such as arthritis and the aftermath of major trauma, as well as disabling chronic respiratory disease, chronic renal failure, and chronic alcoholism. Cardiac disease, especially after a myocardial infarction, frequently interferes with sexual activity.

Physical illness normally causes marked anxiety, anger, grief, and depression, all of which frequently impair sexual function. This is particularly true when illness, trauma, or surgical procedure involves a change in body image or a loss of body parts that have a sexual connotation. For instance, mastectomy and "ostomy" patients are often left with sexual maladjustment, even though they are physiologically intact.

In managing such patients, both organic and psychogenic factors must be assessed, and the impact on the family must be evaluated. Counseling should have a preventive intent wherever possible (e.g., before operation) and should be specific and fitted to the individual. The spouse must be included in the process, because his or her role is crucial to therapeutic success. Treatment is generally behavioral in focus, but can also be educational, informative, and psychotherapeutic where indicated. In some instances, surgical measures play an important role in the treatment of sexual dysfunction with an organic cause, as in the construction of a neovagina, the insertion of a penile prosthesis, or postmastectomy breast reconstruction.

Aging
1. Diokno, A. C., Brown, M. B., and Herzog, A. R. Sexual function in the elderly. *Arch. Intern. Med.* 150:197, 1990.
   In a survey of individuals aged 60 and over, 73 percent of married men and 55 percent of married women were sexually active. For unmarried men and women, the proportions were 31 and 5 percent, respectively.
2. Mooradian, A. D., and Greiff, V. Sexuality in older women. *Arch. Intern. Med.* 150:1033, 1990.

In the absence of disease and with the availability of a sexually active partner, a woman's overall sexual behavior does not necessarily change with age.

3. Keogh, E. J. The male menopause. Fact or fancy? *Aust. Fam. Physician* 19:833, 1990.
   Potential side effects of long-term androgen supplements include exacerbation of prostatic hypertrophy or prostate cancer, polycythemia, and an atherogenic lipid profile. Testicular atrophy inevitably accompanies effective androgen therapy.

4. Schiavi, R. C., et al. Healthy aging and male sexual function. *Am. J. Psychiatry* 147:766, 1990.
   There was a significant negative relationship between age and sexual desire, and between arousal and activity, and an increasing prevalence of sexual dysfunction with age but no age-related difference in terms of sexual enjoyment and satisfaction.

5. Gupta, K. Sexual dysfunction in elderly women. *Clin. Geriatr. Med.* 6:197, 1990.
   Neither aging men nor aging women can afford long, continued periods of coital continence if they are to continue as physically effective sexual partners.

6. Weiss, J. N., and Mellinger, B. C. Sexual dysfunction in elderly men. *Clin. Geriatr. Med.* 6:185, 1990.
   The effects of estrogen on female sexual activity are largely unknown. In both sexes, testosterone has a positive effect on sexual motivation but does not affect sexual function.

Drugs

7. Drugs that cause sexual dysfunction. *Med. Lett. Drugs Ther.* 29:65, 1987.
   Includes a list of 92 medications reported to adversely affect sexual function.

8. Shen, W. W., and Sata, L. S. Inhibited female orgasm resulting from psychotropic drugs: A five-year, updated, clinical review. *J. Reprod. Med.* 35:11, 1990.
   Iatrogenic sexual dysfunction is a major reason for noncompliance with antihypertensive and antipsychotic agents.

9. Segraves, R. T. Reversing anorgasmia associated with serotonin uptake inhibitors. *J.A.M.A.* 266:2279, 1991.
   The serotonin reuptake blocker, fluoxetine, which is used in the treatment of depression, may impair libido or orgasmic capacity in both sexes. This side effect may be counteracted by cyproheptadine, an anticholinergic and antiserotoninergic medication.

10. Urman, B., Pride, S. M., and Yucan, B. H. Elevated serum testosterone, hirsutism, and virilism associated with combined androgen-estrogen hormone replacement therapy. *Obstet. Gynecol.* 77:595, 1991.
    Although the addition of androgens for hormone replacement therapy may be beneficial in countering problems of sexual dysfunction, great care must be exercised to avoid overdosage, as the virilizing effects may be irreversible.

Diseases

11. Whitehead, E. D. Diabetes-related impotence and its treatment in the middle-aged and elderly: Part II. *Geriatrics* 42:77, 1987.
    Before specific therapy is instituted, diabetes should be controlled and nutritional problems dealt with, genital and urinary infections should be treated, and the use of medications and substances such as smoking, drug abuse, and alcohol should be discontinued—all factors that might contribute to or cause the dysfunction.

12. Schover, L. R. Sexual Rehabilitation of the Patient with Gynecologic Cancer. F. N. Rutledge, R. S. Freedman, and D. M. Gershenson (eds.), *Gynecologic Cancer: Diagnosis and Treatment Strategies*, Austin: University of Texas Press, 1987.
    Short-term counseling can help, and includes information on anatomic alterations and erroneous beliefs, along with recommendations on when and how to resume intercourse and ways to minimize the physical effects of cancer on sexual function.

13. Morokoff, P. J., and Gilliland, R. Stress, sexual functioning, and marital satisfaction. *J. Sex Res.* 30:43, 1993.

Marital satisfaction was found to be closely related to several aspects of sexual functioning.

14. Mahlstedt, P. P. The psychologic component of infertility. *Fertil. Steril.* 43:335, 1985.
    The focus on sex for procreation in the management of infertility may lead to sexual dysfunction.

15. Papadopoulos, C., et al. Sexual concerns and needs of the postcoronary patient's wife. *Arch. Intern. Med.* 140:38, 1990.
    If the patient can walk rapidly for 10 minutes and then climb two flights of steps in 10 seconds without symptoms then sexual intercourse should not place undue stress on the heart.

16. Saxton, M. Reclaiming sexual self-esteem—peer counseling for disabled women. *West. J. Med.* 154:629, 1991.
    The severely disabled are underserved by mental health providers because of inadequate training, attitudinal barriers, and inaccessible programs, particularly regarding sexual issues.

17. Wellisch, D. E., et al. Psychosocial outcomes of breast cancer therapies: lumpectomy versus mastectomy. *Psychosomatics* 30:365, 1989.
    Lumpectomy fosters a more intact body image, but no surgical procedure either produces or inhibits psychologic symptomatology.

18. Wright, L. K. The impact of Alzheimer's disease on the marital relationship. *Gerontologist* 31:224, 1991.
    Major sources of stress for spouses of Alzheimer's victims include loss of sexual activity and a decline in companionship.

19. Shain, R. N., Miller, W. B., and Holden, A. E. C. Impact of tubal sterilization and vasectomy on female marital sexuality. *Am. J. Obstet. Gynecol.* 164:763, 1991.
    No detrimental effects on female marital sexuality were observed and perhaps there were some short-term benefits.

20. Meyer-Bahlburg, H. F. L., et al. Sexual function in HIV+ and HIV− injected drug–using women. *J. Sex Marital Ther.* 19:56, 1993.
    There was a relatively high prevalence of problems observed in all phases of the sexual response cycle, with a significantly higher rate in human immunodeficiency virus–positive women, even at an early stage of disease progression.

76. INHIBITED FEMALE SEXUAL DESIRE, EXCITEMENT, AND ORGASM
Michel E. Rivlin

Sexual response is described in terms of three related phases—desire, excitement, and orgasm. Sexual dysfunction may affect one or another of these phases without affecting the others. Sexual desire appears to be a centrally situated appetite, part of the brain system responsible for emotion and reproduction. There appears to be an exciting center (dopamine sensitive) in balance with an inhibitory center (serotonin sensitive). Testosterone may be responsible for programming these centers in prenatal life. During the excitement phase, there is vascular engorgement and increased muscular tension. Vasocongestion results in vaginal lubrication by means of fluid transudation, as well as in clitoral tumescence and expansion of the upper vagina. This phase is primarily under parasympathetic control, with afferent fibers originating from the clitoris and anterior labia and efferent fibers coming from the pelvic nerve. Marked extragenital reactions also take place, including tachycardia, tachypnea, increased blood pressure, and a "sex flush," or a red rash that covers the chest, neck, and face. In the orgasmic phase, uterine contractions occur and the muscles around the vagina, anus, and uterus undergo a series of reflex clonic contractions while extragenital reactions reach their maximum. Orgasm is primarily under sympathetic control, with afferent fibers originating from the clitoris and labia and efferent fibers traveling via the pelvic plexuses and via the pudendal nerve to striated muscles. The sexual response cycle ends with the phase of resolution. Unlike men, women have no refractory period and may be multiorgasmic; however, their orgasm is reached less directly and more slowly. There does not appear to be a "vaginal," as distinct from a "clitoral," orgasm.

Sexual dysfunction may be primary (never satisfactory), secondary (previously satisfactory), or situational (satisfactory in some circumstances, but not in others). Problems generally affect the orgasmic phase, but, if neglected, may eventually involve the other phases. Primary problems are usually psychogenic in origin; secondary problems may be organic in nature or related to the use of pharmacologic agents. Situational problems are almost always psychogenic or relational in origin. The organic causes of sexual dysfunction include neurogenic and vascular diseases, local pelvic abnormalities, plus endocrine and general medical disorders. The psychologic causes may be intrapersonal, including depression, anxiety, and trauma such as rape or incest; or they may be interpersonal and characterized by poor communication, anger, and resentment. Common disorders include the secondary inhibition of sexual desire, which is usually related to interpersonal strife. *Inhibited sexual excitement* refers to the failure to obtain or maintain genital swelling and lubrication in spite of adequate sexual activity. A delay in, or absence of, orgasm during adequate sexual activity is referred to as inhibited orgasm. Reliable estimates of the prevalence of these disorders may never be attainable.

The primary care physician can deal with many of these problems based on the information obtained during a general and sexual history in conjunction with a full physical and pelvic examination. The finding of severe anxiety, depression, or psychosis necessitates psychiatric referral. A finding of major marital disharmony might prompt referral for sexual and marital therapy. Abnormal medical, surgical, or gynecologic findings would constitute reasons for other relevant referrals. When in doubt, therapy may be started and future management guided by the patient's response. Many concerns can be alleviated by reassuring the patient that certain sexual behaviors are in order (permission) and that such concerns are common. Every effort must be made to remain nonjudgmental and to avoid giving too hasty advice or reassurance regarding specific problems. Education is most important. Misconceptions need to be dispelled by factual information. Many sexual concerns may be prevented, for instance, by careful counseling prior to hysterectomy or mastectomy—procedures commonly attended by sexual dysfunction. Some practitioners may not be comfortable dealing with sexual problems and may wish to refer all such patients.

Sex therapy attempts to initiate or restore previously absent sexual function in an individual or a couple. Most problems have a multifactorial basis. The initial focus of therapy should be on immediate causes, using the behavioral techniques popularized by Masters and Johnson. These include an initial ban on intercourse, with emphasis on nongenital sensual pleasuring (sensate focus exercises), improving interpersonal communication skills, masturbation training, and general sex education. Treatment may be done on an individual or couple basis (the relationship is the "patient"), or it may be dealt with in group therapy. If progress is not made, remote causes may then be sought using a psychodynamically oriented program.

Primary anorgasmy with arousal may result in pelvic congestion and irritability, owing to the nonorgasmic sexual response. Secondary anorgasmy may occur in certain situations but not in others. Medical and gynecologic causes of painful or difficult intercourse may be the source of the problem, or a specific partner may play an important causal role. Therapy for primary anorgasmy includes body acceptance and exploration using self-touching and masturbation techniques, including the use of lubrication jellies and vibrators. Pubococcygeus pelvic muscle exercises enhance sexual function and should be taught and practiced regularly. Once orgasm by self-stimulation is achieved, couple counseling is needed with the intent to lead to orgasm with a partner.

In counseling the couple, discussion of the importance of foreplay and the desire of most women to be courted, plus advice regarding the time, place, and form of sexual contact, are outlined. If the problem is one of orgasm accomplished by clitoral stimulation rather than with intercourse, it may be possible to get the patient to accept the situation as normal. If not, continuation of manual or vibrator masturbation induced by the partner or patient during intercourse may be used as a "bridging" technique until, through the process of experimental learning, orgasm may occur during coitus. In general, better clitoral contact and stimulation are obtained in the female-superior position than in the more generally used "missionary" position.

The treatment of secondary anorgasmy is more complex. There should be an emphasis on the relationship, commitment, trust, and need for honesty about feelings. The female partner needs to communicate what she wants; the male partner must listen without being defensive. "Define what is missing, create an emotionally safe environment for change, add whatever sexual information or technique is required."

No strong claims for the overall effectiveness of directive sex therapies are justified at the present time because of the great difficulties in defining, reporting, and sampling these patients. Undoubtedly, sexual and marital therapy can sometimes bring about an improvement in sexual responses by providing insight into the problems and allowing realistic communication to take place; appropriate home assignments can enhance the process. The intrinsic limitations of therapy must, however, be faced realistically. Sex may often be disruptive, if not more often than it is bonding, in many relationships. A relatively asexual marriage might be more stable than one in which the couple is sexually active. Experience gained from the use of surrogates emphasizes the simple fact that many sexual problems are partner specific—that sexual arousal is a vital element and cannot be evoked simply by reducing anxiety. Sex therapists need to have human nature on their side if they are to succeed.

Reviews
1. Sanderson, M. O., and Maddock, J. W. Guidelines for assessment and treatment of sexual dysfunction. *Obstet. Gynecol.* 73:130, 1989.
   Basic principles of assessing and treating sexual dysfunction are summarized in the form of a grid. The axes represent "problem focus" and "influencing variables."
2. Bachmann, G. A., Leiblum, S. R., and Grill, J. Brief sexual inquiry in gynecologic practice. *Obstet. Gynecol.* 73:425, 1989.
   Anxiety and "spectatoring" (the woman detaches herself from her experience in order to monitor her own performance and responsiveness) are significant barriers to sexual satisfaction.
3. Spector, I. P., and Carey, M. P. Incidence and prevalence of the sexual dysfunctions: a critical review of the empirical literature. *Arch. Sex. Behav.* 19:389, 1990.
   The sexual dysfunctions are classified by the American Psychiatric Association in the Diagnostics and Statistical Manual of Mental Disorders, *which is generally referred to as* DSM.

Physiology, Incidence, Etiology
4. Weisberg, M. Physiology of female sexual function. *Clin. Obstet. Gynecol.* 27:697, 1984.
   The classic works of Masters and Johnson, Human Sexual Response *and* Human Sexual Inadequacy, *are somewhat difficult to read; fortunately, numerous excellent commentaries on them are readily available.*
5. Darling, C. A., Davidson, J. K., and Conwag-Welch, C. Female ejaculation: perceived origins, the Grafenberg spot/area, and sexual responsiveness. *Arch. Sex Behav.* 19:29, 1990.
   Heated controversy has surrounded the existance and nature of the Grafenberg or G spot, a purported major erogenous zone distinct from the clitoris on the anterior vaginal wall, as well as the concept of "female ejaculation."
6. Frank, E., Anderson, C., and Rubinstein, D. Frequency of sexual dysfunction in "normal" couples. *N. Engl. J. Med.* 299:111, 1978.
   The authors suggest that there is an epidemic of sexual dysfunction and unhappiness.
7. Reamy, K., and White, S. E. Sexuality in pregnancy and the puerperium: a review. *Obstet. Gynecol. Surv.* 40:1, 1985.
   Sexual response and expression are altered, and, in general, decreased interest and participation in sexual activity are the norms as pregnancy progresses.

8. Segraves, K. B., and Segraves, R. T. Hypoactive sexual desire disorder: prevalence and comorbidity in 906 subjects. *J. Sex Marital Ther.* 17:55, 1991.
   The prevalence of psychosexual dysfunctions in females is estimated to be as follows: inhibited orgasm, 5 to 30 percent; inhibited sexual desire, 1 to 35 percent; and inhibited sexual excitement, indeterminate.

9. Bozman, A. W., and Beck, J. G. Covariation of sexual desire and sexual arousal: the effects of anger and anxiety. *Arch. Sex Behav.* 20:47, 1991.
   Anxiety was found to impair desire but did not affect arousal, while anger was found to significantly reduce both desire and arousal.

10. Donahey, K. M., and Carroll, R. A. Gender differences in factors associated with hypoactive sexual desire. *J. Sex Marital Ther.* 19:25, 1993.
    There were significant differences in terms of age (men were older), psychologic distress (higher levels in women), relationship satisfaction (females more dissatisfied), levels of stress (no difference), and the duration of another sexual dysfunction (longer in the women).

11. Performance anxiety no longer just a problem for men: parallel problem noted in women. *Contemp. Sex* 22:1, 1990.
    Perimenopausal vaginal dryness resulting in anorgasmy may foster fears that her partner will think she does not care for him. She may fake orgasm, thus impairing her self-image and libido.

Management
12. Kegel, A. Sexual function of the pubococcygeus muscle. *West. J. Surg. Obstet. Gynecol.* 60:521, 1952.
    Performing regular pelvic floor exercises appears to lead to an increase in vaginal perception and sensation during genital intercourse.

13. Russell, L. Sex and couples therapy: a method of treatment to enhance physical and emotional intimacy. *J. Sex Marital Ther.* 16:111, 1990.
    Couples tend to repeat patterns of behavior they have observed while growing up in their families-of-origin. Faulty perceptions are corrected in therapy to improve the quality of the relationship.

14. Hurlbert, D. F. A comparative study using orgasm consistency training in the treatment of women reporting hypoactive sexual desire. *J. Sex Marital Ther.* 19:41, 1993.
    The addition of orgasm consistency training (exercises directed at fulfilling "the ladies come first rule") improved the results of standard therapy for decreased sexual desire.

15. Barry, W., and McCarthy, J. Treating sexual dysfunction associated with prior sexual trauma. *J. Sex Marital Ther.* 16:142, 1990.
    The guiding principles are to teach the person to be a "survivor" rather than a "victim" and to help the couple develop a functional and satisfying sexual style, because "living well is the best revenge."

16. Kilmann, P. R., et al. The treatment of secondary orgasmic dysfunction II. *J. Sex Marital Ther.* 13:93, 1987.
    The prognosis is less positive in patients with secondary orgasmic dysfunction than it is for those with primary anorgasmy because nonsexual relationship problems are likely to be maintaining the orgasmic difficulty.

17. Wakefield, J. C. The semantics of success: do masturbation exercises lead to partner orgasm? *J. Sex Marital Ther.* 13:3, 1987.
    Questions the claim that masturbation exercises assigned in preorgasmic women's groups enable previously nonorgasmic women to achieve orgasms during partner sex.

18. O'Carroll, R. Sexual desire disorders: a review of controlled treatment studies. *J. Sex Res.* 28:607, 1991.
    Reviews the psychologic and medical literature on controlled treatment studies of the hypoactive sexual desire disorder published from 1970 to 1989. A lack of scientifically adequate treatment studies was identified.

19. Katz, R. C., Gipson, M., and Turner, S. Recent findings on the sexual aversion scale. *J. Sex Marital Ther.* 18:141, 1992.

The scale consists of a questionnaire for assessing the sexual fears and phobic avoidance associated with sexual trauma, guilt, social inhibitions, and the fear of acquiring sexually transmitted diseases.

20. Kaplan, H. S. *Sexual Aversion, Sexual Phobias, and Panic Disorder.* New York: Brunner/Mazel, 1987.

   These disorders involve avoidance of almost all genital contact with a sexual partner. Management was enhanced by the concomitant use of antidepressants and sexual therapy.

77. PROBLEMS OF ORGASMIC RESPONSE IN THE MALE
Michel E. Rivlin

The corpora cavernosa of the penis consist primarily of a trabecular network of lacunar spaces composed of smooth muscle and a fibroelastic frame. The walls of the arteries and arterioles that empty into the lacunar spaces are also primarily composed of smooth muscle. Engorgement and erection are due to relaxation of penile smooth muscle, with resulting dilatation of the penile arterial vessels leading to an increase of blood flow to the lacunar spaces. The increased flow expands the trabecular walls against the tunica albuginea, compressing the draining venous plexuses. As a consequence of the diminished venous drainage, there is an increase in pressure in the lacunar spaces, which leads to penile rigidity. Detumescence occurs as a result of penile smooth muscle contraction. Trabecular smooth muscle tone is controlled by three neurologic pathways. First, the adrenergic release of norepinephrine causes corporal smooth muscle contraction. Second, cholinergic stimuli have dilatory effects, as does the third pathway, which is neither cholinergic nor adrenergic but appears to be mediated via an as-yet-unidentified neurotransmitter. The sympathetic pathways travel from T-11 through L-2 to the hypogastric and pelvic plexus, whereas the parasympathetic pathways (nervi erigentes) originate from S2 to S4 via the pelvic plexus; a third innervation comes from S2 to S4 via the pudendal nerve. Thereafter, prostatic secretions, sperm in the vasa and ampulla, and the fructose-rich seminal vesicle content are expressed by contraction of these organs into the posterior urethra (emission). The bladder neck and external sphincter are closed during this phase, resulting in increased urethral pressure; thereafter, rhythmic contractions of the pelvic floor and periurethral muscles, along with intermittent relaxation of the external sphincter and urogenital diaphragm, allow for expulsion of the ejaculate. The male orgasm is the cortical appreciation of the sympathetically and somatically coordinated events of ejaculation.

Impotence, the inability to achieve and maintain an erection sufficient for vaginal penetration and intercourse, may be primary or secondary in origin. The latter always follows a period of normal erectile function. Situational impotence is experienced by all men at one time or another, and is commonly associated with fatigue, stress, and alcohol consumption. The incidence of persistent impotence is about 1 per 1000 at age 20 years and gradually rises to affect 7 percent of men 75 years of age or older.

Organic causes of impotence include neurogenic and vascular diseases as well as well as many drugs, such as abused substances (alcohol and marijuana), antihypertensive agents (diuretics and methyldopa), and psychiatric medications (tricyclics and phenothiazines). Diabetes, probably stemming from both neurogenic and vascular involvement, as well as associated psychogenic factors, is associated with a 35 percent prevalence of impotence. Other endocrine disorders, including hyperprolactinemia, hypogonadism, and thyroid disease, have also been implicated as causal factors. Less common are the end-organ problems such as Peyronie's disease, phimosis, microphallus, and chordee, and almost all pelvic surgical procedures are associated with varying degrees of impotence postoperatively. The prevalence of psychogenic impotence ranges from 14 to 51 percent, so that most impotence would appear to be organic in origin. Most men perceive their loss of erectile potency as a devastating impairment of their fundamental self-concept as men, invariably resulting in vicious cycles of escalating anxiety and pathologic defenses.

Diagnosis depends on a careful history, with particular attention to possible physical factors such as diabetes, alcoholism, and drugs. A detailed psychosexual history is taken, and evidence of a depressive illness must be sought. A history of nocturnal and waking erections, as well as erections elicited by tactile stimulation, may indicate psychologic impotence, whereas a slowly progressive decline in erectile function suggests organic causes. Physical examination is directed specifically at searching for endocrine, neurologic, and vascular abnormalities. Palpation of the testes, penis, and prostate, with assessment of secondary sexual characteristics, is necessary. A minimal neurologic evaluation should include assessment of the cutaneous sensation of the saddle area (S1–S3), as well as testing of the bulbocavernous and lower limb reflexes.

In most instances, a costly detailed evaluation is not necessary and, in general, the workup should be directed toward the individual patient. For instance, a full and maintained erection after the intracavernous injection of vasoactive agents (i.e., papaverine, phentolamine, or prostaglandin E_1) largely rules out the existence of vascular abnormalities. Absence of this response might suggest the need for sophisticated measures of arterial inflow and venous drainage, such as dynamic infusion cavernosometry and cavernosography, duplex sonography, plethysmography, and interval pudendal angiography. Measurement of the brachial and penile blood pressures allows calculation of the penile-brachial index; an index of less than 0.75 suggests the presence of vascular insufficiency. Such studies may identify a group of patients amenable to corrective vascular procedures directed toward either improving arterial inflow or correcting abnormal increased venous leakage. If neurologic disease is suspected, neurologic review, biothesiometry (estimation of the penile vibratory threshold), and perhaps electromyography may be included in the diagnostic assessment.

Endocrine studies must include testing of the glucose tolerance. Thyroid studies, as well as measurement of serum testosterone, prolactin, luteinizing hormone (LH), and follicle-stimulating hormone (FSH) levels, may also be performed, although findings of thyroid disease, hypogonadism, or hyperprolactinemia are uncommon. Psychologic testing may be carried out, or a routine brief psychiatric consultation may be obtained to gauge the extent of the psychic component present. Nocturnal penile tumescence testing may be helpful in differentiating organic from psychic impotence.

Management should include medical, surgical, psychiatric, and sexual treatments, as well as marital counseling, all tailored to the needs of the individual patient. Defective sexual skills owing to either ignorance or misinformation and obsessive concerns over sexual performance are common and require correction through education and counseling. Behavioral alterations directed at removing performance anxiety include the use of self-stimulation, sensate focus exercises, and techniques such as "stuffing" (in which the flaccid penis is literally stuffed into the vagina with no requirement for actual intercourse).

Drug therapy is indicated only for specific reasons. For instance, injections of testosterone can be administered in patients with clinical and biochemical evidence of hypogonadism, or bromocriptine can be given in some impotent men with hyperprolactinemia. The use of androgens in normal men remains highly controversial, and it must be realized that exogenous androgens inhibit spermatogenesis, may elevate cholesterol levels, and may cause polycythemia and cholestatic jaundice. The clinical experience with intracorporeal injections of vasodilators has been encouraging in the treatment of all forms of impotence. However, major complications (priapism, damage to the corpora, and systemic effects) may occur. Mechanical devices that can be used for the management of erectile dysfunction include externally positioned constriction bands, vacuum devices, and penile implants. The implantation of penile prostheses is indicated in those patients with a strong sexual desire in whom other modalities have failed and who understand that this measure will not restore libido, the ability to ejaculate, or penile sensation. There are two types of prostheses: semirigid rods and inflatable devices, each having advantages and disadvantages. Counseling before and after implantation of these devices is important. Satisfaction rates of about 80 percent have been reported for both vacuum constriction devices and implants.

Premature ejaculation is a common problem but difficult to define. In general, ejaculation is considered premature if it occurs before or immediately upon intromission. Lack of control of the ejaculatory response is the critical factor. Organic causes are rare. Proposed psychologic mechanisms include performance anxiety, maturational delay of neurologic control mechanisms (analogous to enuresis), and unresolved marital problems. Faulty learning stemming from initial sexual experiences with furtive masturbation, backseat intercourse, and impatient prostitutes may ultimately cause rapid ejaculation to become a conditioned reflex in response to sexual stimuli. In the marital context, the symptom may be used as a weapon by either partner to serve a destructive function in the transactional relationship of the couple. Not infrequently, the complaint may be secondary to a masked female sexual dysfunction. Sexual counseling of the couple in this instance is usually highly successful. Careful history taking regarding both remote and recent factors that have fostered the condition, together with providing proper information and education, is combined with behavioral techniques aimed at extending voluntary control over the ejaculatory reflex. These include vaginal containment without thrusting (to acclimate the penis) and the "stop-and-go" technique, in which intercourse is deliberately interrupted to allow arousal to diminish. Another valuable technique is firm squeezing of the glans penis to end excitement intermittently.

Inhibited sexual excitement or desire, or both, are common in both men and women. Hormonal factors are rare, and explanations are usually sought in terms of relationship dynamics and family-of-origin theories. Inhibited orgasm (retarded ejaculation and ejaculatory incompetence) is rare in males and is psychogenic in origin. Elements from the treatment of anorgasmic women, including the use of vibrators and behavior maneuvers that are orgasm triggers, have been used with some success in men in these situations.

Reviews
1. Morgentaler, A. Current diagnosis and management of impotence. *Compr. Ther.* 17:25, 1991.
   The source of impotence in many patients is multifactorial; the stereotyped presentation of organic versus psychogenic impotence can be highly misleading.
2. Williams, G. Erectile dysfunction—advances. *Practitioner* 235:117, 1991.
   Many men, irrespective of the course of their erectile dysfunction, have some form of psychologic, marital, or social problem. Firmer erections are rarely, if ever, the sole solution to a deteriorating relationship.

Etiology
3. Maatman, T. J., Montague, D. K., and Martin, L. M. Erectile dysfunction in men with diabetes mellitus. *Urology* 29:589, 1987.
   The glucose metabolism was abnormal in 32 percent of the 497 men with erectile dysfunction studied; 91 percent of these had organic pattern impotence.
4. Richardson, J. D. Medical causes of male sexual dysfunction. *Med. J. Aust.* 155:32, 1991.
   The word impotence is also a mnemonic that stands for its various causes: Inflammatory, Mechanical, Postsurgical, Occlusive vascular disease, Traumatic, (lack of) Endurance, Neurological, Chemical, Endocrine.
5. Weiss, R. J. Effects of antihypertensive agents on sexual function. *Am. Fam. Physician* 44:2075, 1991.
   Alpha-adrenergic blockers, angiotensin-converting enzyme inhibitors, and calcium channel blockers have little adverse effect on sexual function.
6. Lue, T. F. Impotence after radical pelvic surgery: physiology and management. *Urol. Int.* 46:259, 1991.
   Transurethral prostatic resection does not decrease potency in 85 to 95 percent of the cases, but perineal procedures or lower abdominal operations may damage either nerves or vessels, which can lead to erectile incompetence.

Diagnosis
7. Jeffcoate, W. J. The investigation of impotence. *Br. J. Urol.* 68:449, 1991.
   There is no clear way of identifying psychologic impotence; it is a diagnosis by exclusion.
8. Benson, G. S. The clinical evaluation of the patient presenting with erectile dysfunction: what is reasonable? *Semin. Urol.* 8:94, 1990.
   Some workers believe that prolactin levels should be measured only if there are clinical grounds for suspicion.
9. Morales, A., Condra, A., and Reid, K. The role of nocturnal penile tumescence monitoring in the diagnosis of impotence: a review. *J. Urol.* 143:441, 1990.
   Normally, men have several firm erections during rapid-eye-movement sleep; absence of such erections indicates a probable organic cause of impotence.
10. Rosen, M. P., et al. Radiographic assessment of impotence: angiography, sonography, cavernosography, and scintigraphy. *Am. J. Roentgenol.* 157:923, 1991.
    Evaluation of vasculogenic factors was carried out with infusion cavernosometry and cavernosography, duplex color sonography, and internal pudendal angiography. Scintigraphic studies may also yield further information.
11. Kaufman, J. M., et al. Evaluation of erectile dysfunction by dynamic infusion cavernosometry and cavernosography: multi-institutional study. *Urology* 41:445, 1993.
    Accurate preoperative evaluation is needed to identify candidates for revascularization procedures for the treatment of cavernosal artery insufficiency and corporeal venoocclusive dysfunction.
12. Baskin, H. J. Endocrinologic evaluation of impotence. *South. Med. J.* 82:446, 1989.
    Hormonal screening of impotent men should include measurement of the serum prolactin and testosterone levels.

Treatment
13. Cumming, J., and Pryor, J. P. Treatment of organic impotence. *Br. J. Urol.* 67:640, 1991.
    Repeated failure at sexual intercourse due to organic impotence leads to frustration and the anticipation of further failure. A psychologic factor then acts synergistically to worsen the problem.
14. Reid, K., et al. Double-blind trial of yohimbine in treatment of psychogenic impotence. *Lancet* 2:421, 1987.
    Yohimbine is an alpha-adrenergic receptor blocker; 46 percent of the patients treated with it reported a positive response—a rate similar to that previously obtained in patients with organic impotence.
15. Witherington, R. Mechanical devices for the treatment of erectile dysfunction. *Am. Fam. Physician* 43:1611, 1991.
    Most external vacuum constriction devices consist of a vacuum chamber, a pump, and penile constriction bands. The satisfaction rate is 80 percent.
16. Lakin, M. M., et al. Intracavernous injection therapy: analysis of results and complications. *J. Urol.* 143:1138, 1990.
    Absence of a sustained erection after the injection of vasoactive drugs usually indicates penile vascular insufficiency.
17. Katlowitz, N. M. Potentiation of drug-induced erection with audiovisual sexual stimulation. *Urology* 41:431, 1993.
    The use of audiovisual stimulation improved erection in 52 percent of the patients.
18. Kabalin, J. N., and Kessler, R. Penile prosthesis surgery: review of ten-year experience and examination of reoperations. *Urology* 33:17, 1989.
    Patient and partner satisfaction with a penile prosthesis appears to be uniformly about 80 percent. Difficulties include permanent erection, urethral erosion, and concealment problems with the rods; mechanical failure occurs with the inflatable devices, which also cost more.
19. Levine, F. J., and Goldstein, I. Vascular reconstructive surgery in the management of erectile dysfunction. *Int. J. Impotence Res.* 2:59, 1990.

Surgical measures are directed at penile artery revascularization or at the prevention of venous leak, depending on the nature of the vascular problem.

20. Leiblum, S. R., and Rosen, R. C. Couples therapy for erectile disorders: conceptual and clinical considerations. *J. Sex Marital Ther.* 17:147, 1991.
    The authors identify four key relationship variables (status and dominance, sexual attraction, intimacy and trust, and sexual scripts) of special importance in the management of erectile problems.

Abnormalities of Ejaculation
21. Murphy, J. B., and Lipshultz, L. I. Abnormalities of ejaculation. *Urol. Clin. North Am.* 14:583, 1987.
    Premature ejaculation is a problem only if the couple sees it as such. Seventy-five percent of men ejaculate within 2 minutes of beginning intercourse.
22. Kaplan, H. S. *How to Overcome Premature Ejaculations.* New York: Brunner/Mazel, 1989.
    It is theorized that individuals vary in the amount of genital stimulation they can tolerate before the orgasmic reflex is triggered, and that the threshold in premature ejaculators may be low.
23. Strassberg, D. S., et al. The role of anxiety in premature ejaculation. *Arch. Sex. Behav.* 19:251, 1990.
    Most of these men report shorter ejaculatory latencies, even with masturbation and usually with all partners and under all circumstances, suggesting that performance anxiety may not be the critical factor.
24. Shaw, J. Play therapy with the sexual workhorse: successful treatment with twelve cases of inhibited ejaculation. *J. Sex Marital Ther.* 16:159, 1990.
    Erection may coexist with lack of arousal and desire, hostility, resentment, frustration, disappointment, and a compulsive need to please a partner sexually.

78. DYSPAREUNIA AND VAGINISMUS
Michel E. Rivlin

Dyspareunia may be defined as persistent and recurrent genital pain experienced during intercourse. The *Diagnostic and Statistical Manual of Mental Disorders* includes dyspareunia under the classification of psychosexual disorders. Dyspareunia and vaginismus are linked; either may be the cause of the other. The difference between the two is that, while intromission is usually painful in women with dyspareunia, it is virtually impossible in women with vaginismus because of the muscle spasm involved. If vaginismus is the cause of dyspareunia, the primary diagnosis is vaginismus. Dyspareunia and anorgasmy are often, but not always, linked. Primary dyspareunia exists throughout the patient's sexual lifetime, whereas secondary dyspareunia develops in a patient who had once enjoyed pain-free intercourse. The problem may be complete, that is, present under *all* circumstances, or selective, that is, occurring only in specific situations. In women with superficial dyspareunia, the pain is perceived at the introitus or in the vagina; in those with deep dyspareunia, the pain is experienced in the lower abdominal area.

The incidence of dyspareunia is not known, but it is thought to be one of the most common sexual dysfunctions and the most common in women of lower socioeconomic status. The literature presents two viewpoints regarding the etiology. In one, psychogenic or functional dyspareunia is considered uncommon; in the other, organic factors are regarded as usually temporary and easily correctable and rare as a cause of longstanding disorder. A recommended approach to adopt in such patients is to regard the causality on a continuum as primarily physical or psychogenic, with the potential for both to be equal contributors. Thus, an integrated diagnostic and therapeutic approach requires the careful evaluation of the emotional and psychologic aspects as well as the physical.

The physical causes of superficial pain on entry include vulvovaginitis, urethritis and urethral syndrome, cystitis or interstitial cystitis, vulvar vestibulitis, and bartholinitis. Postoperative tender or contracted scars, especially those resulting from episiotomy or vaginal surgical repair, are common causes. In older women, lack of estrogen or vulvar dystrophy frequently leads to discontinuation of intercourse because of pain. In younger patients, a rigid hymen or a developmental anomaly of the vagina may be another obvious etiologic factor. Traumatic factors include errors in sexual technique, such as an absence of foreplay, leading to poor lubrication. Allergic reactions to contraceptive chemicals, feminine sprays, and vaginal douches are also possible causes.

The physical causes of deeply situated coital pain include endometriosis and pelvic inflammatory disease stemming from inflammation, adhesions, and adnexal masses. The pain that may follow pelvic operations can be due to adhesions or scarring, or may result from an ovary that has become adherent to the vaginal cuff. Radiation therapy and radical pelvic operations or pelvic neoplasms may produce sufficient anatomic distortion as to cause dyspareunia and even apareunia (absent intercourse). Whereas a retrodisplaced uterus is a frequently encountered normal variation, occasionally, an ovary displaced to the cul-de-sac or a tender retroflexed uterine fundus may lead to "deep thrust" dyspareunia. Cervical lacerations and scars can also be significant etiologic factors. Rectal and orthopedic problems must be ruled out. The myofascial pain syndrome and pelvic varicocele are believed by some to be possible causes of dyspareunia.

During the assessment of dyspareunia, intrapersonal (intrapsychic) and interpersonal (relationship) problems must be sought and identified. In patients with intrapersonal problems, fear, trauma, ignorance, anxiety, and lack of sexual emancipation may be the primary reasons or may have an impact on a physical disorder. Interpersonal problems may be due to conflicts in the areas of contraception, relationship priorities, sexual frequency, sexual timing and technique, and sexual boredom. "Struggle for control" can be an issue and these relationships are often characterized by poor communication in general, particularly with regard to feelings and sexual issues. Often these factors are interrelated; for instance, a physical problem can adversely affect the relationship or may coexist with an intrapersonal problem. Cases are classified according to the most obvious source of the problem. Faulty information and intrapsychic problems are more common in women with primary dyspareunia, and relationship issues may be more important in women with secondary dyspareunia.

The diagnosis depends on the woman's history, with particular reference to the site and duration of pain, and on the findings from physical examination, in which different maneuvers should be used to reproduce the same kind of pain that the patient feels during coitus. Special investigations may be helpful in certain circumstances, particularly laparoscopy, which may be essential in establishing the diagnosis of minimal endometriosis or in confirming the absence of genital pathology. Once the organic and psychologic components of the problem have been identified, therapy is directed toward ameliorating these factors. The patient and, if possible, her partner should be educated and reassured regarding the nature of and prognosis for the problem. Organic disease is dealt with using standard pharmacologic or surgical methods, for instance, estrogen therapy for atrophic vaginitis and hormonal manipulation or surgical ablation for endometriosis. When indicated, marital and sexual therapy should be offered, with particular emphasis on the couple's communication skills, sensate focus exercises, relaxation, and masturbatory techniques. Specific behavioral modifications include changes in coital position, Kegel's pelvic floor exercises, and vaginal self-dilation with lubricated fingers and graduated dilators. Specific surgical procedures indicated for eradicating introital dyspareunia include the excision of painful scars, with resuture in the transverse plane, or hymenotomy for an unruptured or inadequately ruptured hymen. Plastic surgical procedures may be required to correct congenital or surgically acquired disorders of the vulva or vagina (perineoplasty and vaginoplasty), or both, that are not amenable to progressive self-dilation. Specific surgical procedures for the treatment of deep dyspareunia unresponsive to standard therapy include ventral suspension of the retroverted uterus with ovaries prolapsed in the cul-de-sac, or even hysterectomy in a few carefully selected patients with disabling symptomatology who have no wish to conceive. In patients with postoperative adhesions or with ovaries trapped in the cul-de-sac, lysis of the adhesions and removal or resuspension of the ovaries may be indicated. All surgical procedures also require concomitant psychologic, marital, and sexual therapy, as indicated.

Vaginismus is a condition characterized by an involuntary conditioned reflex spasm of the musculature surrounding the vaginal outlet and outer third of the vagina—that is, the perineal and levator muscles and even the adductor muscles of the thighs. The spasm is stimulated by real or imaginary attempts at vaginal penetration of any sort. It has been compared with the blink reflex elicited when corneal contact is anticipated. It is termed *primary* when coitus has never been achieved and *secondary* if successful intercourse has preceded onset of the problem. It is the least common of the female sexual dysfunctions but the most disabling; in the absence of organic pathology, it represents a prime example of a psychosomatic condition consisting of phobic features and somatically expressed vaginospasm. There are varying degrees of severity and it may be absolute or situational in occurrence.

Reported etiologic factors include sexual assault, religious beliefs, sexual misinformation, and anxiety. Often, however, no history of clear trauma can be elicited. Vaginismus and dyspareunia are inevitably linked. Although vaginismus may cause dyspareunia, repeated episodes of dyspareunia may result in secondary vaginismus. An organic cause of vaginismus must always be ruled out before initiating therapy. The most frequent presenting complaints of the condition include unconsummated marriage (primary apareunia), secondary apareunia, an inability to use tampons or undergo pelvic examination, exposure to male sexual dysfunction, and infertility. Low libido may be a factor, but women with vaginismus are at least as frequently able to achieve orgasm as normal women, because the patient usually chooses partners for their passivity, and alternative, noncoital sexual release may be substituted.

Therapy consists of desensitization techniques involving Kegel's exercises and the use of passive vaginal dilatation using either a set of graduated plastic dilators (syringe barrels may be substituted) or the patient's fingers. She is encouraged to observe the pubococcygeal muscle contraction using a mirror and a finger to palpate the contracted muscle. By tightening and relaxing the muscle she is helped to understand the source of the problem. This combined deconditioning of the abnormal physical response and the behavior modification techniques then progress to include the partner and the eventual attempt at male passive coitus in the female-superior position. Because vaginismus is a hysterical condition and a type of conversion reaction, management of the phobic element is essential. Both partners must be involved and must be instructed in normal sexuality and the nature of their problem. Surgical defloration, in the absence of organic pathology, is contraindicated, because muscle spasm, not an imperforate hymen, is usually the problem. Treatment takes about 6 to 8 weeks and usually yields good results. If progress is limited after three or four treatment sessions, psychiatric or psychologic referral to deal with patient resistance should be considered.

Reviews
1. DeWitt, D. E. Dyspareunia. Tracing the cause. *Postgrad. Med.* 89:67, 1991.
   A proper assessment requires careful consideration of the intrapsychic and relationship factors, as well as a physical assessment.
2. Sarazin, S. K., and Seymour, S. F. Causes and treatment options for women with dyspareunia. *Nurse Pract.* 16:30, 1991.
   Inhibited sexual desire can forestall normal physiologic response, leading to failure to lubricate. When the vagina is dry, penile thrusting is painful.

Dyspareunia
3. Glatt, A. E., Zinner, S. H., and McCormack, W. M. The prevalence of dyspareunia. *Obstet. Gynecol.* 75:433, 1990.
   Of 324 women who responded to questionnaires, 61 percent reported current or previous episodes of dyspareunia; less than half of these women had consulted a health-care practitioner.

4. Schover, L. R., Youngs, D. D., and Cannata, R. Psychosexual aspects of the evaluation and management of vulvar vestibulitis. *Am. J. Obstet. Gynecol.* 167:630, 1992.
   A combined surgical and psychologic treatment program was critical in addressing the multiple factors responsible for promoting and maintaining vulvar vestibulitis.
5. Brashear, D. B., and Munsick, R. A. Hymenal dyspareunia. *J. Sex Educ. Ther.* 17:27, 1991.
   Hymenectomy in combination with perineoplasty is performed to eliminate dyspareunia related to a tender, inadequately ruptured hymen.
6. Yoong, A. F. Laparoscopic ventrosuspensions. A review of 72 cases. *Am. J. Obstet. Gynecol.* 163:1151, 1990.
   The success of laparoscopic ventrosuspension for the treatment of deep dyspareunia or pelvic pain in association with a retroverted uterus varies from 18 to 42 percent. Prior use of a Hodge pessary did not predict success of the procedure.
7. Samuel, A. W. Coccydynia and dyspareunia. *Br. J. Obstet. Gynaecol.* 11:365, 1991.
   One of the causes of dyspareunia is coccydynia. If local steroid injections are unsuccessful, coccygectomy may be necessary.

Vaginismus
8. Silverstein, J. L. Origins of psychogenic vaginismus. *Psychother. Psychosom.* 52:197, 1989.
   Some women with vaginismus admit to fearing pregnancy, childbirth, and penetration pain. Many experience shame, conflict, and guilt about their genitals due to early learning.
9. Lamont, J. A. Dyspareunia and Vaginismus. In J. J. Sciarra (ed.), *Gynecology and Obstetrics,* Vol. 6. Hagerstown, MD: Harper & Row, 1992.
   The term apareunia refers to the inability to experience vaginal containment of the penis.
10. Scholl, G. M. Prognostic variables in treating vaginismus. *Obstet. Gynecol.* 72:231, 1988.
    The worst prognostic sign was a fixed belief on the woman's part that her vagina was anatomically abnormal. Previous attempts to correct the vaginismus surgically were particularly detrimental to the success of sex therapy.
11. Elkins, T. E., et al. Interactional therapy for the treatment of refractory vaginismus. *J. Reprod. Med.* 31:721, 1986.
    Interactional, or family, therapy focuses on the possibilities that a dysfunction is a means of avoiding intimacy, of expressing hostility, of maintaining control in the relationship, or of retaliating for other grievances in the relationship. A failure to assess such factors may lead to treatment failure.

79. RAPE, INCEST, AND ABUSE

Michel E. Rivlin

Sexual assault may be defined as any sexual act committed by one person on another without that person's consent, using either force or the threat of force. The inability to give appropriate consent, because of age or mental condition, is deemed to be a lack of appropriate consent (statutory rape). The presence of semen is not necessary. Common situations include abduction rape, spousal rape, date rape, and rape of the most vulnerable, including children, the elderly, and those with physical or mental disabilities. Males may also be rape victims. Sexual molestation is a noncoital sexual contact performed without consent.

Rape is reported to be the fastest growing violent crime in the United States. In 1987, the annual incidence was 73 per 100,000 females. It is estimated that ten times that number go unreported. Rape victims are generally young, unmarried women, many of them younger than 18 years of age. A substantial number are prepubertal. Adult women tend to be raped at home—60 percent by a stranger. A weapon is used in approximately one third of the alleged assaults, and about 1 percent of the victims require hospitalization. The assault generally occurs in the late night or early morning hours. Physical injury is present in 8 to 45 percent of the victims. The average rapist commits about 12 offenses before being caught. Rapists are mostly male (98%), and come from all walks of life. The personality and character traits of rapists are separate and distinct from their sexual orientation and interests. The rapist does not want consensual sex; because of anger, his wish is to overpower, humiliate, and degrade the victim. Most follow certain patterns in their assaults; the conclusion of sexual activity, generally in the first 10 minutes, is usually followed by further physical and psychologic abuse lasting for another 45 minutes on average. In offender programs, it has been found that it takes rapists approximately 1 year to believe that they are indeed rapists or child molesters. Rape has far-reaching effects on the victim and her family; about half of married rape victims are divorced within 1 to 2 years of the assault.

Those involved in any kind of trauma—war, floods, fires, and the like—tend to experience similar reactions afterward. Symptoms can arise both immediately after the event and later, and often last for years. This kind of reaction is called posttraumatic stress disorder. Sexual assault can produce similar effects, which have been described as the rape trauma syndrome. Reactions can be divided into two phases. An acute phase, lasting for hours or days, is associated with disorganization of usual behavior patterns as well as emotional and somatic symptoms. In the expressed style, fear and anxiety are manifested through crying, restlessness, or tenseness. In the controlled style, a subdued affect masks the victim's true feelings. Somatic reactions include headaches, fatigue, sleep disturbances, and urinary and bowel upset. Emotional reactions include anger, self-blame, fear, and humiliation. The long-term second phase starts 2 to 3 weeks after the trauma. It consists of reorganization with return toward normal function. Dreams and nightmares, fears, phobias, and sexual anxieties are common. Major life-style changes may be instituted. Some victims never fully recover; they suffer chronic stress disorders and loss of security, with a significant long-term morbidity.

In evaluating the patient, medical concerns include documentation of the pertinent history, physical examination, prompt treatment of any physical injuries, and psychologic support and follow-up. Laboratory specimens must be collected and preserved so they may be used in court, and prophylaxis against venereal disease and pregnancy must be offered. Informed consent is necessary to permit the examination to be performed, and also to allow the alleged assault to be reported and the records and specimens released to law enforcement authorities. In practice, a careful protocol should be available at a center such as a large emergency room, where office-based physicians can refer rape victims to avoid the legal, social, and psychologic consequences of an inappropriate work-up.

The history includes the specifics of the alleged assault, and information on the last voluntary sexual experience, drug use, contraceptive practice, and the menstrual record. The physical examination includes determination of the patient's mental status, relevant photographs, and collection of significant stains and clothing. Combing of the pubic hairs can yield foreign material, and the pelvic examination should include rectal examination. Wet samples from the vagina, rectum, and mouth should be examined for the presence of motile sperm, as indicated by the patient's history. If no sperm are seen, the acid phosphatase level should be checked. A saliva sample for the determination of blood group antigens is obtained to see whether the victim is a secretor or not (85% secrete blood type in all body fluids). Drug screening, blood typing, serology, and serum pregnancy tests are carried out. The specimens obtained must conform to legal protocol, known as the chain of evidence, with documentation of acceptance and transference of materials.

The risk of acquiring gonorrhea ranges from 6 to 12 percent and of syphilis up to 3 percent. Because 40 to 90 percent of the patients are lost to follow-up, treatment should be given presumptively and be sufficient to cure persistent gonorrhea, incubating syphilis, and *Chlamydia* infection. Because patients may not take oral medications, some authorities recommend the parenteral administration of ceftriaxone, followed by a 7-day course of oral doxycycline. Endocervical sampling and serology should be repeated at 6 weeks. Acquired immunodeficiency syndrome testing should be offered. Although pregnancy resulting from rape is rare (the probability of pregnancy resulting from any one unprotected coital act is 4%), pregnancy prophylaxis should be offered. Two 50-μg estrogen-containing combination oral contraceptive tablets given initially, and taken again in 12 hours, if carried out within 72 hours of intercourse, have a 1 percent failure rate and are used in preference to high-dose estrogens, which are associated with nausea and the risk of causing fetal injury in the event of failure. Some women may prefer to wait and, if pregnancy occurs, may then elect termination. In either event, a follow-up pregnancy test should be performed. Subsequent visits at 1 and 6 weeks should be scheduled so that the patient's emotional condition and the need for further counseling or psychiatric intervention can be assessed, in addition to the general medical follow-up.

Child sexual abuse includes rape, incest, and molestation. The latter two are grossly underreported. An estimated 2 percent of natural fathers and 17 percent of stepfathers are likely to have sexual contact with their daughters. In all cases of sexual abuse, the appropriate authorities (e.g., Child Protective Service) must be notified immediately.

A sexual offense is the performance of any sexual act prohibited by law. Sexual deviation (perversion) is a predominant and unconventional sexual interest in a particular activity, object, or individual. These activities are currently referred to as paraphilias. Deviations may not be offenses, as in the case of habitual cross-dressing (transvestism), or they may be, as in the case of pedophilia, in which adult males are attracted to and sexually abuse young boys. Some authorities maintain that sexual offenders can be treated just as successfully as alcoholics, and that effective treatment reduces the rate of recidivism. Treatment includes the administration of drugs such as medroxyprogesterone acetate, behavior modification, and psychologic counseling or therapy. It is often necessary to institutionalize or incarcerate some offenders.

In 85 percent of child sexual assault cases, the molester is known to the child and has an important relationship with the child (e.g., a child care provider). The history is frequently difficult to obtain, and it may be advisable to work with the child protection agency. Although occasional "coaching" by a parent or guardian may be evident, in general, false reporting is uncommon. The medical examination performs an important psychologic function and helps to allay unrealistic fears and fantasies in the child. After the examination, the parents need to be informed of the findings and plan, keeping the discussion open and nonjudgmental.

Incest and molestation differ from rape in that the abuse often takes place over a period of years and the victim has an ongoing relationship with the assailant. Frequently, other adults give covert permission to the activity. The clinical presentation is often typical, and consists of sexually transmitted disease, pregnancy, and various emotional and social disorders. A child who is physically abused may also be a victim of sexual abuse. Physical examination may reveal the existence of signs such as a spacious introitus in a premenstrual child or the presence of healed lacerations, leukorrhea, and cervicitis. Frequently, child assailants were themselves assaulted as children, and child victims of sexual abuse, when adult, often experience difficulty in establishing stable relationships. Nevertheless, with proper intervention and help, most children can recover from the adverse experience; even adults who were abused as children can benefit from treatment and overcome their long-standing problems. Generally, the more trusted the assailant, the more damaging the experience. The reaction of other adults is also important in determining the degree of guilt felt by the child.

Sexual abuse is a specific area of the larger problem of physical violence. Up to 25 percent of the injured women seen in emergency rooms are victims of domestic battering. Physicians treating these patients recognize the presence of physical abuse only 3 percent of the time, and often their approach to treatment consists only of prescribing pain medications or psychiatric referral. There are an estimated 500,000 to 2.5 million cases of abuse of an elderly person annually. This exceeds other forms of violence against the unprotected, and this problem will escalate as the numbers of elderly increase. The most common abuser is an adult child with whom the parent lives. One must be aware of the possibility when interviewing elderly patients who exhibit strange behaviors and apparently irrational fears. If suspected, community resources should be involved to remove the victims and counsel the abuser.

Review

1. Beebe, D. K. Emergency management of the adult female rape victim. *Am. Fam. Physician* 43:2041, 1991.
   In obtaining the "chain of evidence," each separate piece of evidence should be marked with the patient's name, hospital number, date, physician's name, and type of specimen. Each person in the chain must document acceptance and transference of material.

2. Sexual Assault. *ACOG Tech. Bull.* No. 172, September 1992.
   The physician's legal responsibilities include the accurate recording of events, documentation of injuries, collection of samples, and reporting to authorities, as required.

The Rapist

3. Kalichman, S. C. Affective and personality characteristics of MMPI profile subgroups of incarcerated rapists. *Arch. Sex. Behav.* 19:443, 1990.
   Rape, although a sexual offense, is mainly concerned with anger, rage, revenge, power, and punishment. Sex is used as a weapon, and the assailant seldom experiences sexual gratification.

4. Fuller, A. K. Child molestation and pedophilia. An overview for the physician. *J.A.M.A.* 261:602, 1989.
   A single child molester may commit hundreds of sexual acts on hundreds of children.

5. Nutter, D. E., and Kearns, M. E. Patterns of exposure to sexually explicit material among sex offenders, child molesters, and controls. *J. Sex Marital Ther.* 19:77, 1993.
   This study provided no evidence that sexually explicit material is a cause of offending behavior.

6. Puxon, M. Rape. *Practitioner* 226:296, 1982.
   Explores the myths related to rape, urges that sexual offenders and their victims should not be stereotyped, and states that, by far, the largest number of sexual offenders should be dealt with by purely penal methods.

The Victim

7. Ramin, S. M., et al. Sexual assault in postmenopausal women. *Obstet. Gynecol.* 80:860, 1992.
   Postmenopausal women are more likely to sustain genital trauma than younger victims. Almost one case in four in this series was severe enough to require surgical repair.

8. Satin, A. J., et al. Sexual assault in pregnancy. *Obstet. Gynecol.* 77:710, 1991.
   Less physical trauma was incurred in pregnant rape victims than in nonpregnant ones, and there was little immediate effect on pregnancy outcome.

9. Marchbanks, P. A., Liu, K. J., and Mercy, J. A. Risk of injury from resisting rape. *Am. J. Epidemiol.* 132:540, 1990.
   Whether physical resistance alters the victim's chances of being injured is not well established and requires further study before recommendations can be made to potential victims.

10. Jones, R. F. Domestic violence—an epidemic. *Int. J. Gynecol. Obstet.* 41:131, 1993.
    In the United States, wife beating results in more injuries that require medical treatment than do rape, auto accidents, and muggings combined.

Psychology
11. Burgess, A. W., and Holmstrom, L. L. Rape trauma syndrome. *Am. J. Psychiatry* 131:9, 1974.
    Two states were described: (1) an immediate, acute phase in which there were either expressed or controlled emotional responses to a life-threatening situation, and (2) a long-term phase of reorganization, accompanied by changes in life-style, phobic reactions, dreams, and nightmares.
12. Duddle, M. Emotional sequelae of sexual assault. *J. R. Soc. Med.* 84:26, 1991.
    Immediate support seems to be a factor in alleviating later symptoms. There appears to be significantly more related distress in those women who did not receive help until later.
13. Moscarello, R. Psychological management of victims of sexual assault. *Can. J. Psychiatry* 35:25, 1990.
    During the first 6 weeks or so of disorganization, victims need someone to listen to their problems over and over again without getting impatient, as close friends and relatives often do.

Statutory Rape
14. Committee on Child Abuse and Neglect. American Academy of Pediatrics: guidelines for the evaluation of sexual abuse of children. *Pediatrics* 87:254, 1991.
    A comprehensive evaluation requires the experience of many professionals representing the areas of child protection, mental health, and law enforcement. Physicians should form an integral part of the investigational team in their community.
15. De Jong, A. R., and Finkel, M. A. Sexual abuse of children. *Curr. Probl. Pediatr.* 20:491, 1990.
    Treatment of the entire family is essential, especially if incest is a factor. Therapy is frequently not wanted, and the family may choose to "forget it," as the problem is so difficult to face.
16. Adams, J. A., Harper, K., and Knudson, S. A proposed system for the classification of anogenital findings in children with suspected sexual abuse. *Adolesc. Pediatr. Gynecol.* 5:73, 1992.
    Normal anatomy and normal variations must be understood in order to determine whether a given finding is abnormal. However, clear guidelines as to the significance of anogenital findings with respect to sexual abuse have yet to be developed.
17. Pokorny, S. F., Pokorny, W. J., and Kramer, W. Acute genital injury in the prepubertal girl. *Am. J. Obstet. Gynecol.* 166:1461, 1992.
    The most dangerous injuries were the penetrating ones that were symmetric and transected the hymen.
18. Yordan, E. E., and Yordan, R. A. Sexually transmitted diseases and human immunodeficiency virus screening in a population of sexually abused girls. *Adolesc. Pediatr. Gynecol.* 5:187, 1992.
    Sexually transmitted diseases have been diagnosed in approximately 10 percent of the children suspected to be victims of sexual abuse.

Laboratory Evidence
19. Young, W. W., et al. Sexual assault: review of a national model protocol for forensic and medical evaluation. *Obstet. Gynecol.* 80:878, 1992.
    The object of such a protocol is to minimize the physical and psychologic trauma while maximizing the probability of collecting and preserving physical evidence for potential use in the legal system.
20. Chakraborty, R., and Kidd, K. The utility of DNA typing in forensic work. *Science* 254:1735, 1991.
    Extremely small samples, even if decomposed, can be used for analysis. DNA typing is almost absolutely exclusionary and, if a match occurs, there is a high probability that the evidence was left by the suspect.
21. Kamenev, L., Leclercq, M., and Francois-Gerard, C. Detection of P30 antigen in sexual assault case material. *J. Forensic Sci. Soc.* 30:193, 1990.
    P30 is a prostatic antigen; its presence is regarded as conclusive evidence of semen whereas the acid phosphatase test is considered only a presumptive test.

Medical Management

22. Schwarcz, S. K., and Whittington, W. L. Sexual assault and sexually transmitted diseases: detection and management in adults and children. *Rev. Infect. Dis.* 6:S682, 1990.

The risk of acquiring a viral sexually transmitted disease may be less than the risk of a bacterial infection because of the episodic nature of viral shedding.

23. Slaughter, L., and Brown, C. R. V. Colposcopy to establish physical findings in rape victims. *Am. J. Obstet. Gynecol.* 166:83, 1992.

This study revealed that mounting injuries are common and may be detected and documented through colposcopic photography to provide valuable medicolegal information.

24. Yuzpe, A. A., Smith R. P., and Rademaker, A. W. A multicenter clinical investigation employing ethinyl estradiol combined with dl-norgesterol as postcoital contraceptive agent. *Fertil. Steril.* 37:508, 1982.

The 1 percent failure rate and teratogenicity of postcoital medications should be explained to the patient. All interventions are ineffective after 72 hours.

XV. GYNECOLOGIC ENDOCRINOLOGY

80. AMENORRHEA
Cecil A. Long

Amenorrhea is defined as the complete absence of vaginal bleeding in a woman of reproductive age, but this is a symptom, and not a diagnosis. Lack of menstruation is considered to be normal and physiologic before puberty, during pregnancy and lactation, and after menopause. Primary amenorrhea, or delayed puberty, pertains to those females who fail to undergo menarche or the development of secondary sexual characteristics by age 14, or who have no menstrual period by age 16 regardless of the presence of secondary sexual characteristics. Secondary amenorrhea is defined as the absence of menstrual periods for 6 months, or a span of time equivalent to three normal menstrual cycles.

For normal menstruation to take place, it is necessary for four conditions to exist: (1) a patent reproductive outflow tract; (2) ovaries with follicles that have the capability to synthesize and secrete 17-beta-estradiol; (3) a pituitary gland that synthesizes and secretes follicle-stimulating hormone (FSH) and luteinizing hormone (LH); and (4) a functional gonadotropin-releasing hormone (GnRH) "pulse generator." The cells that secrete GnRH are located in the arcuate nucleus of the hypothalamus. Abnormalities in any of these compartments will result in amenorrhea.

Disorders of the reproductive outflow tract that lead to amenorrhea include congenital and acquired abnormalities of the uterus, cervix, and vagina. Congenital structural anomalies associated with incomplete canalization of the reproductive tract can spawn a variety of disorders, including complete absence of the vagina and uterus (müllerian agenesis, and the Mayer-Rokitansky-Küster-Hauser syndrome), a transverse vaginal septum, and an imperforate hymen. These defects are usually discovered in adolescence when the female patient seeks medical care because of primary amenorrhea. Defects such as a transverse vaginal septum or imperforate hymen require surgical correction. In the case of müllerian agenesis, a vaginal pouch can be formed by applying progressive pressure to dilate the vaginal dimple or by surgically creating a neovagina.

There are two situations in which disorders of the reproductive outflow tract can be acquired. The first is cervical stenosis, which may follow chronic cervical infections, cervical conization or cauterization, cryosurgery, laser surgery, and irradiation of the cervix. In the second situation, intrauterine adhesions (Asherman's syndrome) may result from the use of intrauterine instrumentation or from infection.

The malformation of androgen receptors in the presence of normal male testosterone levels leads to the androgen insensitivity syndrome. This disorder is inherited as an X-linked recessive trait and the patients have XY karyotypes. Because the normally functioning fetal testes produce testosterone and müllerian inhibitory factor, the lack of response to dihydrotestosterone (which stimulates the differentiation of normal male external genitalia) causes female external genitalia to develop, but the uterus is absent.

Attenuated ovarian function may also lead to amenorrhea. Chronic anovulation resulting in amenorrhea arises from a variety of disorders, including the polycystic ovarian syndrome (the most common cause of chronic anovulation), hyperprolactinemia, thyroid dysfunction, Cushing's syndrome, congenital adrenal hyperplasia, androgen-secreting ovarian and adrenal tumors, psychogenic causes (including anorexia nervosa), and obesity. Gonadal agenesis and dysgenesis is the physical absence of functioning gonads in the female, and is characterized by the existence of bilateral rudimentary (streak) gonads, resulting in sexual infantilism, primary or secondary amenorrhea, and elevated gonadotropin levels. Turner's syndrome (karyotype, 45,XO) is the most common form of female phenotypic gonadal dysgenesis. Features of this syndrome include short stature, webbed neck, coarctation of the aorta, high arched palate, cubitus valgus, a broad shieldlike chest with widely spaced nipples, low hairline on the neck, short fourth and fifth metacarpal bones, and renal abnormalities. Other varieties of gonadal dysgenesis may also be observed, and include Turner's mosaic (46,XX/45,XO), pure gonadal dysgenesis (46,XX), and Swyer's syndrome (46,XY). In patients with the last condition (gonadal dysgenesis with a Y chromosome; 46,XY) gonadectomy is recommended to eliminate the malignant potential. Premature ovarian failure is defined as a cessation of ovarian function before age 40. The reason for this failure in most patients is unknown; however, resistant ovarian syndrome, caused by LH and FSH receptor abnormalities (the Savage syndrome), has been proposed. Because of the association with autoimmune processes, evaluation of the thyroid gland and adrenal gland is essential in such patients.

Disorders of the pituitary gland leading to amenorrhea include tumors either arising from the pituitary or near the gland. Tumors of the pituitary are classified according to their secretory products. Prolactinomas (lactotroph adenomas) are by far the most common type. Pituitary insufficiency resulting in decreased secretion of gonadotropins by the gland may also lead to amenorrhea. The most common form of pituitary insufficiency in the female is postpartum pituitary necrosis (Sheehan's syndrome), resulting from obstetric hemorrhage. In general, loss of pituitary function follows an orderly pattern (prolactin, gonadotropins, growth hormone, thyroid-stimulating hormone, and then corticotropin). The empty sella syndrome is a condition in which the diaphragm that separates the pituitary from the hypothalamus is either absent or discontinuous. This may be congenital or surgically induced; it may arise after radiation therapy, or it may be due to tumor infarction. Pressure exerted by the cerebrospinal fluid flattens the pituitary gland against the sellar floor, and this is seen as an apparent absence of the gland on computed tomographic (CT) or magnetic resonance (MRI) studies. In most cases, this condition is benign and does not progress to pituitary failure.

Hypothalamic disorders that lead to amenorrhea may be divided according to functional or nonfunctional causes of hypogonadotropic hypogonadism. Functional causes include exercise, stress, weight loss, anorexia nervosa, pseudocyesis, post-pill amenorrhea, and drug-induced amenorrhea. In general, these conditions alter the GnRH pulse generator, leading to alterations in the secretion of FSH and LH. A body fat content that constitutes approximately 17 percent of the total body weight is necessary for initiating menarche, and a body fat content of 20 to 25 percent is necessary for the maintenance of menses. Pseudocyesis, on the other hand, presents as a willful alteration of reproductive function. In affected women, there is hypersecretion of prolactin and pituitary LH. Both estradiol and progesterone levels are increased and the elevated levels of prolactin and LH are enough to maintain luteal function and produce galactorrhea. On discontinuation of the birth control pill, 80 percent of the women resume ovulation within 3 to 6 months, 90 percent within the first year, and only 1 percent experience long-term amenorrhea.

Nonfunctional hypogonadotropic hypogonadism may be caused by a space-occupying lesion or by Kallmann's syndrome. Space-occupying lesions comprise tumors such as cranial pharyngiomas, germinomas, and gangliomas; infiltrative conditions such as tuberculosis or sarcoidosis; and other lesions that may compress or partially destroy the hypothalamus, resulting in decreased GnRH secretion with subsequent hypogonadotropic function. Kallmann's syndrome is characterized by primary amenorrhea, anosmia, and an infantile sexual development. Amenorrhea results from deficient GnRH secretion and is thought to have an X-linked or autosomal dominant inheritance pattern.

Evaluation of the amenorrheic patient begins with obtaining historical information, including developmental data, the nutritional history, the family history, the existence of skin lesions, and the presence of symptoms that may arise from systemic endocrine disorders (e.g., diabetes or thyroid disorders). Menarche should be documented, as well as the existence of secondary sexual characteristics. During physical examination, a thorough neurologic evaluation and pelvic evaluation, which identifies problems in the reproductive tract, are important. Laboratory evaluation of the amenorrheic patient is critical. The major objectives are to rule out pregnancy and to screen for the presence of a central nervous system (CNS) tumor. The measurement of serum human chorionic gonadotropin as well as human gonadotropin and prolactin levels, plus thyroid function tests, are suggested for all patients with amenorrhea. Increased gonadotropin levels indicate ovarian failure, whereas low gonadotropin

levels indicate either a hypothalamic or pituitary defect. In patients with low gonadotropin levels, imaging of the head (CT or MRI) is essential to rule out CNS
lesions. In the patient with symptoms of androgen excess in association with amenorrhea, testosterone and dehydroepiandrosterone sulfate (DHEA-s) levels may be determined. In general, the testosterone level reflects the androgen productivity of the
ovary, while DHEA-s is produced almost exclusively by the adrenal gland. A progestin challenge test (withdrawal bleeding follows the administration of a progestational agent if there is adequate estrogen, a functional endometrium, and a patent
outflow tract) not only can establish the existence of adequate levels of circulating
estradiol, but can also confirm the intactness of the lower reproductive tract.

Chromosomal evaluation should be entertained in the patient with premature
ovarian failure that occurs under the age of 30, as indicated by elevated gonadotropin
levels, and in the patient with altered secondary sexual development and a blind
vaginal pouch. The specific treatment of patients with amenorrhea depends primarily
on the diagnosis. Once pregnancy and CNS lesions are ruled out, the major treatment
for hypothalamic, pituitary, or gonadal deficiency disorders includes combined estrogen and progestin therapy. Patients with ovarian failure and those with müllerian
agenesis should be counseled as to their reproductive potential.

General

1. Doody, K. M., and Carr, B. R. Amenorrhea. *Obstet. Gynecol. Clin. North Am.*
   17:361, 1990.
   A general review of the topic of amenorrhea.
2. Mashchak, C. A., et al. Clinical and laboratory evaluation of patients with primary amenorrhea. *Obstet. Gynecol.* 57:715, 1981.
   A review of the laboratory evaluation for patients with amenorrhea.
3. Rojers, J. Menstruation and systemic diseases. *N. Engl. J. Med.* 259:721, 1958.
   A review of the influence of systemic diseases on the menstrual cycle.
4. Reindollar, R. H., Byrd, J. R., and McDonough, P. G. Delayed sexual development: a study of 252 patients. *Am. J. Obstet. Gynecol.* 140:371, 1981.
   A review of the topic of delayed puberty.
5. Griffin, J. E., and Wilson, J. D. The syndromes of androgen resistance. *N. Engl.
   J. Med.* 302:198, 1980.
   A review of the subject of androgen insensitivity syndromes.

Hypothalamic Disorders

6. Lambalk, C. B., et al. The frequency of pulsatile luteinizing hormone–releasing
   hormone treatment and luteinizing hormone and follicle-stimulating hormone
   secretion in women with amenorrhea of suprapituitary origin. *Fertil. Steril.*
   51:416, 1989.
   *The pituitary needs to be stimulated in a pulsatile fashion by LH-releasing hor-
   mone to maintain LH and FSH secretion.*
7. Frisch, R. E., and Revell, R. Height and weight at menarche and a hypothesis of
   menarche. *Arch. Dis. Child.* 46:695, 1971.
   Impact of weight on the establishment of menarche.
8. Vigersky, R. A., et al. Hypothalamic dysfunction in secondary amenorrhea associated with simple weight loss. *N. Engl. J. Med.* 297:1141, 1977.
   *A detailed investigation of the hypothalamic alterations associated with weight
   loss.*
9. Jonnavithula, S., et al. Bone density is compromised in amenorrheic women despite return of menses: a 2-year study. *Obstet. Gynecol.* 81:669, 1993.
   *Bone mineral density was measured by single- and dual-photon absorptiometry
   in the spine, wrist, and foot.*
10. Warren, M. P., and Vande Wiele, R. L. Clinical and metabolic features of ano-
    rexia nervosa. *Am. J. Obstet. Gynecol.* 117:435, 1973.
    A comprehensive review of the topic of anorexia nervosa.
11. Tagatz, G., et al. Hypogonadotropic hypogonadism associated with anosmia in
    the female. *N. Engl. J. Med.* 282:1326, 1970.

A review of Kallmann's syndrome as a cause of primary amenorrhea.

12. Berga, S. L., et al. Neuroendocrine aberrations in women with functional hypothalamic amenorrhea. *J. Clin. Endocrinol. Metab.* 68:301, 1989.
    Reproductive quiescence is associated with the existence of unfavorable environments.

Pituitary Disorders

13. Sheehan, H. L. Simmonds' disease due to postpartum necrosis of the anterior pituitary gland. *Q. J. Med.* 8:277, 1939.
    Original description of postpartum pituitary necrosis.

Ovarian Disorders

14. Kazer, R. R., Kessel, B., and Yen, S. S. C. Circulating luteinizing hormone pulse frequency in women with polycystic ovary syndrome. *J. Clin. Endocrinol. Metab.* 65:233, 1987.
    A discussion of the role of LH in polycystic ovarian syndrome.
15. Rosenfeld, R., and Grumbach, M. M. (eds.). *Turner Syndrome.* New York: Marcel Dekker, 1990.
    An in-depth review of Turner's syndrome.
16. Mignot, M. H., et al. Premature ovarian failure: the association with autoimmunity *Eur. J. Gynecol. Reprod. Biol.* 30:59, 1989.
    This discusses the autoimmune disorders that result in premature ovarian failure.
17. Corenblum, B., Rowe, T., and Taylor, P. J. High-dose, short-term glucocorticoids for the treatment of infertility resulting from premature ovarian failure. *Fertil. Steril.* 59:988, 1993.
    Results of treatment were best in women with ovarian failure of less than 2 years' duration and with concomitant autoimmune thyroid disease.

Outflow Tract Disorders

18. Frank, R. I. The formation of an artificial vagina without operation. *Am. J. Obstet. Gynecol.* 35:1053, 1938.
    This describes treatment of the blind vaginal pouch with progressive dilatation.
19. Jones, H. W., and Rock, J. A. *Reparative and Constructive Surgery of the Female Genital Tract.* Baltimore: Williams & Wilkins, 1983.
    A useful reference that details the diagnosis and surgical correction of mullerian anomalies.
20. Asherman, J. G. Traumatic intrauterine adhesions and their effects on fertility. *Int. J. Fertil.* 2:49, 1957.
    This discusses amenorrhea related to the use of intrauterine instrumentation.

81. HYPERPROLACTINEMIA
Cecil A. Long

Prolactin is a polypeptide hormone made up of 198 amino acids. There are several biologic forms of prolactin secreted that possess different molecular sizes; however, the small form (22,000 daltons) is the active hormone and represents approximately 80 percent of the molecules secreted. Prolactin is secreted by lactotropic cells located in the lateral wings of the anterior pituitary gland. The half-life of prolactin is approximately 20 minutes.

Prolactin is secreted in a sleep-related circadian rhythm. The level is highest between 3 and 5 A.M. and is also increased in the early afternoon. The secretion of prolactin from the anterior pituitary gland is controlled mainly by the inhibitory action of dopamine. Depending on individual laboratory methodology, the upper limits of prolactin levels range between 20 and 25 ng/ml.

Prolactin promotes lactogenesis. The concentration may increase 10- to 20-fold during pregnancy; however, it returns to baseline levels within approximately 6 weeks in nonnursing mothers and within 6 to 8 months in lactating mothers. Prolactin levels are also affected by various environmental factors, including nipple stimulation, the ingestion of food, and stress. The use of certain medications, such as antihypertensive agents, antidepressants, psychotropic drugs, sex steroids, and antiemetics, may lead to elevated prolactin levels. Inhibitors of prolactin secretion include dopamine and bromocriptine (Parlodel).

Prolactin secretion is sensitive to alterations of the hypothalamic-pituitary axis. Pathologic factors affecting the secretion of prolactin include endocrine disorders, prolactin-secreting adenomas, and nonpituitary tumors that interfere with the transport of hypothalamic hormones and with neural transmitters, resulting in pituitary dysfunction. Primary hypothyroidism results in elevated prolactin levels accompanied by galactorrhea in approximately 3 percent of all patients. These patients have a low serum thyroxine concentration that causes an increased secretion of thyroid-releasing hormone (TRH) from the hypothalamus. The TRH then overstimulates the thyrotropes and the lactotropes in the anterior pituitary gland, causing an increase in both the thyroid-stimulating hormone (TSH) and prolactin levels.

Another common cause of hyperprolactinemia is a prolactin-secreting pituitary adenoma (prolactinoma). Most patients with pituitary prolactinomas have galactorrhea and prolactin levels approaching 100 ng/ml. As these tumors grow, they compress the pituitary stalk, leading to interruption of inhibitory dopamine action. When the tumor is 1 cm or greater, this is a macroadenoma; if less than 1 cm, it is a microadenoma.

Nonpituitary tumors can also affect prolactin secretion. Craniopharyngiomas arise from epithelial remnants of Rathke's pouch. These types of tumors, along with other space-occupying lesions, including germinomas and gliomas as well as infiltrative processes (tuberculosis, sarcoidosis, and histiocytosis), lead to a loss of the inhibitory control exerted by dopamine by compressing on the pituitary stalk. A variety of other disorders may also be responsible for hyperprolactinemia. These include chronic disease processes such as renal failure, adrenal insufficiency, and acromegaly.

Sheehan's syndrome is the only known entity that involves lower-than-normal prolactin levels. The insult to the pituitary gland that precipitates Sheehan's syndrome usually arises from hemorrhage in the immediate postpartum period. This results in ischemia of the lateral pituitary gland, which damages the lactotropes. These women may also have blunted luteinizing hormone (LH), follicle-stimulating hormone (FSH), and TSH responses.

Hyperprolactinemia should be suspected in the patient who presents with galactorrhea (>50%) and oligo- or amenorrhea (20%). Hyperprolactinemia may also be responsible for a subtle ovulation dysfunction, manifested by an inadequate luteal phase. These patients typically have shortened luteal phases and lowered mid–luteal phase progesterone levels. Disruption of gonadotropin secretion from the anterior pituitary resulting from elevated prolactin levels is thought to be the source of anovulation and luteal-phase defects in these women.

Prolactin levels should be measured in all patients seen because of menstrual cycle irregularities or galactorrhea. Because of the intricate relationship between prolactin and TSH secretion, thyroid evaluation (TSH and thyroid hormone levels) should also be carried out. The best time to collect serum for prolactin measurements is between 8 and 12 A.M. Elevated prolactin levels indicate the need for evaluation of the sella turcica. Magnetic resonance imaging (MRI) or computed tomography are the most reliable methods for this purpose

There are four indications for treatment of the patient with hyperprolactinemia: (1) progressive pituitary enlargement (macroadenoma, ≥1 cm in diameter), (2) persistent galactorrhea, (3) hypoestrogenemia, and (4) ovulation dysfunction in the patient who desires pregnancy. For these patients, bromocriptine is the treatment of choice. The oral administration of this agent produces nausea and vomiting in greater than 50 percent of patients. These side effects usually subside; however, in some women, the treatment has to be discontinued. When this situation arises, the vaginal administration of bromocriptine may be substituted, which reduces the gastrointestinal side effects. Patients with pituitary macroadenomas usually respond well to bromocriptine therapy. Therapy must be continued indefinitely because discontinuation usually results in the return of hyperprolactinemia as well as growth of the adenoma. In patients who do not respond to bromocriptine, surgical management may be required. Overall, there is an approximately 50 percent recurrence of pituitary adenomas after surgical ablation.

An understanding of the natural history of prolactinomas is evolving. In general, prolactin-secreting microadenomas progress in less than 10 percent of the cases; the balance of the tumors either remain the same or, in some cases, spontaneously reduce. There is only a minimal risk of complications from prolactinomas during pregnancy. Once pregnancy is confirmed, bromocriptine should be discontinued. Evaluation during pregnancy should be reserved for the patient who starts to experience headaches or exhibit focal neurologic defects, indicating progression of the tumor. Imaging of the sella turcica is required when these symptoms develop. In the event of tumor progression in the setting of pregnancy, bromocriptine treatment may be restarted. Medical management with bromocriptine can be extremely effective and most women have a successful pregnancy outcome.

Prolactin Physiology
1. Hwang, P., Guyda, H., and Friesen, H. Purification of human prolactin. *J. Biol. Chem.* 247:1955, 1972.
   This describes the biochemistry of prolactin.
2. Zacur, H. A., et al. Multifactorial regulation of prolactin secretion. *Lancet* 1:410, 1976.
   This is a review of the numerous factors that stimulate or suppress prolactin secretion.
3. Sassin, J. F., et al. Human prolactin: 24 hr pattern with increased release during sleep. *Science* 177:1205, 1972.
   Reviews the circadian secretion of prolactin.
4. Robyn, C., et al. *Physiological and Pharmacological Factors Influencing Prolactin Secretion and Their Relation to Human Reproduction.* London: Academic Press, 1977.
   The role of prolactin in reproduction.
5. Kletzky, O. A., et al. Prolactin synthesis and release during pregnancy and puerperium. *Am. J. Obstet. Gynecol.* 136:545, 1980.
   This discusses the topic of prolactin production in pregnancy.
6. Noel, G. L., Suh, H. K., Frantz, A. G. Prolactin release during nursing and breast stimulation in postpartum and non-postpartum subjects. *J. Clin. Endocrinol. Metab.* 38:413, 1974.
   Postpartum prolactin secretion.
7. Okatani, Y., and Sagara, Y. Role of melatonin in nocturnal prolactin secretion in women with normoprolactinemia and mild hyperprolactinemia. *Am. J. Obstet. Gynecol.* 168:854, 1993.
   Melatonin, a pineal gland secretion, can stimulate prolactin release and may be involved in the nocturnal increase in prolactin secretion noted in normal and mildly hyperprolactinemic women.

Management
8. Brant-Zawadski, M., et al. Magnetic resonance imaging of the brain: the optimal screening technique. *Radiology* 152:71, 1984.
   This discusses the applications of MRI to pituitary evaluation.
9. Thorner, M. O., et al. Rapid regression of pituitary prolactinomas during bromocriptine treatment. *J. Clin. Endocrinol. Metab.* 51:438, 1980.
   Bromocriptine therapy for pituitary prolactinomas.
10. Kletzky, O. A., and Vermesh, M. Effectiveness of vaginal bromocriptine in treating women with hyperprolactinemia. *Fertil. Steril.* 51:269, 1989.
    This article considers the efficacy of vaginally administered bromocriptine in the treatment of hyperprolactinemia.
11. Lengyel, A.-M. J., et al. Long-acting injectable bromocriptine (Parlodel LAR)

in the chronic treatment of prolactin-secreting macroadenomas. *Fertil. Steril.* 59:980, 1993.
Monthly injections were well tolerated and highly effective.

12. Schlechte, J., et al. The natural history of untreated hyperprolactinemia: a prospective analysis. *J. Clin. Endocrinol. Metab.* 68:412, 1989.
Thirty women were observed for an average of 5.2 years. Disease progression is unlikely and improvement may occur.

13. Serri, O., et al. Recurrence of hyperprolactinemia after selective transsphenoidal adenomectomy in women with prolactinoma. *N. Engl. J. Med.* 309:280, 1983.
This discusses the recurrence of prolactin-secreting tumors after surgical ablation.

14. Bergh, T., Nillius, S. J., and Wide, L. Clinical course and outcome of pregnancies in amenorrheic women with hyperprolactinemia and pituitary tumors. *Br. Med. J.* 1:875, 1978.
The clinical course of prolactinomas during pregnancy is considered.

82. PRECOCIOUS PUBERTY
Harriette L. Hampton

The development of the capacity for reproduction commences in utero and continues through puberty. During the fetal stage, gonadotropin secretion increases progressively, with patterns and levels comparable to those that occur with the onset and during the first half of puberty. Gonadal steroidogenesis increases and the episodic release of gonadotropins indicates that negative feedback mechanisms and differentiation of the hypothalamic-pituitary-gonadal axis are functional. During the neonatal phase, hormonal secretion is greater than that during childhood. For a few weeks, secretion persists at pubertal levels but without causing overt physical changes. In the childhood phase, down-regulation results in hormone levels equivalent to those in hypogonadotropic hypogonadal adults. The low levels of secretion are a function of decreased hypothalamic stimulation, which is governed by the central nervous system (CNS). The final phase of development is puberty, which is marked by a resurgence of gonadotropin and sex steroid secretion. This begins with pulsatile, sleep-coincident, pituitary gonadotropin release. With further maturation, the pattern becomes regularly episodic over the entire 24-hour period.

In girls, normal puberty is accompanied by an acceleration of growth and by breast development (thelarche). Pubic and axillary hair then develop (adrenarche), followed by menses (menarche). In true or central precocious puberty, gonadotropin-dependent changes follow the production of gonadotropins with sex hormone elaboration, and the normal clinical sequence of pubertal changes is preserved. In the setting of peripheral or gonadotropin-independent precocious puberty (precocious pseudopuberty), primary disease of the gonads or adrenals is implicated. Alterations in the normal sequence of pubertal changes may occur. A change consistent with the sex of the individual is called isosexual precocity; heterosexual precocity indicates the presence of virilization in the female. Those disorders in which the development is mild or not progressive, including precocious thelarche and adrenarche, are sometimes termed incomplete sexual precocity.

Puberty begins in 95 percent of normal girls between the ages of 9 and 13, and in 95 percent of normal boys, between the ages of 10 and 14. To avoid performing unnecessary medical investigations in those children at the extremes of the normal distribution, a practical definition for precocious puberty is required. Sexual maturation below age 8 in a female or below age 9 in a male warrants evaluation in the North American population. The onset of puberty is frequently later in children suffering from chronic illness or malnutrition. However, contrasexual development requires evaluation regardless of the age of presentation.

In approximately 75 percent of the cases of female precocious puberty, the cause is idiopathic. A thorough evaluation must be performed, however, to rule out the existence of gonadal, adrenal, or CNS dysfunction. The early development of secondary sexual characteristics may be the source of psychosocial problems for the child, and these should be carefully addressed. Typically, these girls are taller than their peers due to estrogen stimulation of long-bone growth, but become short adults secondary to the premature fusion of the long-bone epiphyses. The radiologic determination of bone age is an important adjunct in the classification of precocious sexual development.

Various classification systems are proposed for female precocious puberty. For the purposes of this discussion, premature thelarche, premature adrenarche, luteinizing hormone releasing hormone (LHRH)–dependent precocious puberty, and LHRH–independent precocious puberty are considered.

Isolated breast development, premature thelarche, usually presents in a female child aged 3 years or younger and arrests at Tanner stage III. The purpose of a careful history and physical examination is to identify other features of puberty that would suggest the diagnosis is not simply one of premature thelarche. These findings include the presence of pubic or axillary hair, vaginal bleeding, a growth spurt, or acne and body odor. With confirmation of isolated thelarche and normal bone age, careful follow-up at 3- to 6-month intervals is appropriate until the child's lack of progression confirms the presumptive diagnosis of premature thelarche. Any progression of pubertal events should prompt a more complete evaluation.

Precocious isolated pubic hair development, premature adrenarche, usually results from early maturation of the adrenal androgen pathways. Adrenal maturation normally begins at age 4 to 7 and ends at age 15 to 20. Isolated pubic hair development can also be associated with late-onset 21-hydroxylase deficiency, or rarely 11-hydroxylase deficiency. The diagnosis of premature pubarche due to 21-hydroxylase deficiency is confirmed by an elevated early morning serum 17-OH progesterone (17-OHP) level. Dehydroepiandrosterone-sulfate (DHEA-s) in the early to mid-adrenarchal range (60–200 μg/dl) confirms that adrenarche is in progress. With this finding, it is appropriate to make a presumptive diagnosis of premature adrenarche and to reevaluate the child carefully every 3 to 6 months until a typical pattern of premature adrenarche confirms the diagnosis. If the plasma DHEA-s concentration is either preadrenarchal or above the adult range, further diagnostic studies are called for to determine whether the child has adrenal hyperplasia or tumor.

Female isosexual development can be either LHRH dependent or independent. To determine whether there has been pubertal activation of LHRH secretion, an LHRH stimulation test must be performed. A prepubertal response (no luteinizing hormone [LH] release after LHRH stimulation) indicates that hypothalamus-pituitary maturation (puberty) has not occurred. A pubertal response, LH elevation, should be followed by evaluation of the pituitary and hypothalamus using computed tomography or magnetic resonance imaging. Midline CNS tumors may cause sexual precocity by impinging on the hypothalamus, resulting in gonadotropin-releasing hormone activation. Craniopharyngiomas and hamartomas are the most common CNS tumors to prematurely activate puberty. Negative scan findings imply the existence of idiopathic precocious puberty.

The evaluation of LHRH-independent precocity includes imaging of the adrenals and gonads to search for possible neoplasia. It is necessary to measure the serum levels of 17-OHP and human chorionic gonadotropin (hCG) to exclude 21-hydroxylase (or 11-hydroxylase) deficiency or an hCG-secreting neoplasm. Thyroid function tests are appropriate when primary hypothyroidism is suspected.

All forms of LHRH-dependent precocious puberty can be treated effectively with LHRH agonists. Treatment options include deslorelin (4 μg/kg body weight/day, subcutaneously), histrelin (10 μg/kg/day, subcutaneously), or depot leuprolide (0.3 mg/kg every 2 weeks, intramuscularly for the first month, then 0.3 mg/kg every 3 to 4 weeks thereafter).

Precocious puberty resulting from an LHRH-independent mechanism requires treatment tailored to the particular case. Adrenal and gonadal tumors are treated surgically. Congenital adrenal hyperplasia due to 21-hydroxylase deficiency is treated conventionally with glucocorticoid and mineralocorticoid replacement.

The infrequent finding of sexual precocity warrants a thorough history, physical examination, and laboratory studies to distinguish benign from serious, even fatal, causes. Appropriate therapy ensures suppression of the pituitary gonadal axis and allows long-bone growth to progress at the normal rate.

General
1. Cutler, G. B., Jr. Precocious Puberty. In J. W. Hurst, et al. (eds.). *Medicine for the Practicing Physician*, 3rd ed. Woburn, MA: Butterworth, 1992.
   A well-written, clinically oriented chapter on the evaluation and treatment of precocious puberty.
2. Styne, D. M., and Grumbach, M. M. Puberty in the male and female: its physiology and disorders. In S. S. C. Yen and R. B. Jaffe (eds.). *Reproductive Endocrinology: Physiology, Pathophysiology and Clinical Management*, 3rd ed. Philadelphia: Saunders, 1991.
   A comprehensive chapter prepared by leading authorities.

Normal Puberty
3. Tanner, J. M. (ed.). *Growth at Adolescence*, 2nd ed. Oxford: Blackwell, 1962.
   The Tanner stage I to V classification categorizes the changes of puberty, including breasts and pubic hair, with stage I constituting infantile and stage V adult appearance and, the other stages describing intermediate morphology.
4. Marshall, W. A., and Tanner, J. M. Variations in pattern of pubertal changes in girls. *Arch. Dis. Child.* 44:291, 1969.
   Pubertal sexual development progresses in a predictable way; any deviation from this sequence may indicate abnormal development.
5. Tanner, J. M., and Davies, P. S. W. Clinical longitudinal standards for height and height velocity for North American children. *J. Pediatr.* 107:317, 1985.
   The peak height velocity is attained in the majority between ages 11 and 14. The average girl grows 2 to 3 inches (5–7.5 cm) during the 2 years after menarche.
6. Goji, K. Pulsatile characteristics of spontaneous growth hormone (GH) concentration profiles in boys evaluated by an ultrasensitive immunoradiometric assay: evidence for ultradian periodicity of GH secretion. *J. Clin. Endocrinol. Metab.* 76:667, 1993.
   Human growth hormone secretion could exhibit an ultradian rhythm, with periodicities of 100 to 120 minutes under physiologic conditions.
7. Lee, P. A. Pubertal neuroendocrine maturation: early differentiation and stages of development. *Adoles. Pediatr. Gynecol.* 1:3, 1988.
   The nature of the neuroendocrine mechanism that initiates puberty at the appropriate time is not known.
8. Oerter, K. E., et al. Gonadotropin secretory dynamics during puberty in normal girls and boys. *J. Clin. Endocrinol. Metab.* 71:1390, 1990.
   This provides normative data for spontaneous and LHRH-stimulated gonadotropin levels during puberty.

Abnormal Pubertal Development
9. Van Winter, J. T., et al. Natural history of premature thelarche in Olmsted County, Minnesota, 1940 to 1984. *J. Pediatr.* 116:278, 1990.
   Idiopathic premature thelarche, in the absence of a source of exogenous estrogen, is usually a benign self-limiting disorder, and, in general, no therapy is indicated.
10. Ibanez, L., et al. Natural history of premature pubarche: an auxological study. *J. Clin. Endocrinol. Metab.* 74:254, 1992.
    Controversies surround the etiology and diagnostic approach to the child with isolated pubic hair development. Premature adrenarche may be a normal variant of puberty.
11. White, P. C., New, M. I., and Dupont, B. Congenital adrenal hyperplasia. *N. Engl. J. Med.* 316:1519, 1987.
    A comprehensive review.
12. Foster, C. M., et al. Absence of pubertal gonadotropin secretion in girls with McCune-Albright syndrome. *J. Clin. Endocrinol. Metab.* 58:1161, 1984.

Polycystic fibrous dysplasia (McCune-Albright syndrome) may be associated with precocious puberty. The disorder is characterized by long-bone cysts and café au lait spots.

13. Navarius, C., et al. Paraneoplastic precocious puberty. Report of a new case with hepatoblastoma and review of the literature. *Cancer* 56:1725, 1985.
   Tumors that secrete hCG can cause precocious puberty. The hCG stimulates the gonads directly.

14. Cook, C. D., McArthur, J. W., and Berenberg, W. Pseudoprecocious puberty in girls as a result of estrogen ingestion. *N. Engl. J. Med.* 248:671, 1953.
   Estrogen-containing medications, including skin care products and therapeutic estrogen cream for vulvar agglutination can cause premature thelarche.

15. Hochman, H. I., Judge, D. M., and Reichlin, S. Precocious puberty and hypothalamic hamartoma. *Pediatrics* 67:236, 1981.
   Other CNS disorders associated with precocious puberty include Von Recklinghausen's disease (neurofibromatosis), which is characterized by café au lait spots and subcutaneous neurofibromas.

16. Sonis, W. A., et al. Behavior problems and social competence in girls with true precocious puberty. *J. Pediatr.* 106:156, 1985.
   The psychosocial consequences of early physical maturation are discussed.

Diagnosis and Treatment

17. Wilkins, L. (ed.). *The Diagnosis and Treatment of Endocrine Disorders of Childhood and Adolescence,* 3rd ed. Springfield: Charles C Thomas, 1965, p. 223.
   A classic textbook with clinical insights.

18. Pescovitz, O. H., et al. The NIH experience in precocious puberty: diagnostic subgroups and the response to short-term LHRH analogue therapy. *J. Pediatr.* 108:47, 1986.
   This describes a large series of patients referred to the National Institutes of Health after the institution of LHRH agonist treatment.

19. Pescovitz, O. H., et al. Premature thelarche and central precocious puberty: the relationship between clinical presentation and the gonadotropin response to LHRH. *J. Clin. Endocrinol. Metab.* 67:474, 1988.
   This discusses the diagnosis and mechanisms of premature thelarche.

20. Counts, E. R., and Cutler, G. B., Jr. Precocious puberty: pathogenesis and treatment. *Curr. Opin. Pediatr.* 4:674, 1992.
   A brief review of the recent literature on the topic.

21. Laue, L., et al. Treatment of familial male precocious puberty with spironolactone, testolactone, and deslorelin. *J. Clin. Endocrinol. Metab.* 76:151, 1993.
   Spironolactone is an antiandrogen, testolactone is an aromatase inhibitor that blocks the conversion of androgen to estrogen, and deslorelin is an LHRH agonist.

83. HIRSUTISM AND VIRILIZATION
Bryan D. Cowan

The masculine distribution of hair in a girl or woman represents a cosmetic catastrophe that is a source of emotional trauma for the patient and often creates anguish for her family. Excess growth of hair on the body surface of a woman where hair growth is ordinarily absent is known as hirsutism. When clitoral hypertrophy, varying degrees of suppression of cephalic hair, deepening of the voice, increased muscle mass, and amenorrhea are present in conjunction with hirsutism, the symptom complex is called virilism. Virilism is almost always the accompaniment of pathologic processes in which androgens are produced to extreme excess.

The human hair follicle lies more or less dormant until puberty, and then becomes fully activated only under the stimulation of androgenic hormones. In women, androgen production is biglandular, and these hormones are produced in roughly equal amounts by the adrenal glands and ovaries. The most important androgens are testosterone, dihydrotestosterone, androstenedione, dehydroepiandrosterone, and dehydroepiandrosterone-sulfate (DHEA-s).

Approximately 25 percent of the circulating testosterone in normal women is produced directly by the ovary; an additional 25 percent is produced directly by the adrenal gland; and the remaining 50 percent is produced through the peripheral conversion of testosterone precursors. At target sites for androgen utilization (genital skin and hair follicles), the enzyme 5-alpha-reductase converts testosterone to the potent hormone 5-alpha-dihydrotestosterone (DHT). Both testosterone and DHT interact with androgen receptors to promote the androgen-mediated cellular response. However, DHT has a much greater affinity for the receptor and, hence, is the more potent of the two predominant androgens.

The clinician often views every female with excess hair as having an endocrine problem. Such a conclusion is essentially correct if the hair follicle is regarded as an end-organ influenced and stimulated by androgens. However, many (if not most) hirsute females do not manifest any obvious disorder of endocrine homeostasis. Secondary sexual characteristics such as body contour, breast development, muscle mass, and fat deposits are completely normal. The menstrual cycles in these women may be regular and ovulatory, and the ability to bear children may not be impaired at all. Factors that can stimulate excess hair growth in the female who has no pathologic endocrine condition include increased sensitivity of the pilosebaceous apparatus to androgens, abnormal distribution of circulating androgens (steroid bindings; see later discussion), and certain drugs.

Except for direct effects at the site of production, androgens are transported by plasma to target tissues before they can express a biologic effect. In plasma, most androgens are bound to one of two proteins: albumin or sex hormone–binding globulin (SHBG). Albumin has a low affinity for testosterone, whereas SHBG has a high affinity for testosterone. Only about 1 to 2 percent of the measurable testosterone in the circulation is free; the remainder is bound to protein. SHBG is synthesized by the liver, and its plasma levels are determined by the balance between estrogens and androgens, thyroid hormone, and liver function. Abnormalities in SHBG function or production can affect the free testosterone concentration in plasma and produce clinical androgen excess without causing demonstrable biochemical abnormalities in the total testosterone concentrations.

Women with abnormal hair growth can be classified into three groups. The first group is composed of women with pathologic androgen excess; this is associated with ovarian and adrenal tumors, congenital adrenal hyperplasia (CAH), or Cushing's syndrome. The second group constitutes those women with nonpathologic androgen excess, which is seen in the many variant forms of the polycystic ovarian syndrome (PCOS). Patients with idiopathic or unexplained hirsutism, the third group, have no detectable hormonal abnormalities but do exhibit excess hair growth.

The most important task of the physician caring for a patient with hirsutism or virilization, or both, is to disprove the presence of a pathologic condition producing androgen excess. Tumors of the adrenal gland are rare, and the incidence of the malignant form approaches only 2 per one million population per year. These neoplasms can arise at any age of life, and the average age of diagnosis in one large series was 34 years. Unfortunately, only 10 to 25 percent of the patients with adrenal carcinomas exhibit evidence of endocrine dysfunction. Of these, approximately two fifths of the patients demonstrate virilization; the remainder have signs of Cushing's syndrome.

Virilizing ovarian tumors, like adrenal tumors, are uncommon. Although the true incidence and prevalence of such tumors are unknown, they constitute much less than 1 percent of all ovarian tumors. The findings revealed by the pelvic examination are of fundamental importance in arriving at the diagnosis of androgen-secreting ovarian tumors. Approximately 80 percent of patients with androgen-secreting ovarian tumors have palpable adnexal abnormalities discovered by bimanual examination. An elevated serum testosterone level greater than 2 ng/ml or a palpable adnexal mass, or both, are found in most women with a functional androgen-secreting ovarian tumor. Furthermore, pelvic sonography can identify the abnormality in that small residual group of patients with ovarian enlargement not detectable by pelvic examination. There are several varieties of histologically definable tumors of the ovaries that secrete androgens. These tumors are usually of stromal cell origin. The most common gonadal stromal tumors are thecoma and fibrothecoma. These lesions are almost always unilateral and benign. The androblastoma (arrhenoblastoma and gynandroblastoma) is also a gonadal stromal tumor. These tumors are principally benign, but can be associated with the Peutz-Jeghers syndrome or mucinous cystadenoma. Sertoli cell tumors in the female do not produce virilization, but the Sertoli-Leydig cell tumor is associated with androgen excess.

Besides an ovarian or adrenal tumor, CAH is also a source of pathologic androgen excess. Three inheritable enzymatic defects are recognized, all of which lead to a decrease in cortisol biosynthesis (and hence an increase in pituitary adrenocorticotropic hormone [ACTH] release). The most common is the 21-hydroxylase deficiency, which is referred to as the salt-losing form. The next most common defect is the 11-beta-hydroxylase deficiency, and this is referred to as the hypertensive form. The rarest form of all is 3-beta-ol-dehydrogenase deficiency. The source of androgen excess in each form of CAH is the excess production of adrenal androgens, which is driven by excess pituitary ACTH production. The diagnosis is confirmed by the detection of pathologic elevations in the levels of the precursor steroid hormone, which is normally converted by the enzyme in question.

Cushing's syndrome represents a systemic illness associated with myriad clinical and metabolic abnormalities and pathologic androgen excess. This syndrome develops from the excess adrenal production of glucocorticoids and androgens. Endogenous hypercortisolism results from one of three disorders: (1) ACTH excess stemming from hypothalamic or pituitary disease (referred to as Cushing's disease); (2) autonomous hypercortisolism resulting from an adrenal neoplasm (Cushing's syndrome); or (3) the ectopic production of ACTH from a tumor (ectopic ACTH syndrome). Specific features of Cushing's syndrome consist of central obesity, pigmented stria, muscle weakness, hypokalemia, and ecchymosis. Diagnostic tools to determine whether the patient has pituitary, adrenal, or ectopic ACTH Cushing's syndrome include the overnight 1-mg dexamethasone suppression test (screening), measurement of the urinary free cortisol levels, low- and high-dose dexamethasone suppression tests, and measurement of the plasma ACTH level.

In the course of evaluating affected women, any menstrual irregularity should be noted. Of significance is the finding that the menstrual irregularities are new in onset. In women with idiopathic hirsutism or PCOS, or both, the onset of hirsutism and menstrual irregularities is associated with menarche. Women with pathologic ovarian or adrenal tumors report that the onset of hair growth and menstrual irregularities is new. On physical examination, the location and extent of terminal hair on the face, neck, chest, upper back, upper abdomen, lower abdomen, and perineum should be determined. Clitoral inspection should be performed, and a clitoral index can serve as a good marker for the presence of androgen excess. A pelvic examination should be performed, and blood pressure should be recorded.

Women with clinically significant hirsutism or minimal hirsutism associated with changes in menstrual patterns, infertility, or pelvic masses, as well as women with infertility and anovulatory cycles, should undergo serum androgen determinations. To properly evaluate patients with clinical signs and symptoms of androgen excess, the measurement of androgen hormone levels and interpretation of their significance are essential. The most useful measurements for determining the status of androgen production in women are the serum testosterone and DHEA-s levels. The purpose of the testosterone measurement is to determine the likelihood of an androgen-producing ovarian tumor. If the testosterone concentration is greater than 2 ng/ml, the likelihood of an ovarian tumor is increased. DHEA-s is a steroid whose concentration reflects the status of adrenal androgen production. Greater than 90 percent of the circulating DHEA-s is produced by the adrenal gland, and measurements of this steroid display little diurnal variation. A value of greater than 8000 ng/ml is highly suggestive of an adrenal neoplasm as the source of androgen excess.

Treatment of a pathologic androgen excess should be directed at correcting the pathologic condition responsible for the aberrant hormone production. The treatment of androgen excess owing to PCOS or idiopathic causes is governed somewhat by the short- and long-term goals of each patient. In general, combined pharmacologic and cosmetic treatments offer the most effective therapy. Pharmacologic options include oral contraceptives to reduce ovarian androgen production, glucocorticoids to reduce adrenal androgen secretion, and androgen receptor antagonists (spironolactone). In addition, gonadotropin-releasing hormone (GnRH) agonists have demonstrated remarkable efficacy in reducing ovarian androgen production. Cosmetic adjuncts include shaving, waxing, depilatories, and electrolysis. These treatments are effective in most patients but often do not achieve optimal results. New hair growth can be halted, but the involution of established hair follicles is a slow process.

Androgen Production and Metabolism

1. Wajchenberg, B. L., et al. The source(s) of estrogen production in hirsute women with polycystic ovarian disease as determined by simultaneous adrenal and ovarian venous catheterization studies. *Fertil. Steril.* 49:56:1988.
   The major source of estradiol in women with PCOS is the ovary, whereas the major source of estrone is the peripheral conversion of androstenedione.

2. Loric, S., et al. Determination of testosterone in serum not bound by sex-hormone–binding globulin: diagnostic value in hirsute women. *Clin. Chem.* 34:1826, 1988.
   Androgens are bound to testosterone-binding globulin. Only free, unbound testosterone stimulates excessive hair growth and produces virilization.

3. Ruvtiainen, K., et al. Androgen parameters in hirsute women: correlation with body mass index and age. *Fertil. Steril.* 50:255, 1988.
   Both age and body mass affect the "normal values" of testosterone and SHBG.

4. Kirschner, M. A., Samojlik, E., and Szmal, E. Clinical usefulness of plasma androstanediol glucuronide measurements in women with idiopathic hirsutism. *J. Clin. Endocrinol. Metab.* 65:597, 1987.
   Twenty-eight women with idiopathic hirsutism exhibited abnormal androstanediol glucuronide levels.

Congenital Adrenal Hyperplasia

5. Bongiovanni, A. M., and Root, A. W. The adrenogenital syndrome. *N. Engl. J. Med.* 268:1283, 1963.
   A comprehensive review of the topic of CAH.

6. Givens, J. R., et al. Adrenal function in hirsutism. I. Diurnal change and response of plasma androstenedione, testosterone, 17-hydroxyprogesterone, cortisol, LH and FSH to dexamethasone and 1/2 unit of ACTH. *J. Clin. Endocrinol. Metab.* 40:988, 1975.
   The basis for dexamethasone therapy in adrenal hyperplasia is described.

7. Baskin, H. G. Screening for late-onset congenital adrenal hyperplasia in hirsutism or amenorrhea. *Arch. Intern. Med.* 147:847, 1987.
   Describes the method and utility of the short ACTH stimulation test for the assessment of late-onset CAH.

Polycystic Ovarian Disease

8. Stein, I. F., and Leventhal, M. L. Amenorrhea associated with bilateral polycystic ovaries. *Am. J. Obstet. Gynecol.* 29:181, 1935.
   The original description of PCOS.

9. Gindoff, P. R., and Jewelewicz, R. Polycystic ovarian disease. *Obstet. Gynecol. Clin. North Am.* 14:931, 1987.
   A contemporary review of PCOS.

10. Grasinger, C. C., Wild, R. A., and Parker, I. J. Vulvar acanthosis nigricans: a marker for insulin resistance in hirsute women. *Fertil. Steril.* 59:583, 1993.
    The association between hyperandrogenism, insulin resistance, and acanthosis nigricans (a thickened pigmented skin lesion) was first described in this article, and designated the HAIR-AN syndrome.

11. Wajchenberg, B. L., et al. Free testosterone levels during the menstrual cycle in obese versus normal women. *Fertil. Steril.* 51:535, 1989.

Even moderate obesity was associated with alterations in testosterone binding and in elevated free testosterone levels.

12. Rittmaster, R. S., and Givner, M. L. Effect of daily and alternate day low dose prednisone on serum cortisol and adrenal androgens in hirsute women. *J. Clin. Endocrinol. Metab.* 67:400, 1988.

    There was no advantage to alternate-day therapy, but the adrenal androgen levels were suppressed easily by the nocturnal administration of prednisone (100 μg/kg).

13. Pache, T. D., et al. Association between ovarian changes assessed by transvaginal sonography and clinical and endocrine signs of the polycystic ovary syndrome. *Fertil. Steril.* 59:544, 1993.

    This represents an additional tool for the diagnosis and treatment of PCOS.

14. Faure, N., and Lemay, A. Ovarian suppression in polycystic ovarian disease during 6 month administration of a luteinizing hormone–releasing hormone (LH-RH) agonist. *Clin. Endocrinol.* 27:703, 1987.

    It is possible to selectively inhibit ovarian steroid production with a GnRH agonist.

Treatment

15. Givens, J. R., et al. Dynamics of suppression and recovery of plasma FSH, LH, androstenedione, and testosterone in polycystic ovarian disease using an oral contraceptive. *J. Clin. Endocrinol. Metab.* 38:727, 1974.

    This describes the basis for the therapy of PCOS using oral contraceptives.

16. Lobo, R. A., et al. The effects of two doses of spironolactone on serum androgens and anagen hair in hirsute women. *Fertil. Steril.* 43:200, 1985.

    A discussion of the uses and effectiveness of spironolactone for treating hirsutism.

Androgen Excess Disorders in Childhood

17. Rittmaster, R. S., and Thompson, D. L. Effect of leuprolide and dexamethasone on hair growth and hormone levels in hirsute women: the relative importance of the ovary and the adrenal in the pathogenesis of hirsutism. *J. Clin. Endocrinol. Metab.* 70:1096, 1990.

    The ovary is the major source of androgens in the setting of PCOS.

18. Bates, G. W. Hirsutism and androgen excess problems in childhood and adolescence. *Pediatr. Clin. North Am.* 28:513, 1981.

    This provides a comprehensive review of the pediatric androgen-excess disorders, along with discussion of treatment.

19. Serafini, P., and Lobo, R. A. Increased 5 alpha-reductase activity in idiopathic hirsutism. *Fertil. Steril.* 43:74, 1985.

    The authors report on a new biochemical link to the understanding of idiopathic hirsutism.

20. Emans, S. J., et al. Treatment with dexamethasone of androgen excess in adolescent patients. *J. Pediatr.* 112:821, 1988.

    The free testosterone levels reflect the efficacy of therapy.

84. DYSFUNCTIONAL UTERINE BLEEDING
Bryan D. Cowan

Cyclic menstruation is the culmination of the programmed hormonal stimulation of the endometrium. This orchestrated event is referred to as the ovarian-menstrual cycle. In the course of a normal ovulatory cycle, follicle-stimulating hormone (FSH) stimulates the maturation of an ovarian follicle. The responding ovarian follicle secretes increasing quantities of estradiol-17β (E^2) during the proliferative phase of the menstrual cycle. When the plasma concentration of E^2 reaches the threshold level necessary to induce a luteinizing hormone (LH) surge, ovulation follows and the follicle is transformed into a corpus luteum.

In response to increasing ovarian E^2 secretion, the endometrial epithelium proliferates, the stroma thickens and becomes compact, and the endometrial glands increase in number and length. If estrogen secretion were to continue unopposed by the action of progesterone, the endometrium would proliferate until eventually it would outgrow its blood supply and slough away from the myometrium. In the normal ovulatory cycle, however, ovulation is followed by the formation of a corpus luteum at the site of the ovarian follicle, and the corpus luteum begins secreting progesterone. Progesterone acts on the endometrium to suppress the mitogenic action of E^2 and converts the proliferative endometrium into secretory endometrium. The straight, narrow endometrial glands become tortuous and dilated, and the endometrial stroma is transformed to decidua. If fertilization and implantation of the ovum do not occur, the corpus luteum fails approximately 12 days after it is formed. With corpus luteum regression, E^2 and progesterone production decline, hormonal stimulation of the endometrium is withdrawn, and menstruation begins. After hormone withdrawal from the endometrium at the end of corpus luteum function, the concentrations of prostaglandins (PGE_2 and PGF_2) increase. The prostaglandins induce spiral arteriolar vasomotor responses, which, in turn, induce epithelial ischemia with subsequent necrosis and shedding.

The ovarian-menstrual cycle is repeated 10 to 13 times a year in nonpregnant, sexually mature women. The repetitive nature of the cycle depends on changes in the levels of the two pituitary gonadotropins, FSH and LH, and the two ovarian steroid hormones, E^2 and progesterone. If the concentrations of any one of these four hormones becomes tonically elevated or suppressed, anovulation results. Uterine bleeding that is acyclic and associated with anovulation is termed dysfunctional uterine bleeding (DUB). Such endometrial sloughing can be focal, resulting in frequent episodes of vaginal spotting, or it can be extensive, resulting in frank menorrhagia. DUB should respond to appropriate steroid hormone therapy, which either corrects the hormonal aberration of the menstrual cycle or directly affects the endometrium.

Various times or conditions in which anovulation can lead to DUB are (1) puberty, (2) climacteric, (3) polycystic ovarian syndrome (PCOS), and (4) obesity. At the time of puberty, the cyclic hormonal interactions are not fully established. Estradiol secretion is continuous, and irregular uterine bleeding can occur. In the climacteric, the FSH and LH levels become tonically elevated, E^2 secretion becomes tonically low, ovulation fails, and irregular uterine bleeding ensues. In PCOS, the LH and estrone concentrations are tonically elevated, the endometrium is continuously stimulated by estrogens, ovulation fails, and the endometrium sloughs at irregular intervals. In the setting of obesity, estrone and LH levels are tonically elevated, the endometrium is continuously stimulated by estrogens, as in PCOS, and irregular uterine bleeding results.

In each of these conditions, the endometrium is stimulated by estrogens, without the suppressive action of progesterone and without the withdrawal of progesterone that initiates cyclic bleeding. Thus, the usual treatment of DUB should be directed at the endometrium to suppress the action of unopposed estrogens.

Before therapy for DUB can be instituted, organic disease of the uterus, cervix, or endometrium must be ruled out. In the adolescent girl, it would be unusual to find an organic disease of the reproductive tract, but organic disease is not unusual in the sexually mature woman. Because continuous estrogen stimulation of the endometrium is often associated with endometrial polyps and endometrial hyperplasia, either endometrial sampling (by biopsy or curettage) or visualization (hysteroscopy) should be considered as part of the diagnostic evaluation. Pelvic examination may disclose uterine tumors (fibroids), another cause of pathologic uterine bleeding.

After an organic cause for irregular uterine bleeding has been ruled out, a regimen of medical therapy directed at suppressing chronic estrogen stimulation and restoring the cyclic interactions between the pituitary gland and ovaries is begun. For a woman who is actively bleeding, medroxyprogesterone acetate (MPA; 10 mg daily for 5 to 10 days) is administered. MPA is an orally active synthetic progestin and, like progesterone, can transform proliferative endometrium into secretory endometrium. When the MPA is discontinued, withdrawal uterine bleeding will ensue 2 to 14 days later. Women treated with MPA should be forewarned of this withdrawal bleeding;

otherwise, they may think that the treatment has failed. After the dysfunctional uterine bleeding has been controlled by MPA therapy, the physician should develop a long-term therapeutic plan.

Adolescent girls can usually be reassured that the problem is self-limiting and will remit spontaneously when ovulatory cycles are established. Likewise, perimenopausal women can be reassured that irregular bleeding will subside with menopause (although other hormonal management may be required). Obese women of all ages should be encouraged to reduce their body weight to near ideal size. A spontaneous resumption of ovulatory cycles often follows weight reduction. PCOS, especially in nonobese women, tends to be chronic and requires long-term medical management in accordance with the patient's treatment goals. If control of irregular bleeding is the desired therapeutic goal, long-term ovarian suppression with an oral contraceptive agent can control the bleeding and suppress the excess androgen secretion associated with PCOS. If fertility is the desired goal, ovulation induction with clomiphene citrate is indicated.

Occasionally, young women suffer severe bleeding and significant anemia (hematocrit, $<25\%$) as a result of anovulatory dysfunctional uterine bleeding. This medical emergency usually requires hospitalization for treatment of the bleeding and anemia. High-dose estrogen treatment is usually efficacious as the first treatment before progestin therapy is started. We recommend a dosage consisting of 25 mg of conjugated equine estrogens (Premarin) given intravenously every 4 hours for three doses, or until the bleeding stops. Once the bleeding is stopped, progestin therapy must be initiated to mature and then slough the endometrium.

Management of chronic unopposed estrogen stimulation of the endometrium, such as that seen in the setting of PCOS or obesity, may require intermittent progestin therapy maintained for years. In these patients, we prescribe 10 mg of MPA to be taken on cycle days 16 to 25 during each or every other month. In addition, the use of a menstrual calendar greatly facilitates patient compliance with therapy and the interpretation of clinical responses.

Normal Menstrual Cycle
1. Speroff, L. Regulation of the Menstrual Cycle. In L. Speroff, R. H. Glass, and N. G. Kase (eds.), *Clinical Gynecologic Endocrinology and Infertility* (4th ed.). Baltimore: Williams & Wilkins, 1989.
   A comprehensive and clear presentation of the endocrine events that take place in the normal menstrual cycle.
2. Sherman, B. W., and Korenman, S. G. Hormonal characteristics of the human menstrual cycles throughout reproductive life. *J. Clin. Invest.* 55:699, 1975.
   A longitudinal study of the dynamics of gonadotropin and sex-steroid hormones during the reproductive years.

Variations in Gonadotropin and Steroid Hormone Secretion
3. Noyes, R. W., Hertig, A. T., and Rock, J. Dating the endometrial biopsy. *Fertil. Steril.* 1:3, 1950.
   The classic description of the dynamic events that take place during endometrial maturation.
4. Boyar, R. M., et al. Anorexia nervosa: immaturity of the 24-hour luteinizing hormone secretory pattern. *N. Engl. J. Med.* 291:861, 1974.
   In this disorder, the pituitary gonadotropin secretory pattern reverts to a prepubertal state.
5. Sherman, B. M., West, J. H., and Korenman, S. G. The menopausal transition: analysis of LH, FSH, estradiol, and progesterone concentrations during menstrual cycles in older women. *J. Clin. Endocrinol. Metab.* 42:629, 1976.
   An analysis of the gradual hormonal changes occurring in the late reproductive years.
6. Grodin, J. M., Siiteri, P. K., and MacDonald, P.C. Source of estrogen production in postmenopausal women. *J. Clin. Endocrinol. Metab.* 36:207, 1973.
   Discusses the mechanism that underlies estrogen production in menopausal women.

7. Nappi, C., et al. Plasma β-endorphin levels in obese and nonobese patients with polycystic ovarian disease. *Eur. J. Obstet. Gynecol. Reprod. Biol.* 30:151, 1989.
These authors suggest that the elevated endorphin levels often found in patients with PCOS are related to obesity and not to the pathogenesis of the syndrome.

8. Berga, S. L., and Yen, S. S. C. Opioidergic regulation of LH pulsatility in women with polycystic ovary syndrome. *Clin. Endocrinol.* 30:177, 1989.
The apparent opioidergic impairment in women with PCOS represents a functional state that is due to ovarian acyclicity rather than to an inherent hypothalamic defect.

9. Gidwani, G. P. Vaginal bleeding in adolescents. *J. Reprod. Med.* 29:417, 1984.
A careful elimination of organic causes is necessary before the diagnosis of DUB can be made in adolescents.

10. Greydanus, D. E., and McAnarney, E. R. Menstruation and its disorders in adolescence. *Curr. Probl. Pediatr.* 12:1, 1982.
A review of menstrual disorders that affect adolescents.

Management of DUB

11. Zimmermann, R. Dysfunctional uterine bleeding. *Obstet. Gynecol. Clin. North Am.* 15:107, 1988.
The judicious use of hysteroscopy to evaluate patients with DUB adds a new dimension in handling this often perplexing problem.

12. McLachlan, R. I., Healy, D. L., and Burger, H. G. Clinical aspects of LHRH analogues in gynaecology: a review. *Br. J. Obstet. Gynaecol.* 93:431, 1986.
Gonadotropin-releasing hormone analogues promise to have a profound impact on the management of a diverse range of estrogen-dependent gynecologic diseases.

13. Bayer, S. R., and DeCherney, A. H. Clinical manifestations and treatment of dysfunctional uterine bleeding. *J.A.M.A.* 269:1823, 1993.
Contains a useful algorithm detailing the evaluation of the patient with DUB.

14. Kase, N. G. Dysfunctional Uterine Bleeding. In L. Speroff, R. H. Glass, and N. G. Kase (eds.), *Clinical Gynecologic Endocrinology and Infertility* (4th ed.). Baltimore: Williams & Wilkins, 1989.
An overview of the clinical problem, with suggestions for therapy.

15. DeVore, G. R., Owens, O., and Kase, N. Use of intravenous Premarin in the treatment of dysfunctional uterine bleeding—a double-blind randomized control study. *Obstet. Gynecol.* 59:285, 1982.
Bleeding stopped in 72 percent of the women who received intravenous Premarin, compared with 38 percent in those who received placebo.

16. Wilansky, D. L., and Greisman, B. Early hypothyroidism in patients with menorrhagia. *Am. J. Obstet. Gynecol.* 160:673, 1989.
Fifteen of 67 apparently euthyroid menorrhagic women with normal uteri were found to have early hypothyroidism. The menorrhagia in these women was cured by thyroxine administration.

17. Cowan, B. D., and Morrison, J. C. Management of abnormal genital bleeding in girls and women. *N. Engl. J. Med.* 324:1710, 1991.
A review of the etiology and management of DUB.

18. Valle, R. F. Endometrial ablation for dysfunctional uterine bleeding: role of GnRH agonists. *Int. J. Gynecol. Obstet.* 41:3, 1993.
Hormonal thinning of the endometrium before surgical intervention simplifies the procedure, decreases blood loss, and improves the overall success rates.

85. PREMENSTRUAL SYNDROME

Michel E. Rivlin

Premenstrual syndrome (PMS) may be defined simply as a mixture of physical and emotional symptoms occurring during the week before menstruation that are so severe as to interfere with a woman's life-style or work. Psychiatrists have included PMS in the *Diagnostic and Statistical Manual of Mental Disorders (DSM)* as the "late luteal-phase dysphoric disorder." The *DSM* diagnostic criteria require that the symptoms occur in the last week of the luteal phase in most cycles during the previous year and that they remit within a few days after the onset of the follicular phase. The diagnosis is not based on the existence of specific symptoms, but on the timing of the symptoms.

A useful working definition of PMS is the occurrence of a marked change in the intensity of symptoms, measured daily from day 5 to 10, compared with the intensity within 6 days before menses for at least two consecutive cycles. Molimina, the nondistressing but perceived physical and emotional changes occurring before normal menses, is identical to PMS in terms of the kind of symptoms and the timing, but differs in intensity. It is estimated that 20 to 40 percent of all women experience some difficulty with PMS, but only about 5 percent report a significant impact on work or life-style. PMS was thought to be more common in women 30 to 40 years old than in those aged 20 to 30 years, but it may be that women do not seek treatment for PMS until they are older. In Europe, law courts have accepted PMS as a disease affecting the mind, but, in the United States, it has been effectively argued that, although the symptoms are real, they do not sufficiently justify or excuse uncontrollable behavior.

PMS symptoms are highly variable, and more than 150 have been reported. The most common are the typical psychologic symptoms of irritability, aggression, depression, tension, anxiety, poor coordination, and clumsiness. There are also the typical somatic or physical symptoms, including bloating, distention, feeling of weight gain, edema, breast swelling, headache, and others. Some clinicians believe that PMS may be best understood as a variety of subsyndromes that have been misleadingly classified under one name. One such classification is as follows: PMT (premenstrual tension)-A—nervous tension, mood swings, irritability, and anxiety; PMT-H—weight gain, breast tenderness, swelling of the extremities, and abdominal bloating; PMT-C—headaches, a craving for sweets, increased appetite, heart pounding, and fatigue; and PMT-D—depression, insomnia, forgetfulness, crying, and confusion. It is postulated that the various symptom clusters each have a unique etiology and that women whose symptoms fall under different categories would respond differently to particular therapeutic interventions. However, although women may experience one subsyndrome most clearly, they often have symptoms that are classified under another subsyndrome.

The cause, or causes, of PMS are unknown. Because treatment consisting of a specific agent or approach connotes a mechanism of action, the mechanisms and treatment may be considered together. Flattened glucose tolerance test results have been reported in patients with PMS, and hypoglycemia has been thought to be a possible cause of the headaches, fainting, and food cravings typical of the syndrome. Although this has not been proved, dietary changes that are recommended include a low intake of refined sugar and salt, meals eaten in six small portions throughout the day, and the avoidance of methylxanthine-containing substances such as coffee, tea, or chocolate. Substance abuse is not uncommon and, if present, requires therapy. Alcohol consumption frequently increases in the premenstruum, and this tendency should be discouraged. Vitamin B_6 (pyridoxine) in doses of 200 to 800 mg daily is also a common therapy, although its effectiveness is uncertain and overdosage may cause neuropathy. Fluid retention is a favorite hypothesis for explaining many of the symptoms, such as weight gain and bloating. Increased levels of estrogen and progesterone can lead to increased aldosterone plasma concentrations. Estrogen stimulates angiotensin synthesis, and progesterone exerts a natriuretic action, leading to a compensatory aldosterone response. The luteal-phase increase in the aldosterone level provides a rationale for diuretic therapy with spironolactone (an aldosterone antagonist diuretic). However, studies have not demonstrated the existence of either premenstrual water retention or weight gain. Attempts have therefore been made to attribute the symptoms to fluid redistribution, gut distention owing to progesterone's relaxing effect on smooth muscle, and a psychologic cause similar to the overestimation of body size seen in anorexia nervosa.

For many years, PMS was postulated to be the result of an impaired corpus luteal function, and therapy with synthetic or natural progesterone has been widely used, but has not yielded results better than those observed for placebo therapy. In fact, when patients and controls have been compared, no differences in the levels or patterns of secretion of progesterone, estradiol, gonadotropins, androgens, prolactin, or cortisol have been observed for the various phases of the menstrual cycle, suggesting that PMS represents an abnormal response to normal endocrine levels. Another etiologic hypothesis proposes a role for endorphins, the endogenous opioids. Because endorphin levels peak during the luteal phase and decline with menses, it has been suggested that PMS is a consequence of endogenous narcotic withdrawal.

Cyclic PMS symptoms may resemble a bipolar affective disorder. Excessive norepinephrine activity, such as is thought to occur in manic states, is diminished by the use of clonidine. Opiate withdrawal results in norepinephrine release, which then produces withdrawal symptoms. Clonidine has therefore been used with success in treating manic states, opiate withdrawal, and PMS. By contrast, lithium has not proved useful in the management of PMS. Some PMS symptoms are associated with prostaglandin-induced dysmenorrhea. Treatment with an inhibitor of prostaglandin synthesis may therefore ameliorate the associated symptoms as well as the cramps. Prolactin levels are higher in the luteal phase than the follicular phase; however, although bromocriptine can relieve the mastalgia, other symptoms are not alleviated. Because PMS is characteristically associated with mood, cognitive, and behavioral disturbances, a special relationship with psychiatric disorders has been postulated. About 80 percent of the patients who complain of PMS, but who do not have PMS, suffer depression; about 40 percent of the patients investigated for PMS have had some affective disorder. Menstrual cycle–related events may modulate or exacerbate a preexisting psychopathologic condition, and the often complex interweaving of a neurotic disorder and PMS makes it difficult to determine which came first in individual cases.

Dysfunction of serotoninergic transmission may be involved in the pathogenesis of several neuropsychiatric disorders, including anxiety and depression. Central serotonin systems also regulate many functions, such as appetite. It is therefore possible that derangements in serotonin activity may be important in the pathophysiology of PMS, as there is a relationship between ovarian steroids and serotoninergic function. Pharmacologic agents that influence serotonin activity have therefore been used for the treatment of PMS and have yielded good results. These agents include clomipramine, buspirone, d-fenfluramine, and fluoxetine. Although the improvement obtained is maximal with regard to behavioral symptoms, somatic problems are also frequently relieved.

The premenstrual syndromes are associated with cyclic ovarian activity and do not occur before puberty, during pregnancy, or after menopause. Menstruation itself is incidental, as the cyclic symptoms continue after hysterectomy if ovarian function has been preserved. The corollary of considering cyclic ovarian activity as fundamental in the etiology of PMS is that the suppression of ovulation should therefore abolish the PMS symptoms. Anovulation may be achieved pharmaceutically through the use of estrogen-progestin combinations, gonadotropin agonists, or danazol, or by surgical means (oophorectomy). In practice, however, the outcome of therapy is by no means predictable, and, in the instance of oral contraceptive agents, although some women may experience improvement, the condition in many may deteriorate or PMS symptoms may even be precipitated by the medication. In the rare patient undergoing oophorectomy, hysterectomy should also be performed, as estrogen replacement is usually well tolerated, but symptoms may recur if a progestin is added.

The first step in diagnosis is to recognize that the woman has a genuine disorder related to biologic events. She is not imagining her symptoms. The next step is to rule out other physical causes. This requires a full physical and gynecologic examination, including a Papanicolaou smear, complete blood count, chemistry screen, fasting blood glucose determination, and thyroid studies. The importance of a thorough evaluation is obvious when considering the common physical complaints: fatigue, headaches, bowel problems, and abdominal bloating. Numerous previously undetected diseases may be diagnosed in this way. A psychiatric diagnostic interview is also required if an emotional illness is suspected that may be exacerbated premenstrually. It is important to document that the symptoms are related to the menstrual cycle, rather than to other factors such as family or work stress. This is done by having the patient keep a daily diary of her symptoms for at least three cycles. Several PMS charts and calendars are available for this purpose. If records show that a marked increase in symptoms takes place premenstrually for two consecutive cycles, then a diagnosis of PMS is made at the end of 3 months' charting. For formal psychologic testing, the Minnesota Multiphasic Personality Inventory (MMPI) is ideal because of its ability to detect attempts by a patient to make herself appear emotionally "healthier" or "more disturbed" than she actually is. The MMPI is administered to the patient in both the follicular and luteal phases, and the results are compared as an aid to diagnosis and therapy.

Because no single cause is known, there is no routine treatment. While arriving at a diagnosis, however, treatment is begun, because many women gain a sense of control as they chart their daily changes and identify and quantify their symptoms. Education and support are necessary in helping the woman modify her life-style so that she can plan her activities to free the premenstruum from as much external stress as possible. Physical exercise increases self-esteem, reduces stress, and enhances a feeling of well-being, so that a regular program of exercise should be encouraged. Dietary changes have already been mentioned. Conservative measures are probably successful in about a third of the patients; the remainder require more extensive management, probably either with the help of ancillary services or at a PMS clinic. Thus, the patient may be offered a combination of the following therapies: education; medication; peer support groups; individual psychotherapy; group psychotherapy in such areas as stress management, impulse control, or assertiveness training; and sex or marital therapy, or family therapy. Help in these areas is directed at interrupting the cycle in which premorbid personality characteristics and the psychosocial consequences of premenstrual symptoms act as stresses that exacerbate the severity of symptoms.

Both the physician and the patient should be aware of the placebo effect. PMS shows a strong response to placebo, often quoted as 50 to 60 percent, but rates as high as 94 percent have been reported. The duration of the placebo response varies, but the patient is generally back to a pretreatment intensity of symptoms by 6 months. The psychosocial and subjective components of medical care make the placebo process a legitimate part of every patient-physician interaction. It is likely that successful therapy of PMS, regardless of the agent or method used, depends to a significant degree on the placebo process.

Reviews
1. Tucker, J. S., and Whalen, R. E. Premenstrual syndrome. *Int. J. Psychiatry Med.* 21:311, 1991.
   PMS symptoms include mood (irritability, depression, mood swings, and hostility), somatic complaints (mastalgia, bloating, headache, fatigue, insomnia, appetite changes, and hot flashes), cognitive problems (confusion and poor concentration), and behavioral symptoms (hyperphagia, social withdrawal, and arguing).
2. Johnson, S. R. Clinician's approach to the diagnosis and management of premenstrual syndrome. *Clin. Obstet. Gynecol.* 35:637, 1992.
   There are three key elements of the diagnosis: (1) a symptom complex consistent with the diagnosis, (2) a luteal-phase pattern, and (3) severity sufficient to disrupt the woman's life.

Pathophysiology
3. Rabin, D. S., et al. Hypothalamic-pituitary-adrenal function in patients with premenstrual syndrome. *J. Clin. Endocrinol. Metab.* 71:1158, 1990.
   The authors attempt to explain the regular cycles seen in PMS patients with the irregular cycles associated with depression, anorexia nervosa, and chronic strenuous exercise.
4. Backström, T. Neuroendocrinology of premenstrual syndrome. *Clin. Obstet. Gynecol.* 35:612, 1992.

Several areas within the brain are affected by ovarian steroids. Some of the effects might be mediated via the gamma butyric acid receptor, and others via the genome; other mechanisms are also possible.

5. Chuong, C. J., and Dawson, E. B. Critical evaluation of nutritional factors in the pathophysiology and treatment of premenstrual syndrome. *Clin. Obstet. Gynecol.* 35:679, 1992.
Nutritional supplements can only be considered empiric therapy for PMS.

6. Rapkin, A. J. The role of serotonin in premenstrual syndrome. *Clin. Obstet. Gynecol.* 35:629, 1992.
Many studies have identified a deficiency in the whole-blood serotonin, cerebrospinal fluid serotonin metabolite, and brain serotonin contents, as well as in the platelet uptake of serotonin, in various abnormal behavioral states in which the salient characteristics are depression, anxiety, and aggression.

7. Schmidt, P. J., et al. Thyroid function in women with premenstrual syndrome. *J. Clin. Endocrinol. Metab.* 76:671, 1993.
Irrespective of the role that thyroid axis dysregulation may play in PMS, the use of thyroid hormone in the absence of hypothyroidism in treating PMS is not indicated.

8. Reading, A. E. Cognitive model of premenstrual syndrome. *Clin. Obstet. Gynecol.* 35:693, 1992.
Cognitive therapy creates an awareness of habitual self-defeating thoughts and exchanges them for more constructive alternatives.

9. Yonkers, K. A., and White, K. Premenstrual exacerbation of depression: one process or two? *J. Clin. Psychiatry* 53:8, 1992.
Is PMS an entity distinct from other psychiatric disorders? This study suggests that PMS changes, including dysphoria and irritability, can continue despite effective treatment of major depression.

10. Ramcharan, S., et al. The epidemiology of premenstrual symptoms in a population-based sample of 2650 urban women: attributable risk and risk factors. *J. Clin. Epidemiol.* 45:377, 1992.
The results of this study suggest that severe PMS is not the extreme manifestation of a physiologic gradient of severity in the population but is a discrete disorder affecting a small subgroup, with an actual prevalence of about 1 percent.

11. Hammarbäck, S., Ekholm, U. B., and Bäckström, T. Spontaneous anovulation causing disappearance of cyclical symptoms in women with the premenstrual syndrome. *Acta Endocrinol. (Copenh.)* 125:132, 1991.
This describes significant worsening of symptoms during ovulatory cycles and disappearance of symptoms in anovulatory cycles. Suggests PMS is related to corpus luteum factors.

12. Osborn, M. F., and Gath, D. H. Psychological and physical determinants of premenstrual symptoms before and after hysterectomy. *Psychol. Med.* 20:565, 1990.
PMS symptoms were reduced after hysterectomy even though ovarian function continued normally, suggesting a major role for psychologic factors in many patients.

13. Freeman, E. W., Sondheimer, S. J., and Rickels, K. Effects of medical history factors on symptom severity in women meeting criteria for premenstrual syndrome. *Obstet. Gynecol.* 72:236, 1988.
Stress arising from disagreement on sexual matters aggravates other premenstrual symptoms, which, in turn, exacerbate sexual conflicts. Inclusion of the husband early in the consultation is of great benefit.

14. Bancroft, J., et al. Perimenstrual complaints in women complaining of PMS, menorrhagia, and dysmenorrhea: toward a dismantling of the premenstrual syndrome. *Psychosom. Med.* 55:133, 1993.
The three groups of disorders (PMS, menorrhagia, and dysmenorrhea) showed considerable overlap in a number of symptoms.

Management

15. Allen, S. S., McBride, C. M., and Pirie, P. L. The shortened premenstrual assessment form. *J. Reprod. Med.* 36:769, 1991.

The MOOS Menstrual Distress Questionnaire (MMDQ) and the premenstrual assessment form (PAF) are widely used for assessing premenstrual distress. They are long and require extensive time to complete.

16. Prior, J. C., et al. Conditioning exercise decreases premenstrual symptoms: a prospective, controlled 6-month trial. Fertil. Steril. 47:402, 1987.
Moliminal symptoms were found to decrease in association with increasing exercise, without the development of anovulatory cycles, loss of body weight, or measured decreases in gonadal steroid levels.

17. Graham, C. A., and Sherwin, B. B. A prospective treatment study of premenstrual symptoms using a triphasic oral contraceptive. J. Psychosom. Res. 36:257, 1992.
Premenstrual mastodynia and bloating were significantly reduced in patients treated with triphasic oral contraceptives, but there were no significant changes in any of the mood symptoms.

18. Burnet, R. B., et al. Premenstrual syndrome and spironolactone. Aust. N.Z. J. Obstet. Gynaecol. 31:366, 1991.
In those patients who did respond to spironolactone treatment, there was a significant difference in the androgen levels from the follicular to the luteal phase of the cycle, versus those before treatment was initiated.

19. Mortola, J. F., Girton, L., and Fischer, U. Successful treatment of severe premenstrual syndrome by combined use of gonadotropin-releasing hormone agonist and estrogen/progestin. J. Clin. Endocrinol. Metab. 72:252A, 1991.
The addition of sequential estrogen-progestin did not significantly reduce the effectiveness of the agonist, but did prevent the undesirable consequences of ovarian steroid deficiency.

20. Kleijnen, J., Ter Riet, G., and Knipschild, P. Vitamin B_6 in the treatment of the premenstrual syndrome—a review. Br. J. Obstet. Gynaecol. 97:847, 1990.
The evidence of positive effects from this therapy is weak. A sensory neuropathy may occur even with low-dose pyridoxine. Physicians should tell their patients about appropriate precautions.

21. Giannini, A. J., et al. Clonidine in the treatment of premenstrual syndrome: a subgroup study. J. Clin. Psychiatry 49:62, 1988.
Good results are claimed for this drug, which is an alpha$_2$-agonist that decreases the amount of norepinephrine released at presynaptic sites.

22. Wood, S. H., et al. Treatment of premenstrual syndrome with fluoxetine: a double-blind, placebo-controlled, crossover study. Obstet. Gynecol. 80:339, 1992.
Fluoxetine, a specific serotonin uptake inhibitor, was a highly effective treatment for both the psychologic and physical symptoms in women with no concomitant history of a psychiatric disorder.

23. Chuong, C. J., et al. Clinical trial of naltrexone in premenstrual syndrome. Obstet. Gynecol. 72:332, 1988.
An oral opioid agonist (naltrexone), given before the periovulatory beta-endorphin peak and before withdrawal to maintain a constant level of beta-endorphin, proved helpful in the patients in this study.

24. Glick, R., et al. Treatment of premenstrual dysphoric symptoms in depressed women. J. Am. Med. Wom. Assoc. 46:182, 1991.
Most women with atypical depression who responded to phenelzine or imipramine also found their premenstrual dysphoric symptoms were alleviated.

86. MENOPAUSE
Cecil A. Long

Menopause is defined as the cessation of menstruation due to failure of ovarian follicular development in a woman who had previously had regular menstrual cycles. The average age of menopause in the United States is approximately 51 years old, with a range between ages 45 and 55 years. If a female ceases menstruation before the age of 40, the condition is labeled premature ovarian failure. If this occurs before the age of 30, such patients should undergo karyotyping. The presence of mosaicism with a Y chromosome indicates the need for gonadectomy to prevent the malignant change of testicular components within the gonads. The chance of such malignant tumor transformation approximates 25 percent. Because of the association of premature ovarian failure with autoimmune disorders, evaluation of thyroid and adrenal function as well as selective laboratory tests for the detection of autoimmune disease are indicated.

During embryologic and fetal development, germ cells migrate from the yolk sac to the genital ridge. By 20 weeks of gestation, 6 to 7 million oogonia are present. From this point on, there is a rapid depletion of oogonia by atresia, leaving approximately 1 to 2 million follicles at the time of birth. By puberty, the number of follicles has been reduced to approximately 400,000. By the age of 50 years, the store of oogonia approaches exhaustion.

Symptomatic features of menopause include hot flushes, night sweats, insomnia, and hypoestrogenic changes of the urogenital tract. Hot flushes occur in 50 to 75 percent of the women who reach the age of menopause. The hot flush is characterized by a sensation of intense warmth, especially of the upper body, usually following a prodrome. Episodes can last from 30 seconds to 5 minutes, and rarely even longer. The vasomotor flush is due to an abrupt withdrawal from estrogen. The hot flush coincides with a luteinizing hormone surge. The most valuable laboratory value to determine whether menopause is taking place is an elevated follicule stimulating hormone level (>40 mIU/ml).

The long-term effects of estrogen deprivation in a postmenopausal female include osteoporosis and an increased risk of cardiovascular disease. To counteract these events, estrogen replacement therapy is recommended in all postmenopausal women in whom there is no absolute contraindication to it.

In the United States, approximately 1.5 million fractures (primarily spinal and hip fractures) occur annually as a result of osteoporosis. This translates into approximately 7 to 8 billion dollars spent annually for the health-care costs related to osteoporosis. Menopausal women experience bone loss at the rate of up to 2.5 percent per year after menopause. Black women have greater bone density, and thus osteoporosis does not develop as rapidly in them as it does in Caucasian women. The minimum dosage of estrogen needed to prevent osteoporosis is 0.625 mg of conjugated estrogen or 1 mg of micronized estradiol. Calcium replacement (1500 mg of calcium per day) is also indicated. The combination of estrogen and calcium reduces bone resorption and stimulates osteoblastic activity in the bone. Synthetic calcitonin has also been used for the treatment of osteoporosis. Its mechanism of action is primarily a reduction of osteoclastic activity. However, tolerance to calcitonin develops in 25 to 50 percent of patients. This, combined with the cost of calcitonin, limits its widespread use for the treatment of osteoporosis.

Estrogen has also been found to protect against cardiovascular disease. The results of studies have indicated that doses as low as 0.625 mg of conjugated estrogen daily significantly lower low-density lipoprotein levels and increase high-density lipoprotein levels. Epidemiologic studies have demonstrated that estrogen use decreases the relative risk of ischemic heart disease by approximately 50 percent.

Estrogen for replacement therapy is available in several forms, and several regimens have been developed for administration. The dose and form of estrogen depend on the reason for estrogen replacement, as well as the age at which estrogen replacement is required. Younger women who need estrogen replacement because of surgical castration or premature ovarian failure need much higher doses than do women who reach menopause. These groups of younger patients need up to 2.5 mg of conjugated estrogen or 2 to 3 mg of micronized estrogen per day in order to achieve symptomatic relief of the hypoestrogenic effects. In the menopausal patient, a daily estrogen dose of 0.625 mg of conjugated estrogen or 1 to 2 mg of micronized estrogen (estradiol) confers both bone and cardiovascular protection. The doses must be titrated in order to completely resolve other symptoms of menopause, including hot flushes and insomnia, and to counteract atrophy of the urogenital tract. In women who have a uterus, it is important to add progestin to the estrogen replacement regimen to counteract the effects of unopposed estrogen on the endometrium, as endometrial hyperplasia and, ultimately, adenocarcinoma may ensue in the patient who receives estrogen only. Medroxyprogesterone acetate (10 mg), taken for 7 days, reduces these changes to approximately 3 percent. Treatment with progestin for 10 to 13 days reduces the incidence to essentially zero. The regimen most widely recommended for menopausal women consists of 25 days of estrogen therapy combined with 10 days of progestin therapy. Some dosages used consist of daily estrogen therapy, with 10 days of progestin therapy starting on the first of each month. Other authors advocate continuous progestin therapy (2.5 to 5.0 mg per day) throughout the entire cycle. Parenteral forms of replacement include transdermal estrogen therapy as well as transvaginal delivery, and both provide protection against osteoporosis and vascular disease.

Adverse effects of estrogen replacement therapy include gallbladder disease, thromboembolic disease, and a potential increased risk of breast cancer. Estrogen replacement has been found to double the incidence of gallbladder disease. Estrogen therapy is also associated with thromboembolic changes that exhibit a dose-response relationship. However, several studies have shown there is no increase in the incidence of thrombosis when minimal estrogen doses are used (0.625 mg of conjugated estrogen or 1 mg of micronized estradiol). Use of the vaginal and transdermal routes of delivery avoids the hepatic "first pass" effect. There is much controversy surrounding a potential increased incidence of breast cancer associated with estrogen replacement. Most studies have shown this is not so, though smoking appears to potentiate all the adverse effects of estrogen replacement therapy. Contraindications to estrogen replacement include unexplained vaginal bleeding, breast cancer, endometrial carcinoma, estrogen-related thromboembolic processes, and active liver failure. Estrogen replacement may be considered if these disorders resolve or if the patient with endometrial or breast cancer survives more than 2 years with no evidence of disease recurrence. For all patients, the known risks and potential benefits must be carefully weighed.

Many women undergo a perimenopausal period lasting from 2 to 5 years before menopause. In this period, a woman begins to experience a change in the length of her cycles as well as the effects of estrogen deprivation. For these women, provided they are nonsmokers, the newer low-dose oral contraceptive pills have proved to be effective in this transitional period. Not only do they provide adequate estrogen replacement, but they also offer a method of contraception. Once the patient reaches the menopausal age, she may switch to conventional estrogen-progestin replacement.

General
1. Erlik, Y., Meldrum, D. R., and Judd, H. L. Estrogen levels in postmenopausal women with hot flashes. *Obstet. Gynecol.* 59:403, 1982.
   The pathophysiology of hot flashes in postmenopausal women is discussed.
2. Brenner, P. F. The menopausal syndrome. *Obstet. Gynecol.* 77:6S, 1988.
   A current review of the menopausal syndrome.
3. Gambrell, R. D., Jr. The menopause: benefits and risks of estrogen-progestogen replacement therapy. *Fertil. Steril.* 37:457, 1982.
   Hormonal replacement therapy in the form of continuous estrogen-progestin treatment is discussed.
4. Willett, W., et al. Cigarette smoking, relative weight, and menopause. *Am. J. Epidemiol.* 117:651, 1983.
   The negative effects of smoking in the menopausal patient are considered.
5. Session, D. R., Kelly, A. C., and Jewelewicz, R. Current concepts in estrogen replacement therapy in the menopause. *Fertil. Steril.* 59:277, 1993.
   The daily administration of an estrogen and progestin eliminates the withdrawal bleeding and increases patient compliance.

Osteoporosis
6. Lindsay, R. The menopause: sex steroids and osteoporosis. *Clin. Obstet. Gynecol.* 30:847, 1987.

This describes the changes in serum sex steroid levels that lead to osteoporosis in the postmenopausal female.

7. Raisz, L. G. Local and systemic factors in the pathogenesis of osteoporosis. *N. Engl. J. Med.* 318:818, 1988.
   A comprehensive review of osteoporosis.
8. Field, C. S., et al. Preventive effects of transdermal 17β-estradiol on osteoporotic changes after surgical menopause: a two-year placebo-controlled trial. *Am. J. Obstet. Gynecol.* 168:114, 1993.
   Transdermal estrogen is a safe and effective regimen for preventing bone loss in recently postmenopausal women.
9. Kiel, D. P., et al. Hip fracture and the use of estrogens in postmenopausal women. The Framingham study. *N. Engl. J. Med.* 317:1169, 1987.
   A follow-up of the Framingham study on the role of estrogens in the prevention of hip fracture.
10. Civitelli, R., et al. Bone turnover in postmenopausal osteoporosis. Effect of calcitonin treatment. *J. Clin. Invest.* 82:1268, 1988.
    The effects of calcitonin therapy for the treatment of postmenopausal osteoporosis are discussed.

Arteriosclerosis
11. Witteman, J. C. M., et al. Increased risk of atherosclerosis in women after the menopause. *Br. Med. J.* 298:642, 1989.
    Women with a natural menopause were found to face a 3.4 greater risk of atherosclerosis than did premenopausal women; women who had undergone a bilateral oophorectomy had a 5.5 times greater risk.
12. Sullivan, J. M., et al. Postmenopausal estrogen use and coronary atherosclerosis. *Ann. Intern. Med.* 108:358, 1987.
    Postmenopausal women who receive estrogens have a reduced risk of coronary artery disease.
13. Paganini-Hill, A., Ross, R. K., and Henderson, B. E. Postmenopausal oestrogen treatment and stroke: a prospective study. *Br. Med. J.* 2:519, 1988.
    The risk of stroke in women receiving estrogen is reduced compared with that in women not taking estrogens.

87. GONADAL DYSGENESIS
Stephen R. Lincoln

Gonadal dysgenesis is described as the involution of germ cells soon after migration into the undifferentiated gonad early in embryonic life, resulting in fibrous streaks where the ovaries are usually found. Loss or mutation of the genetic material essential for gonadal development is the cause of the dysgenesis, and a wide range of karyotypes can be found in affected patients. The most common group includes phenotypic females who display the short stature, webbed neck, primary amenorrhea, and sexual infantilism originally described by Turner. Other forms of gonadal dysgenesis may be categorized as mosaic chromosome abnormalities, structured abnormalities of the second sex chromosome, or pure gonadal dysgenesis.

Reportedly, one X chromosome is completely absent in half of the patients with gonadal dysgenesis, resulting in the 45X karyotype referred to as Turner's syndrome. The most common feature encountered is shortness of stature, with virtually all patients less than 60 inches tall. A variety of other anomalies may be present, including a short webbed neck, shielded chest with wide-set nipples, a low hairline, a high-arched palate, epicanthal folds, cubitus valgus (a wide carrying angle of the arms), hypoplastic nail beds, shortening of the fourth or fifth metacarpals, and renal anomalies. Cardiac anomalies may also occur, including coarctation of the aorta, atrial septal defects, and valvular defects. Lymphedema of the extremities can occur (30%) at birth, which may be referred to as Bonnevie-Ullrich syndrome.

Treatment of these individuals is focused on obtaining maximum height followed by the development of secondary sexual characteristics. If large doses of cyclic steroid hormones are given before the total height has been reached, premature closure of the epiphysis may occur. For this reason, only small doses of estrogen (0.3 mg/day on days 1 to 21) are given, together with cyclic medroxyprogesterone acetate (5 mg/day on days 12 to 21), beginning at the usual age of menarche (12–13 years), and maximum growth is thereby achieved. After a year or more of low-dose estrogen therapy, total replacement doses of estrogen and progesterone are given in a cyclic manner to maximize breast development and genital tract maturation.

Synthetic growth hormone, produced by recombinant DNA technology beginning in 1985, has been used successfully to augment growth in patients with Turner's syndrome. Dosages vary between 0.5 and 1.0 IU/kg/week, given subcutaneously in three divided doses beginning around age 12. The long-term effects of growth hormone given at an earlier age are currently under investigation. In addition to hormonal therapy, patients with Turner's syndrome should undergo a thorough cardiac and renal evaluation because of the increased risks of anomalies in these organs. Other disorders may occur later in life, including diabetes, hypertension, and inflammatory bowel disease.

A second group of patients with the stigmata of gonadal dysgenesis are sex chromatin positive and have some form of mosaicism or structural abnormality of the X chromosome. Deletion of the short (XXp−) or long (XXq−) arm and an isochrome for the long arm of the X chromosome (XXqi) are the most common structural anomalies, and may exist with or without mosaicism. Interestingly, the stature in patients with deletion of the long arm without mosaicism is normal despite gonadal dysgenesis and sexual infantilism. These findings suggest that stature may be governed by genes on the short arm, while ovarian development may be determined by genes on both the long and short arm of the X chromosome.

Mosaicism, due to a mitotic error, results in the development of two or more cell lines in one individual. The most common form of mosaicism is XO/XX, with resultant sex chromatin–positive material. Varying percentages of the amount of XO mosaicism reflect the varying degrees of physical stigmata characteristic of classic Turner's syndrome. Patients with mosaicism are not always short, may menstruate, and may even become pregnant.

Another form of mosaicism with gonadal dysgenesis exists in patients with sex chromatin–negative studies. This group includes patients with either mosaicism and a normal Y chromosome (such as XO/XY, XO/XYY, or XO/XY/XYY) or those with a structurally abnormal Y chromosome. As a consequence of its effect on gonadal differentiation, a Y-bearing cell line modifies the typical female phenotype of the syndrome by causing a variable degree of masculine differentiation of the genital tract.

Clinically, most patients have at least one fallopian tube and a uterus, and many patients have sexual ambiguity of the genitalia. When a Y chromosome is found in patients with gonadal dysgenesis, there is an approximate 20 percent chance of gonadal malignancy. Gonadoblastoma is the most common neoplasm found. Prophylactic gonadectomy is indicated in patients with streak or dysgenetic gonads who have a Y chromosome.

The disorder in individuals who are phenotypic females with a 46XX or 46XY karyotype, who have rudimentary streak gonads and remain sexually infertile, but are of normal stature and lack the somatic stigmata of Turner's syndrome, is referred to as pure gonadal dysgenesis. These patients often come to medical attention at the time of expected puberty because of primary amenorrhea and are found to have elevated gonadotropin levels, as would individuals with prepubertal castration. The body habitus is eunuchoid. The 46XY gonadal dysgenesis was first described by Swyer and the syndrome is often referred to by his name. Incomplete forms of gonadal dysgenesis result in varying degrees of virilization and sexual ambiguity.

Because of the dysgenetic Y chromosome involved, the incidence of gonadal neoplasms is high and prophylactic extirpation is recommended. The sex rearing of patients with the incomplete form of 46XY gonadal dysgenesis is determined by the extent of genital ambiguity and the age at diagnosis. Patients raised as females should be placed on estrogen replacement therapy at the age of 12 or 13 and eventually cycled with progesterone, as previously outlined. In patients raised as males, testosterone replacement therapy is begun at the age of puberty.

Gonadal Dysgenesis
1. Grumbach, M. M., and Conte, F. A. Disorders of Sexual Differentiation. In J. D. Wilson and D. W. Foster (eds.), *Williams Textbook of Endocrinology*. Philadelphia: Saunders, 1992.
   The section of this chapter entitled The Syndrome of Gonadal Dysgenesis: Turner Syndrome and Its Variants represents a comprehensive review of gonadal dysgenesis.
2. Jaffe, R. B. Disorders of Sexual Development. In S. S. C. Yen and R. B. Jaffe (eds.), *Reproductive Endocrinology* (3rd ed). Philadelpia: Saunders, 1991, Pp. 484–490.
   In the section on "Gonadal Dysgenesis," the topic is comprehensively reviewed.
3. Tsutsumi, O., et al. Y chromosome analysis and laparoscopic surgery in XY pure gonadal dysgenesis: a case report and a review of the literature. *Asia-Oceania J. Obstet. Gynaecol.* 19:37, 1993.
   The sex-determining region Y is a gene located in the sex-determining region of the Y chromosome, which has many of the properties expected of the testis-determining factor.

88. ANDROGEN INSENSITIVITY
Stephen R. Lincoln

Androgen insensitivity results from defects that can occur at any step in the mechanism of action of androgens on their target cells. When androgens cannot effectively induce virilization in a genetic male (46XY), these individuals are termed male pseudohermaphrodites and are phenotypically female. When androgen actions are incompletely impaired, a spectrum of phenotypes may arise, ranging from a severely undervirilized male to a normally virilized male who is only infertile or even a fertile man who is minimally undervirilized.

By understanding the embryology of genital development, the clinician is able to interpret the range of presentations of patients with androgen insensitivity. Until 7 weeks' gestation, the fetal gonad is indifferent and both wolffian (male) and müllerian (female) structures are present. If the testis does not produce testosterone and anti-müllerian substance (AMS), the wolffian structures regress and the müllerian structures form the internal genitalia, including the fallopian tube, uterus, cervix, and upper vagina. When a normal Y chromosome is present, production of the testis-determining factor (TDF) from the long arm of the Y chromosome triggers the differentiation of the gonad into a testis. Recent evidence points to the SRY region of the long arm of the Y chromosome as being responsible for governing TDF production. The Sertoli cells of the testes secrete AMS, thereby inducing regression of the müllerian structures. The Leydig cells of the testis produce testosterone, which directs differentiation of the wolffian structures into the vas deferens, epididymis, and seminal vesicles. Testosterone is also converted intracellularly to dihydrotestosterone (DHT) by the enzyme 5-alpha-reductase. DHT induces virilization of the external genitalia (which in the absence of DHT would develop as female) to produce male genitalia and the prostate.

All patients with androgen insensitivity are genetically 46XY, but the disorder may be grouped into complete and incomplete forms. Individuals with the complete form of androgen insensitivity are phenotypic females who present with primary amenorrhea and normal breast development. These patients have phenotypic female external genitalia, a blind vaginal pouch, absent or vestigial müllerian structures (uterus and tubes), and testes, which are located in the labia, inguinal canal, or intraabdominally. Wolffian duct derivatives are usually absent, but vestiges may exist in a rudimentary or hypoplastic form. Patients with complete androgen insensitivity have little if no pubic, axillary, or facial hair, and this form is often referred to as testicular feminization. Although often missed at birth and early childhood, the diagnosis should be suspected in the phenotypic female infant with an inguinal hernia and a testislike mass in the labia or inguinal region.

The incomplete form of androgen resistance includes a heterogeneous group of 46XY individuals who exhibit variable degrees of masculinization. All affected males lack müllerian structures, and wolffian duct derivatives are sometimes present but usually hypoplastic. The external genitalia may be ambiguous and range in form from a blind vaginal pouch to a hypoplastic male appearance to normal. The most common presentation found in infancy consists of an apparent male but with hypospadias, a small penis, and often cryptorchidism. These patients experience puberty but do not androgenize completely and frequently have gynecomastia. This combination of ambiguous genitalia and only small degrees of androgenization is often referred to as Lub's syndrome, whereas the disorder in phenotypic males whose undervirilization is minimal is referred to as Reifenstein's syndrome.

The androgen insensitivity syndrome is an X-linked recessive disorder. Hormonal profiles in such patients reveal elevated luteinizing hormone (LH) and testosterone, normal follicle-stimulating hormone (FSH), and increased estradiol (for male) levels. The increased secretion of estradiol as well as the peripheral conversion of elevated androgens to estrogens result in the formation of secondary female sexual characteristics.

The cause of the androgen insensitivity can occur at any step of the mechanism of action of androgens on their target cells. The androgen resistance may be due to insufficient numbers of androgen receptors in target tissues, defective receptor function, or a postreceptor defect. The gene responsible for encoding the androgen receptor has been identified on the long arm of the X chromosome. Absence or decreased numbers of androgen receptors may be caused by a deletion, insertion, or mutation in the gene. There may also be normal numbers of the androgen receptors, but the qualitative function of these receptors may be decreased or absent. Hence, this range of defects explains the variety of phenotypes seen, from the complete form of androgen insensitivity with female features to the incomplete form consisting of minimal undervirilization of the male phenotype.

A form of incomplete male pseudohermaphrodism often included in discussions on androgen insensitivity is an entity referred to as 5-alpha-reductase deficiency. These individuals with 46XY chromosomes and ambiguous genitalia are usually found at birth to have a small hypospadiac phallus and blind vaginal pouch. The testes are normally differentiated but located in the labioscrotal folds or inguinal canal. The internal male ducts are fully developed and end either in the vaginal pouch or the perineum. Because of the deficiency in the enzyme that converts testosterone to DHT, the embryologic structures responsive to testosterone (wolffian system) develop normally but the structures responsive to DHT (external genitalia and peripheral target tissues) virilize incompletely. At puberty, these individuals undergo marked, although selective, masculinization, including deepening of the voice, an increase in muscle mass, and enlargement of phallus. This disorder is very similar to the incomplete forms of androgen insensitivity, but gynecomastia does not occur at puberty. The 5-alpha-reductase deficiency syndrome is inherited as an autosomal recessive trait, unlike the X-linked recessive inheritance pattern of androgen insensitivity.

The diagnosis of complete androgen insensitivity can be established after puberty based on clinical criteria alone. An adolescent with breast development, a short, blind-ending vagina without a cervix, amenorrhea, and scant pubic and axillary hair has complete androgen insensitivity that can be confirmed by the finding of a 46XY karyotype. The diagnosis of complete androgen insensitivity in infants younger than 6 months or in children can be made when a 46XY female is found to have an inguinal hernia or labial mass together with elevated LH or testosterone levels, or both, without virilization. Incomplete androgen insensitivity may be more difficult to diagnose. If the methods are available, fibroblast cultures and molecular analysis are helpful for demonstrating androgen receptor defects. Measuring the levels of LH and testosterone (and their precursors) after the administration of human chorionic gonadotropin may also discern androgen insensitivity from other forms of male pseudohermaphrodism, such as 5-alpha-reductase deficiency (discussed already) or defects in testosterone biosynthesis (not discussed). Patients with 5-alpha-reductase deficiency will have elevated testosterone-DHT ratios, whereas patients with defects in testosterone biosynthesis will have elevated levels of precursors (dehydroepiandrosterone sulfate and androstenedione).

The therapy for patients with complete androgen insensitivity centers around reinforcing the female gender and identity. Informing the patient of the genetic karyotype is rarely indicated. The testis should be removed due to the risk of malignancy, but the risk is low before the age of 25. Therefore, surgical correction should generally be delayed until after puberty to allow the formation of secondary sexual characteristics. If the vagina is too short for intercourse, manual dilatation with a prosthesis or surgical repair in the form of a McIndoe vaginoplasty is indicated at the time when adult relationships are expected to begin.

The therapy for incomplete forms of androgen insensitivity depends on the degree of masculinization of the external genitalia. Sex rearing depends on the patient's age at diagnosis and the degree of ambiguity. Patients with minimal degrees of undervirilization are best raised as males, but patients with ambiguous genitalia may best be reared as females because of the varying response to high-dose androgens and the gynecomastia that occurs at puberty. Gonadectomy is often indicated, and plastic repair of the genitalia may also be necessary. If gonadectomy is performed before puberty, estrogen replacement beginning at age 12 to 13 should be instituted to ensure development of female secondary sexual characteristics.

Androgen Sensitivity Syndromes
1. Grumbach, M. M., and Conte, F. A. Disorders of Sex Differentiation. In J. D. Wilson and D. W. Foster (eds.), *Williams Textbook of Endocrinology* (8th ed.). Philadelphia: Saunders, 1992.
2. Santen, R. J. Male Hypogonadism. In S. S. C. Yen and R. B. Jaffe (eds.), *Reproductive Endocrinology—Physiology, Pathophysiology and Clinical Management* (3rd ed.). Philadelphia: Saunders, 1991.
3. Jaffe, R. B. Disorders of Sexual Development. In S. S. C. Yen and R. B. Jaffe (eds.), *Reproductive Endocrinology—Physiology, Pathophysiology and Clinical Management* (3rd ed.), Philadelphia: Saunders, 1991.
   The above three works are comprehensive reviews of androgen insensitivity, including the complete and incomplete forms as well as 5-alpha-reductase deficiency.
4. Griffin, J. E., et al. The syndromes of androgen resistance. *N. Engl. J. Med.* 302:198, 1980.
   A review of the spectrum of androgen resistance.
5. Lee, P. A., Brown, T. R., and La Torre, H. A. Diagnosis of the partial androgen insensitivity syndrome during infancy. *J.A.M.A.* 25:2207, 1986.
6. Nagel, B. A., Lippe, B. M., and Griffen, J. E. Androgen resistance in the neonate: use of hormones of hypothalamic-pituitary-gonadal axis for diagnosis. *J. Pediatr.* 109:486, 1986.
   These two articles review the diagnosis of androgen insensitivity in infants and children.
7. Castro-Magana, M., Angulo, M., and Uy, J. Male hypogonadism with gynecomastia caused by late-onset deficiency of testicular 17-ketosteroid reductase. *N. Engl. J. Med.* 328:1297, 1993.
   A late-onset form of testicular 17-ketosteroid reductase deficiency can cause gynecomastia and hypogonadism in men.

Molecular Genetics of the Androgen Receptor
8. Brown, C. J., et al. Androgen receptor locus in the human X chromosome: regional localization to Xq11−12 and description of a DNA polymorphism. *Am. J. Hum. Genet.* 44:264, 1989.

9. French, F. S., et al. The molecular basis of androgen insensitivity. *Recent Prog. Horm. Res.* 46:1, 1990.
   Two articles reviewing the findings from recent research into the DNA sequencing of the androgen receptor to the X chromosome.
10. McPaul, M. J., et al. The spectrum of mutations in the androgen receptor gene that causes androgen resistance. *J. Clin. Endocrinol. Metab.* 76:17, 1993.
    This discusses the findings from the molecular biologic analysis of androgen receptor gene mutations. The phenotypic abnormalities are the result of receptor function impairment or decreases in receptor abundance, or both.

Mechanisms of Sexual Differentiation
11. Jost, A., et al. Studies on sex differentiation in mammals. *Recent Prog. Horm. Res.* 29:1, 1973.
    A classic review of the role of the gonad in sexual differentiation.
12. Wilson, J. D. Testosterone uptake by the urogenital tract of the rabbit embryo. *Endocrinology* 92:1192, 1973.
13. Wilson, J. D., et al. The role of gonadal steroids in sexual differentiation. *Recent Prog. Horm. Res.* 37:1, 1981.
    The author of the above two articles discusses the molecular and biochemical aspects of sex differentiation.
14. Koopman, P., et al. Male development of chromosomally female mice transgenic for SRY. *Nature* 351:117, 1991.
    The reports on recent evidence indicating that the location of the testis-determining factor on the Y chromosome is in the SRY region.

XVI. GYNECOLOGIC ONCOLOGY

89. NONNEOPLASTIC AND INTRAEPITHELIAL NEOPLASTIC VULVAL CONDITIONS
Michel E. Rivlin

Primary vulvar disease may be congenital, inflammatory, or dermatologic, owing to abnormal epithelial growth (dystrophy), or it may result from a neoplastic change. The vulva is a mucocutaneous structure, and the vulvar dermatoses are a heterogeneous group of disorders linked simply by their common location. They cannot properly be distinguished in terms of color, vesiculation, or the presence of erosions or ulcerations because these overlap in many diseases. A definitive diagnosis is mandatory, even though the treatment is often similar, so that therapeutic and prognostic guidelines can be devised. Biopsy findings frequently provide or support a diagnosis, and the procedure should not be long delayed.

Eczematous dermatitis refers to a category of diseases characterized by scaly or vesicular red papules or plaques that often itch or burn. Allergic contact dermatitis resulting from sensitization to a particular allergen is a member of this group. Exposure may exist for years before the allergy develops. Acute cases are treated with wet-to-dry dressings using Burow's solution in conjunction with the topical application of steroids. Chronic contact dermatitis responds best to an ointment-based midpotency topical steroid. Irritant dermatitis results from contact with an irritating substance, commonly urine and feces, soap residues, or rough clothing. Treatment in this instance focuses on removal of the irritant and the institution of local hygiene, including cleaning the genital area with warm water and patting it dry with a soft towel. Topical low-potency steroids are also helpful.

In contrast to the aforementioned rashes that itch, lichen simplex chronicus (neurodermatitis) is an itch that becomes a rash. Irritant dermatitis may progress to lichen simplex chronicus as a result of prolonged scratching or rubbing, leading to epidermal hyperplasia and increased sensitivity. Penetrating the thickened epidermis that forms requires a moderate-strength topical steroid, and several months of therapy may be necessary to effect cure.

The papulosquamous dermatoses, including psoriasis and seborrhea, vary in appearance in different parts of the body. On glabrous (smooth and bare) skin, the lesions are raised (papular) and scaly (squamous). In the intertriginous areas, scale does not accumulate and the lesions appear shiny and red. Psoriasis is an inherited disorder in which there are discrete scaling plaques, usually affecting extensor surfaces. Inverse psoriasis involves the axillae, vulva, and umbilicus. Prolonged treatment may be necessary using a midpotency steroid. Because psoriasis is a hyperplastic disorder, steroid atrophy is not a problem. Seborrheic dermatitis of the intertriginous areas, including the vulva, is manifested as red, moist, and poorly marginated plaques. The differential diagnosis includes the eczematous dermatoses and candidiasis. Response to low-potency steroid creams is excellent.

Whatever topical steroid is used, it should be applied in a thin coat so that the skin just glistens. Two major factors account for potency. First is the chemical composition—potency is greatly increased by fluorination. Second is the base—the more occlusive, the more steroid is absorbed; thus, ointments are excellent for the management of thick chronic dermatitis but are poor choices for the treatment of inflamed skin that requires lotions or creams. Both 1% and 2.5% hydrocortisone are examples of a low-potency steroid cream; 0.1% triamcinolone acetonide is an example of a midpotency steroid cream; and 0.5% triamcinolone acetonide is an example of a high-potency steroid cream. Because itching is often worse at night and scratching is more possible in bed, a dose of diphenhydramine or hydroxyzine is useful at bedtime.

The vulvar dystrophies are chronic disorders of epithelial growth that may cause overt changes in the appearance of the vulvar skin. The disorder may be either localized or generalized, resulting in thickening or thinning and changes in color. The International Societies of Gynecologic Pathologists and for the Study of Vulvar Disease have classified the dystrophies as either hyperplastic, lichen sclerosus, or mixed, with or without cellular atypia. Atypia is classified as mild, moderate, or severe. More recently, the term *hyperplastic dystrophy* was replaced by *squamous cell hyperplasia*. The term *mixed dystrophy* was abandoned in favor of the recognition that cases of lichen sclerosus may have hyperplastic areas without the presence of another disease. Cases in which atypia is present are now all classified as vulvar intraepithelial neoplasia (VIN), but both diagnoses should be reported.

Squamous cell hyperplasia (hyperplastic dystrophy) tends to be symmetric. The skin in this disorder appears coarse or thickened and white. Microscopically, epithelial thickening (hyperplasia), thickening of the keratin layer (hyperkeratosis), elongation and widening of the epithelial rete ridges (acanthosis), the retention of nuclear material in the keratin layer (parakeratosis), and varying degrees of chronic inflammation within the dermis are seen. Some lesions that exhibit inflammatory changes fulfill the criteria for lichen simplex chronicus and should not be confused with squamous cell hyperplasia. If atypia is present, it begins in the deeper layers and becomes more severe as the process extends superficially. In the absence of atypia, relief of pruritus is the major objective of treatment. A fluorinated compound in a cream or ointment base applied twice daily should cause the lesion to regress within 4 to 8 weeks. Combining the steroid with crotamiton (Eurax) in a cream base is a particularly effective treatment.

Lichen sclerosus is the most common form of white vulvar lesions. It can appear on areas such as the neck and trunk but is usually confined to the anogenital area. It commences with discrete maculopapular lesions that gradually coalesce and destroy the vulvar structures. In the later stages, there is loss of architecture and it exhibits a white atrophic cigarette-paper appearance, often in an hourglass distribution. Symptoms include burning, itching, dryness, and dyspareunia, which may be intermittent or unremitting. Microscopically, hyperkeratosis and epithelial thinning are seen, and a pink-staining acellular collagenous layer appears under the epidermis. The elastic fibers are absent, and a band of chronic inflammatory cells can be seen in the middermal area. Although the etiology of lichen sclerosus is unknown, there is evidence suggesting a familial incidence and an underlying autoimmune disorder. Hormonal status appears to play a role, and it is most common in postmenopausal women, although it does occur in prepubescent girls and its male equivalent, balanitis xerotica obliterans, is most often seen in prepubescent boys. The most successful treatment consists of 2% testosterone ointment, which is applied twice daily until the disease is under control, then weekly, and often indefinitely, although the disease may resolve spontaneously. The testosterone may produce troublesome masculinizing side effects; if these are severe, progesterone cream may be a helpful alternative. If severe pruritus is present, a corticosteroid preparation can also be used and alcohol injections may be considered for the more intractable cases. Women with squamous cell hyperplasia occurring in the setting of lichen sclerosus (mixed dystrophy) constitute a distinct group of patients who are at higher risk of developing invasive cancer, and, for this reason, require regular histologic assessment. Both corticosteroid and testosterone preparations may be used in a combined or alternate-day regimen for the management of mixed lesions. Once the hyperplastic lesions have receded, the testosterone treatment should be continued. Vulvar dystrophies without atypia are benign lesions whose primary treatment is medical. Recurrence follows surgical treatment in at least half of the patients who undergo vulvectomy, usually with no attendant change in symptomatology. A high incidence of recurrence has also been noted in association with laser therapy.

VIN is classified as I through III (severe atypia and carcinoma in situ [CIS]), in a manner similar to the system used for classifying cervical intraepithelial neoplasia (CIN). The incidence of VIN has increased sharply, and the mean age of affected women has decreased from over 50 years to under 38 years. There is an association between VIN and sexually transmitted infections and other forms of genital tract neoplasia. Of patients with VIN III, 30 percent have synchronous or metachronous neoplasia at another genital site. At least 20 percent of women with VIN III have associated CIN III. The tendency for multicentric disease to develop obviously influences management. The etiology of VIN is unknown, but the increased incidence parallels the increase in the incidence of genital infections with human papillomavirus (HPV). Molecular hybridization studies have shown HPV deoxyribonucleic acid (DNA) in 70 percent of the patients with VIN III and in 50 percent of those with vulvar carcinomas.

A continuum from preinvasive to invasive vulval neoplasia has not been clearly established, and the malignant potential is uncertain. The disease is as likely to regress as to progress, although the risk of progression is probably less than 5 percent. In older women, VIN tends to be unifocal and the malignant potential appears to be greater. Immunosuppressed women also seem to be at higher risk of rapid progression. Most VIN III lesions show an aneuploid DNA content, suggesting a malignant potential. About half of the patients are asymptomatic. Pruritus, burning, and pain are the most common complaints in the remainder. The appearance is variable: 60 percent are white plaques and about 15 percent are hyperpigmented. The cytologic changes that take place in mild atypia include enlarged hyperchromatic nuclei; in moderate atypia, there is coarse chromatin clumping. In the moderate form, the increased cellularity and cellular disarray are confined to the inner two thirds of the epithelium. In severe atypia, more than two thirds are involved, cells of the parabasal type are found near the surface, and chromatin clumping is moderately coarse and irregular. CIS is characterized by full-thickness cellular disorientation (with the exception of the most superficial keratinized layers), in conjunction with giant cells, multinucleated cells, individual cell keratinization, corps ronds formation (a pale halo of cytoplasm around a pyknotic nucleus), abnormal mitoses, and squamous "pearls" at the tips of the rete pegs. Parakeratosis and hyperkeratosis may be present, and there is usually an inflammatory response in the dermis.

The study of biopsy specimens obtained for diagnosis is aided by the use of a nuclear stain, 1% toluidine blue. The dye is applied, allowed to set, and then decolorized with 1% acetic acid. The nonulcerated areas that remain blue are probably parakeratotic and, thus, atypical. Although helpful, there are unfortunately high false-positive and false-negative rates associated with this technique. Colposcopy, following the application of 5% acetic acid, is more accurate. Biopsy specimens are taken from "acetowhite" areas using a Keyes punch or biopsy forceps under local anesthesia.

The three preferred treatments for VIN are wide local excision, carbon dioxide laser vaporization, and, in unusual circumstances, a skinning vulvectomy with a split-thickness skin graft. Laser ablation is well adapted to hairless areas and surgical excision, to hairy sites; the two procedures may thus be combined to advantage. Recurrence of VIN is common regardless of the therapy, but can be managed again using conservative therapy.

The symptom complex of chronic burning vulvar discomfort is termed vulvodynia. In some cases, point tenderness that is localized within the vestibule, together with severe pain in response to vestibular touch and physical findings confined to vestibular erythema, is termed the vulvar vestibulitis syndrome, a form of vulvodynia. In general, no obvious physical cause should be found, thus ruling out the presence of vulvar dermatoses, cyclic candidiasis, and squamous cell hyperplasia. Some cases may be associated with a subclinical HPV infection. Because of the lack of physical signs, many of these women are told that their problem is psychogenic, especially when dyspareunia is a major component. Response to therapy has been variable, with good results claimed for both laser therapy and surgical excision of the vulvar tissue containing the vestibular glands.

Squamous Cell Hyperplasia/Lichen Sclerosus
1. Report of the Committee on Terminology. New nomenclature for vulvar disease. *Am. J. Obstet. Gynecol.* 160:769, 1989.
   What's in a name? In this context, it can mean the difference between treatment using an ointment and a vulvectomy.
2. Soper, J. T., and Creasman, W. T. Vulvar dystrophies. *Clin. Obstet. Gynecol.* 29:431, 1986.
   Two percent testosterone propionate in a petroleum ointment is not commercially available but can be compounded by mixing 3 ml of 100 mg/ml of testosterone propionate in sesame oil with 12 gm of petrolatum.
3. Ridley, C. M. Lichen sclerosus et atrophicus. *Arch. Dermatol.* 123:457, 1987.

The classic features comprise homogenized collagen with an underlying bandlike lymphocytic infiltrate.

4. Micheletti, L., et al. Cellular atypia in vulvar dystrophies. *J. Reprod. Med.* 33:539, 1988.
The total frequency of this finding was 9.4 percent. Atypia was found almost exclusively in hyperplastic areas. Epithelial changes suggestive of HPV were found in 14.2 percent of the cases of atypical dystrophy.

5. Ayhan, A., et al. Vulvar dystrophies: an evaluation. *Aust. N.Z. J. Obstet. Gynaecol.* 29:250, 1989.
Medical treatment should not be used in those patients with findings of atypia on biopsy specimens; these patients require surgical intervention.

6. Leibowitch, M., et al. The epithelial changes associated with squamous cell carcinoma of the vulva: a review of the clinical, histological and viral findings in 78 women. *Br. J. Obstet. Gynaecol.* 97:1135, 1990.
Lichen sclerosus was found in 61 percent of the patients and half of these also had VIN III. Epithelial hyperplasia was noted in 25 percent of the women with lichen sclerosus.

7. Dalziel, K. L., and Wojnarowska, F. Long-term control of vulval lichen sclerosus after treatment with a potent topical steroid cream. *J. Reprod. Med.* 38:25, 1993.
This treatment proved safe and effective with no long-term cutaneous side effects.

8. Helm, K. F., Gibson, L. E., and Muller, S. A. Lichen sclerosus et atrophicus in children and young adults. *Pediatr. Dermatol.* 8:97, 1991.
The condition resolved in 44 percent of the 52 patients who were observed for 7.5 years.

Vulvar Intraepithelial Neoplasia

9. Park, J. S., et al. HPV-16 viral transcripts in vulvar neoplasia: preliminary studies. *Gynecol. Oncol.* 42:250, 1991.
Specific HPV types are strongly associated with intraepithelial neoplasia and invasive cancer of the cervix. In contrast, the role of HPVs in the pathogenesis of vulvar carcinoma is poorly understood.

10. Woodruff, J. D. Carcinoma in situ of the vulva. *Clin. Obstet. Gynecol.* 34:669, 1991.
VIN rarely progresses to cancer in patients under 50 unless they are immunosuppressed; in women in the seventh and eighth decades, VIN lesions are precursors of invasive cancer.

11. Hoffman, M. S., et al. Laser vaporization for vulvar intraepithelial neoplasia III. *J. Reprod. Med.* 37:135, 1992.
Complications such as bleeding, pain, and scarring are uncommon, but recurrence and the need for repeated treatments are common. Laser vaporization is particularly useful for the treatment of multifocal lesions.

12. Thuesen, B., Andreasson, B., and Bock, J. E. Sexual function and somatopsychic reactions after local excision of vulvar intra-epithelial neoplasia. *Acta Obstet. Gynaecol. Scand.* 71:126, 1992.
Local excision results in better-preserved sexual function, causes fewer psychologic problems, and yields a better cosmetic result than does simple vulvectomy, which should be used, if possible, only in the older patient who is no longer sexually active.

Vulvodynia and the Vulvar Vestibulitis Syndrome

13. Mann, M. S., et al. Vulvar vestibulitis: significant clinical variables and treatment outcome. *Obstet. Gynecol.* 79:122, 1992.
Evidence of HPV and candidiasis should be sought in such patients; laser ablation has proved disappointing; perineoplasty provides good results in properly selected cases.

14. Goetsch, M. F. Vulvar vestibulitis: prevalence and historic features in a general gynecologic practice population. *Am. J. Obstet. Gynecol.* 164:1609, 1991.
A single practitioner sought evidence of the syndrome in 210 consecutive patients in her practice and found that 31 women (15%) met the clinical criteria.

15. Scrimin, F., et al. Vulvodynia and selective IgA deficiency. Case reports. *Br. J. Obstet. Gynaecol.* 98:592, 1991.
    These authors report on two patients with vulvodynia and selective immunoglobulin A deficiency. They suggest a possible immunologic basis for the condition.
16. McKay, M. Dysesthetic ("essential") vulvodynia. Treatment with amitriptyline. *J. Reprod. Med.* 38:9, 1993.
    Sorting out "itches that rash" from "rashes that itch" is complicated by the multifactorial nature of vulvar disease.

90. CARCINOMA OF THE VULVA
Michel E. Rivlin

Ninety-five percent of the invasive vulvar carcinomas are of the squamous cell type and account for about 5 percent of the malignancies of the female genital tract. There is often a background of chronic vulvar dystrophy or vulvar intraepithelial neoplasia (VIN) in these patients. However, progression from VIN to carcinoma in a manner analogous to that noted in the cervix has not been shown. Vulvar carcinoma is a disease of older women, with a peak incidence in the seventh decade. Seventy percent of the tumors develop anteriorly on the labia majora, although sites on the labia minora, clitoris, and perineum also occur. The usual symptoms consist of pruritus, an ulcer or nodule, and bleeding with pain. Although often well localized, these lesions may be extensive, as they are frequently neglected for prolonged periods. Grossly, the lesion assumes the appearance of an indurated ulcer with raised, rolled edges. Histologically, they are well differentiated as a rule, although anaplastic varieties occur in 5 to 10 percent of the cases. Cords of squamous cells extend into the dermis and subcutaneous tissue, forming keratinizing epithelial pearls. Rare adenosquamous variants occur. The cancer then spreads directly to adjacent vulvar, perineal, and perianal areas. Metastasis to the lymph nodes is common and often takes place early. Lymphatic spread is predictable, first to the inguinal nodes (superficial, then deep) and then to the femoral and deep pelvic nodes. Midline tumors may drain to contralateral nodes. Large or poorly differentiated tumors are more likely to metastasize to lymph nodes. The 5-year survival rate in affected patients after treatment is quoted to be 70 percent, which rises to 90 percent if lymph nodes are not involved, falls to 65 percent if inguinal nodes are involved, and decreases further to 10 to 15 percent if metastases are present in deep pelvic nodes.

The revised International Federation of Gynecology and Obstetrics (FIGO, 1988) staging system for vulvar cancer has changed from a clinical to a surgical system because the clinical assessment of groin nodes is often in error. The staging includes designations regarding the primary tumor (T), regional lymph nodes (N), and distant metastases (M). Stage 0 (Tis) indicates an intraepithelial carcinoma. A stage 1 (T1 N0 M0) tumor is confined to the vulva or perineum, or both, is 2 cm or less in its greatest dimension, and nodes are not palpable. A stage II (T2 N0 M0) tumor is confined to the vulva or perineum, or both, is more than 2 cm in its greatest dimension, and nodes are not palpable. A stage III (T3 N0 M0) tumor is a lesion of any size showing (1) adjacent spread to the lower urethra and/or vagina, or the anus (T3 N1 M0) and/or (2) unilateral regional lymph node metastasis (T1 N1 M0; T2 N1 M0). A tumor is classified as stage IVA if it has invaded any of the following: the upper urethra, bladder, rectum, or pelvic bone, and/or shows bilateral nodal metastases (T1–4 N2 M0). A stage IVB tumor constitutes any distant metastases, including the pelvic nodes (any T, any N, M1).

There appears to be an interrelationship between the human papillomaviruses and the development of lower genital tract intraepithelial and invasive neoplasia. A high proportion of the cases of intraepithelial neoplasia in the lower genital tract are multicentric. Carcinoma of the vulva is therefore frequently found in association with intraepithelial carcinoma of the vagina and cervix. Papillomavirus infections of the male partner may also be found. Diagnosis is based on biopsy findings, often with the aid of colposcopic findings or toluidine blue staining. The differential diagnosis includes the vulvar dystrophies and sexually transmitted ulcerative or condylomatous lesions, as discussed in Chapter 57. The preoperative workup may include lymphangiography or computed tomography (CT) or magnetic resonance imaging (MRI), with or without needle biopsy, to demonstrate whether groin or deep pelvic lymph nodes are involved. Associated cervical or vaginal disease should be sought and assessed if present.

Obesity, hypertension, diabetes, and arteriosclerosis are common in these patients, which, together with their advanced age, complicates therapy. Nevertheless, the majority of patients are sufficiently healthy to permit definitive therapy, which is generally surgical, as radiotherapy and chemotherapy are relatively unsuccessful in the treatment of vulvar cancer.

For many years, radical vulvectomy with bilateral inguinal lymphadenectomy was the standard surgical approach for the treatment of vulvar carcinoma. The procedure removes the tumor along with the lymphatics and nodes en bloc. The presence of tumor in Cloquet's node (the deepest femoral node in the femoral canal) was an indication to proceed to deep pelvic lymphadenectomy. This radical procedure brought about dramatically improved survival rates, but was associated with significant mortality and morbidity and severe damage to sexual function, and hence the patient's self-image. As a result, there has been a trend toward using more conservative approaches in the management of early forms of this disease. In more advanced malignancies, the combination of surgical removal plus radiotherapy or radiotherapy alone has been used. The main source of postoperative morbidity is breakdown of the groin wound, though the use of myocutaneous flaps in some cases has decreased the incidence of this complication. Wound sloughs over the femoral vessels were sometimes complicated by heavy bleeding, but this problem is now eliminated by the routine transplantation of the sartorius muscles over the femoral vessels. A common difficulty after vulvectomy, stress urinary incontinence and vaginal wall prolapse, may also be avoided by the use of appropriate repair procedures at the time of vulvectomy. Persistent lymphedema of the legs, another significant problem, is managed by elevation of the legs and prompt treatment of cellulitis, and preservation of the saphenous veins during groin dissection also helps to minimize the problem.

The incidence of intraepithelial and invasive neoplasia of the vulva may be increasing, especially in young women. If it were possible to identify a microinvasive stage at which there is little risk of nodal involvement, less aggressive therapy could be considered. There is no universally accepted definition for *microinvasive carcinoma* of the vulva. In the definition proposed by the International Society for the Study of Vulvar Disease, the diameter of the lesion should be less than 2 cm and the depth of invasion under 1 mm. These patients might be treated by wide local excision together with ipsilateral lymphadenectomy. However, many clinicians believe that this and other conservative approaches should still be considered experimental at this time.

Malignant melanoma accounts for less than 10 percent of all vulvar malignancies, occurring as a rule in the sixth or seventh decade of life. It is the second most common vulvar cancer, however, so it is advised that any suspicious pigmented nevus on the vulva should be excised. Neither the FIGO vulvar cancer staging system nor the Clark classification of malignant melanomas is appropriate for classifying vulvar melanoma; other systems provide better prognostic information. The overall prognosis in these patients is poor, and, because radical resection does not appear to confer any greater benefit in terms of local control, a disease-free interval, or patient survival, versus a less extensive resection, it seems likely that, as in the treatment of anorectal melanoma, the less radical resection should be the usual therapy. Verrucous carcinoma is an unusual variant of squamous cell carcinoma. It presents postmenopausally as a large fungating, locally invasive tumor with well-differentiated squamous epithelium and little cellular atypia. Wide local excision is sufficient, as nodal metastasis is rare. Radiotherapy is contraindicated. Basal cell carcinoma is a localized tumor seen in postmenopausal women; typically it has the appearance of a slightly raised, ulcerated nodule with rolled margins. Downgrowths of cells from the basal layer of the epidermis are apparent. The tumor is only locally invasive, and wide local excision to negative margins is therapeutic, although 20 percent recur after removal. Bartholin's gland tumors are rare, occur in persons aged 40 to 70 years, and may be either adenocarcinoma (46%) or squamous cell carcinoma (40%). Like squamous cell cancer, metastasis to regional and distant nodes occurs. Paget's disease of the vulva is frequently associated with other malignancies, including underlying intraepithelial adenocarcinoma (20% of cases) and other vulvar cancers. Furthermore, there is a strong potential for a second urogenital primary to develop, and thus thorough urogenital evaluation and follow-up are indicated.

The size of the tumor is not always an accurate guide to the presence of groin metastasis (10% of the lesions <2 cm have nodal involvement), and clinical assessment of the lymph nodes is incorrect in 13 to 39 percent of cases. If the tumor is confined to the vulva, a corrected 5-year survival rate of 86 percent may be expected; if the superficial nodes are involved, this rate falls to 55 percent; and if deep nodes are involved, the rate falls to 12.5 to 50 percent.

At present, it appears that a certain degree of individualization in therapy is possible without compromising the good results obtained in the past.

Reviews
1. Franklin, E. W., III, and Weiser, E. B. Surgery for vulvar cancer. *Surg. Clin. North Am.* 71:911, 1991.
   The problem is to define the subset of cases that can be treated by conservative procedures without sacrificing the improved survival provided by radical operations.
2. Gordon, A. N. Current concepts in the treatment of invasive vulvar carcinoma. *Clin. Obstet. Gynecol.* 34:587, 1991.
   Radical vulvectomy with inguinal-femoral lymphadenectomy is frequently complicated by wound breakdown, prolonged hospitalization, and other problems, including lymphedema and dyspareunia.

Etiology
3. Andersen, W. A., et al. Vulvar squamous cell carcinoma and papillomaviruses: two separate entities? *Am. J. Obstet. Gynecol.* 165:329, 1991.
   In younger women, sexual factors, cigarette smoking, and human papillomaviruses infection are significant associations; in older women, vulvar inflammatory diseases (dystrophies) are associated. These findings confirm the diverse nature of vulvar cancer.
4. Parazzini, F., et al. Determinants of invasive vulvar cancer risk: an Italian case-control study. *Gynecol. Oncol.* 48:50, 1993.
   No association with reproductive history, sexual habits, or smoking was detected.
5. Crum, C. P. Carcinoma of the vulva: epidemiology and pathogenesis. *Obstet. Gynecol.* 79:448, 1992.
   A substantial proportion of vulvar cancers may not be related to a venereally transmitted agent.

Pathology
6. Homesley, H. D., et al. Assessment of current International Federation of Gynecology and Obstetrics staging of vulvar carcinoma relative to prognostic factors for survival (a Gynecologic Oncology Group study). *Am. J. Obstet. Gynecol.* 164:997, 1991.
   The 5-year survival rates were found to be 98 percent, 85 percent, 74 percent, and 31 percent for stages I, II, III, and IV, respectively.
7. Wilkinson, E. J. Superficially invasive carcinoma of the vulva. *Clin. Obstet. Gynecol.* 34:651, 1991.
   There is likely no nodal involvement when tumors are confined to the vulva with less than 1 mm of invasion, but there can be significant nodal metastasis as the depth of invasion increases beyond 1 mm.
8. Frankman, O. Stage III squamous cell carcinoma of the vulva. Results of a Swedish study. *J. Reprod. Med.* 36:108, 1991.

The 5-year survival was 89 percent if there were no groin metastases and 36 percent if there were.

Treatment

9. Stehman, F. B., et al. Early stage I carcinoma of the vulva treated with ipsilateral superficial inguinal lymphadenectomy and modified radical hemivulvectomy: a prospective study of the Gynecologic Oncology Group. *Obstet. Gynecol.* 79:490, 1992.
   Inherent in any conservative approach is the fact that the benefits gained from the conservative procedure, versus the radical approach, in terms of the lessened risks of morbidity and mortality outweigh the risks of recurrence of the cancer treated conservatively.
10. Hoffman, M. S., et al. A comparative study of radical vulvectomy and modified radical vulvectomy for the treatment of invasive squamous cell carcinoma of the vulva. *Gynecol. Oncol.* 45:192, 1992.
   There have been many variations on the classic trapezoid or butterfly-shaped incision, including the use of separate incisions, skin grafts, and myocutaneous flaps.
11. Grimshaw, R. N., Murdoch, J. B., and Monaghan, J. M. Radical vulvectomy and bilateral inguinal-femoral lymphadenectomy through separate incisions—experience with 100 cases. *Int. J. Gynecol. Oncol.* 3:18, 1993.
   Radical vulvectomy with bilateral lymphadenectomy represents the "gold standard" to which any modification of treatment should be compared.
12. Calame, R. J. Pelvic relaxation as a complication of the radical vulvectomy. *Obstet. Gynecol.* 55:716, 1980.
   Pelvic relaxation complicated 17 percent of 58 cases; the author recommends preventive or reconstructive procedures to be performed during the primary operation.
13. Anderson, B. L., and Hacker, N. F. Psychosexual adjustment after vulvar surgery. *Obstet. Gynecol.* 62:457, 1983.
   Radical surgical removal may alter the woman's body image and threaten her self-esteem. Sexual function is seldom impaired, but desire may be altered.
14. Homesley, H. D., et al. Radiation therapy versus pelvic node resection for carcinoma of the vulva with positive groin nodes. *Obstet. Gynecol.* 68:733, 1986.
   In patients with positive groin nodes, adjunctive groin and pelvic irradiation proved superior to pelvic node resection.
15. Berek, J. S., et al. Concurrent cisplatin and 5-fluorouracil chemotherapy and radiation therapy for advanced-stage squamous carcinoma of the vulva. *Gynecol. Oncol.* 42:197, 1991.
   Data are presented supporting the use of concurrent chemoradiation therapy, sometimes followed by surgical treatment, as an alternative to primary radical surgery to treat advanced-stage vulvar cancer.

Other Vulvar Malignancies

16. Japaze, H., Van Dinh, T., and Woodruff, J. D. Verrucous carcinoma of the vulva: study of 24 cases. *Obstet. Gynecol.* 60:462, 1982.
   Verrucous carcinoma is histologically similar to condyloma acuminatum. It occurs in the oral cavity as well as on the genitalia.
17. Hoffman, M. S., Roberts, W. S., and Ruffolo, E. H. Basal cell carcinoma of the vulva with inguinal lymph node metastases. *Gynecol. Oncol.* 25:113, 1988.
   This is the third well-documented case with nodal metastases reported in the literature.
18. Copeland, L. J., et al. Bartholin gland carcinoma. *Obstet. Gynecol.* 67:794, 1986.
   Wide excision or radical hemivulvectomy together with ipsilateral inguinal lymphadenectomy and adjunctive irradiation to the vulva and regional nodes provided an 84 percent survival rate despite there being a nearly 50 percent frequency of nodal metastasis.
19. Trimble, E. L., et al. Management of vulvar melanoma. *Gynecol. Oncol.* 45:254, 1992.
   These authors recommend radical local excision in those patients who have more

than a superficially invasive lesion; inguinal lymph node dissection is also indicated.

20. Curtin, J. P., et al. Paget's disease of the vulva. *Gynecol. Oncol.* 39:374, 1990.
    The authors recommend local excision based on the findings from frozen-section margin evaluation in patients with superficial Paget's disease. Associated adenocarcinoma (14% in this series) requires radical surgery.

91. CERVICAL INTRAEPITHELIAL NEOPLASIA
Michel E. Rivlin

The junction between the squamous epithelium lining the ectocervix and the columnar epithelium lining the endocervix is called the *squamocolumnar junction* or *transitional zone* (TZ). In young adults, it is usually located on the ectocervix and may enlarge and become more distally located during pregnancy (ectopy). After menopause, the junction usually recedes and is frequently located in the endocervical canal. Throughout reproductive life, the more fragile red columnar glandular epithelium is gradually replaced by the more resistant pink squamous epithelium, a process termed squamous metaplasia. The significance of these observations is that all grades of cervical neoplasia originate in the TZ. Normal epithelial maturation proceeds outward from the basal cells on the basement membrane, and minor lesions involve this zone only.

All grades of abnormal epithelial maturation may evidence abnormalities in either the deoxyribonucleic acid (DNA) content or chromosome number. Various degrees of cytologic and histologic dedifferentiation are seen, and cytologic cervical smears (Papanicolaou [Pap] smears) as well as cervical biopsy specimens are graded according to the degree and extent of the cellular abnormalities found. The size, configuration, denseness of the chromatin, number of mitoses, pleomorphism, and percentage of abnormal cells form the basis for the cytologic and histologic grade of the lesions. If the undifferentiated neoplastic cells extend through the full thickness of the epithelium but do not penetrate the basement membrane, the lesion is called carcinoma in situ (CIS).

Mild, moderate, and severe cervical dysplasia, together with CIS, represent stages along a continuum of preinvasive lesions of the epithelium of the uterine cervix. These lesions differ in the degree of cellular abnormalities seen and in the thickness of the epithelium involved. In an alternative terminology, the term cervical intraepithelial neoplasia (CIN) is used, such that CIN I represents mild; CIN II, moderate; and CIN III, severe dysplasia and CIS. Unlike invasive cancer, these lesions are reversible or may arrest, and this is especially true of the earlier changes seen in the setting of CIN I and II.

Intraepithelial neoplasia of the cervix occurs mainly in young women. Furthermore, the frequency of the diagnosis is increasing in this group, with a peak in the age incidence of the milder lesions in women in their late twenties and of the more severe lesions in those in their midthirties. The incidence is approximately twice as high in black women as in white. The cause of cervical neoplasia is not known, but potential epidemiologic risk factors include early intercourse (before age 18), multiple sex partners, a history of sexually transmitted diseases, and low socioeconomic status. Other possible risk factors include cigarette smoking, oral contraceptive use, and intrauterine diethylstilbestrol exposure. Male factors include a "high-risk" consort—one whose previous female partners have either developed cervical neoplasia or have had many sex partners. Because many of the epidemiologic factors have a venereal association, sperm and sexually transmitted viruses (human papillomavirus [HPV], herpes simplex II, and cytomegalovirus) have been proposed as mutagens in this condition. At present, attention is focused on the distinct cellular changes, the most characteristic of which is koilocytosis (perinuclear cavitation), that are frequently identified in areas of CIN. Through the technique of molecular hybridization of HPV DNA, many types of HPV have been identified. Those associated with neoplasia are types 16, 18, and 31. The link with neoplasia is suggestive but has not been proved. Koilocytes may be found in the epithelium of all grades of CIN. Diploidy is usual in condylomata, polyploidy in CIN I, and aneuploidy in CIN III. The specific viral DNA of HPV 16 has been discovered in 60 percent of the cases of invasive genital cancer. It appears that initial infection with an oncogenic virus, if accompanied by appropriate cofactors, will eventually lead to further epithelial alterations that can develop into invasive cancer.

Cervical cytologic study is basic to the diagnosis of dysplasia. A properly taken Pap smear must sample both the endocervix and ectocervix. False-negative rates vary from 20 to 40 percent, but the repetition of smears over time markedly improves the rates of pick-up. Historically, Pap test results were reported as class I to V; class I being negative; class II, inflammation; and classes III, IV, and V, increasing grades of dysplasia. Since 1988, however, "The Bethesda System" has been adopted for the reporting of cervical and vaginal cytologic findings. This system introduced the term *low-grade squamous intraepithelial lesion* (SIL), to include cellular changes consistent with HPV infection with or without mild dysplasia (CIN I). Moderate dysplasia (CIN II), severe dysplasia, and CIS (CIN III) are now reported as a high-grade squamous intraepithelial lesion. The system also requires a comment regarding the adequacy of the smear and includes the categories of abnormal squamous cells of uncertain significance (AS-CUS) and abnormal glandular cells of uncertain significance (AGCUS) to include those smears in which the nature of the cells is unclear to the cytologist. Similar changes in histopathologic reporting may follow these changes in the cytologic nomenclature. The prevalence of dysplasia found by cytologic examination varies from 5 to 65 per 1000, depending on the population group being screened. The American College of Obstetricians and Gynecologists recommends annual Pap smears starting at age 18, or at the age when sexual activity starts, if this is before 18 years of age.

Cervical cytologic study is a screening process only; definitive diagnosis requires tissue sampling. Colposcopy can delineate the extent of the cervical lesion and direct biopsy to the worst areas. If colposcopy is unavailable, biopsy of areas that do not stain with iodine (Schiller's test) may be the diagnostic technique used, although it is not a very reliable method and, frequently, cone biopsy becomes necessary. Cone biopsy is also required if the colposcopic examination is deemed unsatisfactory for any of the following reasons: the entire TZ cannot be seen, the colposcopic biopsy reveals a lesser grade of disease than the smear, or the endocervical curettage finding is positive. Cone biopsy is used for therapy as well as for diagnosis.

The treatment of CIN must be individualized according to the extent and grade of the lesion, the age and parity of the patient, the presence or absence of pregnancy, and her desire for future childbearing. The patient's suitability for surgery, her reliability with regard to regular follow-up, and the cost of therapy must also be taken into account.

In general, less extensive and less severe lesions are treated on an outpatient basis using local methods, such as eradication of infections known to cause inflammatory cellular atypia (*Trichomonas*), cryosurgery, electrocautery, and laser therapy. The loop electrosurgical excision procedures, also referred to as loop excision of the transformation zone (LETZ), have largely replaced the laser methods because they are faster and less expensive. Both laser ablation and LETZ may be used for local destruction or cone biopsy, although the heat-induced artifact may make subsequent histologic interpretation difficult. More severe and more extensive lesions are usually treated by cone biopsy and, occasionally, especially if other indications exist in patients who have completed their families, by hysterectomy. A concomitant pregnancy poses a problem, and, if possible, treatment is postponed until after pregnancy in these women. Cone biopsy may be performed during pregnancy, if necessary. Generally, the initial follow-up examination is performed 4 months after therapy and repeated every 6 months for 2 years before reverting to an annual basis. CIN can recur many years after therapy, and, although the risk is small (3%), recurrence is more common in patients who have had high-grade lesions, emphasizing the importance of more intensive and prolonged follow-up for these patients.

Reviews
1. 1988 Bethesda System for Reporting Cervical/Vaginal Cytological Diagnoses. National Cancer Institute Workshop. *J.A.M.A.* 262:931, 1989.
   A system of terminology and classification for cervical and vaginal cytology that is currently the standard method, but which has provoked considerable controversy and will probably require modification.
2. Wilkinson, E. J. Pap smears and screening for cervical neoplasia. *Clin. Obstet. Gynecol.* 33:817, 1990.
   The causes of false-negative cytologic findings include sample error (cells not on slide), screening error (cells missed by the cytotechnologist), and interpretative error (the pathologist misjudged the cells).

Epidemiology
3. Eddy, D. M. Screening for cervical cancer. *Ann. Intern. Med.* 113:214, 1990.
   Indirect evidence indicates that cervical cancer screening should reduce the incidence and mortality of invasive cervical cancer by about 90 percent.
4. Hayward, R. A., et al. Who gets screened for cervical and breast cancer? Results from a new national survey. *Arch. Intern. Med.* 148:1177, 1988.
   The authors concluded that being older, uninsured, and in a lower socioeconomic bracket are independent risk factors for receiving less preventive care.

Etiology and Pathogenesis
5. Panazzini, F., et al. Risk factors for cervical intraepithelial neoplasia. *Cancer* 69:2282, 1992.
   Women who experienced their first intercourse before age 18 and who smoked were at significantly higher risks for CIN and invasive cervical cancer.
6. Singer, A. Sex and genital cancer in heterosexual women. *J. Reprod. Med.* 28:109, 1983.
   The number of sex partners reported by men represented a significant risk factor for their wives (of the order of 7.8-fold for 15 or more partners).
7. Gram, I. T., Macaluso, M., and Stalsberg, H. Oral contraceptive use and the incidence of cervical intraepithelial neoplasia. *Am. J. Obstet. Gynecol.* 167:40, 1992.
   A weak positive association was found; however, confounding sexual behavior and detection bias have yielded conflicting results, so that a definite causal association has not yet been established.
8. Marte, C., et al. Papanicolaou smear abnormalities in ambulatory care sites for women infected with the human immunodeficiency virus. *Am. J. Obstet. Gynecol.* 166:1232, 1992.
   The rates of abnormal smear findings were increased and a significant correlation with CD4 counts was observed in human immunodeficiency virus–infected women at ambulatory care sites.
9. Stanbridge, C. M., et al. A cervical smear review in women developing cervical carcinoma with particular reference to age, false negative cytology and the histologic type of the carcinoma. *Int. J. Gynecol. Cancer* 2:92, 1992.
   A significant abnormality was found in 89 percent of the women under 40 years of age up to 6 years before diagnosis. The preinvasive phase of cervical cancer may be briefer in younger women.
10. Montz, F. J., et al. Natural history of the minimally abnormal Papanicolaou smear. *Obstet. Gynecol.* 80:385, 1992.
    Most women will experience complete regression over a short interval (53.8% over 9 months).
11. Syrjänen, K., et al. Natural history of cervical human papillomavirus lesions does not substantiate the biologic relevance of the Bethesda System. *Obstet. Gynecol.* 79:675, 1992.
    All six HPV types (6, 11, 16, 18, 31, and 33) as well as double infections were encountered in both the low-grade and high-grade cases of SIL; however, HPV 16

infections have a fivefold risk for progression, versus the risk observed for HPV 6 or 11 lesions.

Diagnosis

12. Cox, J. T., et al. An evaluation of human papillomavirus testing as part of referral to colposcopy clinics. *Obstet. Gynecol.* 80:389, 1992.
    Suggests that Vira Pap tests for HPV infection, together with the cytologic findings, may help to limit the number of women referred to already overburdened colposcopy services.
13. Helmerhorst, Th. J. M. Clinical significance of endocervical curettage as part of colposcopic evaluation. A review. *Int. J. Gynecol. Cancer* 2:256, 1992.
    This meta-analysis of the literature data revealed that the clinical application of endocervical curettage is limited.
14. Orr, J. W., Jr., et al. The efficacy and safety of the cytobrush during pregnancy. *Gynecol. Oncol.* 44:260, 1992.
    Innovative techniques for endocervical cytologic sampling increase the endocervical cell yields, thus decreasing the prevalence of inadequate smears, and may improve the detection of abnormal smears.
15. Skehan, M., et al. Reliability of colposcopy and directed punch biopsy. *Br. J. Obstet. Gynaecol.* 97:811, 1990.
    Laser and electrosurgical excisional therapy techniques provide a histopathologic quality control of colposcopic biopsy findings. The data indicate that biopsy is relatively unreliable and management should include consideration of the cytologic and colposcopic findings.
16. Saunders, N., et al. Unsatisfactory colposcopy and the response to orally administered oestrogen: a randomized double blind placebo controlled trial. *Br. J. Obstet. Gynaecol.* 97:731, 1990.
    Satisfactory colposcopic inspection of the TZ was possible in a significantly greater proportion of the estrogen-treated group (70% versus 23%).
17. Adachi, A., et al. Women with human immunodeficiency virus infection and abnormal Papanicolaou smears: a prospective study of colposcopy and clinical outcome. *Obstet. Gynecol.* 81:372, 1993.
    Cytologic examination was reliable, and rapid progression after standard care had been carried out for early lesions was not seen.

Treatment

18. Benedet, J. L., Miller, D. M., and Nickerson, K. G. Results of conservative management of cervical intraepithelial neoplasia. *Obstet. Gynecol.* 79:105, 1992.
    Both cryosurgery and laser surgery were found to be simple and effective methods for the treatment of CIN.
19. Bigrigg, M. A., et al. Colposcopic diagnosis and treatment of cervical dysplasia at a single clinic visit: experience of low-voltage diathermy loop in 1000 patients. *Lancet* 336:229, 1990.
    These authors attempt to use wire-loop excision as both a diagnostic and therapeutic tool. The majority opinion, however, favors initial diagnosis based on the colposcopic biopsy findings before instituting therapy.
20. Hellberg, D., and Nilsson, S. 20-year experience of follow-up of the abnormal smear with colposcopy and histology and treatment by conization or cryosurgery. *Gynecol. Oncol.* 38:166, 1990.
    The authors cite a cure rate of 87 percent achieved by cryosurgery, 96 percent by conization, and 97 percent by hysterectomy. Most treatment failures occurred within the first 5 years.
21. Killackey, M. A., Jones, W. B., and Lewis, J. L., Jr. Diagnostic conization of the cervix: review of 460 consecutive cases. *Obstet. Gynecol.* 67:766, 1986.
    Problems sometimes encountered with cone biopsy include postoperative hemorrhage, unclear surgical margins, and adverse effects on future fertility. Advantages include definitive histologic diagnosis and retention of fertility in most cases.
22. LaPolla, J. P., O'Neill, C., and Wetrich, D. Colposcopic management of abnormal cervical cytology in pregnancy. *J. Reprod. Med.* 33:301, 1988.

These authors describe their experience with 265 cases; 23 patients underwent cone biopsy, of whom 16 had persistent dysplasia postpartum, including 4 with microinvasion.

23. Campion, M. J., et al. Psychosexual trauma of an abnormal cervical smear. *Br. J. Obstet. Gynaecol.* 95:175, 1988.
    This study revealed a significantly decreased frequency of intercourse, decreased vaginal lubrication, decreased sexual arousal, and decreased frequency of orgasm after the diagnosis and treatment of CIN.

24. Cullimore, J. E., et al. A prospective study of conization of the cervix in the management of cervical intraepithelial glandular neoplasia (CIGN)—a preliminary report. *Br. J. Obstet. Gynaecol.* 99:314, 1992.
    CIGN comprises cervical glandular atypia and adenocarcinoma in situ. The finding from this study suggest that further surgical treatment is unnecessary if the cone specimen margins are free of disease, but recommends close follow-up with cytologic studies and colposcopy.

25. Hubley, J. E., and Hopkins, M. P. An analysis of residual disease in hysterectomy specimens after cone biopsy. *J. Gynecol. Surg.* 9:17, 1993.
    The authors suggest that mild to moderate disease, regardless of the cone margins, and severe disease with free margins are associated with a low rate of residual disease in the cervix.

92. CARCINOMA OF THE CERVIX
Michel E. Rivlin

Widespread cytologic screening has had a major impact on the earlier detection and associated decrease in the incidence and mortality associated with cervical cancer. However, delay by some women in seeking health care will contribute significantly to the estimated 13,500 new cases and 4400 deaths from the disease expected in the United States for 1992. Cervical cancer is the third most common female pelvic cancer, endometrial cancer being the most common. The average age at diagnosis is 45 years. Epidemiologic data indicate that the major risk factors for acquiring the disease include early age at first intercourse and multiple sexual partners. These patterns suggest a venereal form of transmission. There is a strong association between infection with human papillomavirus type 16 or 18 and the development of cervical dysplasia and carcinoma. If left untreated, carcinoma in situ can develop into frankly invasive cancer over a period of from 3 to 20 years in 70 percent of patients. Squamous cell carcinoma accounts for about 87 percent of the cases, and adenocarcinoma for about 13 percent. Of the epidermoid cancers, 65 percent are large-cell nonkeratinizing, 23 percent are large-cell keratinizing, and 17 percent are small cell. Based on the degree of differentiation, the cancers are further graded I, II, or III, depending on whether they are well, moderately, or poorly differentiated.

It is important to estimate the extent of the disease as an aid to determining the prognosis, planning therapy, and comparing therapeutic approaches. The pretreatment clinical evaluation and staging of the cancer are based on the findings at pelvic examination. The remainder of the evaluation includes a chest x-ray study, intravenous pyelogram, and barium enema. Cystoscopy or sigmoidoscopy, or both, are indicated in patients with advanced-stage disease or with symptoms referable to those organs. Computed tomography (CT) and magnetic resonance imaging (MRI) scans, as well as lymphangiography, may provide further information, especially in regard to lymph node involvement. Staging is usually reported using the International Federation of Gynecology and Obstetrics (FIGO) definitions. In stage I, disease is confined to the cervix. Stage IA lesions are diagnosed only on the basis of microscopy findings, preferably using a cone biopsy specimen: stage IA1 indicates minimal stromal invasion and stage IA2 signifies a depth of invasion less than 5 mm from the base of the epithelium with a horizontal spread of less than 7 mm. These latter two patterns are often referred to as microinvasion, and, in this respect, there is much disagreement. In the United States, microinvasion is usually diagnosed only if the depth of invasion is 3 mm or less, so that the criterion of 5 mm represents the European viewpoint. Stage IB includes larger lesions than those in stage IA2. In stage II carcinoma, the disease extends beyond the cervix and may involve the upper two thirds of the vagina. In stage IIA, there is a lack of parametrial involvement, but, in stage IIB, there is obvious parametrial spread. In stage III, there is no cancer-free space between the tumor and pelvic wall or the tumor involves the lower third of the vagina. In stage IIIA, the extension has not reached the pelvic wall; in stage IIIB, there is extension to the wall, as evidenced by ureteric obstruction together with hydronephrosis or a nonfunctioning kidney. Stage IV carcinoma extends beyond the true pelvis and involves the bladder or rectal mucosa, with spread to adjacent organs classified as stage IVA, and to distant organs, stage IVB. Lymphatic spread is to the regional pelvic nodes (parametrial, hypogastric, obturator, and external iliac). Stage I cancers involve regional nodes in 15 to 20 percent of cases; stage II, 30 to 40 percent (10 percent of these patients have paraaortic node involvement as well). The paraaortic nodes are involved in 45 percent of the stage III cancers. Blood-borne metastases are rare but may affect the lungs, brain, and bone. Unfortunately, it has been found that clinical understaging occurs in 30 to 40 percent of the cases; however, thorough surgical staging has had no clear impact on survival, such that staging laparotomy is not a routine procedure in patients with locally advanced disease, although many clinical trials have included this procedure. By convention, however, all cases retain their original clinical staging for the purpose of comparative data, even though the treatment may be altered by the surgical findings.

Intermenstrual, postcoital, and postmenopausal bleeding are the most common symptoms of invasive cancer, and a vaginal discharge is usually present. Pelvic pain, often unilateral and radiating to the hip or thigh, indicates late disease. Physical examination may reveal an exophytic or ulcerative growth with a firm consistency that is usually friable and hemorrhagic. A rectovaginal examination may reveal infiltration with nodular thickening of the uterosacral and cardinal ligaments. Urinary or fecal fistulas, or both, may be present with stage IV disease. Diagnosis in patients with a gross lesion is based on the findings yielded by a cervical punch biopsy specimen. Colposcopic and cone biopsies are indicated for patients with abnormal cytology and no gross lesion.

The treatment of microinvasive disease depends on the depth of stromal penetration. If it is no more than 3 mm, the probability of lymphatic involvement is under 2 percent, so that simple hysterectomy and, in rare instances where fertility is a factor, even cone biopsy is regarded as acceptable management. Cancer cure should approach 100 percent in this stage. If the depth of penetration exceeds 3 mm, the risk of nodal involvement rises to 5 to 10 percent, so radical hysterectomy and pelvic lymphadenectomy or radiotherapy is indicated. Stages IB and IIA disease can be treated either with radical hysterectomy and pelvic lymphadenectomy or with radiotherapy, which comprises a combination of external-beam irradiation and brachytherapy (the temporary insertion of intrauterine and vaginal colpostats that are loaded with a radioisotope, usually cesium 137). Surgical treatment is usually selected for younger women to preserve ovarian function and avoid vaginal irradiation. Radiotherapy is used for older patients or those with medical contraindications to surgery. Results for both approaches are equivalent, with a 60 to 90 percent survival rate. The prognosis has as much to do with the nodal status as it does with the stage, such that, when the stage is disregarded, there is an 80 percent survival rate for patients without lymphatic involvement, versus 20 percent if the nodes are involved. Most patients with stage IIB or III lesions are treated with external-beam irradiation (total dose, 45–55 Gy), followed by intracavitary brachytherapy. Survival rates of 60 to 70 percent for stage IIB and 33 to 50 percent for stage III disease can be expected. Those patients with locally advanced disease at presentation (stage IVA) or locally recurrent cervical cancer after radiotherapy may be candidates for pelvic exenteration (surgical removal of the entire contents of the pelvis). Survival rates of 12 percent are quoted for stage IV disease. The overall cure rate for all stages is about 50 to 60 percent. Chemotherapy is used when radiation ports cannot encompass the extent of disease or when cancer recurs outside the pelvis. Cervical cancer is resistant to chemotherapy; the best single-agent treatment has proved to be cisplatin, with response rates of about 38 percent. Combination therapy has been somewhat more successful, but the median survival has not been improved and toxicity is more severe. To achieve optimal results from radiotherapy may require the concurrent use of a radiosensitizing agent (e.g., hydroxyurea). Surgery, radiotherapy, and chemotherapy are discussed in greater detail in Chapters 98 through 100.

The recommended follow-up after therapy comprises history, physical examination, and vaginal cytologic studies performed at 4-month intervals for 2 years, then every 6 months for 3 years, and then annually. Chest x-ray studies and intravenous pyelograms are obtained only in symptomatic patients. Recurrences appear within 2 years in 80 percent of the patients; half of these are asymptomatic. The classic triad of recurrence consists of pain, unilateral leg edema, and ureteral obstruction. It is often difficult on clinical grounds to distinguish recurrence from radiation-induced changes. A tissue biopsy specimen should be obtained, and this may require surgical exploration if needle techniques are unsuccessful. Unfortunately, most recurrences are amenable to palliation only. Pain relief, using neurosurgical procedures where necessary, is an important aspect of therapy.

Occasionally, the patient with cervical cancer is pregnant, and management depends on the extent of the tumor and the duration of the pregnancy. Before 24 weeks' gestation, the pregnancy may be disregarded and treatment with external irradiation commenced. Abortion generally follows in 4 to 5 weeks, allowing internal therapy to be carried out; if not, hysterotomy can be performed. In some pregnancies of more than 24 weeks' duration, fetal viability may be awaited, followed by cesarean delivery and the initiation of therapy. Surgical treatment may be chosen in place of irradiation, as in the nonpregnant woman.

Reviews
1. Orr, J. W., Jr., and Holloway, R. W. Surgical aspects of cervical cancer. *Surg. Clin. North Am.* 71:1067, 1991.
   Summarizes all aspects of preinvasive and invasive disease.
2. Anton-Culver, H., et al. Comparison of adenocarcinoma and squamous cell carcinoma of the uterine cervix: a population-based epidemiologic study. *Am. J. Obstet. Gynecol.* 166:1507, 1992.
   There appeared to be little difference in survival between patients with adenocarcinoma and those with squamous cell carcinoma of the cervix, suggesting that these two tumors should be treated similarly.
3. Copeland, L. J., et al. Superficially invasive squamous cell carcinoma of the cervix. *Gynecol. Oncol.* 45:307, 1992.
   The definition of microinvasion based on a depth of less than 3 mm is practical, and conservative treatment of these cases almost always results in cure.

Epidemiology
4. Benedet, J. L., Anderson, G. H., and Matisic, J. P. A comprehensive program for cervical cancer detection and management. *J. Obstet. Gynecol.* 166:1254, 1992.
   Comprehensive cytology and colposcopy programs reduce the incidence and mortality of cervical cancer and also the rates of in situ disease.
5. Mandelblatt, J., et al. Clinical implications of screening for cervical cancer under Medicare. *Am. J. Obstet. Gynecol.* 164:644, 1991.
   Women over age 65 account for nearly half of the cervical cancer deaths. The extension of Medicare coverage to include cervical cancer screening provides the potential for a marked improvement in this age group.
6. Sebbelov, A. M., et al. The prevalence of human papillomavirus type 16 and 18 DNA in cervical cancer in different age groups: a study of the incidental cases of cervical cancer in Norway. *Gynecol. Oncol.* 41:141, 1991.
   Human papillomavirus infection was not found to relate to the stage of disease, age, or 5-year survival. Type 16 was five times more common than type 18 in this study.

Diagnostic Evaluation

7. Sironi, S., et al. Invasive cervical carcinoma: MR imaging after preoperative chemotherapy. *Radiology* 180:719, 1991.
   MRI is somewhat better than CT in delineating the pelvic tumor and is comparable to CT in the evaluation of lymph node metastases.
8. Camilien, L., et al. Predictive value of computerized tomography in the presurgical evaluation of primary carcinoma of the cervix. *Gynecol. Oncol.* 30:209, 1988.
   Neither CT nor MRI significantly improves on the physical findings when it comes to determining the presence of parametrial involvement.
9. Herd, J., et al. Laparoscopic para-aortic lymph node sampling: development of a technique. *Gynecol. Oncol.* 44:271, 1992.
   Intraperitoneal or retroperitoneal lymph node sampling may increase the enteric complication rate associated with standard or extended radiation fields. Node sampling by laparoscopy warrants further investigation.
10. Johnson, D. W., et al. The use of para-aortic radiation therapy based on lymphangiogram interpretation in uterine cervical carcinoma. *Gynecol. Oncol.* 16:326, 1983.
    Lymphangiographic findings were useful, second only to the stage, in predicting prognosis. Extended radiotherapy based on these findings did not lead to an improved outcome, and therefore was not recommended.
11. Peters, R. K., et al. Invasive squamous cell carcinoma of the cervix after recent negative cytologic tests results—a distinct subgroup? *Am. J. Obstet. Gynecol.* 158:926, 1988.
    Does not appear to differ etiologically from the usual carcinoma; failure of screening was probably due to rapid progression or failure to shed cancer cells in sufficient quantity for detection.

Treatment

12. Perez, C. A., et al. Radiation therapy alone in the treatment of carcinoma of the uterine cervix: a 20-year experience. *Gynecol. Oncol.* 23:127, 1986.
    If the clinical staging is incorrect, such that tumor is actually present outside radiation fields, standard radiotherapy will be unsuccessful.
13. Lee, Y.-N., et al. Radical hysterectomy with pelvic lymph node dissection for treatment of cervical cancer: a clinical review of 954 cases. *Gynecol. Oncol.* 32:135, 1989.
    The authors suggest that radical hysterectomy is the treatment of choice in younger women with early invasive cancers because ovarian and vaginal function are preserved.
14. Massi, G., Savino, L., and Susini, T. Schauta-Amreich vaginal hysterectomy and Wertheim-Meigs abdominal hysterectomy in the treatment of cervical cancer: a retrospective analysis. *Am. J. Obstet. Gynecol.* 168:928, 1993.
    The extended vaginal hysterectomy (Schauta) yielded a high cure rate for stages IB and IIA cases, and may be indicated in the presence of obesity or elevated surgical risk.
15. Miller, B. E., et al. Carcinoma of the cervical stump. *Gynecol. Oncol.* 18:100, 1984.
    The survival rates were the same as those in patients with an intact uterus.
16. Hopkins, M. P., and Morley, G. W. The prognosis and management of cervical cancer associated with pregnancy. *Obstet. Gynecol.* 80:9, 1992.
    The prognosis was not altered by pregnancy or the trimester at diagnosis.
17. Coleman, D. L., et al. Patterns of failure of bulky-barrel carcinomas of the cervix. *Am. J. Obstet. Gynecol.* 166:916, 1992.
    Bulky-barrel cervical cancers carry a worse prognosis than do smaller lesions of equivalent stage. The addition of extrafascial hysterectomy to radiation therapy did not lead to improved survival in this series.
18. Ayhan, A., Kücüközkan, T., and Tuncer, Z. S. Management of invasive cervical cancer in patients initially treated by simple hysterectomy. *Eur. J. Surg. Oncol.* 18:177, 1992.

In patients who have undergone "cut-through" hysterectomy, possible adjuvant treatments include radiation therapy and secondary radical surgery. Cure rates ranging from 40 to 65 percent may be obtained if adequate therapy is given within 4 months postoperatively.

19. Curtin, J. P., and Morrow, C. P. Therapy of patients with positive nodes. *Clin. Obstet. Gynecol.* 33:883, 1990.
    It is unclear whether resection of positive nodes improves disease control or whether these patients benefit from chemotherapy in addition to radiotherapy.

Recurrent Disease

20. McDonald, T. W., et al. Role of needle biopsy in the investigation of gynecologic malignancy. *J. Reprod. Med.* 32:287, 1987.
    Positive results can rule out the need for surgical exploration. Negative results still require surgical validation. Very helpful in discriminating between radiation-induced fibrosis and persistent or recurrent neoplasm after completion of radiotherapy.

21. Larson, D. M., et al. Diagnosis of recurrent cervical carcinoma after radical hysterectomy. *Obstet. Gynecol.* 71:6, 1988.
    Ninety percent of the patients who suffer recurrent carcinoma after radical hysterectomy do so within 2 years of surgery, and must be monitored during this critical period.

22. Carlson, J. A., Jr. Chemotherapy of cervical cancer. *Clin. Obstet. Gynecol.* 33:910, 1990.
    Although the results of chemotherapy for recurrent disease are poor, there may be a place for chemotherapy in the initial treatment of individuals at high risk for relapse.

23. Smith, H. O., et al. Treatment of advanced recurrent squamous cell carcinoma of the uterine cervix with mitomycin-C, bleomycin and cisplatin chemotherapy. *Gynecol. Oncol.* 48:11, 1993.
    Combination mitomycin-C, bleomycin, and cisplatin chemotherapy is shown to have some activity against previously untreated local disease, and also metastatic disease, with acceptable toxicity.

93. ENDOMETRIAL HYPERPLASIA
Michel E. Rivlin

Prolonged stimulation by either endogenous or exogenous estrogen, in the absence of progesterone, leads to endometrial hyperplasia in some premenopausal or postmenopausal women. Possible mechanisms responsible for this abnormal response include an abnormal estrogen metabolism, reduced levels of sex hormone–binding globulin leading to a greater concentration of circulating steroid, and increased sensitivity of the endometrium. It is unclear why only some women respond in this manner. Hyperplasia may be defined as an abnormal increase in the amount of proliferative endometrium that exhibits varying degrees of architectural and cytologic atypia. There are three distinct forms: simple, complex, and atypical. Simple hyperplasias (cystic hyperplasia) are the most common. These conditions are characterized by the formation of dilated glands lined by cuboidal or tall columnar epithelium, producing the typical "swiss cheese" appearance. The malignant potential is less than 1 percent in such patients and most cases regress spontaneously. The complex hyperplasias (adenomatous hyperplasia and moderate adenomatous hyperplasia) are so named because of the complex architectural pattern involved, in which the glands become numerous and crowd the intervening stroma. The malignant potential of this entity is estimated at 1 to 4 percent. Atypical hyperplasias (severe adenomatous hyperplasia, adenomatous hyperplasia with atypia, and carcinoma in situ) are characterized by the existence of more glands, such that they are almost back-to-back; there is also cellular atypia (the cells display increased proliferation, enlarged vesicular nuclei, prominent nucleoli, and altered staining characteristics) and no separating stroma. An estimated 23 percent of these cases progress to cancer at a mean of 4 years. Adenocarcinoma is distinguished from atypical hyperplasia by the invasion of tumor cells into the stroma.

The risk factors for endometrial hyperplasia and endometrial cancer appear to be the same. There is overwhelming evidence that the unopposed effects of estrogen can bring about progression from normal proliferative endometrium through hyperplasia to malignant endometrium. The incidence of endometrial hyperplasia and malignancy is increased 2- to 10-fold in women treated with exogenous estrogens. The risk is related to both the dose and duration of exposure and diminishes with cessation of estrogen use. Anovulation may result from primary ovarian dysfunction, as it does in the setting of functioning ovarian tumors (e.g., granulosa cell tumor), or from disturbances in the neuroendocrine regulation of ovarian function, such as polycystic ovarian syndrome, with a consequent increased risk of hyperplasia and carcinoma. Other risk factors include nulliparity, early age of menarche, and late age at menopause. Obesity, hypertension, and diabetes are commonly associated with estrogen excess, and this is probably related to the conversion of adrenal androstenedione to estrone in adipose tissue. Progesterone-progestins oppose the mitogenic and proliferative stimuli of estrogen by suppressing deoxyribonucleic acid synthesis and the actions of the nuclear estradiol receptors. They also accelerate the conversion of estradiol to estrone by means of enzyme induction and stimulate inactivation of estrogen through the process of sulfurylation. The risk of hyperplasia and carcinoma in patients treated with exogenous estrogens for the alleviation of menopausal symptoms or as replacement therapy, such as for gonadal dysgenesis, can therefore be neutralized by the addition of progestin, given in a dosage and duration appropriate to those of the estrogen replacement therapy.

The sporadic bleeding that typically precedes menopause can make it difficult to know whether a full patient workup is necessary. Yet, because older women are at high risk for hyperplasia, any bleeding cannot be ignored. The most common definition of postmenopausal bleeding (PMB) is that which occurs more than 12 months after the last normal period. Hormonal correlates of the menopause include a level of follicle-stimulating hormone greater than 40 mU/ml; estradiol, less than 25 pg/ml; and progesterone, less than 0.5 ng/ml. No matter how minimal or remote the PMB occurs from the time of examination, it should always be investigated, as endometrial cancer has been associated with all types of bleeding patterns. The causes of PMB include gynecologic malignancies in 10 to 20 percent of the cases. The most common finding is endometrial atrophy, discovered in 60 to 80 percent of the cases; vaginal atrophy may be the cause in about 15 percent of the cases. Hyperplasia causes 5 to 10 percent of the cases of PMB, and endometrial polyps, between 2 to 12 percent. The exogenous estrogens responsible for causing PMB vary with the population studied. Therefore, detailed questioning is vital to elicit information on the past or current use of estrogen medication. Gastrointestinal or urinary bleeding may be confused with vaginal bleeding and should be kept in mind.

The standard investigation of perimenopausal and postmenopausal bleeding includes a history directed at eliciting relevant risk factors, the bleeding pattern, and exogenous sources of estrogen. In the pelvic examination, obvious lesions and pelvic masses are sought and uterine size is evaluated. Special studies include cervical cytology, biopsy of any visible lesions, urinalysis, the stool guaiac test, hematocrit, and, in most instances, endometrial sampling. The Papanicolaou (Pap) smear is positive in only 50 percent of the patients with invasive endometrial lesions, and, although the results of endometrial cytology are more reliable, they are insufficient for establishing a diagnosis in more than a third of the cases. The two usual methods for obtaining a histologic sample are (1) fractional dilatation and curettage (D&C), in which first the endocervix and then the endometrium are curetted; and (2) the endometrial aspiration biopsy. The former is usually a hospital-based procedure and therefore an expensive one; it carries about a 10 percent false-negative rate. The latter procedure is inexpensive and can be performed in the physician's office, although it is often uncomfortable for the patient; it provides results similar to those yielded by D&C. Office sampling is appropriate as a first-step evaluation, but may prove inadequate in older patients with cervical stenosis or in women with an enlarged or irregular uterus or fibroids. D&C is probably indicated in these patients. If hyperplasia is found, D&C should be performed to rule out the existence of adjacent foci of invasive disease. If atrophic endometrium is found, the patient should be closely monitored for the recurrence of bleeding.

In about half of the women with atrophic endometrium, no tissue is obtained; such patients may require a D&C or hysterectomy, although some clinicians would await bleeding recurrence. Hysteroscopy is an important aid in the evaluation of abnormal bleeding and can be carried out as an ambulatory procedure with a paracervical block. Failure rates of less than 5 percent have been achieved for this procedure, and failure is due to unsatisfactory visualization of the endometrial cavity. Recurrent bleeding requires further evaluation with D&C, hysteroscopy, and pelvic ultrasound, as indicated in the individual patient, to rule out extrauterine malignancy. Hysterectomy is indicated in most women requiring a second curettage. Younger patients with endometrial hyperplasia who desire children may be treated with ovulation induction. If attempts at ovulation induction fail and the hyperplasia persists, progesterone therapy followed by further attempts at ovulation induction should be tried. If atypical hyperplasia is present, hysterectomy is generally advisable. Management in older, morbidly obese, or other patients with major surgical risk factors can consist of a progestational agent such as medroxyprogesterone acetate. Careful monitoring with endometrial biopsies is essential.

Endometrial cancer is the most common reproductive cancer in the United States and the fourth most common cancer in women. Three fourths of the cases are diagnosed in postmenopausal women at an average age of 61 years. The incidence of endometrial carcinoma in women on combined estrogen-progestin regimens is not only reduced, compared to the incidence in those on unopposed estrogen replacement, but it is also below that observed in untreated women. Some clinicians therefore recommend the performance of a progesterone challenge test in postmenopausal women. If withdrawal bleeding occurs, they recommend a monthly dosage with progestin to eliminate an unopposed estrogen action. If the progestin challenge yields negative results, the existence of endometrial atrophy and the absence of estrogen stimulation is presumed and the progestin therapy is discontinued.

In general, there may be two different types of endometrial cancer: one arising from the endometrial hyperplasia and associated with hyperestrogenism, either endogenous or exogenous, and another (40–50%) arising from an inert or atrophic endometrium and associated with compromised immune function secondary to aging. Of the two, the hormonally influenced group appears to be the less aggressive and to have a better prognosis.

Reviews
1. Norris, H. J., Connor, M. P., and Kurman, R. J. Preinvasive lesions of the endometrium. *Clin. Obstet. Gynecol.* 13:725, 1986.
   Squamous metaplasia or acanthosis (replacement of glandular cells by squamous cells) may be present. This change is found in normal endometrium but is more common (9.8%) in hyperplastic endometrium. This metaplastic squamous epithelium is capable of undergoing the same dysplastic and invasive changes as cervical, vaginal, or vulvar squamous epithelium.
2. Fu, Y. S., Gambone, J. C., and Berek, J. S. Pathophysiology and management of endometrial hyperplasia and carcinoma. *West. J. Med.* 153:50, 1990.
   Review article with 125 references.

Etiology
3. McDonald, T. W., Malkasian, G. D., and Gaffey, T. A. Endometrial cancer associated with feminizing ovarian tumor and polycystic ovarian disease. *Obstet. Gynecol.* 49:654, 1977.

Endometrial cancer associated with a coexistent endogenous estrogen stimulus is usually low grade, low stage, and superficial, with a good prognosis.

4. Coulam, C. B., Annegers, J. F., and Kranz, J. S. Chronic anovulation syndrome and associated neoplasia. *Obstet. Gynecol.* 61:403, 1983.
   Women who do not ovulate are at increased risk for breast cancer, endometrial cancer, and pituitary adenoma.
5. Wolf, D. M., and Jordan, V. C. Gynecologic complications associated with long-term adjuvant tamoxifen therapy for breast cancer. *Gynecol. Oncol.* 45:118, 1992.
   Tamoxifen is used as an antiestrogen in women with breast cancer, but also acts as a partial estrogen receptor agonist. Long-term therapy can therefore be associated with endometrial hyperplasia, polyps, and cancer.
6. Vitoratos, N., et al. The role of androgens in the late-premenopausal woman with adenomatous hyperplasia of the endometrium. *Int. J. Gynecol. Obstet.* 34:157, 1990.
   An increased availability of the precursor hormone androstenedione or an increased capacity for the extraglandular conversion of androstenedione to estrone occurs in older, obese women—the same population at high risk for endometrial neoplasia.
7. Lobo, R. A., and Whitehead, M. Too much of a good thing? Use of progestogens in the menopause: an international consensus statement. *Fertil. Steril.* 51:229, 1989.
   High doses of progestin cause depression, anxiety, breast tenderness, backache, abdominal cramps, edema, and irritability in some users. They should be given in the smallest dose and shortest duration required for endometrial protection.
8. The Cancer and Steroid Hormone Study of the Centers for Disease Control and the National Institute of Child Health and Human Development. Combination oral contraceptive use and the risk of endometrial cancer. *J.A.M.A.* 257:796, 1987.
   Use of oral contraceptives for 12 months or longer conferred protection against all subtypes of endometrial cancer.

Pathology
9. Ayhan, A., Yarali, H., and Ayhan, A. Endometrial carcinoma: a pathologic evaluation of 142 cases with and without associated endometrial hyperplasia. *J. Surg. Oncol.* 46:182, 1991.
   The presence of endometrial hyperplasia was significantly associated with better-differentiated tumor that exhibited less myometrial invasion and lymph node involvement.
10. Thornton, J. G., Quirke, P., and Wells, M. Flow cytometry of normal, hyperplastic, and malignant human endometrium. A study of ploidy and proliferative indices including comparison with in vitro S-phase labeling. *Am. J. Obstet. Gynecol.* 161:87, 1989.
    This describes novel laboratory indices that are under investigation as predictors of tumor behavior.
11. Ferenczy, A., and Gelfand, M. The biologic significance of cytologic atypia in progestogen-treated endometrial hyperplasia. *Am. J. Obstet. Gynecol.* 160:126, 1989.
    The presence of cytologic atypia in combination with a failure to respond to medroxyprogesterone acetate connoted a significant elevation in cancer risk.
12. Van Bogaert, L.-J. Clinicopathologic findings in endometrial polyps. *Obstet. Gynecol.* 71:771, 1988.
    Endometrial polyps may be the site of various types of hyperplasia and may also contain foci of carcinoma or accompany carcinoma elsewhere in the endometrium.

Diagnosis
13. Cherkis, R. C., et al. Significance of atypical endometrial cells detected by cervical cytology. *Obstet. Gynecol.* 69:786, 1986.

Endometrial pathology is common in this context, and endometrial sampling is therefore mandatory.

14. Kaunitz, A. M., et al. Comparison of endometrial biopsy with the endometrial Pipelle and Vabra aspirator. *J. Reprod. Med.* 33:427, 1988.
    The Pipelle, like the Vabra aspirator, can obtain a histologic sample. The correct diagnosis was made in 89 percent of the patients sampled using either instrument.

15. Gimpleson, J. R., and Rappold, H. O. A comparative study between panoramic hysteroscopy with directed biopsies and dilatation and curettage: a review of 276 cases. *Am. J. Obstet. Gynecol.* 158:489, 1988.
    Submucous myomata, endometrial atrophy, and polyps were often missed by D&C and diagnosed by hysteroscopy.

16. Toppozada, M. K., et al. Progesterone challenge test and estrogen assays in menopausal women with endometrial adenomatous hyperplasia. *Int. J. Gynaecol. Obstet.* 26:115, 1988.
    Serum estrogen levels and the progesterone challenge test can be used as screening tools to identify postmenopausal women with endometrial adenomatous hyperplasia, and thus at greater risk for carcinoma.

17. Alberico, S., et al. A clinical and epidemiological study of 245 postmenopausal metrorrhagia patients. *Clin. Exp. Obstet. Gynecol.* 16:113, 1989.
    Twenty-four percent of the patients had adenocarcinoma or atypical hyperplasia; in patients over age 60, this increased to 44 percent.

18. Malpani, A., et al. Endometrial hyperplasia: value of endometrial thickness in ultrasonographic diagnosis and clinical significance. *J. Clin. Ultrasound* 18:173, 1990.
    There is a significant difference in the sonographic appearance of normal and hyperplastic endometrium. Sonography may be helpful in the investigation of women with abnormal bleeding.

19. Syrop, C. H., and Sahakian, V. Transvaginal sonographic detection of endometrial polyps with fluid contrast augmentation. *Obstet. Gynecol.* 79:1041, 1992.
    Injection of the endometrial cavity with isotonic solutions during transvaginal sonography was used to diagnose endometrial polyps, with good results.

Management

20. Kistner, R. W. Treatment of hyperplasia and carcinoma in situ of the endometrium. *Clin. Obstet. Gynecol.* 25:63, 1982.
    In the postmenopausal patient, hysterectomy is indicated when any degree of endometrial hyperplasia is detected. In patients with major surgical risk factors, progestin therapy should be maintained for at least a year.

21. Gal, D. Hormonal therapy for lesions of the endometrium. *Sem. Oncol.* 13:33, 1986.
    The higher the grade, the higher the percentage of patients who develop cancer and the shorter the transition time. Progestin therapy should be continued indefinitely, as it does not abolish the continuous extraglandular estrogen production.

22. Soh, E., and Sato, K. Clinical effects of danazol on endometrial hyperplasia in menopausal and postmenopausal women. *Cancer* 66:983, 1990.
    An effective alternative to progesterone for the treatment of endometrial hyperplasia.

23. Whitehead, M. I. Prevention of endometrial abnormalities. *Acta Obstet. Gynaecol. Scand.* 134:81, 1986.
    The incidence rate for endometrial cancer in an untreated population was 242 per 100,000 women; in those treated with combined estrogen-progestin therapies, it was 70.8 per 100,000 women.

24. Persson, I., et al. Risk of endometrial cancer after treatment with oestrogens alone or in conjunction with progestogens: results of a prospective study. *Br. Med. J.* 298:147, 1989.
    Estrogens alone are associated with a two- to threefold increase in the risk of neoplasia; the addition of progestins either removes this increased risk or delays its onset. Continuing follow-up is essential.

94. ENDOMETRIAL CARCINOMA
Michel E. Rivlin

Endometrial carcinoma is the most common female pelvic malignancy in the United States. It is estimated that 32,000 women will develop this cancer and that 5600 deaths will result from the disease in 1992. Carcinoma of the uterine corpus appears to be hormonally dependent, and epidemiologic factors are known. In obese women, androstenedione is converted to estrone in fatty tissue, and the resulting unopposed action of estrogen leads to a several-fold increase in the risk of endometrial cancer. Most estrogen-related cancers are well differentiated and superficially invasive, with an excellent prognosis. However, there is no room for complacency concerning endometrial cancer, because the overall survival rate is lower in these women than in those with other early stage gynecologic malignancies. The peak incidence occurs in those aged 58 to 60 years; only 10 percent of the cases arise in women younger than 50 years. Nulliparity, obesity, hypertension, and diabetes are frequently associated findings.

The malignant epithelial tumors of the endometrium are usually classified using the World Health Organization (WHO) or International Federation of Obstetricians and Gynecologists (FIGO) systems. The two most common subtypes, adenocarcinoma and adenoacanthoma (adenocarcinoma with squamous metaplasia), have the best prognosis and constitute approximately 80 percent of the cases. Other subtypes, including papillary, adenosquamous, glassy cell, and clear cell carcinoma, are associated with a much less favorable outcome. The tumors are graded according to the degree of histologic differentiation and nuclear atypia. Well-differentiated growths are designated grade 1 and less well differentiated tumors are downgraded (G1 to G3). The less differentiated the tumor, the higher the incidence of deep myometrial penetration and of lymph node metastasis, and thus the worse the prognosis. The gross appearance is usually that of a friable tumor mass with areas of necrosis and hemorrhage. The tumor invades the myometrium and cervix. Lymphatic spread is to the pelvic nodes and then to the aortic nodes, although rarely direct spread to the aortic nodes may occur. Vaginal metastases are found in about 10 percent of the cases; hematogenous spread (to the lungs) occurs with advanced disease.

Abnormal bleeding occurs in about 80 percent of the cases. About 20 percent of the patients with postmenopausal bleeding have underlying cancer, and this increases to 50 to 60 percent after age 80. About 10 percent of the patients complain of uterine cramping and pain. If the uterine contents become infected, a pyometra develops and signs of sepsis may supervene. The findings from physical examination are usually noncontributory unless the disease is advanced.

The revised system for staging endometrial cancer (FIGO, 1988) is based on the findings obtained at surgical exploration. Stage IA tumors are limited to the endometrium; stage IB tumors invade less than half the myometrium; and stage IC tumors invade more than half the myometrium. Stage IIA represents endocervical glandular involvement, and stage IIB indicates cervical stromal invasion. In stage IIIA, tumor invades the serosa, or adnexa, or both, and peritoneal cytologic findings that are positive also place the patient in this stage. Stage IIIB represents vaginal metastases, and stage IIIC, metastasis to the pelvic or paraaortic lymph nodes, or both. In stage IVA, there is invasion of the bladder or bowel, or both, and in stage IVB, distant metastases, including the intraabdominal or inguinal nodes, or both. In those patients (usually about 10% of the cases) who do not undergo surgical exploration because of medical contraindications to operation, the older FIGO (1979) clinical staging is used.

Screening and initial diagnosis can be accomplished by either cytologic or histologic sampling (Papanicolaou smears are negative in 50% of the cases); however, fractional dilatation and curettage (D&C; with the endocervix sampled before the endometrium) is the most reliable method. Hysterography and hysteroscopy have also proved to be useful diagnostic adjuncts in skilled hands. The search for metastases includes chest x-ray studies and intravenous pyelography or, where available, computed tomography or magnetic resonance imaging. Thin-needle biopsy may then be used to sample suspicious areas and determine the presence of disseminated disease. However, clinical staging correlates poorly with surgical staging and may be incorrect in as much as 50 percent of the women. Surgical evaluation includes removal of the uterus, tubes, and ovaries, sampling of the pelvic and paraaortic nodes, and cytologic examination of the washings from the pelvic cavity. Histopathologic evaluation of the depth of the myometrial invasion, the presence or absence of occult cervical and/or lymph nodes metastasis, the presence or absence of hormone receptors, and tumor grading complete the assessment for high-risk disease.

Approximately 75 percent of the cases are in clinical stage I when diagnosed. Management of these women is primarily surgical, and often includes adjuvant radiotherapy in selected cases, given either before or after the operation. Stage I, grade 1 adenocarcinomas with less than one-third myometrial invasion and negative cytologic findings are generally managed by extrafascial hysterectomy and adnexectomy. Features indicating a high likelihood of lymph node metastasis include grade 3 lesions, deep myometrial penetration, histologic cervical involvement, and a clear cell, serous papillary, or adenosquamous histology. In these patients, selective pelvic and aortic node dissection is indicated. If the nodes contain cancer, postoperative pelvic and possibly also aortic radiation therapy (4500 cGy) is administered. This "tailoring" of therapy to the individual patient avoids the use of unnecessary radiation treatment in the low-risk patient while providing the best available therapy for high-risk patients. Stage II carcinoma is diagnosed only if the histopathology indicates cervical stromal invasion, not only on an endocervical curettage containing floating fragments of adenocarcinoma. Treatment is the same as that for cervical cancer, with a choice between radical radiotherapy, radical surgery, and combinations of surgery and radiotherapy. Patients with stage III disease are not predictably cured of their disease. In them, both external and brachytherapy are usually administered; hysterectomy is occasionally used, especially if disease has responded well to irradiation. High-dose progestational agents and chemotherapy may help in palliation. The overall response rate associated with progestin therapy has been reported to be 33 percent for patients with well-differentiated lesions and 10 percent for those with poorly differentiated lesions. Lesions with a high steroid receptor content respond more favorably than do those with a low-receptor content. Tamoxifen is another hormonal agent, with response rates approximating 30 percent. Nonhormonal single cytotoxic agents that yield response rates of up to 42 percent include doxorubicin, cyclophosphamide, cisplatin, and hexamethylenamine. Combination regimens containing cisplatin have shown overall response rates up to 60 percent. Combining hormonal and cytotoxic chemotherapy does not appear to improve response. Five-year survival rates are 75 percent for patients in stage I; 50 percent, in stage II; 30 percent, in stage III; and 9 percent, in stage IV.

Review
1. Creasman, W. T. (ed.). Endometrial cancer. *Clin. Obstet. Gynecol.* 13:1, 1986.
   Ten chapters cover various aspects of this by no means benign disease.

Diagnosis
2. Stovall, T. G., et al. Pipelle endometrial sampling in patients with known endometrial carcinoma. *Obstet. Gynecol.* 77:954, 1991.
   This soft plastic catheter device proved to be an accurate method for endometrial sampling in an office setting.
3. Hricak, H., et al. MR imaging evaluation of endometrial carcinoma: results of an NCI cooperative study. *Radiology* 179:829, 1991.
   Magnetic resonance imaging was better than sonography for the evaluation of myometrial invasion, but is probably not sufficiently accurate to justify the cost.
4. Bourne, T. H., et al. Detection of endometrial cancer by transvaginal ultrasonography with color flow imaging and blood flow analysis: a preliminary report. *Gynecol. Oncol.* 40:253, 1991.

There is a strong correlation between the thickness of the ultrasonic endometrial stripe and the endometrial pathology, with measurements over 5 mm suggesting an endometrial abnormality.

5. Dorum, A., et al. Evaluation of endometrial thickness measured by endovaginal ultrasound in women with postmenopausal bleeding. *Acta Obstet. Gynecol. Scand.* 72:116, 1993.
   Using a 5-mm end point, the sensitivity and negative predictive value of ultrasound evaluation were not high enough to warrant its replacing endometrial biopsy in excluding endometrial abnormalities, including cancer.

Treatment

6. Vardi, J. R., et al. The value of exploratory laparotomy in patients with endometrial carcinoma according to the new International Federation of Gynecology and Obstetrics staging. *Obstet. Gynecol.* 80:204, 1992.
   Surgical staging defined the true extent of disease and identified 20 percent of the cases that might otherwise have gone without effective treatment.

7. Belinson, J. L., et al. Clinical stage I adenocarcinoma of the endometrium—analysis of recurrences and the potential benefit of staging lymphadenectomy. *Gynecol. Oncol.* 44:17, 1992.
   All patients with positive paraaortic nodes died. In no patient who received vaginal or pelvic irradiation, or both, did disease recur in the pelvis. The authors concluded that a staging lymphadenectomy would not have improved the outcome of these patients.

8. Rubin, S. C., et al. Management of endometrial adenocarcinoma with cervical involvement. *Gynecol. Oncol.* 45:294, 1992.
   The preferred treatment of stage II disease has not been established. Some advocate primary radical hysterectomy and others primary radiotherapy. Currently, an approach combining external and internal irradiation with surgery has yielded good results.

9. Bloss, J. D., et al. Use of vaginal hysterectomy for the management of stage I endometrial cancer in the medically compromised patient. *Gynecol. Oncol.* 40:74, 1991.
   The usual reasons for using the vaginal approach are obesity and coexistent medical problems. Careful case selection is the key to good results.

10. Aalders, J. G., Abeler, V., and Kolstad, P. Stage IV endometrial carcinoma: a clinical and histological study of 83 patients. *Gynecol. Oncol.* 17:75, 1984.
    The sites of extrapelvic extension of stage IV disease, in descending order of frequency, were the lungs (36%), multiple sites (23%), the lymph nodes (13%), and the bladder (13%).

11. Gallagher, C. J., et al. A new treatment for endometrial cancer with gonadotrophin releasing–hormone analogue. *Br. J. Obstet. Gynaecol.* 98:1037, 1991.
    Six of 17 women with recurrence experienced complete or partial remission for a median of 20 months with no adverse effects; this treatment warrants comparison with progestin therapy.

12. DeOliviera, C. F., et al. Phase II study of cyclophosphamide, Adriamycin, and cisplatin in recurrent or advanced endometrial cancer. *Proc. A.S.C.O.* 5:123, 1986.
    Multidrug regimens are generally reserved for those patients with poor differentiation, absent progesterone receptors, and reduced performance status.

Pathology and Prognosis

13. Abeler, V. M., Kjørstad, K. E., and Berle, E. Carcinoma of the endometrium in Norway: a histopathological and prognostic survey of a total population. *Int. J. Gynecol. Cancer* 2:9, 1992.
    Poor prognostic indicators included deep myometrial invasion, vascular invasion, advanced age, and grade 3 histopathologic features.

14. Larson, D. M., Johnson, K., and Olson, K. A. Pelvic and paraaortic lymphadenectomy for surgical staging of endometrial cancer: morbidity and mortality. *Obstet. Gynecol.* 79:998, 1992.

Lymphadenectomy did not lead to an increase in morbidity or mortality when compared to the results of standard surgery alone for the treatment of endometrial cancer.

15. Wolfson, A. H., et al. The prognostic significance of surgical staging for carcinoma of the endometrium. *Gynecol. Oncol.* 45:142, 1992.
    Surgical staging is the strongest predictor of survival. The role of adjunctive radiotherapy in stage I disease is not yet clarified.
16. Deligdisch, L. When endometrial carcinoma is not a good cancer. *Rev. Fr. Gynecol. Obstet.* 85:513, 1990.
    The author identified a group of patients who were often older, rarely obese, and often multiparous, with no history of estrogen intake and no evidence of endometrial hyperplasia. The endometrial cancers in these women exhibited greater virulence than did the more common "hormonally-dependent" ones.
17. Milosevic, M. F., Dembo, A. J., and Thomas, G. M. The clinical significance of malignant peritoneal cytology in stage I endometrial carcinoma. *Int. J. Gynecol. Cancer* 2:225, 1992.
    Malignant cytology is usually associated with other adverse prognostic factors that dominate the clinical course of the disease. Routine adjuvant treatment for this finding alone is therefore probably not justified.
18. Cormier, P., et al. Results of assays of estrogen, progesterone and androgen receptors in stage I and stage II adenocarcinoma of the endometrium. *Rev. Fr. Gynecol. Obstet.* 86:491, 1991.
    These hormone assays did not provide any further information on which to base the prognosis of endometrial cancers.
19. Aalders, J. G., Abeler, V., and Kolstad, P. Recurrent adenocarcinoma of the endometrium: a clinical and histopathological study of 379 patients. *Gynecol. Oncol.* 17:85, 1984.
    Local recurrences occurred in 50 percent; distant metastases, in 28 percent; and simultaneous local and distant metastases, in 21 percent.

95. UTERINE SARCOMA
Michel E. Rivlin

Uterine sarcomas constitute 1 to 3 percent of all uterine malignancies (approximately 1000 cases per year). From a clinical point of view, the uterine sarcomas can be divided into three major groups: leiomyosarcomas, endometrial and stromal sarcomas, and mixed mesodermal (müllerian) sarcomas. However, more specific, although often confusing, histogenetic systems of classification are frequently referred to in the literature. Thus, pure uterine sarcomas contain only one cell type and mixed uterine sarcomas contain more than one. Each of these categories is either homologous (all tissue elements are native to the uterus) or heterologous (e.g., striated muscle, cartilage, or bone). All myometrial sarcomas are leiomyosarcomas, whereas endometrial sarcomas may contain one or more types of malignant connective tissue, often also with glandular or squamous carcinoma interspersed. Because the endometrium is derived from mesodermal coelomic epithelium with its underlying mesenchyme, endometrial sarcomas may be termed mesenchymal, mesodermal, or müllerian. The carcinosarcomas may include homologous or heterologous elements.

Abnormal uterine bleeding is the most common symptom (80%) of uterine sarcoma; abdominal pain or discomfort occurs in about 15 to 50 percent of the patients; and about 10 percent are aware of an abdominal mass. Approximately 30 percent of the patients complain of gastrointestinal or genitourinary symptoms. There may be a history of previous pelvic irradiation in as much as 10 percent of the patients. Uterine sarcomas are classified using the International Federation of Obstetricians and Gynecologists (FIGO) staging system for uterine cancer: stage I, tumor confined to the corpus; stage II, tumor involving the cervix; stage III, tumor extending outside the uterus but confined to the pelvis; and stage IV, tumor extending beyond the pelvis or distant metastases. Leiomyosarcoma occurs in younger age groups, with a median age about 50 years; mixed mesodermal sarcoma afflicts older patients, usually in the sixth and seventh decades; and endometrial stromal sarcomas typically arise in patients between the ages of 30 and 75 years, with a mean of 45 years. Mixed mesodermal sarcomas represent 60 percent of the cases; leiomyosarcoma, 30 percent; and other sarcomas, 10 percent.

The preoperative diagnosis is often missed because deep-seated tumors cannot be detected by diagnostic dilatation and curettage (D&C). Most cases are diagnosed at operation performed for the treatment of "fibroids." The main treatment modality is surgical, and usually consists of total abdominal hysterectomy combined with bilateral salpingo-oophorectomy. This also provides information regarding the histologic nature and the extent of disease. Surgery alone carries a high risk of local recurrence and distant metastasis. Adjuvant radiation therapy enhances the pelvic control rate by sterilizing the primary tumor but has little influence on the final outcome because most patients succumb to distant metastases within a short period. Prophylactic chemotherapy reduces the incidence of metastasis, but effects no difference in survival.

Leiomyosarcoma arises from the myometrial smooth muscle, and originates from a fibroid in approximately 5 to 10 percent of the cases. The mitosis count (mitotic index) is helpful in distinguishing sarcoma from cellular smooth muscle tumors and is also a guide to prognosis, as there is an inverse relationship between the mitotic index and the prognosis. When there are more than 10 mitoses per 10 high-power fields (hpf), the tumor is malignant; if there are less than five mitoses, the tumor is benign; and, when there are five to nine mitoses, the tumor is malignant if cellular atypia is also present. Extension beyond the uterus is evidence of malignancy regardless of the mitosis count or pleomorphism. Spread occurs by means of local extension, vascular invasion, and peritoneal implantation. Distant metastases occur to the lung, kidney, liver, brain, and bone. After operation, neither radiotherapy nor chemotherapy has proved to be of added value in the management of this disease; however, adjuvant therapy is recommended if the tumor was not confined to the uterus or if the mitosis count is greater than 10 per 10 hpf. Other unusual smooth muscle tumors of the uterus include intravenous leiomyomatosis, in which fibrous extensions into vessels occur, sometimes involving the iliac veins, vena cava, and right heart. Most patients are premenopausal, and hormonal manipulation may be helpful in management. Because of their benign histology and slow growth, repeated local excision is helpful. Benign metastasizing leiomyoma produces pulmonary metastases, which also appear to be hormonally influenced, as they progress more rapidly in premenopausal than in postmenopausal women. Leiomyomatosis peritonealis disseminata features multiple peritoneal tumors. Chiefly found in blacks, it is often associated with pregnancy and usually regresses when the hormonal stimulus is removed.

Stromal sarcoma, arising from undifferentiated endometrial stromal cells, is the rarest of the three major uterine sarcomas. The diagnosis can be made based on the D&C findings in 75 percent of the patients. There are three distinct variants, based on the morphology, mitosis counts, and biologic behavior. The stromal nodule, with a mitosis count under five, is considered benign; the endolymphatic stromal myosis is a low-grade infiltrating sarcoma that is also referred to as stromal endometriosis, stromatosis, or endolymphatic stromal myosis. This tumor is characterized by infiltrating margins, myometrial invasion, and a mitosis count less than 10 per 10 hpf. Extension into lymphatic and venous channels is common. The tumor is associated with slow progression and late recurrences, with long-term survival the rule, as repeated local excision can often control the disease. Endometrial stromal sarcomas are high-grade malignancies with mitosis counts above 10 per 10 hpf. Pelvic irradiation improves local control and is warranted even when the disease is confined to the uterus. The prognosis in these patients is poor.

Mixed mesodermal sarcomas characteristically occur in postmenopausal women, with the exception of embryonal rhabdomyosarcoma of the cervix or vagina (sarcoma botryoides), which afflicts infants and children. A significant number of patients may

h...
tions. ...
ponent. T...
exhibits a ma...
spindle cell or fus... diation for the treatment of benign or malignant conditions. The sarcoma may be the major component... in the carcinoma or the sarcoma may be the major component in this instance. It is... the carcinoma or the sarcoma may be the major com... prognosis than those com... endometrial and grade 2 or 3. The entire group composed of malignant gland... ma, usually in the form of an undifferentiated the tumor is endometrial in origin... is counts are not useful in predicting outcome 75 percent of the cases. In most inst... native tissues. Metastases are usually orrhagic, necrotic tumor, and, in up to a t... elements may also be found. Because the time of diagnosis. The standard therapy is... de based on D&C findings in up to diotherapy; combination chemotherapy is given i... is is filled with fungating, hemtastases, with response rates as low as 10 percent. ... llowed by whole-pelvis raextent of the tumor, with minimal survival likely if extr... trol of recurrence or meplace. The exception is sarcoma botryoides, in which combina... nosis depends on the of surgery, irradiation, and chemotherapy has considerably impro... spread has taken may be associated with a good prognosis. ... the outlook and

The overall 3-year survival rate for women with uterine sarcomas is 20 to 50 percent. The survival rate in patients with stage I disease is better (50–60%). Once a tumor extends to the cervix or outside the uterus, the survival rate decreases to about 10 to 15 percent; thus, the disease extent at diagnosis is the most important prognostic factor.

Review
1. Oláh, K. S., et al. Retrospective analysis of 318 cases of uterine sarcoma. *Eur. J. Cancer* 27:1095, 1991.
   The overall 5-year survival was 31 percent; a major prognostic indicator was tumor stage; and the ratio of distant to pelvic recurrence was 3:1.
2. Echt, G., et al. Treatment of uterine sarcomas. *Cancer* 66:35, 1990.
   Adjuvant radiotherapy eliminated locoregional disease but failed to effect an improved overall disease-free survival.

Classification
3. Ober, W. B., and Tovell, H. M. M. Mesenchymal sarcomas of the uterus. *Am. J. Obstet. Gynecol.* 77:246, 1959.
   It is often difficult histologically to distinguish benign from malignant mesenchymal neoplasms.
4. Kempson, R. L., and Bari, W. Uterine sarcomas. Classification, diagnosis and prognosis. *Hum. Pathol.* 1:331, 1970.
   This describes a modification of Ober's classification that is histogenetically correct and clinically applicable.

Pure Sarcomas
5. Leibsohn, S., et al. Leiomyosarcoma in a series of hysterectomies performed for presumed uterine leiomyomas. *Am. J. Obstet. Gynecol.* 162:968, 1990.
   The incidence of leiomyosarcoma in fibroids is estimated at 0.13 to 0.29 percent. Conservative therapy of fibroids can delay the diagnosis of leiomyosarcoma.
6. Berchuck, A., et al. Treatment of uterine leiomyosarcoma. *Obstet. Gynecol.* 71:845, 1988.
   Many of the responses to chemotherapy are only partial and temporary. Combination regimens are not superior and produce more severe toxicity.
7. Nordal, R. N., et al. Leiomyosarcoma (LMS) and endometrial stromal sarcoma (ESS) of the uterus. A survey of patients treated in the Norwegian Radium Hospital 1976–1985. *Int. J. Gynecol. Cancer* 3:110, 1993.
   Despite the widespread use of chemotherapy, the prognosis was not improved.
8. Chang, K. L., et al. Primary uterine endometrial stromal neoplasms. A clinicopathologic study of 117 cases. *Am. J. Surg. Pathol.* 14:415, 1990.

The 5- and 10-year survival for stage 1 disease was 98 and 89 per

9. El-Naggar, A. K., et al. Uterine stromal neoplasms: a clinico
   flow cytometric correlation. *Hum. Pathol.* 22:897, 1991.
   The proliferative index yielded by flow cytometry may ...vic irradiation.
   predicting the aggressive potential of a subset of low

Mixed Sarcomas

10. Meredith, R. F., et al. An excess of ute... *...radiation for malignancy*
    Cancer 58:2003, 1986. ...s, *compared with those who had*
    In this study, women who had pre... *conditions.*
    tended to have advanced, aggres... tumors of the uterine corpus: a review.
    previously undergone irradi...

11. Ali, S., and Wells, M. Mi...copathologic features, prognosis, and treatment, as
    Int. J. Gynecol. Oncol...re.
    A critical account ...
    derived from the ...rognostic value of peritoneal washings in patients with ma-

12. Geszler, G.,...d müllerian tumors of the uterus. *Am. J. Obstet. Gynecol.* 155:83,
    lignant ...
    1996.
    The ...ical *course in pathologic stage I patients with positive washings was simi-*
    lar to that in patients with more advanced disease.

13. Podczaski, E. S., et al. Management of malignant, mixed mesodermal tumors of
    the uterus. *Gynecol. Oncol.* 32:240, 1989.
    The surgical extent of the disease was a major prognostic factor. Cisplatin was
    moderately active with mild toxicity.

14. Costa, M. J., Khan, R., and Judd, R. Carcinosarcoma (malignant mixed müller-
    ian [mesodermal] tumor) of the uterus and ovary. Correlation of clinical, patho-
    logic, and immunohistochemical features in 29 cases. *Arch. Pathol. Lab. Med.*
    115:583, 1991.
    There was no prognostic difference between the homologous or the heterologous
    tumors.

15. Gordon, A. N., and Montag, T. W. Sarcoma botryoides of the cervix: excision
    followed by adjuvant chemotherapy for preservation of reproductive function.
    Gynecol. Oncol. 36:119, 1990.
    The botryoid type is a variant of embryonal rhabdomyosarcoma with a "grapelike"
    appearance. Excision with chemotherapy may be sufficient treatment for localized
    disease.

Treatment and Prognosis

16. Thigpen, J. T., et al. Phase II trial of cisplatin as a first-line chemotherapy in
    patients with advanced or recurrent uterine sarcoma: a Gynecologic Oncology
    Group study. *J. Clin. Oncol.* 9:1962, 1991.
    Cisplatin has definite activity for mixed mesodermal sarcomas but little for leiom-
    yosarcoma. The converse is found with doxorubicin.

17. Sutton, G. P., et al. Phase II trial of ifosfamide and mesna in leiomyosarcoma of
    the uterus: a Gynecology Oncology Group study. *Am. J. Obstet Gynecol.* 166:556,
    1992.
    Ifosfamide, an alkylating agent similar to cyclophosphamide, exhibits modest ac-
    tivity for leiomyosarcoma and mixed mesodermal sarcomas.

18. Levenback, C., et al. Resection of pulmonary metastases from uterine sarcomas.
    Gynecol. Oncol. 45:202, 1992.
    In a carefully selected group, a 35 percent 10-year survival was achieved.

19. Malmström, H., et al. Flow cytometric analysis of uterine sarcoma: ploidy and S-
    phase rate as prognostic indicators. *Gynecol. Oncol.* 44:172, 1992.
    DNA ploidy showed a significant prognostic value even when adjusted for stage,
    grade, and mitotic index.

20. Wade, K., et al. Uterine sarcoma: steroid receptors and response to hormonal
    therapy. *Gynecol. Oncol.* 39:364, 1990.

The tumors are estrogen receptor positive in 48 percent and progesterone receptor positive in 30 percent; neither the receptor status nor the use of adjuvant hormonal therapy affected survival.

BENIGN OVARIAN NEOPLASMS

Norma Rivlin

tered in the ... differentiated from normal ovarian cysts are the most common adnexal masses encoun-teum cysts are rarely larger. Their significance lies in the fact that they must be mobile. There may be associated ... ovarian or tubal lesions. Follicular and corpus lu-rhage, torsion, or rupture of a cyst may ... in diameter, and they are unilateral and freely Observation, or a short course of oral contraceptive ... abnormalities. Uncommonly, hemor-appearance of the cysts, which are dependent ... an acute abdominal condition. lutein cysts are usually large and bilateral. They res... gonadotropin stimulation. Theca chorionic gonadotropin (hCG), commonly stemming from trophoblastic disease. They may also form after the use of ovulation-inducing agents such as clomiphene. Invo-lution occurs once the hormonal stimulus is removed.

Most ovarian neoplasms (70%) are derived from the coelomic germinal surface epi-thelium. This epithelium is of paramesonephric (müllerian) origin, so these tumors contain epithelium similar to that lining adult müllerian structures (e.g., the endo-cervix, endometrium, and endosalpinx) and are named mucinous, endometrioid, or serous neoplasms, respectively. Serous cystadenomas account for 25 percent of the benign ovarian tumors. In general, these neoplasms arise in the reproductive years. They may occur as unilateral, unilocular cysts, termed simple cystomas, but serous cystadenomas are usually multilocular and may have papillary excrescences; 20 per-cent may be bilateral. The papillary cystadenoma is the most likely to undergo ma-lignant change. Symptoms depend on the size of the tumor and whether accidents, such as rupture or torsion, occur. They are treated by conservative surgical treatment in younger women and by removal of the uterus and adnexa in older women.

Mucinous cystadenomas account for 15 percent of the benign ovarian tumors. Ma-lignant change occurs in about 5 percent. They are multilocular tumors containing a thick mucinous substance secreted by the columnar epithelium lining the cyst. They are usually unilateral (bilateral in 10%) and can become very large. Papillary excres-cences may develop and increase the malignant potential. The clinical picture and management of the mucinous cystadenomas are similar to those for serous tumors.

The remaining benign epithelial tumors are uncommon. Endometrioid and meso-nephroid (clear cell) cysts are included in this category and are extremely rare. The Brenner tumor, composed of nests of epithelial cells in a fibrous stroma, accounts for 1 percent of the ovarian tumors. Usually found in postmenopausal women, the malig-nant potential is low. The tumor may also occur in conjunction with mucinous or dermoid cysts. Management usually consists of removal of the uterus and adnexa because of the patient's age.

About 20 percent of the primary ovarian neoplasms are derived from germ cells. The mature cystic teratoma (dermoid), the most common tumor of young women, is second only to the serous tumor in frequency in all age groups. The tumor may con-tain tissues derived from all three germ layers, although ectodermal elements (par-ticularly sebaceous fluid and hair) usually predominate. In 15 percent, functional or nonfunctional thyroid tissue may be present. The tumor is mobile and may lie ante-rior to the uterus. Malignant change is rare. Symptoms are uncommon unless a com-plication (usually torsion) occurs. Dermoids display a characteristic sonographic pattern of sharply defined fluid levels, dense echoes, and cystic areas. The approach to management is generally conservative surgical treatment consisting of ovarian cystectomy and careful examination of the opposite ovary, as 15 percent are bilateral. In older patients, the uterus and adnexa should be removed.

Approximately 5 percent of the primary ovarian neoplasms are derived from sexually undifferentiated mesenchymal tissue. The fibroma, a connective tissue tumor composed of fibroblasts and collagen, is relatively common and accounts for 20 percent of the solid ovarian tumors. The tumors vary greatly in size, and are bilateral in 10 percent of the patients. Generally symptomless, or exerting pressure effects, large, about 75 percent have a degree of ascites, whereas 3 percent exhibit syndrome (hydrothorax with ascites). The average age of patients at __ younger years; the usual approach to therapy is hysterectomy with rem__ hemangioma, although malignant change is rare and oophorectomy is s__ patient. Other supporting tissue tumors, such as myxom__ from specialized gonadal are occasionally seen, but all are rare.

An additional 5 percent of ovarian tumors __). These are "functioning" tumors stroma (sexually differentiated mesenchyme__ulosa-theca cell) or androgen (Sertoli-capable of producing either estrogema). The majority of these tumors are potentially Leydig cell), or both (gynandrol__' __ therefore are not regarded as benign.

tially malignant, however __u
Generally, most ovarian neoplasm__ __e clinically silent, except for pressure symptoms such as urinary freque__-y, constipation, and pelvic heaviness. Very large tumors cause abdomi__ swelling and discomfort and might be confused with pregnancy. Pain may be felt, owing either to stretching of the ovarian capsule or to torsion, rupture, or intracystic hemorrhage. If the tumors are functional, menstrual abnormalities may occur.

On physical examination, most of the ovarian tumors will be found lying behind the uterus or they will have ascended into the abdomen, although dermoids may be anteriorly placed. Benign tumors tend to be unilateral, cystic, movable, and symmetrical; there is no ascites. By contrast, malignant growths are usually bilateral, solid, fixed, and nodular, and there is ascites.

Diagnostic evaluation should include sonography, chest and abdominal x-ray examination, as well as intravenous pyelography. Further investigations depend on the individual case and may include bowel x-ray studies and laparoscopy. Estimation of the CA 125 levels, which are elevated in many cases of serous ovarian cancers, may be helpful, although many benign conditions exhibit this elevation as well. Alternative imaging techniques, including computed tomography (CT) and magnetic resonance imaging (MRI), are also being used more frequently in the assessment of pelvic masses. The differential diagnosis of adnexal masses includes benign ovarian tumors, functional ovarian cysts, ovarian malignancies, parovarian cysts (benign lesions in the broad ligament), endometriosis, acute and chronic inflammatory masses, ectopic gestation, pedunculated fibroids, congenital uterine anomalies, and gastrointestinal masses. Careful history, physical examination, and relevant ancillary investigations are essential to ensure adequate management.

Women between the ages of 15 and 45 years who have clinically benign ovarian cysts less than 6 cm in diameter may be observed on a monthly basis for a short time, but premenarchal and postmenopausal females are both at high risk for malignancy, and early diagnosis is thus essential. Cysts greater than 10 cm in diameter are probably neoplastic and require immediate evaluation and probable excision. Almost all solid ovarian tumors are neoplastic (with the exception of the rare luteoma of pregnancy) and mandate aggressive evaluation and therapy. If a cyst persists or enlarges during a period of observation, one should proceed with evaluation and probably surgical excision. If it persists but gets smaller, the patient may be observed through a second cycle.

When laparotomy is indicated, it is performed as soon as diagnostic procedures are completed. If malignancy is a possibility, bowel preparation should precede operation. Features of benign disease include a unilateral, freely mobile, smooth cyst with no ascitic fluid, and smooth peritoneal surfaces. If there is any doubt, frozen sections should be obtained. In older patients, total abdominal hysterectomy with bilateral salpingo-oophorectomy is the treatment of choice, even in patients with benign neoplasms. In younger patients with benign disease, conservative surgical treatment is the rule. Ovarian cystectomy or unilateral salpingo-oophorectomy, performed with great care to determine whether there is disease in the remaining ovary, is the usual procedure. Because the lesions are benign, the prognosis is excellent.

If the diagnostic investigation reveals findings that are overwhelmingly in favor of benign disease, many clinicians currently approach the surgery of adnexal disease, including ovarian masses, laparoscopically. Because of the risk of mismanagement of a malignant growth, however, it should be used only in a highly select group of women and only performed by clinicians with special expertise in its application.

Functional Cysts
1. Spanos, W. J. Preoperative hormonal therapy of cystic adnexal masses. *Am. J. Obstet. Gynecol.* 116:551, 1973.
   No patients with cysts that persisted for 6 weeks while they were on oral contraceptives proved to have functional cysts.
2. Lanes, S. F., et al. Oral contraceptive type and functional ovarian cysts. *Am. J. Obstet. Gynecol.* 166:956, 1992.
   The protective effect of oral contraceptives against functional ovarian cysts, reported previously for high-dose monophasic pills, may be attenuated with newer pills of lower hormonal potency.
3. Ito, M., et al. Theca lutein cysts with maternal virilization and elevated serum testosterone in pregnancy. *Acta Obstet. Gynecol. Scand.* 66:565, 1987.
   Another benign ovarian cyst that can cause virilization during pregnancy is the benign luteoma of pregnancy. As with theca lutein cysts, they regress after delivery.

Neoplasms Derived from Coelomic Epithelium
4. Woodruff, J. D., and Novak, E. R. Papillary serous tumors of the ovary. *Am. J. Obstet. Gynecol.* 67:1112, 1954.
   A fourth of the papillary serous cystadenomas contain microscopic calcospherites (psammoma bodies), which may show up on x-ray studies.
5. Chaitin, B. A., Gershenson, D. M., and Evans, H. L. Mucinous tumors of the ovary. A clinicopathologic study of 70 cases. *Cancer* 55:1958, 1985.
   Mucinous tumors are frequently associated with other cystomas, particularly serous and Brenner tumors, as well as with teratomas. Malignancy occurs in 5 to 10 percent of the patients with primarily benign mucinous cysts.
6. Kahn, M. A. and Demopoulos, R. I. Mucinous ovarian tumors with pseudomyxoma peritonei: a clinicopathological study. *Int. J. Gynecol. Pathol.* 11:15, 1992.
   Rupture of a mucinous tumor can lead to diffuse intraperitoneal spread, a syndrome called pseudomyxoma peritonei.
7. Yoonessi, M., and Abell, M. R. Brenner tumors of the ovary. *Obstet. Gynecol.* 54:90, 1979.
   Three in 24 cases were malignant.

Neoplasms Derived from Germ Cells
8. Williams, S. D. Germ cell tumors. *Hematol. Oncol. Clin. North Am.* 6:967, 1992.
   Teeth are present in nearly 50 percent of the benign cystic teratomas and can be visualized on x-ray films. A nodule, Rokitansky's protuberance, may be noted within the cyst wall.
9. Kempers, R. D., et al. Struma ovarii-ascitic, hyperthyroid, and asymptomatic syndromes. *Ann. Intern. Med.* 72:883, 1970.
   The term struma ovarii *is applied when thyroid tissue is the predominant tissue in a dermoid.*
10. Lee, C. H., Raman, S., and Sivanesaratnam, V. Torsion of ovarian tumors: a clinicopathological study. *Int. J. Gynecol. Obstet.* 28:21, 1989.
    A third of the tumors were dermoids. Pain was the major symptom, and an abdominal mass was palpable in 79 percent of the patients.
11. Kawai, M., et al. Seven tumor markers in benign and malignant germ cell tumors of the ovary. *Gynecol. Oncol.* 45:248, 1992.

These tumor markers include alpha-fetoprotein in yolk sac tumor and immature teratoma, lactate dehydrogenase in dysgerminoma, CA 19-9 in teratomatous growths, and CA 125 in all tumor types except mature cystic teratoma.

Neoplasms Derived from Nonspecific Mesenchyme

12. Dockerty, M. B., and Masson, J. C. Ovarian fibroma: a clinical and pathological study of 283 cases. Am. J. Obstet. Gynecol. 47:741, 1944.
The ovarian fibroma is not easily distinguishable from the thecoma, either clinically or histologically.

13. Meigs, J. V. Fibroma of the ovary with ascites and hydrothorax—Meigs' syndrome. Am. J. Obstet. Gynecol. 67:962, 1954.
This change occurs in less than 5 percent of the fibromas.

Diagnosis

14. Hernandez, E., and Miyazawa, C. K. The pelvic mass. Patients' ages and pathologic findings. J. Reprod. Med. 33:361, 1988.
Of 100 women operated on for pelvic adnexal masses, the most frequent diagnoses, by age group, were cancer in 56 percent older than 50 years, endometriosis in 27 percent 30 to 49 years of age, and dermoid in 33 percent younger than 30 years.

15. Ghossain, M. A., et al. Epithelial tumors of the ovary: comparison of MR and CT findings. Radiology 181:863, 1991.
The accuracy of MRI and CT in the identification of benign versus malignant tumors was 86 percent and 92 percent, respectively.

16. Gadducci, A., et al. The concomitant determination of different tumor markers in patients with epithelial ovarian cancer and benign ovarian masses: relevance for differential diagnosis. Gynecol. Oncol. 44:147, 1992.
The application of monoclonal antibody technology has led to the identification of new tumor-associated antigens. Multiple tumor markers may prove more useful than single markers in the management of ovarian masses.

17. Chalas, E., et al. The clinical significance of thrombocytosis in women presenting with a pelvic mass. Am. J. Obstet. Gynecol. 166:974, 1992.
The positive predictive value of platelet counts over 400,000, in association with an elevated CA 125 level, was 95 percent in the setting of ovarian cancer.

18. Timor-Tritsch, I. E., et al. Transvaginal ultrasonographic characterization of ovarian masses by means of color flow–directed Doppler measurements and a morphologic scoring system. Am. J. Obstet. Gynecol. 168:909, 1993.
This method can detect the low-resistance intratumoral blood vessels characteristic of malignant tumors.

Management

19. Killackey, M. A., and Neuwirth, R. S. Evaluation and management of the pelvic mass: a review of 540 cases. Obstet. Gynecol. 71;319, 1988.
These authors state that patients with a pelvic or adnexal mass who are older than 40 years should undergo a complete evaluation, and should be apprised of the risks of malignancy. A vertical incision should be used, and appropriate surgical and oncologic consultation should be available.

20. Lindeque, B. G., et al. Ultrasonographic criteria for the conservative management of antenatally diagnosed fetal ovarian cysts. J. Reprod. Med. 33:196, 1988.
Routine antenatal ultrasonography can detect fetal ovarian cysts. The majority are benign and functional. Conservative management during the neonatal period is recommended.

21. Lim-Tan, S. K., Cajigas, H. E., and Scully, R. E. Ovarian cystectomy for serous borderline tumors: a follow-up study of 35 cases. Obstet. Gynecol. 72:775, 1988.
Suggests that young women wishing to preserve their fertility may undergo conservative surgical treatment for serous borderline ovarian tumors, in view of the relatively good prognosis associated with these lesions.

22. El-Yahia, A. R., et al. Ovarian tumours in pregnancy. Aust. N.Z. J. Obstet. Gynaecol. 31:327, 1991.
Cysts larger than 10 cm in diameter should be removed in the second trimester.

Urgent laparotomy is indicated if torsion, rupture, or obstructed labor occurs. Cysts between 5 and 10 cm can be managed conservatively, if they are simple, but they should be removed if they contain septae or nodules or are solid.

23. Fleischer, A. C., et al. Transvaginal sonography of postmenopausal ovaries with pathologic correlation. *J. Ultrasound Med.* 9:637, 1990.
    In the evaluation of an ovarian mass, the positive predictive value of transvaginal sonography was 94 percent and the negative predictive value was 92 percent. Other workers have suggested that, if the lesion is seen to be less than 5 cm and is cystic on an ultrasound image, malignancy is unlikely.

24. Lack, E. E., Young, R. H., Scully, R. C. Pathology of ovarian neoplasms in childhood and adolescence. *Pathol. Annu.* 27:281, 1992.
    Although rare, they can be malignant; the most common are germ cell tumors. Surgical treatment, if indicated, should be conservative (cystectomy or unilateral oophorectomy) whenever feasible.

25. Parker, W. H. Management of adnexal masses by operative laparoscopy. Selection criteria. *J. Reprod. Med.* 37:603, 1992.
    This identifies a population of women at low risk for malignancy who may be appropriate candidates for laparoscopic adnexal surgery.

26. Hulka, J. F., et al. Management of ovarian masses. AAGL 1990 survey. *J. Reprod. Med.* 37:599, 1992.
    An overall incidence of 4 per 1000 cases of ovarian cancer was found, and about 70 percent were managed by laparoscopy alone.

27. Ng, P. H., and Hewson, A. D. The residual adnexa syndrome. *Aust. N.Z. J. Obstet. Gynaecol.* 33:71, 1993.
    Removal may be difficult, placing the ureters and great vessels at risk of injury.

97. OVARIAN CARCINOMA
Michel E. Rivlin

Cancer of the ovary is the second most common gynecologic malignancy. In 1992, 21,000 new cases were expected in the United States, with 13,000 deaths. The mortality associated with it is greater than that for cervical and endometrial cancers combined. One in 70 girls born in the United States each year will suffer ovarian cancer. The largest number of new cases affect women between the ages of 50 and 59 years. The mean age at onset is 62 years; the mean age at death is 63 years. U.S. age-specific data for both ovarian cancer and endometrial cancer are difficult to interpret because the denominator cannot be accurately estimated due to the high rate of hysterectomy and oophorectomy performed in the United States. However, as with breast cancer, the rate of increase clearly slows down around age 50, suggesting a protective effect of the menopause. The ovarian cancer risk also decreases steadily with increasing parity and with increasing duration of oral contraceptive use. Thus, late menarche, early menopause, pregnancy, and oral contraception all appear to confer a protective effect by effecting ovulation suppression. Hereditary disorders, environmental factors, viral infection, and irradiation have also been implicated in the etiology of ovarian cancer. Although conclusive proof of the influence of these factors is still lacking, clinicians can suggest preventive measures for high-risk women; this includes oral contraception, or, in those with a family history of ovarian cancer, prophylactic oophorectomy after completion of childbearing. The incidence of ovarian cancer is highest in industrialized countries, with the exception of Japan. This finding also holds for breast cancer. However, if native Japanese women emigrate to the United States, their risk becomes higher than that of women relatives remaining at home. Diet and weight may be responsible for these findings because of their effect on the age of menarche and the menstrual cycle.

Ovarian cancer is classified histologically into epithelial, gonadal stromal, and germ cell tumors. Of the malignant tumors, 40 to 45 percent are serous, 5 to 10 percent are mucinous, 15 to 20 percent are endometrioid, and 4 to 6 percent are clear cell. Epithelial adenocarcinomas are further differentiated into borderline and malignant types. Borderline growths display nuclear abnormalities and cellular stratification but lack stromal invasion. Gonadal stromal tumors (e.g., granulosa cell and Sertoli-Leydig cell) constitute 5 to 10 percent of the cases of ovarian cancer. Of the germ cell tumors, dysgerminoma (1–2%), embryonal carcinoma (1–2%), and immature teratoma (1–2%) are the most common. Metastatic tumors (4–8%) are generally derived from the bowel, endometrium, breast, or thyroid. Spread takes place over the surface of the peritoneum and the bowel and then extends to the upper abdomen. If there is nodal involvement, it usually affects the retroperitoneal nodes of the upper abdomen. Iliac nodes are involved about a fourth as often as in cervical cancer. Hematogenous spread is rarely seen clinically, but transdiaphragmatic dispersion is common.

Staging of ovarian cancer is based on the findings noted at laparotomy. In stage IA, growth is limited to one ovary; in stage IB, both ovaries are involved. Stage IC is either stage IA or IB, but tumor is also on the surface of the ovary, the capsule is ruptured, ascites is present, or the cytologic analysis of peritoneal washings yields positive findings. Stage II disease involves one or both ovaries and there is pelvic extension. Stage IIA involves extension or metastases to the uterus or tubes; stage IIB involves extension to other pelvic tissues; and stage IIC is stage IIA or B, plus there is ascites or positive washings, a ruptured capsule, or tumor on the ovarian surface. In stage III, tumor growth extends outside the pelvis with peritoneal implants or positive retroperitoneal or inguinal nodes, or both. Superficial liver metastases are considered stage III, and this stage is further divided into IIIA through IIIC. Stage IV represents distant metastasis and includes pleural effusions with positive cytology and parenchymal liver metastasis.

The detection of a pelvic mass is often the first indication of an ovarian tumor, although many patients experience vague gastrointestinal symptoms for several months before the mass is discovered. Rarely, the endocrine activity of the tumor may lead to menstrual abnormality. Although pelvic findings can be inconclusive, palpation of an irregular, nodular ("a handful of knuckles"), insensitive, bilateral mass in the pelvis strongly suggests the presence of an ovarian tumor. The disease is bilateral in 70 percent of the cases of ovarian carcinomas, compared with 5 percent for benign lesions. Ascites and a right-sided pleural effusion are common findings in advanced disease. Imaging techniques such as computed tomography (CT) and magnetic resonance imaging (MRI) and sonography are more useful for monitoring the course of the disease than for making an early diagnosis.

Serum tumor markers are useful in the diagnosis and management of several types of ovarian tumors. CA 125 levels are elevated in more than 80 percent of the patients with serous epithelial cancers but in only 1 percent of the normal population. Levels of this marker may also be elevated in association with endometriosis, pelvic inflammatory disease, fibroids, and other malignancies, however. Alpha-fetoprotein serum levels are elevated in endodermal sinus tumors and embryonal cell cancers. Levels of human chorionic gonadotropin are elevated in ovarian trophoblastic disease and may be elevated in embryonal cell carcinoma and dysgerminoma. The lactate dehydrogenase level may be elevated in patients with dysgerminoma. CA 19-9 levels may be elevated in the setting of mucinous ovarian and gastrointestinal cancers. Carcinoembryonic antigen levels are sometimes elevated in association with ovarian cancer, but this finding is not specific for this cancer. None of the tumor markers is sensitive or specific enough to be considered for routine screening, but they are helpful in the differential diagnosis of pelvic masses and in the follow-up of treated cases.

Prime indications for exploratory laparotomy include a pelvic mass appearing after menopause; an adnexal mass at any age, progressively enlarging beyond 5 cm in diameter; adnexal masses 10 cm in diameter or larger; and masses that cannot be identified definitely as either fibroid or carcinoma. The preoperative workup should include an upper and lower bowel series, intravenous pyelography, and bowel preparation. This evaluation documents the extent of disease and helps determine whether the cancer is primary or metastatic. The goal of the primary surgical procedure is to remove the entire cancer and, if this is not feasible, to remove as much of the cancer as possible (debulk) without causing excessive morbidity or mortality. The early results of these major procedures have been improved by the liberal use of hyperalimentation, antibiotics, and critical care monitoring techniques. Conservative surgical treatment has no place in patients older than 40 years with epithelial tumors, which account for 90 percent of the ovarian cancers.

After an adequate midline incision has been made, cytologic evaluation of the pelvis, paracolic gutters, and subphrenic areas is carried out. Palpation and inspection of all peritoneal surfaces, including the liver, diaphragm, and pelvic and peri-aortic nodes, are followed by biopsy of suspicious areas. Total hysterectomy, bilateral salpingo-oophorectomy, omentectomy, and appendectomy should then be performed. In young nulliparous patients with stage IA lesions whose gross and microscopic pathologic findings are favorable, unilateral adnexectomy is an option.

Chemotherapy should be administered to patients with stage II, III, or IV tumors. The effect of adjuvant chemotherapy is unclear but can improve the patient's quality of life. The chemotherapy for stage I disease can be either single or multiagent and make use of drugs such as melphalan or cisplatin. The benefit of therapy for low-grade lesions must be weighed against the risk of its causing subsequent acute leukemia. Stage III and IV disease is generally treated with multiagent regimens that include cisplatin and cyclophosphamide (Cytoxan), although a clear-cut advantage over single-agent therapy has not been established. External radiotherapy has been phased out as an adjuvant measure in most centers, with the exception of its use in the treatment of germ cell and gonadal stromal tumors, which are more responsive to this modality. However, in some hands, external radiotherapy has yielded good results and is still used. Another form of adjuvant therapy, the instillation of radioactive phosphorus at the time of operation, has also been used with some success.

After initial or adjunctive therapy in patients with no evidence of disease (NED), many oncologists proceed to second-look surgery, an operation designed to evaluate the presence and extent of residual disease, if present. The techniques of this procedure are similar to those used for the original staging procedure. Chemotherapy may then be discontinued in patients with NED, whereas those found to have disease may receive agents different from those previously administered. However, there are no hard data to prove that the second-look operation has led to improved long-term survival.

Problems to be palliated in patients with advanced ovarian cancer include ascites, pleural effusions, intestinal or urinary tract obstruction, and bowel fistula. Repeated paracentesis, nasogastric intestinal decompression, total parenteral nutrition, and conservative bypass operation all play a role in the management of these difficult situations.

The prognosis varies: approximately 70 percent of stage I, 50 percent of stage II, 15 percent of stage III, and less than 5 percent of stage IV patients survive 5 years. Sixty to 70 percent are either in stage III or IV at the time of initial diagnosis, however, so there is only a 15 to 25 percent overall 5-year survival rate. The cause of death is usually related to diminished immunocompetence (resulting in severe sepsis) and malnutrition (associated with bowel obstruction).

Germ cell cancers are highly malignant and arise predominantly in the second or third decade of life. Characteristically unilateral (66%), the most common is the dysgerminoma, a tumor that is similar to the seminoma and arises from the primitive germ cell. Stage IA dysgerminomas can be treated by unilateral adnexectomy. Recurrences occur in 10 to 20 percent of the cases, but subsequent radiotherapy is successful in controlling disease in 90 percent. Advanced disease is treated by hysterectomy with adnexectomy and postoperative irradiation administered to the pelvic and para-aortic nodes. The embryonal carcinoma and immature teratoma arise from embryonal cells. Patients with these tumors are good candidates for conservative operation, followed by combination chemotherapy, to which they generally respond well. The endodermal sinus tumor and choriocarcinoma are both derived from extraembryonic tissue. The former responds well to combination chemotherapy, and conservative operation is recommended, as up to 75 percent of the cases can be cured even while preserving fertility. Adjuvant chemotherapy is often recommended even for stage IA tumors.

Gonadal stromal malignancies include granulosa and Sertoli-Leydig cell cancers that are usually unilateral with low-grade malignancy; recurrence is typically confined to the pelvis. Late recurrences are not uncommon. Early disease in young patients may be treated conservatively.

The gonadoblastoma is composed of both germ cell and gonadal stromal cell tumors, in varying combinations. Most patients are intersexual, and 90 percent are chromatin negative. The malignant potential is determined by the type of germ cell tumor present. Generally, bilateral gonadectomy is indicated.

Reviews
  1. Richardson, G. S., et al. Common epithelial cancer of the ovary (first of two parts). *N. Engl. J. Med.* 312:415, 1985.
     This article deals with the topics of epidemiology, prognosis, staging, borderline tumors, and surgical therapy.
  2. Richardson, G. S., et al. Common epithelial cancer of the ovary (second of two parts). *N. Engl. J. Med.* 312:475, 1985.
     This article deals with the topics of adjuvant radiotherapy and chemotherapy.
  3. Hand, R., et al. Staging procedures, clinical management, and survival outcome for ovarian carcinoma. *J.A.M.A.* 269:1119, 1993.
     In stage I and II disease, extensive surgical treatment proved to have little impact on survival, but, in stage III disease, extensive surgery and platinum-based chemotherapy improved survival.

Etiology
  4. Greggi, S., et al. Analysis of 138 consecutive ovarian cancer patients: incidence and characteristics of familial cases. *Gynecol. Oncol.* 39:300, 1990.
     There may be a genetic component in some cases of ovarian cancer, and some practitioners recommend prophylactic oophorectomy for women who have two first-degree relatives with the disease.
  5. Heintz, A. P., Hacker, N. F., and Lagasse, L. D. Epidemiology and etiology of ovarian cancer: a review. *Obstet. Gynecol.* 66:127, 1985.
     Sex cord tumors are found in women with Peutz-Jeghers syndrome, ovarian fibromas in those with basal cell nevus syndrome, and dysgerminomas and gonadoblastomas in those with streak (XY) gonads with gonadal dysgenesis.
  6. McGowan, L. Ovarian cancer after hysterectomy. *Obstet. Gynecol.* 69:386, 1987.
     Fourteen percent of the women in this series of ovarian cancers had a prior hysterectomy. However, if bilateral oophorectomy was performed in all patients older than 40 years who undergo operation for benign lesions, 700 women would be castrated for each cancer prevented.
  7. Spirtas, R., Kaufman, S. C., and Alexander, N. J. Fertility drugs and ovarian cancer: red alert or red herring? *Fertil. Steril.* 59:291, 1993.
     White women who had used fertility drugs had three times the risk of epithelial ovarian cancer compared to women without a history of infertility.

Diagnosis
  8. Creasman, W. T., and DiSaia, P. J. Screening in ovarian cancer. *Am. J. Obstet. Gynecol.* 165:7, 1991.
     Data do not yet justify annual screening of CA 125 levels and/or pelvic ultrasound in all women.
  9. Kawai, M., et al. Transvaginal Doppler ultrasound with color flow imaging in the diagnosis of ovarian cancer. *Obstet. Gynecol.* 79:163, 1992.
     The probable nature of ovarian tumors is now diagnosed based on patient age, tumor size, tumor markers, and ultrasound pattern, as well as the observation of hemodynamic characteristics.
 10. Buist, M. R., et al. Radioimmunotargeting in ovarian carcinoma patients with indium-111 labeled monoclonal antibody OV-TL 3 F(ab')2: pharmacokinetics, tissue distribution, and tumor imaging. *Int. J. Gynecol. Cancer* 2:23, 1992.
     The diagnostic accuracy of immunoscintigraphy was compared with that of ultrasound, CT, MRI, and physical examination. This method proved superior in locating abdominal tumor deposits.

11. Rice, L. W., et al. Epithelial ovarian tumors of borderline malignancy. *Gynecol. Oncol.* 39:195, 1990.
    The ovarian epithelial tumors arise from the coelomic epithelium. There are three categories: benign, low malignant potential (borderline), and malignant.
12. Watkin, W., Silva, E. G., and Gershenson, D. M. Mucinous carcinoma of the ovary. *Cancer* 69:208, 1992.
    The clinical stage and stromal invasion are the most important variables. The prognosis in patients with stage I mucinous carcinomas is excellent.
13. Germá, J. R., et al. Malignant ovarian germ cell tumors: the experience at the Hospital de la Santa Creu i Sant Pau. *Gynecol. Oncol.* 45:153, 1992.
    Despite the exquisite radiosensitivity of dysgerminomas, chemotherapy is usually preferred to prevent infertility and because good results can also be expected.
14. Gershenson, D. M., et al. Treatment of metastatic stromal tumors of the ovary with cisplatin, doxorubicin, and cyclophosphamide. *Obstet. Gynecol.* 70:765, 1987.
    Because of their rarity, multiple histologic patterns, and indolent behavior, with a propensity to recur after several years, the appropriate therapy for malignant stromal tumors is still not clear.

Management
15. Petru, E., et al. Abdominopelvic computed tomography in the preoperative evaluation of suspected ovarian masses. *Int. J. Gynecol. Cancer* 2:252, 1992.
    The routine use of CT in the preoperative evaluation did not appear to be justified.
16. Potter, M. E., et al. Primary surgical therapy of ovarian cancer: how much and when. *Gynecol. Oncol.* 40:195, 1991.
    Reoperating on patients considered unresectable at the time of referral did not increase survival over that seen in patients who underwent reoperation after an attempt at chemotherapeutic reduction.
17. Gruppo Interregionale Cooperativo Oncologico Ginecologia. Long-term results of a randomized trial comparing cisplatin with cisplatin and cyclophosphamide with cisplatin, cyclophosphamide, and adriamycin in advanced ovarian cancer. *Gynecol. Oncol.* 45:115, 1992.
    There was no difference in the results among the three arms of the study.
18. Hoskins, P. J., McMurtrie, E., and Swenerton, K. D. A phase II trial of intravenous etoposide (VP-16-213) in epithelial ovarian cancer resistant to cisplatin or carboplatin: clinical or serological evidence of activity. *Int. J. Gynecol. Cancer* 2:35, 1992.
    It is hypothesized that cure is not possible if drug resistance occurs. It is essential, therefore, to include truly non–cross-resistant agents if cure is to be achieved.
19. Potter, M. E., et al. Second-look laparotomy and salvage therapy: a research modality only. *Gynecol. Oncol.* 44:3, 1992.
    Second-look laparotomy does not improve survival in the context of currently existing salvage modalities.
20. Clarke-Pearson, D. L., et al. Surgical management of intestinal obstruction in ovarian cancer. I. Clinical features, postoperative complications, and survival. *Gynecol. Oncol.* 26:11, 1987.
    Of 49 patients, progressive cancer caused intestinal obstruction in 86 percent. The need for clearer preoperative selection criteria is emphasized.

Prognosis
21. Swenerton, K. D., et al. Ovarian carcinoma: a multivariant analysis of prognostic factors. *Obstet. Gynecol.* 65:264, 1985.
    Within each stage, the extent of residual disease, tumor grade, and patient performance status are independent prognostic factors.
22. Mogensen, O. Prognostic value of CA 125 in advanced ovarian cancer. *Gynecol. Oncol.* 44:207, 1992.
    Chemotherapy may be discontinued if CA 125 levels remain high after the third course of therapy and if other curative regimens are not available.
23. Rubin, S. C., et al. Prognostic factors for recurrence following negative second-

look laparotomy in ovarian cancer patients treated with platinum-based chemotherapy. *Gynecol. Oncol.* 42:137, 1991.
*There is a substantial risk of recurrence even after second-look laparotomy yields
negative findings, particularly within the first few years.*

24. Lederman, J. A., et al. Outcome of patients with unfavorable optimally cyto-
reduced ovarian cancer treated with chemotherapy and whole abdominal radiation. *Gynecol. Oncol.* 41:30, 1991.
Radiotherapy may still have a role in the management of ovarian cancer.

25. Hunter, R. W., Alexander, N. D. E., and Soutter, W. P. Meta-analysis of surgery
in advanced ovarian carcinoma: is maximum cytoreductive surgery an independent determinant of prognosis? *Am. J. Obstet. Gynecol.* 166:504, 1992.
*Cytoreductive surgery probably has only a small impact on survival in patients
with advanced ovarian cancer. The type of chemotherapy used is more important.*

26. King, M.-C., Rowell, S., and Love, S. M. Inherited breast and ovarian cancer.
What are the risks? What are the choices? *J.A.M.A.* 269:1975, 1993.
*The role of the BRCA 1 (breast cancer) gene in inherited forms of breast and
ovarian cancer has been determined through the genetic analysis of families with
multiple cases of these cancers.*

27. Lahti, E., et al. Endometrial changes in postmenopausal breast cancer patients
receiving tamoxifen. *Obstet. Gynecol.* 81:660, 1993.
*Long-term tamoxifen treatment has an estrogenic effect on the postmenopausal
uterus that is associated with an increased occurrence of polyps.*

28. Van Dam, P. A., et al. Flow cytometric DNA analysis in gynecological oncology.
Int. J. Gynecol. Cancer 2:37, 1992.
*DNA ploidy and/or the tumor S-phase fraction may be valuable prognostic indi-
cators in patients with ovarian and endometrial cancers.*

98. SURGERY
Michel E. Rivlin

There are three gynecologic procedures specifically used for the management of pelvic malignancies: radical hysterectomy, pelvic exenteration, and staging laparotomy.

Radical hysterectomy (Wertheim) is generally reserved for patients with stage IB
and perhaps early stage IIA cervical carcinoma who have no medical contraindications to surgery. Further indications for this procedure include certain endometrial
stage II cancers, some vaginal cancers, and cervical cancer unresponsive to radiotherapy when surgery is technically feasible.

The results from either surgery or radiotherapy for stage I cervical cancer are essentially comparable. Irradiation offers the major advantage of being useful in most
patients, regardless of their age or medical condition, and is the choice for large cancers. On the other hand, surgery allows the ovaries to be conserved, provides the
diagnostic accuracy of surgical staging, and does not adversely affect vaginal function, which are important advantages, especially for the younger patient. In general,
we are fortunate to have two good methods for treating cervical cancer.

At laparotomy, it is decided whether surgical treatment is feasible. If biopsy specimens and frozen sections of the paraaortic nodes show tumor changes, the procedure
is terminated. However, opinion is divided as to whether the presence of positive
pelvic nodes should be a reason for terminating the procedure or whether it should
still be completed.

Wertheim's operation includes total abdominal hysterectomy and excision of the
upper third to half of the vagina, along with the uterosacral and cardinal ligaments
and the paracervical and paravaginal tissues out to the pelvic sidewalls. Pelvic
lymphadenectomy is nearly always combined with removal of the pelvic nodes to the
aortic bifurcation. The nodes removed include the obturator, hypogastric, and exter-

nal iliac groups. The adnexa are removed in older patients or in those patients who will also receive adjunctive radiotherapy.

The operative mortality is low (0.3–1.7%), but urinary complications are not uncommon, as a major portion of the endopelvic fascia is removed and the bladder and ureters are extensively dissected. Voiding dysfunction and loss of vesical sensation are the most common problems. Rarer, but major, urinary problems are the formation of vesicovaginal or ureterovaginal fistulas (0.7–1.6%), which are especially common in patients who have also been treated with radiotherapy.

Another, not uncommon, surgical complication is the formation of lymphocysts (3–24%). Fortunately, these generally regress, although some, especially if they are infected or produce pressure effects, may require drainage. Other complications are those found with any major surgical procedure, and all are more common in patients treated with radiotherapy. For this reason, most surgeons prefer to avoid irradiation preoperatively, using it postoperatively only if positive pelvic nodes are encountered.

Pelvic exenteration is seldom used as primary therapy. When it is performed, it is usually for recurrence after radiation therapy, generally of cervical cancer. For the procedure to be feasible, it is essential that the tumor be considered completely resectable. This decision is based on the clinical and operative findings. In general, a swollen leg or sciatic nerve pain is indicative of inoperable disease. Metastasis to common iliac or aortic nodes or outside the pelvis also indicates disease that is too extensive for resection.

For those few patients with operable central recurrence, anterior or total exenterations are usually performed, depending on the site of disease. Posterior exenteration is seldom carried out alone, as urinary fistulas frequently form as complications.

Exenteration involves removal of the pelvic lymph nodes, the internal genitalia, and the vagina. Because the bladder and often the rectum are also removed, urinary and fecal diversions become necessary. These generally take the form of ilial or colon conduits in conjunction with the creation of a sigmoid colostomy. A neovagina may also be constructed, either at the same time or at a later procedure.

Several operative techniques have been developed for contending with the resulting large defect in the pelvic floor and the open pelvic cavity, which otherwise predispose to pelvic hematoma, abscess, bowel obstruction, or even evisceration. The other major complications of the procedure involve problems with the urinary anastomoses, especially if irradiated tissues have been utilized.

The operative mortality rate is about 3 to 14 percent, and the overall survival rate is about 25 to 40 percent. Improvements in all aspects of therapy are yielding steadily better outcomes, however. In view of the formidable nature of exenteration, it should be reserved for only those patients who have the physical and psychologic resources to cope with the therapy. Exenteration is not considered a suitable means of palliation.

Exploratory celiotomy performed for the purposes of surgical staging is generally accepted for ovarian cancer and is also becoming a fairly common procedure for endometrial carcinoma, because the operation is generally the primary treatment for patients with these conditions. Since advanced cervical cancer is usually treated by radiotherapy, a staging laparotomy may turn out to be unnecessary surgery, and is therefore still regarded as investigative. Typical risk estimates for periaortic node involvement in the setting of cervical cancer are 6, 20, and 30 percent for stages I, II, and III, respectively.

The underlying rationale for surgical staging to better evaluate the extent of cervical disease is based on the finding that clinical staging is incorrect in more than a third of the patients who come to surgery.

The staging celiotomy is directed primarily at biopsy of the common iliac and aortic lymph nodes. In addition, the pelvic and abdominal cavities are inspected, and perirectal or perivesical biopsy specimens are obtained, if indicated. The pelvic surgery performed is limited, lest it compromise treatment of the primary tumor. Surgery delays definitive therapy an average of about 8 days, and there is an operative mortality rate of about 1 percent.

If the common iliac or aortic nodes are positive (about 20% of the patients), routine radiation fields cannot encompass the disease process, and failure of standard therapy is inevitable. Therefore, treatment should be modified to include the involved areas, if this is technically possible. To justify the surgical staging procedure, treatment modifications should be shown to increase survival. In practice, the major modification consists of extended-field radiation, generally about 4500 cGy to the paraaortic area, in addition to standard pelvic irradiation. The additional therapy seems unsuitable as a routine prophylactic measure, because there is a definite complication rate, related in particular to small bowel problems. These complications, however, have been much reduced through the use of an extraperitoneal approach to node sampling. However, this approach does not permit intraperitoneal disease and visceral metastases to be assessed. The surgical staging for cervical cancer is still considered investigational, because there are as yet no data to support a resulting increase in survival in the patients who undergo it. (Patients with positive aortic nodes often also have uncontrolled pelvic disease or metastasis elsewhere, resulting in a uniformly poor prognosis.)

The development of nonsurgical lymph node sampling techniques may obviate the need for staging laparotomy. Fine-needle aspiration of suspicious lymph nodes under computed tomographic guidance can predict disease if findings are positive, but has a significant false-negative rate of 14 percent with up to 10 percent of the specimens unsatisfactory. Patients with periaortic nodal involvement can be cured, with 5-year survival rates ranging from 10 to 40 percent. The better results are reported for patients with early clinical stage disease and microscopic nodal involvement. Before any form of surgical staging is carried out, the ability of the patient to tolerate the increased risk of extended-field radiotherapy must first be evaluated.

Radical Hysterectomy
1. Webb, M. J., and Symmonds, R. E. Wertheim hysterectomy: a reappraisal. *Obstet. Gynecol.* 54:140, 1979.
   In 610 cases, there was an 86 percent 5-year survival rate for vaginal cancer; this was 78 percent for cervix cancer and 55 percent for endometrial cancer. In patients with cervical cancer, survival was lowered from 83 to 57 percent when lymph nodes were positive.
2. Levrant, S. G., Fruchter, R. G., and Maiman, M. Radical hysterectomy for cervical cancer: morbidity and survival in relation to weight and age. *Gynecol. Oncol.* 45:317, 1992.
   The authors concluded that neither age nor obesity should be a contraindication to radical surgery in appropriately selected patients.
3. Monk, B. J., and Montz, F. J. Invasive cervical cancer complicating intrauterine pregnancy: treatment with radical hysterectomy. *Obstet. Gynecol.* 80:199, 1992.
   Immediate treatment, low morbidity, acceptable survival, and preservation of ovarian function were all advantages of this treatment.
4. Nezhat, C. R., et al. Laparoscopic radical hysterectomy with paraaortic and pelvic node dissection. *Am. J. Obstet. Gynecol.* 166:864, 1992.
   Surgical curiosity or wave of the future?
5. Greer, I. A., and De Swiet, M. Thrombosis prophylaxis in obstetrics and gynecology. *Br. J. Obstet. Gynaecol.* 100:37, 1993.
   The most common methods of prophylaxis used were subcutaneous heparin administration, elastic stockings, intermittent calf compression, and dextran.
6. Ilancheran, A., and Monaghan, J. M. Pelvic lymphocyst—a 10-year experience. *Gynecol. Oncol.* 29:333, 1988.
   A lymphocyst is an accumulation of fluid in the retroperitoneal space at the dissection site that is bounded by the denuded musculature laterally and posteriorly and the peritoneum medially.
7. Bouma, J., and Dankert, J. Infection after radical abdominal hysterectomy and pelvic lymphadenectomy: prevention of infection with a two-dose perioperative antibiotic prophylaxis. *Int. J. Gynecol. Cancer* 3:94, 1993.
   A two-dose regimen is recommended because of the rapid clearance involved, probably due to the high volume of perioperative blood loss.

Exenteration

8. Barber, H. R. K. Pelvic exenteration. *Cancer Invest.* 5:331, 1987.
   Thirty to 40 percent of the vulvar cancers, 60 to 70 percent of the vaginal cancers, 40 to 60 percent of the cervical cancers, 30 percent of the endometrial cancers, and 70 to 80 percent of the ovarian cancers recur and need further treatment. Regardless of the tumor origin or cell type, exenteration should be considered, because, with careful patient selection, a salvage rate of 30 to 40 percent may be achieved. By contrast, repeated irradiation and chemotherapy are rarely curative.

9. Stanhope, C. R., Webb, M. J., and Podratz, K. C. Pelvic exenteration for recurrent cervical cancer. *Clin. Obstet. Gynecol.* 33:897, 1990.
   The reported surgical mortality rate ranges from 5 to 13 percent, with major postoperative complications, including infection, obstruction, or fistula formation in the gastrointestinal or urinary conduits, occurring in 75 to 77 percent.

10. Trelford, J. D., et al. Formation of a vagina at the time of exenteration. *Gynecol. Oncol.* 45:147, 1992.
    Many techniques, including skin grafts, perineal grafts, musculocutaneous gracilis grafts, and intestinal grafts, can be carried out either with the exenteration or as a secondary procedure.

11. Matthews, C. M., et al. Pelvic exenteration in the elderly patient. *Obstet. Gynecol.* 79:773, 1992.
    The morbidity and mortality observed in elderly patients are similar to those in younger patients. Age should not be considered a contraindication to the procedure.

12. Jarrell, M. A., et al. Human dura mater allografts in repair of pelvic floor and abdominal wall defects. *Obstet. Gynecol.* 70:280, 1987.
    An omental pedicle "carpet" is often used to fill the defect after exenteration. The pedicle flap serves as a vascular bed and as a barrier against intestinal prolapse. This report suggests an alternative method.

13. Orr, J. W., Jr., et al. Urinary diversion in patients undergoing pelvic exenteration. *Am. J. Obstet. Gynecol.* 142:883, 1982.
    The use of unirradiated bowel (transverse colon) as the conduit, in conjunction with ureteral stents and gastrointestinal staplers, led to a lessened risk of anastomotic failure, late stenosis, and infection.

14. Anderson, B. L., and Hacker, N. F. Psychosexual adjustment following pelvic exenteration. *Obstet. Gynecol.* 61:331, 1983.
    Reduced frequency, arousal, and satisfaction as well as disrupted sexual confidence and body image affect virtually all patients. The degree of distress depended on the availability of a partner and the patient's own desire regarding continuation of her sexual life.

Staging Laparotomy

15. Herd, J., et al. Laparoscopic para-aortic lymph node sampling: development of a technique. *Gynecol. Oncol.* 44:271, 1992.
    This describes the search for a technique that avoids many of the complications associated with staging laparotomy, while still allowing valuable information to be obtained regarding spread of the disease.

16. Larson, D. M., Johnson, K., and Olson, K. A. Pelvic and para-aortic lymphadenectomy for surgical staging of endometrial cancer: morbidity and mortality. *Obstet. Gynecol.* 79:998, 1992.
    The addition of node sampling did not significantly increase the morbidity or mortality associated with the standard procedure.

17. Heaps, J. M., and Berek, J. S. Surgical staging of cervical cancer. *Clin. Obstet. Gynecol.* 33:852, 1990.
    Major discrepancies exist between the clinical and surgical estimates of disease extent in the setting of cervical, endometrial, and vulvar carcinomas. However, it must be shown that the performance of surgical staging does not increase the complications or decrease the efficacy of subsequent therapeutic interventions.

18. Kohler, M. F., et al. Computed tomography–guided fine-needle aspiration of

retroperitoneal lymph nodes in gynecologic oncology. *Obstet. Gynecol.* 76:612, 1990.
A positive result is significant; negative findings do not rule out nodal involvement (false-negative rate, 14%).

19. Berman, M. L., et al. Survival and patterns of recurrence in cervical cancer metastatic to periaortic lymph nodes. *Gynecol. Oncol.* 19:8, 1984.
Positive nodes were encountered in 16 percent of the cases in this series. The 3-year survival probability of these women was 25 percent. Recurrences were divided equally between the pelvis and distant sites.

20. Rubin, S. C., et al. Para-aortic nodal metastases in early cervical carcinoma: long-term survival following extended-field radiotherapy. *Gynecol. Oncol.* 18: 213, 1984.
Patients with early stage cervical carcinoma can experience significant survival, thus constituting a distinct subgroup in terms of the curability of paraaortic nodal disease.

21. Heintz, A. P. M., et al. The treatment of advanced ovarian carcinoma (II): interval reassessment operations during chemotherapy. *Gynecol. Oncol.* 30:359, 1988.
The rationale for second-look surgery is based on the serious short- and long-term side effects of chemotherapy that can arise and on the impossibility of ruling out residual tumor using noninvasive methods in patients who clinically appear to be free of disease.

22. Podratz, K. C., et al. Recurrent disease after negative second-look laparotomy in stages III and IV ovarian carcinoma. *Gynecol. Oncol.* 29:274, 1988.
Surgical and histologic assessment did not detect persistent disease in 37 percent; however, recurrent cancer was subsequently documented in 30 percent of these patients. All failures occurred within the abdominal cavity or retroperitoneal space.

99. RADIATION THERAPY
Michel E. Rivlin

Radiation therapy is widely used in the treatment of gynecologic cancer, and may be used either as the only therapy or in combination with surgical procedures, chemotherapy, or immunotherapy. Treatment may make use of radioactive isotopes, such as radium or cesium, which are placed locally in the uterine or vaginal cavities, or both (brachytherapy), or it may be administered from an external source. External irradiation (teletherapy) is usually performed with the supervoltage machines that have replaced the earlier orthovoltage instruments. Frequently, local and external therapies are combined, the former delivering the major radiation dosage to the tumor and the latter directed toward the draining lymph nodes.

The radiation therapy dosage is calculated in rads, which are the units of absorbed dosage. Another measurement of the dosage of radiation absorbed by tissue is the gray unit. One gray is equal to 100 rads, such that 1 centigray (cGy) is equal to 1 rad. The dose of radiation delivered to a tumor depends on the energy of the source, the size of the treatment field, and the depth of the tumor beneath the surface. Using computer techniques, the dosimetry can be accurately calculated so that not too much radiation is delivered to normal tissues, while cancericidal doses are administered to the tumor and lymph nodes. Isodose curves are constructed by connecting points that receive equivalent radiation doses. Normal tissues composed of cells that are rapidly dividing, such as the epithelial tissues of the urinary and intestinal tracts, are less able to tolerate radiation than are the more stable tissues, such as those of the vagina and cervix.

Tumors differ in their radiosensitivity, frequently sharing this property with that of the parent tissue. The sensitivity depends on the histology, clinical variety, tumor bed, and oxygen tension. An anoxic tumor is radioresistant, and this is frequently seen in the setting of large or recurrent tumors with an inadequate blood supply. Radiosensitivity is not the same as radiocurability, however, as a well-localized, relatively resistant tumor may be cured, whereas a widespread radiosensitive tumor can usually be controlled only locally.

Radiation acts on cells primarily in the mitosis phase, making rapidly proliferating cells the most radiosensitive, though normal tissue recovers more efficiently than does tumor tissue. A given dose of radiation kills a constant fraction of tumor cells. Tumors consist of a heterogeneous cell population and have variable growth fractions. Large tumors tend to have smaller growth fractions and a higher proportion of cells in the G_0 (resting) phase of the cycle than do small tumors.

Efforts to improve the local control of bulky hypoxic tumors have included combinations of radiotherapy and hyperbaric oxygen or hypoxic cell sensitizers such as hydroxyurea and misonidazole, which mimic oxygen in their ability to sensitize hypoxic cells. (A true radiosensitizer should augment the tumor cell kill without adversely affecting normal tissues.) Refinements in treatment consisting of combinations of surgery, immunotherapy, or chemotherapy in conjunction with irradiation and unconventional radiation techniques are ongoing in an attempt to improve results in patients with advanced disease.

Tolerance to radiation depends on several factors, including the total dosage administered, the period of time over which the dosage is given, and the volume of tissue irradiated. Tolerance is better when the dosage is fractionated and spread over a longer period and when smaller, rather than larger, areas are treated. These factors must be taken into consideration when preparing a radiotherapeutic plan.

The intensity of radiation from a source varies inversely as the square of the distance from the source. For example, in terms of a cervical tumor, the dosage rate at 1 cm from the radium source is nine times that at 3 cm from the source. In this way, the sensitive bladder and rectal tissues receive dosages well within their individual safety margins, whereas 15,000 cGy or more may be delivered to the tumor site. However, it must be emphasized that generalizations regarding tissue tolerance in relation to total dosage must be regarded as only approximations.

Radiation sources are placed in systems designed to fit in the uterine and vaginal cavities. These systems include the uterine applicator (called the tandem) and the vaginal applicator (called the colpostat), which may be inserted with or without the patient under general anesthesia. Vaginal packing and a keel keep the systems stable and in place. Localization films are then taken to ascertain their position and to calculate the isodose curves for various areas in the pelvis. The actual radioactive sources are then inserted once satisfactory application is confirmed. This technique, called afterloading, minimizes the exposure of personnel to radioactivity. Generally, sources are left in situ for 48 to 72 hours, and insertions are carried out 2 to 4 weeks apart. In the treatment of cervical cancer, two applications are usually administered, and these are given before, during, or after a concomitant course of external therapy.

Computerized dosimetry is used to balance the dosage from the external and internal sources. External therapy is generally delivered from megavoltage instruments in doses fractionated over several weeks. The radiation is delivered in measured areas called portal-of-entry fields. The shape and size of the ports vary with the lesions to be treated. In treating the whole pelvis, these ports are generally 15 to 18 × 15 to 18 cm. Radiosensitive tissues may be protected with lead screens during external-beam therapy. For instance, a 4-cm central shield that protects the bladder and rectum may be used during whole-pelvis irradiation. In treating cervical cancer, a customary regimen consists of 4 to 5 weeks of external therapy (180–200 cGy/day), followed by two brachytherapy applications of 48 hours each, with 2 weeks intervening. A dose of 75 to 80 cGy is delivered to point A (2 cm proximal to the cervical os and 2 cm lateral, corresponding to the approximate point where the uterine artery crosses over the ureter) and a dose of 50 to 55 cGy is delivered to point B (3 cm lateral to point A and corresponding to the pelvic nodes). Treatment takes a total of 8 to 10 weeks.

Therapeutic levels of radiotherapy damage cell nuclei and cause an obliterative endarteritis. These effects on normal tissue result in complications that are closely related to the dosage. It is the complication rate, rather than the cure rate, that places limits on the radiation dosage. Local applications tend to cause focal injuries, whereas external therapy produces a more uniformly irradiated field.

Orthovoltage machines have power in the 125,000 to 400,000 electron volt range, whereas megavoltage machines are in the 2 to 35 million electron volt range. Cobalt machines (1.25 MV) and higher-energy machines cause little skin or systemic reactions because the penetration is much greater than that of the older orthovoltage type, which caused marked skin and subcutaneous tissue reactions.

Early side effects of radiotherapy include cystitis and proctosigmoiditis, both of which usually respond to symptomatic treatment. Bone marrow suppression and radiation sickness are rarely encountered. An important early but occasional complication is acute pelvic sepsis, which necessitates termination of therapy until the infection is cleared.

The late complications are much more difficult to deal with and are related to the ischemic and necrotizing effects of excessive ionizing radiation. They may appear months or years after the completion of therapy. Large-bowel complications involving the rectum and sigmoid may consist of hemorrhage, ulceration, fistulas, or stricture. Milder forms may respond to conservative measures, whereas the more severe forms require the creation of a defunctioning colostomy.

Small-bowel problems arise particularly when previous surgical treatment has resulted in loops fixed by adhesions or when small bowel remains relatively immobile, as at the terminal ileum. Enteritis, subacute obstruction, hemorrhage, ulceration, and perforation can all occur. These complications are more common when irradiation has been extended to the upper abdomen. Management is difficult and may involve surgical measures consisting of resection or bypass procedures.

Urinary tract problems involving the bladder and ureters include cystitis, ulceration, hemorrhage, stenosis, and fistula formation. If conservative measures are unsuccessful, surgical diversion of the urinary stream may be necessary.

The vaginal response to radiation consists of epithelial atrophy, erosions, and adhesion formation. Later, there may be stenosis and even complete vaginal obliteration. These changes can be partially prevented by the use of hormones, dilators, and, most important, the resumption of intercourse as soon as possible after therapy. The cervix also commonly becomes stenotic with, occasionally, retention of secretions in the uterine cavity, thus leading to a pyometra that requires drainage. The most serious of the local complications, although fortunately rare, is complete vault necrosis, often with associated urinary or fecal fistulas.

In the management of complications after radiotherapy, it is vital to keep in mind the poor healing powers of irradiated tissue. Frequently, it is difficult to differentiate recurrence from radiation injury and to perform diagnostic procedures, especially biopsies. Great care must be taken to prevent perforation or fistula formation. If surgical intervention is necessary, the poor healing and infection-resistant properties of irradiated tissue must be allowed for in the therapeutic plan.

Complications associated with radiation therapy are, fortunately, uncommon and chiefly afflict patients who receive an increased dosage as a calculated risk in an attempt to cure advanced disease. The incidence of complications from standard regimens in patients with early disease is low, and the cure rate is excellent when the disease is localized.

Treatment should be individualized and a management team made up of a gynecologic oncologist, a chemotherapist, and a radiotherapist should arrive at a treatment plan after accurate staging of the disease. This plan should be reviewed at periodic intervals to assess the patient's response to therapy and the occurrence of complications that might necessitate a change in management.

Radiotherapy is the major form of treatment for cervical cancer. In patients with endometrial cancer, radiotherapy is commonly used in conjunction with surgical measures. Ovarian cancer is now more frequently managed by surgery and chemotherapy, with radiotherapy used only for particularly radiosensitive tumors such as the dysgerminoma. Vaginal cancer is commonly managed by radiotherapy, often in conjunction with surgery. Although recurrent cancer may be treated with radiation therapy, previous treatment often limits the dosage that can be used, so the therapy can only be for palliative purposes, as in the prevention or treatment of hemorrhage or the relief of pain. Further details on irradiation of pelvic cancer can be found in other chapters in this section.

General

1. Brady, L. W. Radiation therapy in gynecologic cancer: future prospects. *Clin. Obstet. Gynecol.* 18:125, 1975.
   Reviews the treatment programs for endometrial, cervical, and ovarian cancer.
2. Bloomer, W. D., and Hellman, S. Normal tissue responses to radiation therapy. *N. Engl. J. Med.* 293:80, 1975.
   The therapeutic ratio is the ratio between the lethal tumor dose and tissue tolerance.
3. Rotmensch, J., et al. Estimates of dose to intraperitoneal micrometastases from alpha and beta emitters in radioimmunotherapy. *Gynecol. Oncol.* 38:478, 1990.
   Investigators have used radiolabeled monoclonal antibodies to treat intraperitoneal metastases.
4. Greer, B. E., et al. Gynecologic radiotherapy fields defined by intraoperative measurements. *Gynecol. Oncol.* 38:421, 1990.
   Data suggest that conventional radiation fields are inadequate and should be based on intraoperative measurements.
5. Portenoy, R. K. Practical aspects of pain control in the patient with cancer. *CA* 38:327, 1988.
   Therapeutic approaches of value in the control of cancer-related pain include pharmacologic, anesthetic, neuroaugmentative, physiatric, neurosurgical, and psychologic measures.
6. Randall, M. E., et al. Interstitial reirradiation for recurrent gynecologic malignancies: results and analysis of prognostic factors. *Gynecol. Oncol.* 48:23, 1993.
   Applicable to patients with medical contraindications to salvage surgery.
7. Nguyen, H. N., et al. Radiosensitization of uterine cancer cell lines by cytotoxic agents. *Gynecol. Oncol.* 48:16, 1993.
   Adriamycin, 5-fluorouracil, cisplatin, and mitomycin C have the potential to be radiosensitizers in uterine cancer cell lines.

Cervical Cancer

8. Photopulos, G. J. Surgery or radiation for early cervical cancer. *Clin. Obstet. Gynecol.* 33:872, 1990.
   Radiation therapy offers the major advantages of being useful in most patients, regardless of age or medical condition, and is the choice for large cancers.
9. Murray, M. J. New techniques in radiation therapy for cervical cancer. *Clin. Obstet. Gynecol.* 33:889, 1990.
   Documents the effectiveness of newer techniques, including high dose–rate brachytherapy; interstitial brachytherapy; altered fractionation schedules; neutron-beam brachytherapy; hypothermia; and irradiation with immunotherapy or chemotherapy.
10. Koa, K., Nakano, T., and Arai, T. Adenocarcinoma of the cervix treated with radiation alone: prognostic significance of S-100 protein and vimentin immunostaining. *Obstet. Gynecol.* 79:347, 1992.
    Disease-free 5-year survival rates for stages I to IV were 63, 58, 30, and 9 percent, respectively. Immunohistochemical findings appeared to be helpful as prognostic indicators.
11. Tattersall, M. H. N., Ramirez, C., and Coppleson, M. A randomized trial comparing platinum-based chemotherapy followed by radiotherapy vs. radiotherapy alone in patients with locally advanced cervical cancer. *Int. J. Gynecol. Obstet.* 2:244, 1992.
    There are three possible strategies for integrating chemotherapy with local treatment: primary chemotherapy prior to local treatment (neoadjuvant), postoperative

*in high-risk cases (adjuvant), and radiosensitizing, in which drugs and irradia-
tion are given together, with the goal to enhance the efficacy of the irradiation.*

Endometrial Cancer

12. Jazy, F. K., et al. Preoperative versus postoperative irradiation in stage I carcinoma of the endometrium. *Clin. Oncol.* 9:281, 1983.
*Preoperative irradiation was claimed to decrease the depth of myometrial inva-
sion, the rate of pelvic recurrence, and the pathology stage, as well as to increase
survival, compared with postoperative irradiation.*

13. Reisinger, S. A., et al. Preoperative radiation therapy in clinical stage II endometrial carcinoma. *Gynecol. Oncol.* 45:174, 1992.
*Good local control was achieved but there was a high failure rate for disease in
the upper abdomen, with poor survival in patients with papillary serous and clear
cell tumors.*

14. Potish, R. A., et al. Para-aortic lymph node radiotherapy in cancer of the uterine
corpus. *Obstet. Gynecol.* 65:251, 1985.
*In contradistinction to the results reported in much of the literature, radiotherapy
in this series salvaged a substantial proportion of patients with paraaortic metastases, the morbidity rates were acceptable, and there was a 5-year relapse-free
survival rate of 47 percent.*

15. Boronow, R. C. Should whole pelvic radiation therapy become past history? A
case for the routine use of extended field therapy and multimodality therapy.
Gynecol. Oncol. 43:71, 1991.
*This author is a proponent of whole-abdomen irradiation together with concomi-
tant chemotherapy after surgery in carefully selected high-risk cases.*

16. Wang, M.-L., et al. Inoperable adenocarcinoma of the endometrium: radiation
therapy. *Radiology* 165:561, 1987.
*Radiotherapy alone can be an effective treatment in patients with stage I or II
endometrial carcinoma who have poor risk factors for surgery. Although only 46
percent of the patients in this series survived for 5 years, more than half the deaths
resulted from intercurrent disease.*

Vaginal and Vulvar Cancer

17. Kucera, H., and Vavra, N. Radiation management of primary carcinoma of the
vagina: clinical and histopathological variables associated with survival. *Gynecol. Oncol.* 40:12, 1991.
*These patients were treated by external and local radiotherapy; outcome was influ-
enced by tumor stage, patient age, lesion location, and tumor differentiation. For
stage I disease, the 5-year survival was 76 percent; stage II, 44 percent; stage III,
31 percent; and stage IV, 18 percent.*

18. Patton, T. J., Jr., et al. Five-year survival in patients given intra-arterial chemotherapy prior to radiotherapy for advanced squamous carcinoma of the cervix
and vagina. *Gynecol. Oncol.* 42:54, 1991.
*Primary carcinoma of the vagina constitutes only 1 to 2 percent of the female geni-
tal tract neoplasms; most patients are over 60 years old; and squamous cell carcinoma is the usual histologic type.*

19. Pao, W. M., et al. Radiation therapy and conservatve surgery for primary and
recurrent carcinoma of the vulva: report of 40 patients and a review of the literature. *Int J. Radiat. Oncol. Biol. Phys.* 14:1123, 1988.
*In general, a conservative operation was combined with preoperative or postopera-
tive irradiation. Results were encouraging, suggesting that irradiation might play
a major role in the management of vulvar cancer.*

20. Kucera, H., and Weghaupt, K. The electrosurgical operation for vulvar carcinoma with postoperative irradiation of inguinal lymph nodes. *Gynecol. Oncol.*
29:158, 1988.
*Vulvectomy, without inguinofemoral lymphadenectomy, followed by postoperative
inguinal irradiation, was well tolerated and yielded a 60 percent absolute 5-year
cure rate in a series of 607 patients.*

Ovarian Cancer

21. Muto, M. G., et al. Intraperitoneal radioimmunotherapy of refractory ovarian carcinoma utilizing iodine-131–labeled monoclonal antibody OC125. *Gynecol. Oncol.* 45:265, 1992.
Radiolabeled monoclonal antibodies raised to tumor-associated antigens make possible selective tumor irradiation, while reducing toxicity to normal tissues.
22. Bruzzone, M., et al. Chemotherapy versus radiotherapy in the management of ovarian cancer patients with pathological complete response or minimal residual disease at second look. *Gynecol. Oncol.* 30:392, 1990.
In this study, chemotherapy proved superior to whole-abdomen radiotherapy.

Complications

23. Montana, G. S., and Fowler, W. C. Carcinoma of the cervix: analysis of bladder and rectal radiation dose and complications. *Int. J. Radiat. Oncol. Biol. Phys.* 16:95, 1989.
These authors report that the point A dose in patients with complications for all stages was greater than that in those without complications.
24. Greven, K. M., et al. Analysis of complications in patients receiving adjuvant irradiation for endometrial carcinoma. *Int. J. Radiat. Oncol. Biol. Phys.* 21:919, 1991.
Young age was associated with a higher complication rate.
25. Lanciano, R. M., et al. Influence of age, prior abdominal surgery, fraction size, and dose on complications after radiation therapy for squamous cell cancer of the uterine cervix. A patterns of care study. *Cancer* 69:2130, 1992.
Prior operation, young age, the use of cesium, a daily fraction size greater than 200 cGy, and a paracentral (point A) dose greater than 7500 cGy were all factors associated independently with complications.
26. Byrne, J., et al. Early menopause in long-term survivors of cancer during adolescence. *Am. J. Obstet. Gynecol.* 166:788, 1992.
The relative risks of early menopause after treatment with either radiation or alkylating agents alone were significantly increased and were even greater when both modalities were employed.
27. Parkin, D. E., Davis, J. A., and Symonds, R. P. Urodynamic findings following radiotherapy for cervical carcinoma. *Br. J. Urol.* 61:213, 1988.
Up to half of the long-term survivors complained of frequency, urgency, and urge incontinence. Detrusor instability was found in nearly all the symptomatic women.
28. Lee, R. A., Symmonds, R. E., and Williams, T. J. Current status of genitourinary fistula. *Obstet. Gynecol.* 72:313, 1988.
The successful repair of fistulas after radiation damage requires carefully planned and timed procedures using nonirradiated tissue to close the defect.
29. Krebs, H. B., and Goperud, D. R. Mechanical intestinal obstruction in patients with gynecologic disease: a review of 38 patients. *Am. J. Obstet. Gynecol.* 157:577, 1987.
In this series, 17 percent of the small bowel and 26 percent of the colon obstructions were associated with radiation therapy–related strictures and adhesions.
30. Allen-Mersh, T. G., et al. The management of late radiation–induced rectal injury after treatment of carcinoma of the uterus. *Surg. Gynecol. Obstet.* 164:521, 1987.
Florid proctitis resolved within 2 years of onset in 33 percent, and surgical treatment was necessary in 39 percent. Cancer-induced symptoms tended to occur after a median of 8 months, compared to radiation-induced symptoms, which appeared at a median of 16 months.
31. Beemer, W., Hopkins, M. P., and Morley, G. W. Vaginal reconstruction in gynecologic oncology. *Obstet. Gynecol.* 72:911, 1988.
Vaginal reconstruction is feasible when the vagina has been obliterated by the irradiation or surgery.
32. Muram, D., et al. Postradiation ureteral obstruction: a reappraisal. *Am. J. Obstet. Gynecol.* 139:289, 1981.

Differentiating periureteral radiation fibrosis from recurrent carcinoma may require laparotomy in some cases.

100. CHEMOTHERAPY IN GYNECOLOGIC CANCER
Michel E. Rivlin

Chemotherapeutic agents affect rapidly dividing cells, such as tumor cells, but spare static cell populations. However, renewing cell populations are also characteristic of some normal cell types, and these too are commonly damaged during cytotoxic drug treatment. Therefore, the bone marrow, mucous membranes, and gastrointestinal tract are frequently injured during chemotherapy, while muscle cells and bone are spared. It is usually this toxicity that dictates the drug dosage and not the tumor response.

The kinetics of individual tumor cells are important factors, as different drugs act at different phases of the cell cycle. The mitotic phase of the cycle is followed by a variable period (G_1), during which protein and ribonucleic acid (RNA) are synthesized. The S phase follows, with new deoxyribonucleic acid (DNA) synthesis; after this comes the G_2 period, which is relatively short and precedes mitosis. The variation in duration of G_1 is central to the proliferative behavior of cell populations. A short G_1 indicates proliferative behavior; if the postmitotic period is very long, it is termed G_0 and represents nonproliferative populations.

Most cytotoxic agents act by disrupting some aspect of DNA, RNA, or protein synthesis, and rapidly dividing cells are the most sensitive to these agents. Certain agents are cell-cycle specific and proliferation dependent (e.g., hydroxyurea and methotrexate); others kill in all phases of the cell cycle and are not too dependent on the proliferative rate (e.g., alkylating agents). Some drugs may have a greater effect on a particular phase of the cell cycle; for instance, doxorubicin (Adriamycin) is most effective in the late S phase, while cells in mitosis seem most sensitive to agents that disrupt the mitotic apparatus, such as vinblastine, vincristine, and taxol.

Cytotoxic agents kill a constant fraction of cells, rather than a constant number. This first-order kinetic concept means that only very large log kills (>99%) with repetitive therapies can be curative. Furthermore, treatment applied early results in more cures than it does when the tumor is large and clinically obvious. Unfortunately, most tumors have already undergone 30 doublings before they are detected, and then are no longer early. In addition, at later stages of growth, only a few doublings markedly enlarge the tumor. However, there are two other factors that influence tumor growth: cell death and the growth fraction. In most tumors, only a fraction of the cells are proliferating and cell losses may range from 70 to 95 percent. It is estimated that the doubling times in human tumors take about 50 days, but the range for individual growths is broad.

The terms *complete remission* and *partial remission* are used to indicate the response to therapy. A complete remission consists of a clinical response plus the disappearance of all objective evidence of tumor. The mean survival is usually prolonged in this setting. Partial remission indicates a 50 percent or greater reduction in the size of measurable lesions, with some clinical response and no new lesions, but the overall mean survival is usually not improved. In planning clinical trials of new agents or drug combinations, phase I trials determine the dosage and toxicity, phase II trials assess antitumor activity, and phase III trials compare the efficacy against that of established regimens. Tumors may be primarily resistant to drug therapy or may develop drug resistance after an initial response. Acquired resistance may be either specific or broadly based to multiple drugs (pleiotropic). The mechanisms of resistance vary and include spontaneous biochemical mutations or the selecting out of resistant cell lines in the original tumor, as most tumors are not composed of homogeneous clonally derived cells with similar features, but of different populations with differing characteristics.

The balance between tumor sensitivity and normal tissue injury may leave only a very narrow safety margin. The most common toxicity affects the bone marrow. Effects generally arise 7 to 10 days after the initial therapy and persist for 3 to 10 days. The toxicity is graded from 0 to 4, and grade 3 or 4 generally requires a delay in further therapy, or a dose modification, or both. In general, treatment is delayed if the leukocyte count is less than $3000/\mu l$ or if the platelet count is less than $100,000/\mu l$. If leukopenia is accompanied by fever, immediate culture and the institution of broad-spectrum antibiotic therapy while awaiting culture results are indicated. These are continued until granulocyte recovery occurs. Similarly, a platelet count of under $20,000/\mu l$ requires platelet transfusion, while a count of under $50,000/\mu l$ requires platelet transfusion only if hemorrhage occurs. Newer approaches to the management of myelosuppression include bone marrow transplantation and the use of hematopoietic growth agents, such as granulocyte colony–stimulating factor. The growth factors, however, have little effect on platelet recovery.

Most agents cause nausea, vomiting, and anorexia. Diarrhea, oral mucositis, esophagitis, and gastroenteritis are also problems. To prevent gastrointestinal toxicities, pretreatment may be required, especially when using drugs with severe emetogenic side effects, such as cisplatin or cyclophosphamide. Useful medications include antihistamines, phenothiazines, steroids, sedation, and the 5-hydroxytryptamine antagonist, ondansetron. Other common adverse effects include alopecia, skin toxicity, neurotoxicity, and genitourinary toxicity. Examples of serious adverse reactions include the leukemogenic effect of the alkylating agents, the irreversible cardiomyopathy seen with cumulative doses of adriamycin, the renal failure and hearing loss associated with cisplatin, the pulmonary fibrosis and death observed with cumulative doses of bleomycin, and the hemorrhagic cystitis that can occur with cyclophosphamide. Moreover, severe skin necrosis with extravasation from the vein can occur when plant alkaloids and antitumor antimetabolites are used, so that special precautions are necessary for their safe administration.

In view of the inevitable minor and major toxicities associated with antineoplastic drugs, the decision to use them is obviously a complex one. Factors related to the patient, the tumor, the chosen regimen, and the available therapeutic facilities must be taken into account. The probability of achieving a useful response must be shared with the patient. In general, with the exception of gestational trophoblastic disease, drug combinations are necessary to prolong survival or cure in patients with most disseminated tumors. The principles governing the use of combination drug therapy include their intermittent use so as to maximize their effect while minimizing toxicity. The drugs must be active as single agents against the tumor and should possess different mechanisms of action so as to diminish drug resistance. They should also have different spectra of toxicity to enable full dosage, and there should be a biochemical basis for additive or synergistic effects.

Combination chemotherapy used from the outset is termed induction chemotherapy. Adjuvant chemotherapy is that given if the risk of recurrence after definitive initial therapy, usually surgery or irradiation, is high. Neoadjuvant (or primary) chemotherapy is that used to treat local disease difficult to manage with other therapeutic modalities. Salvage chemotherapy is intended for palliation rather than cure. Cytotoxic drugs are generally administered parenterally or orally, but may also be given into body cavities, including intraperitoneally. The advantage of this intracavitary treatment is that many agents are cleared more slowly from body cavities than those given systemically. The major application of this approach is in patients with minimal residual disease because of the limited penetration achieved by this route.

The cytotoxic agents used in patients with gynecologic cancer may be classified as alkylating agents, antimetabolites, antitumor antibiotics, plant-derived alkaloids, hormones and antihormones, and, lastly, a miscellaneous group consisting of various agents that do not fit into any of the other classes.

The alkylating agents include melphalan (Alkeran), cyclophosphamide (Cytoxan), and chlorambucil (Leukeran). All three are effective agents in the treatment of ovarian cancer, while Cytoxan is also active for cervical cancer and uterine sarcoma. Chlorambucil is active for gestational trophoblastic neoplasia (GTN). Alkylating agents form an unstable alkyl group that has a radiomimetic effect, resulting in breaks and cross-linkages of DNA, and thus preventing cell division.

Antimetabolites are cycle-specific agents that substitute for normal metabolites. They act on an enzyme regulatory site, bind to inhibitors of vital enzymes, or occupy a catalytic site on vital enzymes, thus interrupting normal DNA or RNA synthesis, or both. Methotrexate, 5-fluorouracil (5-FU), and hydroxyurea are antimetabolites; the first two are used for GTN and ovarian cancers while the third is used as a radiosensitizer in the treatment of cervical cancer.

Antitumor antibiotics are natural isolates of soil fungi. They act by forming complexes with DNA, but there is a narrow therapeutic index. Those used in the practice of gynecology are dactinomycin (Actinomycin D), bleomycin, and doxorubicin (Adriamycin). The first two are useful for ovarian germ cell tumors, while dactinomycin is also used for GTN. Adriamycin is useful for ovarian, endometrial, and sarcomatous lesions.

The Vinca plant alkaloids, derivatives of the periwinkle, arrest cells in metaphase by binding the microtubular protein used in the formation of the mitotic spindle. Vincristine (Oncovin), vinblastin (Velban), and etoposide (VP-16) are useful for germ cell tumors and Velban or VP-16 for GTN. Oncovin is also active against sarcomas.

The hormonal agents include progestational drugs such as medroxyprogesterone acetate (Depo-Provera) and megestrol acetate (Megace), which are used for endometrial cancer, and antiestrogenic drugs such as tamoxifen, which is possibly useful in endometrial cancer, or leuprolide (Lupron), which is used for ovarian and endometrial cancer.

Miscellaneous agents include cis-dichlorodiammineplatinum (cisplatin) and carboplatin, which form the basis of most ovarian cancer regimens and are also active against cervical cancer. Ifosfamide is used for sarcoma and ovarian cancer. Hexamethylmelamine and paclitaxel (taxol) are active against ovarian epithelial cancer. Taxol, which is derived from the needles and bark of the yew tree, is not cross-resistant with cisplatin in ovarian cancer therapy. It is a mitotic spindle poison but has many and novel toxicities, including anaphylaxis, hypotension, and cardiac toxicity, beside the usual toxicities such as myelosuppression. In addition, the need for 24-hour infusion and high costs have militated against its use as first-line therapy.

The chemotherapy for GTN is detailed in Chapter 3; however, the most common use of chemotherapy in gynecologic cancer is as a supplement to surgery in the treatment of epithelial cancer of the ovary. The treatment of choice for ovarian cancer is a cisplatin-based combination of drugs. Patients with minimal residual disease postoperatively respond better than do those with bulkier disease. For the treatment of early stage ovarian cancer, the place of adjuvant chemotherapy is less clear-cut, but it is usually indicated when high-risk findings are present. In squamous cell cervical cancer, cisplatin also appears to show some activity, and the standard therapy for advanced or recurrent disease is single-agent cisplatin. In addition, cisplatin, hydroxyurea, and 5-FU have been used as radiosensitizing agents for this cancer.

For the management of endometrial cancer, progestins, tamoxifen, and Lupron, given as single agents, may be helpful for advanced disease, especially for receptor-positive cases. In the setting of treatment failure or receptor-negative disease, single-agent therapy with either doxorubicin or cisplatin is indicated. Uterine sarcomas may be treated either with doxorubicin (leiomyosarcoma) or with ifosfamide or cisplatin (mixed mesodermal). Adjuvant chemotherapy has not proved helpful. Germ cell ovarian neoplasms respond well to cisplatin-based combination chemotherapy, often with complete response. Adjuvant therapy for early stage disease is of value. The standard chemotherapy for the less common vulvar, vaginal, and tubal cancers is not well established.

Chemotherapeutic agents that might be used in practice by gynecologists include Alkeran, Cytoxan, methotrexate, and hydroxyurea. Only specialists should administer Adriamycin, Actinomycin D, taxol, or combination therapy. Cisplatin, 5-FU, and carboplatin occupy an intermediate position, and their use depends on the experience and facilities available to the individual practitioner.

General
1. Schilsky, R. L. Cancer chemotherapy and pharmacology. *Semin. Oncol.* 20:1, 1993.
   Includes chapters on regional chemotherapy and targeted drug delivery.
2. Perry, M. C. Toxicity of chemotherapy. *Semin. Oncol.* 19:453, 1992.
   Includes a chapter on fertility after chemotherapy.
3. Weiss, R. B. New antitumor drugs in development. *Semin. Oncol.* 19:611, 1992.
   Includes chapters on taxol and on the new platinum analogues.
4. Rolston, K. V. Infections in the neutropenic cancer patient. *Cancer Bull.* 44:226, 1992.
   Provides a useful algorithm for the management of febrile episodes in neutropenic patients.

Carcinoma of the Ovary
5. Thigpen, J. T., Vance, R. B., and Kahnsur, T. Second-line chemotherapy for recurrent carcinoma of the ovary. *Cancer* 71:1559, 1993.
   Suggest the treatment for platinum-resistant cases should consist of one or more drugs, such as taxol, ifosfamide, and hexamethylmelamine.
6. Baker, T. R., Piver, M. S., and Hempling, R. E. The addition of etoposide and ifosfamide to cisplatin as second line therapy in ovarian carcinoma. *Eur. J. Gynaecol. Oncol.* 14:18, 1993.
   No improvement was observed in both platinum-sensitive and -nonsensitive patients.
7. Markman, M., et al. Intraperitoneal chemotherapy in the management of ovarian cancer. *Cancer* 71:1565, 1993.
   A precise role for regional drug delivery in this setting remains to be defined.
8. Sevin, B. U., et al. Chemosensitivity testing in ovarian cancer. *Cancer* 71:1613, 1993.
   In vitro testing of chemosensitivity is performed on fresh tumor tissue to select those drugs to which the cancer is sensitive.
9. Gershenson, D. M. Update on malignant ovarian germ cell tumors. *Cancer* 71:1581, 1993.
   The "gold standard" treatment is the combination of bleomycin, etoposide, and cisplatin, with overall disease-free survival rates greater than 95 percent.

Carcinoma of the Cervix
10. Carlson, J. A., Jr. Chemotherapy of cervical cancer. *Clin. Obstet. Gynecol.* 33:910, 1990.
    Poor results may be due to inherent chemotherapy insensitivity, decreased blood flow in prior treatment fields, a low tumor growth fraction, and patient intolerance to maximum drug dosages.
11. Park, R. C., and Thigpen, J. T. Chemotherapy in advanced and recurrent cervical cancer. *Cancer* 71:1446, 1993.
    Cisplatin, ifosfamide, and dibromodulcitol yielded partial and complete response rates of 23, 22, and 22 percent, respectively, when used as single agents.
12. Macia, M., et al. Neoadjuvant and salvage chemotherapy with cisplatin and 5-fluorouracil in cervical carcinoma. *Eur. J. Gynaecol. Oncol.* 14:192, 1993.
    The use of chemotherapy before surgery or radiotherapy, or both, appeared to lead to promising results in this study. In contrast, salvage therapy, using the same regimen, led to greater toxicity and worse results.

Endometrial Cancer
13. Piver, M. S., et al. A prospective trial of progesterone therapy for malignant peritoneal cytology in patients with endometrial carcinoma. *Gynecol. Oncol.* 47:373, 1992.

None of the 45 women in this study with tumor confined to the uterus and positive peritoneal cytology, who received progesterone therapy, experienced recurrence of their cancer.

14. Levenback, C., et al. Uterine papillary serous carcinoma (UPSC) treated with cisplatin, doxorubicin, and cyclophosphamide (PAC). *Gynecol. Oncol.* 46:317, 1992.
    Despite its histologic and clinical similarities to ovarian carcinoma, UPSC was relatively resistant to cisplatin, doxorubicin, and cyclophosphamide chemotherapy in this study.

15. Rosenberg, P., Boeryd, B., and Simonsen, E. A new aggressive treatment approach to high-grade endometrial cancer of possible benefit to patients with stage I uterine papillary cancer. *Gynecol. Oncol.* 48:32, 1993.
    UPSC patients treated with a combination of radical surgery, pelvic radiotherapy, and four courses of cis-platinum/epirubicin showed significantly better survival than did controls.

Vulvar Carcinoma/Uterine Sarcoma

16. Russell, A. H., et al. Synchronous radiation and cytotoxic chemotherapy for locally advanced or recurrent squamous cancer of the vulva. *Gynecol. Oncol.* 47:14, 1992.
    Initial management with irradiation and chemotherapy has a curative potential for some cases of surgically unresectable or medically inoperable disease.

17. Baker, T. R., et al. Prospective trial of cisplatin, Adriamycin, and dacarbazine in metastatic mixed mesodermal sarcomas of the uterus and ovary. *Am. J. Clin. Oncol.* 14:246, 1991.
    Of the six patients with uterine sarcomas who could be evaluated for their response, one had a complete and one a partial response.

18. Tore, G., et al. The role of adjuvant chemotherapy in the treatment of uterine sarcoma patients. *Eur. J. Gynaecol. Oncol.* 11:307, 1990.
    For the treatment of recurrent or widespread disease, the drug of choice is ifosfamide or cisplatin for carcinosarcoma and is doxorubicin for leiomyosarcoma. The role of adjuvant chemotherapy is unclear.

101. BENIGN BREAST DISORDERS
John A. Hunt

The major importance of benign breast disorders lies in their resemblance to cancer, although four of five breast lumps or mammographic abnormalities are benign. Symptoms include pain, which may be constant, episodic, or cyclic; tenderness; a lump; swelling; bleeding; lactation or discharge from the nipple; or inversion, retraction, or eczema of the nipple. A focused history should include the age, menstrual history and menopausal status, parity, breast-feeding history, relation of pain to menses or the premenstrual syndrome, the use of oral contraceptives or other hormones, ovarian ablation, and a family history of breast cancer. Benign breast disorders occur mostly in women of menstrual age, with fibroadenomas more common in young women and gross cysts in those around the time of the menopause. The known risk factors are not the same as those for breast cancer, some possibly being hormonal, such as irregular menses, spontaneous abortions, lack of oral contraceptive use, small breasts, and late natural menopause. Others are lack of obesity and a family history of benign or malignant breast disease.

Breasts should be carefully examined on a regular basis, even in the absence of symptoms. Physical examination must include palpation of the axillae and supraclavicular fossae for the nodes. If there is nipple discharge or bleeding, an attempt is made to find the origin by compressing the breast radially toward the nipple. If the examination findings are entirely negative, the patient may be reassured, taught how to perform breast self-examination, and placed on appropriate follow-up. If doubt remains, the patient should be reexamined in 2 to 3 weeks at a different phase of the menstrual cycle. Patients over 40 years should have a mammogram.

If a dominant mass can be palpated, the patient should still have a baseline mammogram and undergo ultrasound examination to document the size and nature of the mass and to assess its multicentricity as well as the status of the opposite breast. Fine-needle aspiration is then done under local anesthesia in the physician's office, if a mass can be easily felt. Ultrasound or stereotactic localization, if available, should be used for the aspiration of impalpable lesions. The aspirate is sent for cytologic examination. Core biopsies may also be done. The cyst fluid is only sent for cytologic analysis if it is bloody. The potassium level in the cyst fluid should be determined; a high level indicates an apocrine cyst, which is more prone to recurrence. Air should be introduced after the cysts are emptied to help prevent recurrence and x-ray studies are then repeated. If a mass does not empty, appears malignant on x-ray films, displays positive cytologic findings, or a cyst refills more than three times, the mass should be excised together with adequate surrounding tissue and submitted for frozen section, hormone receptor assay, and permanent section, including assessment of the margins.

The American Cancer Society recommends that all women over the age 20 should perform breast self-examination every month using a three-step method: (1) palpating the breasts in the shower or bath; (2) standing in front of a mirror and raising the arms to check for any changes in the breast contour, nipple, or skin; and (3) palpating each breast again. Women aged 40 years or more should have a baseline mammogram, then one every 2 years from age 40 to 49 years, and annually after age 50 years. Clinical examination should be done at the time of each mammogram and at least annually. With modern screening mammography equipment, the radiation dose is less than 1 rad, with far better resolution, even in younger women. Cancer attributable to the examination has never been documented.

A clearly inflammatory mass, if found during lactation, requires antibiotic treatment and possibly surgical drainage with biopsy of the walls. At other times, an inflammatory cancer should be considered and ultrasound, mammography, and biopsy performed.

Benign breast disorders are best understood by correlating the symptoms, physical findings, and pathology, and consist of the following: (1) physiologic changes—cyclic swelling and tenderness or lactational engorgement that are not disease processes; (2) nodularity—fine or coarse lumpiness, which is cyclic or not; (3) mastalgia or severe pain, which is cyclic or not; (4) dominant masses, including cysts, fibroadenomas, other benign tumors such as papillomas or adenomas, fat necrosis, galactoceles, and proliferative disorders such as ductal, stromal, or lobular hyperplasia; (5) nipple discharge, including intraduct papilloma, duct ectasia, and galactorrhea; (6) inflammation or infection, including subareolar abscess, lactational mastitis or abscess, and inflammation of large cysts; (7) eczematous change of the nipple—considered Paget's disease (intraduct carcinoma) until proven otherwise; and (8) non-breast conditions—Tietze's disease (costochondritis), radiculopathy of C6 or C7 or the upper thoracic nerve roots, and Mondor's disease (thrombophlebitis of the thoracoepigastric vein).

The difference between cyclic physiologic changes and mastalgia or breast nodularity lies in the degree and persistence of discomfort. At least 50 percent of women of menstrual age have breast symptoms at some time, many of them severely disabled by pain and tenderness and worried about palpable masses. There may be pain without lumps, lumpiness without pain, or both together. Symptoms may be cyclic or noncyclic and unilateral or bilateral. There is usually no dominant mass or nipple problem, just diffuse pain, tenderness, fullness, irregularity, lumpiness, or fine nodularity. The pain is not necessarily or usually related to the presence of clinically apparent cysts. The terms *chronic cystic mastitis* and *fibrocystic disease*, often used to describe benign breast pathology, are confusing. These changes are part of physiologic breast aging as a consequence of repeated hormone-induced stimulation and involution during puberty, menstruation, pregnancy, lactation, and menopause.

The treatment of breast pain may be difficult but initially involves understanding, sympathy, and reassurance; the patient should also wear a well-supporting brassiere and receive analgesic therapy. Improvement may come from modifying the hormonal environment, as occurs with pregnancy, the use of oral contraceptives or progesterone, or the menopause. Danazol, bromocriptine, tamoxifen, evening primrose oil, and thyroxin have all been shown to relieve mastalgia, but many patients fear or dislike the side effects associated with some of these agents.

The pathology of benign breast lesions may be described as either nonproliferative or proliferative, with or without atypia. Nonproliferative lesions include cysts, fibroadenomas, papillary apocrine changes, mild hyperplasia, and epithelial-related calcifications, which are usually benign. (However, clustered mammographic microcalcifications are often malignant.) Nonproliferative lesions are not associated with an increased risk of subsequent malignancy, except gross cysts, which carry a 2.4 to 4 times increase in the risk and more when there is a family history of breast cancer. Proliferative disorders without atypia include sclerosing adenosis, duct hyperplasia, and intraduct papilloma. Although sclerosing adenosis may exhibit microcalcifications, form a mass, and mimic cancer, microscopically it is not premalignant. Moderate and florid hyperplasias are the most common proliferative lesions, but without atypia are not premalignant. Solitary papillomas of the large ducts also carry no increase in cancer risk, whereas multiple or peripheral duct papillomas are often premalignant or associated with malignancy. Atypical proliferative lesions of the ductal or lobular epithelium are histologically similar to carcinoma in situ. Such patients face a four to five times, or higher, risk of cancer. If there is a family history of breast cancer, the risk is even greater. Women with such lesions should undergo regular careful follow-up. A "prophylactic subcutaneous mastectomy" should not be done, because of the poor attendant results and the inability to remove all breast tissue, leaving some at risk.

Fibroadenomas are the most common benign tumors, usually occurring in patients under the age of 25. They are estrogen receptor positive and respond to hormones, enlarging premenstrually and during pregnancy. The use of oral contraceptives may reduce their incidence. They are freely mobile, rubbery tumors that are pseudoencapsulated and usually 2 to 4 cm in diameter. Histologically they exhibit both stromal and glandular components. Associated carcinoma in situ occurs rarely. Treatment consists of simple excision.

Adenomas of the nipple may mimic cancer or Paget's disease. These present between 30 and 50 years of age with discharge, irritation, or scaling of the nipple, which may be enlarged and indurated, sometimes with a palpable mass. On cut section, they appear as solid, gray-tan, badly demarcated tumors, deep to the nipple and areola. Histologically they exhibit a glandular appearance, a strong stromal component, and often a papillary pattern. Glandular epithelium may grow out onto the surface of the nipple, causing the reddish, granular appearance. Adequate excision avoids recurrence.

Solitary intraduct papillomas usually present with a bloody or serous nipple discharge in women 30 to 50 years old. They are usually small and impalpable but may be over 3 to 4 cm and felt beneath the areola. They are identified by radial compression toward the nipple and by galactogram. Surgical treatment consists of placing a probe into the involved opening and removing the duct with a core of surrounding tissue. Histologic examination reveals a fibrovascular core covered by columnar or cuboidal epithelium and sometimes myoepithelial cells. These tumors are seldom malignant. Multiple peripheral intraduct papillomas occur in younger patients, usually without nipple discharge, and are often bilateral. These tumors are associated with or frequently become cancers. Wide excision and careful follow-up are needed.

Radial sclerosing lesions or scars mimic cancer on mammograms, as well as clinically and pathologically. They are usually small, stellate, and irregular, gray-white, and hard with a central retraction, like cancers. Histologically, the lesion has a fibroelastic core, glandular elements, epithelial hyperplasia, papillomatosis, and sometimes sclerosing adenosis and apocrine metaplasia. The glandular elements may be confused with cancer. They require wide local excision and follow-up.

Mammary duct ectasia, periductal mastitis, and plasma cell mastitis are interrelated pathologically; they become more common with increasing age and after menopause, and even occur in men. Their etiology is unclear. Their importance lies in the fact that they manifest a clinical syndrome similar to that of cancer—a mass that may be painful or tender, or cause either skin retraction or nipple inversion due to fibrosis and shortening of the involved ducts. In some patients, there is a cloudy or even bloody nipple discharge. Histologically, they are characterized by ductal dilatation with an inspissated content and periductal inflammation, fibrosis, and often a plasma cell infiltrate. Intense inflammation may arise after the escape of duct material into the tissues. Treatment consists of local excision.

Fat necrosis may occur after trauma or spontaneously in women with large pendulous breasts. These areas form firm, often nontender lumps that are attached to skin and produce some retraction, thus mimicking cancer. The masses may enlarge briefly, remain unaltered for years, or resolve slowly. Fat necrosis may also arise after breast operations, with or without radiotherapy. Complete excision is required for the purpose of both diagnosis and reassurance.

Galactoceles are milk-filled cysts that are usually found in women during pregnancy or lactation and sometimes after menopause. They form a mass, are generally nontender, are not associated with gross cysts, and usually respond to repeated aspiration. Excision is rarely required. Galactorrhea, a milky discharge from the nipple, is discussed in Chapter 81.

A chronic recurrent subareolar abscess is as common as lactational mastitis, forms in mature women before menopause, and is difficult to eradicate. There may be a nipple discharge or an areolar fistula. There is squamous metaplasia of the ducts, and extrusion of keratin may cause severe inflammation. Because 50 percent of them may recur, excision of the entire duct system, abscess, and fistula may be needed.

Mondor's disease is a thrombosis and periphlebitis of the thoracoepigastric or lateral thoracic veins. It may occur spontaneously or after trauma and even after plastic or other breast operation or irradiation. It may be painful for a time but the cause is benign. It is diagnosed by putting the vein on stretch, which reveals a groove due to the fibrosis. Treatment consists of reassurance and antiinflammatory drugs.

Adenomas are rare circumscribed tumors composed of epithelial elements similar to those typical of fibroadenomas. They may be either tubular or lactational (nodular hyperplasia), may have a common origin with fibroadenoma, and should be simply excised. Giant and juvenile fibroadenomas are rare variants of common fibroadenomas. The giant type may occupy most of the breast whereas the juvenile form grows rapidly, perhaps doubling in 3 to 6 months and having dilated overlying veins. Both must be differentiated histologically from cystosarcoma phylloides, which has a florid stromal component. Excision constitutes adequate treatment. Juvenile papillomatosis occurs in the teens and twenties and consists of discrete movable masses, like fibroadenomas. They resemble cancer in situ and require careful watching because of their unknown prognosis. The incidence of cancer in relatives and patients may be increased. Tumors derived from other tissues present in the breast are sometimes found, such as hamartomas, lipomas, and hemangiomas. These are mostly benign and require local excision.

There have been 88 cases of autoimmune-type diseases reported in patients who underwent breast augmentation procedures. The surrounding publicity caused the Food and Drug Administration (FDA) to withdraw the silicone gel–filled implants from use, except in patients with cancer who receive them in the context of clinical trials and close observation. So far, the evidence of harm is only anecdotal, considering the more than 1 million women with implants. Recent work shows no direct proof of association, but there is a higher-than-expected incidence of scleroderma as opposed to other autoimmune diseases among the cases reported (31% versus 10%). The question of causation remains unproved.

Review and Reference Textbook
  1. Schnitt, S. J., et al. Benign Breast Disorders. In J. R. Harris, et al. (eds.), *Breast Diseases* (2nd ed). Philadelphia: Lippincott, 1991.
     Excellent review of the history, epidemiology, risk factors, etiology, clinical fea-

*tures, histopathology, and treatment. Emphasizes the importance of precise histo-
logic diagnosis, and recommends abandoning the terms* fibrocystic disease *and*
chronic cystic mastitis.

Hormones and Cancer

2. Dupont, W. D., and Page, D. L. Menopausal estrogen replacement therapy and
   breast cancer. *Arch. Intern. Med.* 151:67, 1991.
   *A meta-analysis of 28 studies. Low-dose therapy consisting of 0.625 mg of conju-
   gated estrogen per day led to no increase in risk while 1.25 mg daily led to an
   increased risk of less than twice the average.*
3. Schildkraut, J. M., Hulka, B. S., and Wilkinson, W. E. Oral contraceptives and
   breast cancer: a case-control study with hospital and community controls. *Obstet.
   Gynecol.* 76:395, 1990.
   *In general, no association between oral contraceptive use and breast cancer was
   observed. The increased risk for nulliparas using oral contraceptives for over 5
   years is 2.3 times that of hospital controls. There is also a positive relationship
   between oral contraceptive use and breast cancer in older premenopausal women.*
4. Romieu, I., Berlin, J. A., and Colditz, G. Oral contraceptives and breast cancer:
   reviews and meta-analysis. *Cancer* 66:2253, 1990.
   *A review of 34 case-control follow-up cohort studies. No overall increase in risk
   was found, but prolonged use, especially before the first pregnancy, was noted to
   carry an increased relative risk of 1.72. Oral contraceptives are probably better
   used for the purpose of spacing pregnancies and not as a long-term method to stop
   reproduction.*

Mastitis

5. Mansel, R. E., and Dogliotti, L. European multicenter trial of bromocriptine in
   cyclical mastalgia. *Lancet* 335:190, 1990.
   *This is the largest trial conducted so far and consisted of 272 patients from 13
   centers. It was placebo controlled. Bromocriptine (not FDA approved) was found
   to significantly reduce the pain and other symptoms and decrease the prolactin
   levels at 3 to 6 months. Improvement was maintained for 6 months after stopping
   the drug. The percentage of patients dropping out of study was 29 percent, but this
   was greater for the placebo group. There were more side effects associated with
   bromocriptine use.*
6. Gateley, C. A., et al. Drug treatments for mastalgia: 17 years experience in the
   Cardiff Mastalgia Clinic. *J. R. Soc. Med.* 85:12, 1992.
   *The study population was made up of 324 cyclical and 90 noncyclical mastalgia
   patients. Responses were seen in 92 percent of the cyclic and 64 percent of the
   noncyclic cases. Danazol produced the best response, at over 75 percent; the responses to bromocriptine and evening primrose oil were about equal, at over 50
   percent. Evening primrose oil produced the fewest side effects.*
7. Fentiman, I. S., et al. Dosage and duration of tamoxifen treatment for mastalgia:
   a controlled trial. *Br. J. Surg.* 75:845, 1988.
   *Tamoxifen remains experimental. Pain relief was achieved in about 90 percent of
   the patients in this study. An adequate dose is 10 mg per day, with a 40 to 50
   percent relapse rate after 3 months of treatment. The percentage of side effects at
   the 10-mg dose per day was 21 percent, versus 64 percent for a 20-mg dose a day.*

Premalignant Potential

8. London, S. J., et al. A prospective study of benign breast disease and the risk of
   breast cancer. *J.A.M.A.* 267:941, 1992.
   *Compared to women with no proliferative disease, the risk of later cancer was 1.6
   for those with proliferative disease and 3.7 for those with atypical hyperplasia.
   Mammography starting at age 30 may be needed in women with a family history
   of breast cancer whose biopsy specimens show atypical hyperplasia.*
9. Leis, H. P., Jr. Gross breast cysts: significance and management. *Contemp. Surg.*
   39:13, 1991.
   Apocrine cysts have a high potassium content and are prone to be multiple and

bilateral, and to recur. They may be markers for later cancer (two to four times the expected risk of cancer) and require close follow-up.

10. Bundred, M. J., et al. Is there an increased risk of breast cancer in women who have had a breast cyst aspirated? *Br. J. Cancer* 64:953, 1991.
   There is no excess risk of cancer in women with benign breast nodularity, but the risk is 4.4 times greater in those who undergo aspiration of cysts, especially multiple ones. Continued surveillance is needed even after the cysts stop forming.

11. Diaz, N. M., Palmer, J. O., and McDivett, R. W. Carcinoma arising with fibroadenomas of the breast: a clinicopathologic study of 105 patients. *Am. J. Clin. Pathol.* 95:614, 1991.
   This is a rare occurrence. Conservative surgical therapy is recommended.

12. Skolnick, M. H., et al. Inheritance of proliferative breast disease in breast cancer kindreds. *Science* 250:1715, 1990.
   Cytology showed proliferative breast disease (PBD) in 35 percent of the clinically normal first-degree relatives of women with breast cancer versus 13 percent of the controls. A genetic susceptibility probably explains both the carcinoma and PBD. The lifetime risk for cancer is probably 52 to 63 percent in women with PBD.

Management

13. Patton, M. L., et al. An improved technique for needle localized biopsy of occult lesions of the breast. *Surg. Gynecol. Obstet.* 176:25, 1993.
   Lesions presenting as calcifications were more likely to be malignant than mass lesions but less likely to be infiltrating than mass lesions.

14. Zurrida, S., et al. Which therapy for unexpected phylloide tumor of the breast? *Eur. J. Cancer* 28:654, 1992.
   Recurrence was observed in 8 percent of the "benign," 19.6 percent of the borderline, and 23 percent of the malignant cases. The authors recommend wide local excision with tumor-free margins, no lymphadenectomy, and very close follow-up.

15. Hartley, M. N., Stewart, J., and Benson, E. A. Subareolar dissection for duct ectasia and periareolar sepsis. *Br. J. Surg.* 78:1187, 1991.
   Antibiotics and adequate surgical treatment are needed.

16. Leis, H. P., Jr. Management of nipple discharge. *World J. Surg.* 13:736, 1989.
   Papilloma was found in 48 percent, fibrocystic change in 33 percent, cancer in 14 percent, and precancerous change in 7 percent of the patients in this study. The cancer risk is higher in women over age 50 who have a unilateral bloody or watery discharge, and a palpable lump. Mammography and cytology have significant false-negative rates.

17. Dent, D. M., and Cant, P. J. Fibroadenoma. *World J. Surg.* 13:706, 1989.
   Fibroadenomas account for 7 to 12 percent of the cases seen at breast clinics. They may regress, stay the same, or enlarge. There is a low malignant potential and they may be watched in patients under age 25.

18. Evers, K., et al. Mammary hamartomas: the importance of radiologic-pathologic correlation. *Breast Dis.* 5:35, 1992.
   In this series, hamartomas made up 9.6 percent of the benign specimens obtained by needle localization. These tumors are often well localized but may be hard to distinguish from carcinoma on mammograms.

19. Painter, R. W., Clark, W. E., and Deckers, P. J. Negative findings on fine needle aspiration biopsy of solid breast masses: patient management. *Am. J. Surg.* 155:387, 1988.
   In the setting of small clinically benign masses, negative x-ray and fine-needle aspiration findings allow observation without biopsy.

20. Nielsen, P. E., Kiley, K. C., and Rosa, C. Resident training in a multidisciplinary breast clinic. *J. Reprod. Med.* 38:278, 1993.
   General surgery, radiology, and pathology as well as gynecology staff and residents attend the clinic.

Silicone Prostheses

21. Balch, C. M., and Spear, S. The controversy about silicone gel–filled prosthesis: what do we tell our patients? (editorial). *Breast Dis. Q.* 3:14, 1992.

Stories of immunologic problems or scleroderma are essentially only anecdotal. No evidence of increased incidence. Close physician follow-up is required.

22. Press, R. I., et al. Antinuclear antibodies in women with silicone breast implants. Lancet 340:1304, 1992.

In 10 of 24 patients with autoimmune disease and breast implants, the antinuclear antibody titers were high, and exhibited specificities similar to those found with idiopathic autoimmune disorders. The proportion of women with scleroderma was three times that expected with the usual autoimmune diseases. Still, no cause-and-effect relationships have been shown.

102. MALIGNANT BREAST DISEASE
John A. Hunt

Breast carcinoma is the most common cancer afflicting women in the United States (32% of the non-skin cancers), with 182,000 new cases and 46,000 deaths due to the cancer expected in 1993. One in nine American women will acquire breast cancer by the age of 85. The breast cancer incidence rates increased about 2 percent per year starting in the early 1970s, but have leveled off at about 107 per 100,000 since 1988. Much of this increase can be attributed to earlier detection. The incidence varies in different countries. In the United States, it is more common in Caucasian women (32% of the cancers, versus 29% in blacks). The disease is usually more advanced at the time of detection in blacks and survival in this group is slightly worse.

Breast cancer is second to lung carcinoma as the source of female cancer deaths (18% of the total versus 22%). It causes more deaths than do ovarian, uterine, and cervical cancer combined. The mortality rate of 27 per 100,000 women has hardly changed for the past 50 years, although the increase in early detection is expected to reduce this rate in time.

The chief risk factor is age, cancer of the breast being increasingly common after age 30, with both the mean and median age being 60 years, and with 78 percent of the deaths occurring after age 55. In 70 percent of the patients, no risk factor other than age can be identified. Other risk factors are prior breast carcinoma in the patient or mammary cancer in the mother or a sister, especially if premenopausal or bilateral; 9 percent of the cases are familial. Further risk factors are obesity, endometrial cancer, previous breast biopsy specimen showing atypical ductal hyperplasia, prior aspiration of breast cysts, menarche before age 12, menopause after age 50, nulliparity, first pregnancy after age 35, late last pregnancy, and possibly prolonged estrogen intake or lengthy oral contraceptive use before the first pregnancy. Risk is reduced by ovarian ablation, but this is nullified by estrogen use. Marked multiparity may also be a protective factor.

There are few early symptoms. Most cancers are found as painless lumps, either by the patient or during routine medical or screening examination. Sinister signs include eczema, elevation, retraction or inversion of the nipple, bloody discharge, skin dimpling, reddening or ulceration, fixation to muscles or skin, and palpable axillary or supraclavicular nodes. At the initial presentation there may even be metastatic complications, such as bone pain or pathologic fractures. In the literature published before the widespread use of mammography, less than 50 percent of the cancers were confined to the breast when detected, but, in the detection projects conducted by the American Cancer Society (ACS) and the National Cancer Institute (NCI), 80 percent were localized, only 19 percent had positive nodes, and 50.6 percent were classified as "minimal breast cancer" of less than 1 cm. The Swedish two-county trial revealed a mortality reduction of 30 percent at 10 years, resulting from the earlier detection of cancers found by mammographic screening. Thus, healthy women should be taught how to perform monthly breast self-examination, undergo annual medical breast examinations, and have mammograms obtained every 2 years from age 40 to 49 and annually after age 50 (ACS recommendations).

Most breast cancers are adenocarcinomas, arising from ductal or lobular epithelium: invasive ductal tumors occur in 70 to 80 percent of the cases, invasive lobular tumors in 6 to 8 percent, medullary tumors in 5 to 8 percent, mucinous or colloid tumors in 2 to 4 percent, tubular tumors in 1 to 2 percent, and papillary tumors in 1 to 2 percent. Noninvasive or in situ ductal and lobular cancers each constitute 2 to 3 percent of the cases. More early lesions are being found by mammography, and, in some series, more than 7 percent are now found to be in situ ductal cancers. Cystosarcoma phylloides, other sarcomas, lymphomas, and carcinosarcomas account for less than 1 percent of the cancers.

The tumor is initially confined to the ductal or lobular epithelium, then may invade the breast tissue, fat, lymphatics, blood vessels, chest wall, and skin. Lymphatic spread is to the axillary or internal mammary nodes, or both, then to the supraclavicular nodes. Distant metastasis is most commonly to bone, lung, or liver, then to the pleura, adrenals, brain, and other sites. Metastatic spread may already be present at the time of treatment or diagnosis, but may only become apparent later, with the cumulative percentage of patients showing metastasis plateauing after 10 years. The individual probability of distant spread depends mainly on the primary tumor size, the number of involved nodes, and the histologic grade. The rate of metastasis at 10 years for tumors under 1 cm in diameter is less than 10 percent. For 1- to 2.5-cm tumors, the incidence at 10 to 20 years is 25 percent; at 3.5 to 5.5 cm, it is 50 percent; and over 5.5 cm, it exceeds 75 percent. Tumor cells can be shown to enter the bloodstream during surgery, but clearly not all patients develop clinically important metastases.

Modern staging and treatment planning are based on the results and findings from many investigations: clinical examination, chest x-ray studies, mammography, liver scan by isotope or computed tomography, bone scan, liver enzyme studies, and alkaline phosphatase and erythrocyte sedimentation rates, together with excisional biopsy or mastectomy, axillary node removal, estrogen and progesterone receptor assay, and histopathology. To help determine a more accurate prognosis and plan treatment, especially for patients with smaller cancers, estimates of deoxyribonucleic acid ploidy and the S-phase fraction are increasingly being obtained.

Other biologic factors now being explored for their prognostic significance include oncogene overexpression, such as HER-2/neu, tumor suppressor gene protein P53, epidermal growth factor receptor, cathepsin D, urokinase-plasminogen activator, and many more. These remain under evaluation and subject to the results of clinical trials before their exact place in prognosis and treatment becomes clear. Accurate staging is needed to plan treatment and meaningful research. The American Joint Committee on Staging recognizes both a clinical and a pathologic TNM system.

It must be specified whether there is histologic confirmation of the findings. In each case, the suffix X means "cannot be assessed," while 0 means "no evidence or not present" (TX, NX, or MX; T0, N0, or M0). In situ noninvasive tumors are staged as Tis; T1 tumors are 2 cm or less, T1a are under 0.5 cm, T1b are 0.5 to 1 cm, and T1c are 1 to 2 cm. T2 tumors are 2 to 5 cm and T3 tumors exceed 5 cm in the greatest dimension. T4 tumors may be any size, with attachment to the chest wall or skin: T4a are attached to the chest wall, T4b display edema or ulceration of the skin, or the presence of satellite skin nodules (confined to the same breast). T4c tumors have the characteristics of both T4a and T4b, and T4d are inflammatory cancer. Involvement of the lymph nodes is denoted as N1 if they are ipsilateral and movable; N2 if fixed to each other or other structures; and N3 when internal mammary nodes are involved. Distant metastases are designated M1, and this includes spread to supraclavicular nodes.

Four stage groupings are recognized. Stages I and II represent early cancer, with no distant metastases. More specifically, stage I tumors are 2 cm or less in diameter with negative axillary nodes, and stage II disease includes primary tumors of 2 cm or less together with clinically positive axillary nodes, as well as tumors of 2 to 5 cm in diameter regardless of the nodal status. Stage III disease is locally advanced and includes large tumors accompanied by local fixation or nodal spread but no distant metastases. It includes both operable and inoperable disease. Stage IV is distant metastatic cancer.

Survival rates at 5 years correlate with the stage of the cancer, being near 100 percent for Tis, 85 percent for stage I, 66 percent for stage II, 41 percent for stage III, and 10 percent for stage IV.

Tests for estrogen and progesterone receptors are positive in approximately half of all the patients with breast carcinomas, while both are negative in a third and, in a majority of the remainder, only the test for estrogen receptor is positive. Positive receptor activity correlates with better histologic differentiation and better survival and response to hormonal therapy. In those patients who are positive for both receptors, 70 to 80 percent respond to hormonal therapy, versus 30 to 40 percent of those who are positive for only one receptor. In those patients who are negative for both receptors, response to hormonal therapy occurs in less than 10 percent. The titer of receptor activity also predicts response. Levels of less than 10 femtomoles are regarded as negative. The response to hormonal therapy increases as the level rises above 10 femtomoles. There is generally good correlation in terms of the receptor status between the primary tumor and metastatic foci. Receptor activity may be lost as the tumor progresses, probably due to the overgrowth of clones of cells resistant to hormones.

The treatment of breast cancer is no longer purely surgical. The concept that the disease may be systemic from the outset, together with the findings from clinical trials showing that less radical procedures may be as effective as radical operations, has encouraged the use of more limited surgical resection, thus allowing breast preservation, and this is combined with adjuvant radiotherapy, chemotherapy, or hormone treatment.

Fine-needle aspiration biopsy or cytology should be attempted in the office for palpable lesions, or under stereotactic or ultrasound control for those that are not, where facilities for this exist. A positive result aids in treatment planning and discussion. Excisional biopsy and histologic confirmation by frozen or routine section must be done before definitive surgical treatment is carried out. A one cubic centimeter piece of fresh tissue is needed for hormone receptor studies, but newer techniques may soon allow better estimates to be performed on standard slide material. Wide local excision should be done along with the biopsy to avoid the need for two separate operations. If a lesion found by x-ray study cannot be felt, a marking mammogram with needle localization of the suspect area enables accurate excision along with a core of surrounding tissue. If rapport with the patient is good and she understands and elects a particular course of therapy, appropriate surgery may be done immediately after a positive biopsy result is obtained, but it is common to allow a week to elapse after biopsy to permit consideration of treatment options or the acquisition of a second opinion. This step may be modified if the findings from fine-needle aspiration are positive.

The treatment options for stage I disease are (1) wide local excision with axillary node dissection and breast irradiation or (2) modified radical mastectomy, which includes axillary dissection with pectoral muscle preservation but no irradiation, as is done for stage II disease. For more advanced disease, treatment is modified as needed. Radical and ultraradical procedures are rarely used or indicated; thus, skin grafts are not needed and incisions may be transverse with better preservation of appearance. The axillary vein is no longer cleared as fully as it was in the classic Halstead radical mastectomy, so the lymphedema is less. Breast reconstruction by means of myocutaneous flaps or prosthetic implants is now often done at the time of cancer surgery, improving both the patient's psychology and acceptance. This does not compromise oncologic principles or interfere with cure of the cancer.

Radiation therapy may be used in any stage of breast cancer. Its use is carefully individualized, with the dosage, source, and technique varying with the therapeutic objective—adjuvant treatment for early cancer, definitive treatment, or therapy for advanced, metastatic, or recurrent disease. The photon sources must be megavoltage, with electron beam, interstitial implants, and orthovoltage used for boost therapy. A dose of 45 to 50 Gy, given about 5 weeks postoperatively, is adequate for the treatment of subclinical disease, but higher doses are needed when there is greater tumor bulk or residual disease in the breast. Use of chest wall and internal mammary irradiation after mastectomy was out of favor, but may be returning as locoregional therapy has been found to increase disease-free interval. Irradiation has been used to ablate the ovaries, but its effect is slow and it has generally been replaced by tamoxifen therapy for this purpose.

Most patients with early stage disease benefit from adjuvant therapy, with some exceptions, including (1) a minimal or low-risk subset of node-negative stage I patients in whom the value of therapy is unproved, and (2) some elderly patients (>70 years) with node-negative, receptor-positive cancer whose medical condition may preclude chemotherapy.

Good-risk stage I patients with tumor diameters of 1 to 2 cm and low histologic and nuclear grades are treated with tamoxifen, regardless of whether they are pre- or postmenopausal.

High-risk stage I patients with estrogen receptor–negative tumors of 1 cm or greater, estrogen receptor–positive tumors greater than 2 cm, or poor nuclear grade tumors should receive systemic adjuvant therapy. If patients are premenopausal, they should receive chemotherapy, with those who are receptor positive also receiving tamoxifen. In postmenopausal patients who are estrogen receptor positive, tamoxifen is the principal therapy, but there is increasing evidence that additional adjuvant chemotherapy improves the outcome and should be given.

Elderly high-risk, node-negative patients benefit from tamoxifen therapy, regardless of the receptor status. Patients in good health may also be given chemotherapy.

All patients with node-positive cancer should receive adjuvant therapy. In premenopausal patients this should consist of chemotherapy, possibly along with tamoxifen in receptor-positive cases. In postmenopausal receptor-positive patients, tamoxifen is the accepted treatment. There is increasing evidence that additional chemotherapy augments the benefit. Postmenopausal node-positive, receptor-negative patients are appropriately treated with adjuvant chemotherapy. The addition of tamoxifen therapy in this group is under investigation.

After initial treatment, patients should be seen every 3 months for 3 years, then every 6 months for 5 years, and then annually. During the first 5 years, each visit should include breast examination and an alkaline phosphatase estimation. Chest x-ray studies, mammography, and bone scanning are recommended annually for the first 5 years. Mammography and clinical examination should be continued for life.

Inflammatory carcinoma constitutes 1 to 4 percent of the breast cancers, with symptoms consisting of rapidly evolving redness, warmth, enlargement, induration, and peau d'orange, often without a palpable mass. Receptors are usually negative and tumor cells are demonstrable in the lymphatics of the dermis. The tumors are classified as stage IIIB T4d and are initially considered inoperable, with a more than 50 percent chance of local recurrence. Induction chemotherapy should be used first, followed by aggressive, high-dose radiation therapy. This treatment can yield more than 75 percent local control. Surgical measures may be used later. Further chemotherapy, with or without hormonal therapy, is usually added. A 5-year survival of up to 50 percent has been reported for such an aggressive multimodality approach.

About 1 to 2 percent of the breast cancers occur in women during pregnancy or lactation, or about 1 in 3500 pregnancies. The diagnosis is often delayed owing to the reluctance of patients to report it, the difficulty of palpating engorged breasts, and the hesitation of physicians to perform biopsy. Breasts must be examined early in pregnancy before congestion conceals lumps and makes mammography unhelpful. Large, late-stage tumors are more common during pregnancy and lactation. The prognosis depends on the stage; there is about a 70 percent 5-year survival rate for patients with localized disease, and this decreases to 30 to 40 percent if the nodes are positive. This is slightly worse than the situation in nonpregnant patients. Because of the potential fetal damage caused by chemotherapy or irradiation, a modified radical mastectomy should be done in patients with operable disease so that pregnancy is not interrupted. In the setting of inflammatory, advanced, or aggressive cancer, multidisciplinary treatment is urgent and an informed decision must be made concerning termination of pregnancy. Radiation may endanger the fetus. Not enough is known about the effects of chemotherapy in pregnancy, but fetuses may survive with growth retardation, subtle changes, and an unknown prognosis. Intuitively, chemotherapy should be avoided.

In the past, pregnancy after the treatment of breast cancer was discouraged. Currently, the survival rate in patients who become pregnant after the treatment of breast cancer appears better than that in age-matched and stage-matched controls. The reason for this is unknown. After breast cancer, it is desirable to avoid pregnancy for 2 to 3 years until after the danger of early recurrence has passed. Pregnancy should be prevented in women with advanced cancer. If cancer recurs during pregnancy, it should be terminated unless the pregnancy is near term.

Metastatic breast cancer may respond to chemotherapy, irradiation, or hormone manipulation, thus affording the opportunity for repeated or prolonged remissions. In the past, oophorectomy, adrenalectomy, or hypophysectomy were performed sequentially to obtain repeated remissions of disease. Such procedures were often very successful and were a mainstay of treatment for years, but, currently, drugs are used instead, usually tamoxifen, megestrol acetate, or aminoglutethimide plus hydrocortisone. These agents are used sequentially to prolong or induce remissions. Various therapeutic combinations are given as circumstances dictate. Pathologic fractures require internal fixation and radiation therapy, while bone pain responds to local irradiation. Pleural effusions respond to sclerosis with tetracycline and brain metastases respond to steroid therapy and irradiation. Eventually, pain control becomes important and hospice referral is of great help to both the patient and her relatives.

Patients with metastatic disease who originally responded well to chemotherapy and new patients with advanced disease may be candidates for high-dose chemotherapy and stem cell rescue (autologous bone marrow transplantation). This method is still investigational and exceedingly expensive, at between $50,000 and $100,000 per patient, and the long-term benefit to the patient is unknown. Because about 50 percent of the patients with breast cancer will die of their disease, such efforts will no doubt continue, with further attempts being made to improve results and reduce cost.

Reference Textbook
  1. Fowble, B., et al. *Breast Cancer Treatment. A Comprehensive Guide to Management.* St. Louis: Mosby, 1991.
     This reference text contains much useful information.

Large Reviews and Meta-Analyses
  2. Miller, B. A., Feuer, E. J., and Harkey, B. F. Recent incidence trends for breast cancer in women and the relevance of early detection: an update. *CA Cancer J. Clin.* 43:27, 1993.
     These authors predict lower mortality in the future due to an increase in early cancer detection.
  3. Harris, J. R., et al. Breast cancer (3-part review). *N. Engl. J. Med.* 327:319; 390; 473, 1992.
     The most authoritative multiauthored review available, with 429 references. Every aspect is covered, from epidemiology to reconstruction.
  4. Wood, W. C., et al. NIH Consensus Development Conference. Treatment of early stage breast cancer. *J.A.M.A.* 265:391, 1991.
     In the estimate for 1990, there would be 150,000 new patients, 75 to 80 percent would have stage I or II disease, and 50 percent of the total cases would be node negative. The authors recommend no adjuvant treatment if hormone receptors are positive, the nuclear grade is low, the histology is favorable, and the S phase is under 10 percent.
  5. Auquier, A., et al. Post-mastectomy megavoltage radiotherapy: the Oslo and Stockholm trials. *Eur. J. Cancer* 28:433, 1992.
     Adjuvant radiation therapy was found to significantly improve the metastasis-free rate and metastasis-free survival. There was a marginally significant improvement in absolute survival.
  6. Early Breast Cancer Trialists Collaborative Group. Systemic treatment of early breast cancer by hormonal, cytotoxic or immune therapy. *Lancet* 339:1; 71, 1992.
     This article describes the findings from an analysis of 133 randomized trials involving 75,000 women, 31,000 recurrences, and 24,000 deaths. It offers the most

solid, statistically valid data quantifying marked improvement associated with chemotherapy, ovarian ablation, and tamoxifen therapy.

7. Tubiana, M., and Koscielny, S. Natural history of breast cancer: recent data and clinical implications. *Breast Cancer Res. Treat.* 18:125, 1991.
   A superb thoughtful paper. "Must" reading. It describes the mathematical modeling of data from 3000 patients without chemotherapy who were followed for 15 to 30 years. Tumors acquire the potential for metastasizing to the lymph nodes before the bloodstream, and change during the patient's life span to become more aggressive. The size, grade, lymph node metastasis, and S-phase fraction are all vitally important variables. Mammography clearly detects earlier tumors.

Mammography

8. Tabar, L., et al. Update of the Swedish two county program of mammographic screening for breast cancer. *Radiol. Clin. North Am.* 30:187, 1992.
   Screened patients exhibited a relative mortality of 0.7, compared to nonscreened patients. Tumors under 1.5 cm are associated with a survival of 95 percent at 9 years. Early cases are probably not all metastatic from the outset.

9. Robertson, F. M., et al. Effect of mass screening mammography on staging of carcinoma of the breast in women. *Surg. Gynecol. Obstet.* 171:55, 1990.
   In the 3 years before the screening program was implemented, 84 percent of the tumors were found by patients and 6 percent by mammograms. In the 3 years after the start of the program, 46 percent were found by patients and 48 percent by mammography. Screening led to improved staging, in that 41.5 percent were detected while in stage I after screening, versus 16.4 percent before screening.

Carcinoma In Situ

10. Ward, B. A., McKhann, C. F., and Ravikumar, T. S. Ten year follow-up of breast carcinoma in-situ in Connecticut. *Arch. Surg.* 127:1392, 1992.
    There was an increase in the total number of breast cancers and in the proportion of ductal carcinomas in situ (DCIS) of from 1.8 percent in 1978 to 7.4 percent in 1988. Of 217 DCIS patients, 22 percent had bilateral breast involvement with either DCIS or cancer. Unrelated cancers were found in 16.8 percent of the DCIS cases, versus 5.9 percent in cases of lobular carcinoma in situ.

11. Bland, K. I., and Frykberg, E. R. Selective management of in-situ carcinoma of the breast. *Breast Dis. Q.* 3:11, 1992.
    The article considers the topics of contrast lobular (LCIS) and ductal (DCIS) carcinoma in situ. Both show multicentricity and bilaterality and may predict the existence of invasive cancer. LCIS is more of a marker and less malignant, plus requires less aggressive therapy and no contralateral breast biopsy. DCIS must be treated as real cancer with at least lumpectomy plus radiation therapy, and possibly mastectomy. Both need life-long, detailed follow-up.

Early Cancer: Prognosis and Treatment

12. McGuire, W. L., and Clark, G. M. Prognostic factors and treatment decisions in axillary node-negative breast cancer. *N. Engl. J. Med.* 326:1756, 1992.
    The benefits of adjuvant therapy are small, so many patients would be exposed to needless risk. Good-risk patients who do not need adjuvant therapy are those with good histology, tumor less than 1 cm in diameter, diploidy, low S-phase fraction, nuclear grade I, or a 1- to 3-cm tumor with "good" features.

13. Boyages, J., et al. Early breast cancer: predictors of breast recurrence for patients treated with conservative surgery and radiation therapy. *Radiother. Oncol.* 19:29, 1990.
    An extensive intraductal component at any age explained most of breast recurrences. This finding is more common in patients under 34 years of age. Recurrences near the site of excision were the most common and occurred earlier than others.

14. Ball, A. B. S., et al. Radical axillary dissection in the staging and treatment of breast cancer. *Ann. R. Coll. Surg. Engl.* 74:126, 1992.
    This study of 237 cases shows the need for adequate clearance. This procedure

permits staging and complete axillary treatment. Wound complications were encountered in 8 percent; axillary recurrence, in 12 percent; and there was minimal arm edema.

15. Fisher, B., et al. Significance of ipsilateral breast tumor recurrence after lumpectomy. *Lancet* 338:327, 1991.
    At 9 years, 57 percent of the lumpectomy patients were free of breast recurrence, versus 88 percent after added irradiation. There were no differences in terms of either survival or distant disease–free survival among all groups.

16. Bates, T., et al. Breast cancer in elderly women: a cancer research campaign trial comparing treatment with tamoxifen and optimal surgery with tamoxifen alone. *Br. J. Surg.* 78:591, 1991.
    Suggests survival and quality of life may be equal in the two groups. Patients receiving tamoxifen therapy sometimes had to undergo surgical removal because of progression of disease.

17. Ganz, P. A., et al. Breast conservation versus mastectomy: is there a difference in psychological adjustment or quality of life in the year after surgery? *Cancer* 69:1729, 1992.
    No difference in the quality of life, mood disturbance, performance status, or global adjustment was observed for the patients in this study. The major patient concerns are survival and cure. The timing of reconstruction is important for body image.

Advanced Disease and Bone Marrow Transplantation

18. Henderson, I. C., et al. Comprehensive management of disseminated breast cancer. *Cancer* 66:1439, 1990.
    Treatment goals are palliation of symptoms and improvement in quality of life. An excellent review.

19. Arriagada, R., et al. Alternating radiotherapy and chemotherapy in non-metastatic inflammatory breast cancer. *Int. J. Radiat. Oncol. Biol. Phys.* 19:1207, 1990.
    Five-drug chemotherapy and high-dose irradiation without surgery constituted the approach to treatment. The overall 4-year survival was 55 percent; local control was achieved in 72 percent but 53 percent had distant metastases. Surgery could perhaps be avoided when distant metastases are so frequent.

20. Eddy, D. M. High dose chemotherapy with autologous bone marrow transplantation for the treatment of metastatic breast cancer. *J. Clin. Oncol.* 10:657, 1992.
    There were a higher number of total responses (36% versus 8%) and overall responses (70% versus 39%) seen in these patients. The median survival (16 versus 16.6 months) and 2-year overall survival (43% versus 39%) were similar, and there was worse mortality (5–15% versus 1%), plus toxicity was seen in 30 percent and all suffered side effects.

Miscellaneous Topics

21. Johnson, C. H., et al. Oncological aspects of immediate breast reconstruction following mastectomy for malignancy. *Arch. Surg.* 124:819, 1989.
    Patient acceptance of this treatment was good and self-image was improved. There were savings in both time and money. It does not compromise subsequent resection, adjuvant therapy, or the treatment of recurrent disease.

22. Senie, R. T., et al. Timing of breast cancer excision during the menstrual cycle influences duration of disease-free survival. *Ann. Intern. Med.* 115:337, 1991.
    Surgery in the follicular phase carried a risk of recurrence of 43 percent, versus 29 percent when performed in the latter half of the cycle. This effect was mostly seen in patients with positive nodes and with smaller tumors (<2 cm).

23. Mueller, D. B. The disease-free interval in breast cancer trials: scientific or spurious. *Surgery* 110:629, 1991.
    The author expresses the contrary view that only the disease-free interval is improved in patients who receive adjuvant chemotherapy. Overall survival is not changed. After adjuvant chemotherapy, death occurs more rapidly after recurrence and tumors become more resistant to treatment. Why treat all women, pro-

ducing discomfort and potential harm in 93 percent, for the apparent benefit of only 7 percent?

24. King, M.-C., Rowell, S., and Love, S. M. Inherited breast and ovarian cancer. What are the risks? What are the choices? *J.A.M.A.* 269:1975, 1993.

The role of the BRCA 1 (breast cancer) gene in inherited breast and ovarian cancer has been determined by genetic analysis of families with multiple cases of these cancers.

25. Lahti, E., et al. Endometrial changes in postmenopausal breast cancer patients receiving tamoxifen. *Obstet. Gynecol.* 81:660, 1993.

Long-term tamoxifen treatment has an estrogenic effect on the postmenopausal uterus, associated with an increased occurrence of polyps.

26. Vern, A. Causes of breast cancer malpractice litigation: a 20-year civil court review. *Arch. Surg.* 127:542, 1992.

To minimize the threat of malpractice suits, physicians must maintain a high index of suspicion for breast cancer and follow-up well, especially in young patients.

INDEX

Abdominal pregnancy, 10
ABO incompatibility, and hemolytic disease of the newborn, 98
Abortion, 5–7
  cervical cancer and, 431
  defined, 5
  fibroids and, 227
  habitual, 6
  induced, 6–7
  infected, 5–6
  spontaneous
    causes, 5
    incidence, 5
    in IUD users, 323
    maternal age and, 89–90
    in multiple gestations, 94
  uterine bleeding and, 5
Abruptio placentae, 22–24
  causes, 23
  characteristics, 22–23
  classification, 23
  defined, 22
  diagnosis, 23
  DIC due to, 23–24
  for eclampsia, 40
  hemorrhage in, 23
  hypertension and, 29
  incidence, 22–23
  maternal hypertension in, 23
  motor vehicle accidents in pregnancy and, 123–124
  premature ruptured membranes and, 113
  treatment, 24
Abscess
  pelvic, 307–308. See also Pelvic abscess
  subareolar, 471
Abuse, physical, in pregnancy, 124
Acetaminophen, for hyperthyroidism in pregnancy, 77
Acquired immunodeficiency syndrome, 289–292. See also Human immunodeficiency virus infection
  in adolescents, 358
  causes, 290–291
  described, 290
  diagnosis, 291
  drug abuse and, 290, 291
  genital tuberculosis and, 311
  HIV infection and, progression of, 291–292
  incidence, 57

Pneumocystis carinii pneumonia in, 58, 65
  populations at risk for, 290–291
  in pregnancy, 47
  transmission of, 47–48
  prevalence in women, 290, 291
  testing for, in rape victims, 378
  treatment, 292
Acromegaly, hyperprolactinemia due to, 389
Actinomyces infection, IUDs and, 322
Actinomycin D. See Dactinomycin
Acyclovir
  for HSV infection, 279
  for neonatal herpetic encephalitis, 47
  for varicella pneumonia, 65
Adenocarcinoma
  of the breast, 475
  clear cell, in children, 252
  epithelial, in ovarian cancer, 450
Adenoma
  described, 471
  of the nipple, 470
  pituitary, oral contraception and, 318
Adenomyosis, described, 246
Adenosine arabinoside, in neonatal herpetic encephalitis, 47
Adhesion, labial, described, 251
Adnexal mass
  differential diagnosis, 446
  in small bowel obstruction in pregnancy, 123
Adolescents
  AIDS in, 358
  changes in, stages of, 357
  contraceptive use in, 358
  counseling for, 359
  dysfunctional uterine bleeding in, 400
  PID in, 358
  pregnancy in, 85–87
    adolescent fathers, 87
    complications, 85–86
    health care for, 86–87
    hypertension in, 85
    incidence, 85
    long-term consequences of, 86, 87
    nutritional demands, 86
    obstetric complications, 85–86
    prevention, 87
    psychologic factors for, 85
    psychologic ramifications of, 86
    social complications, 85–86

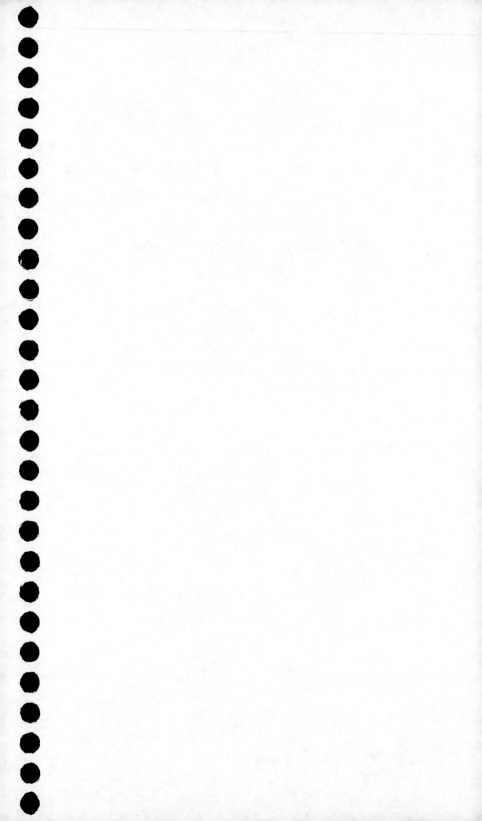

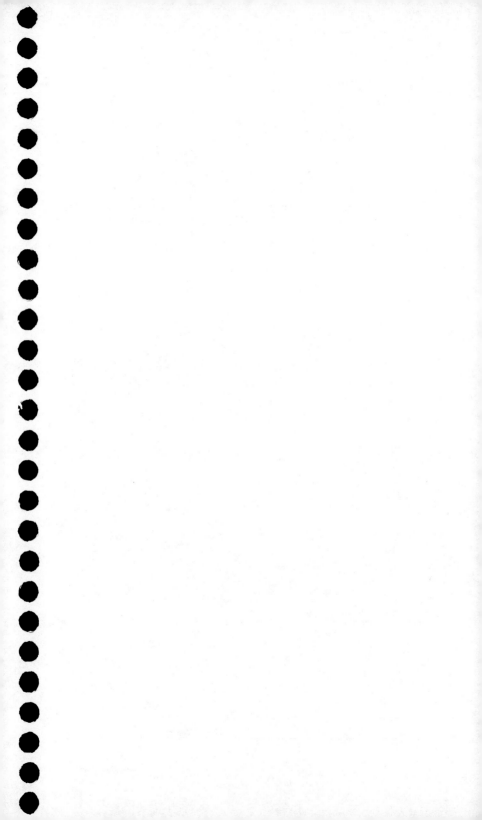

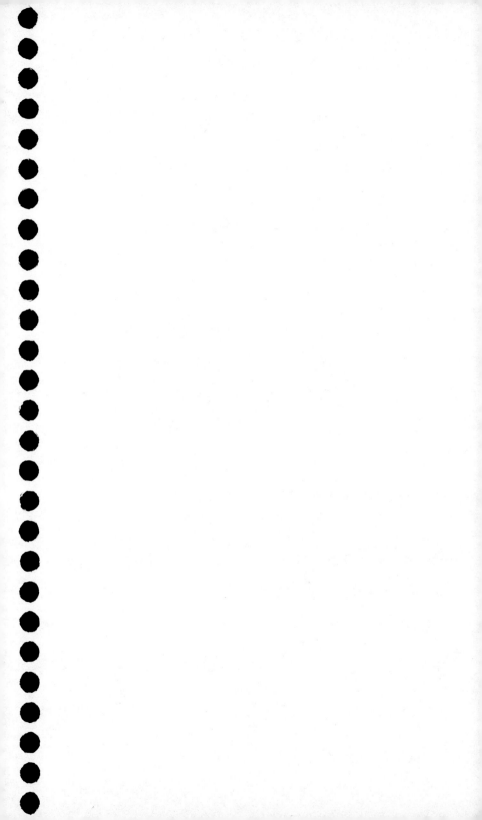

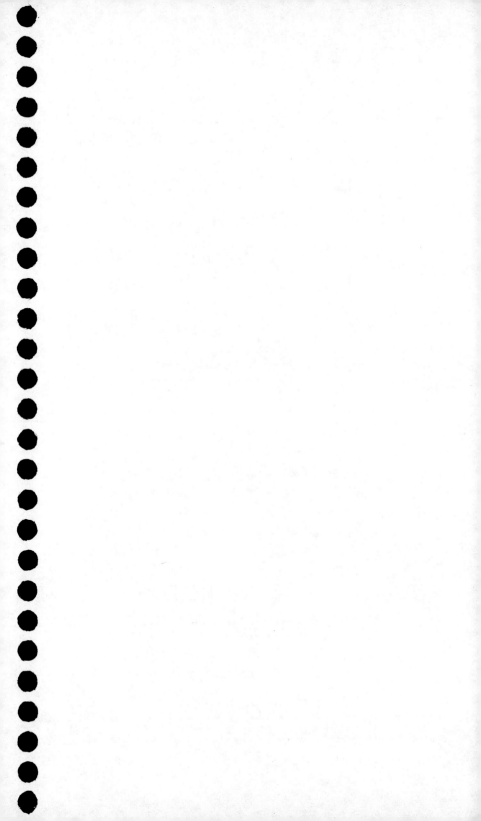

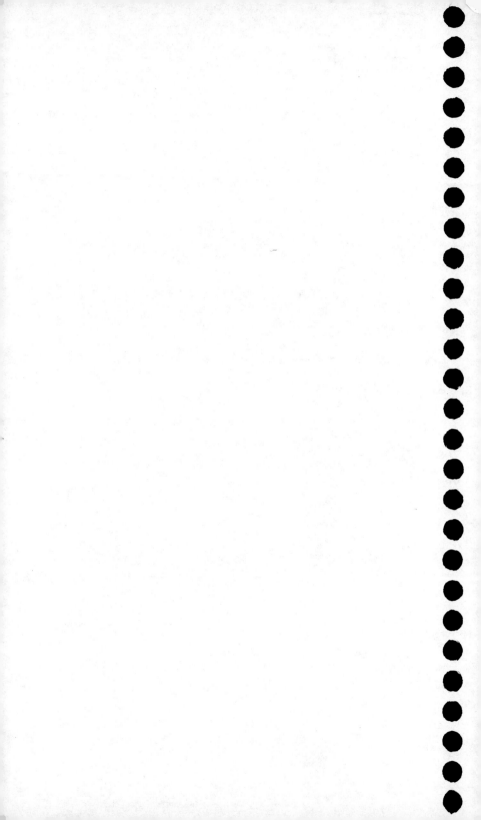

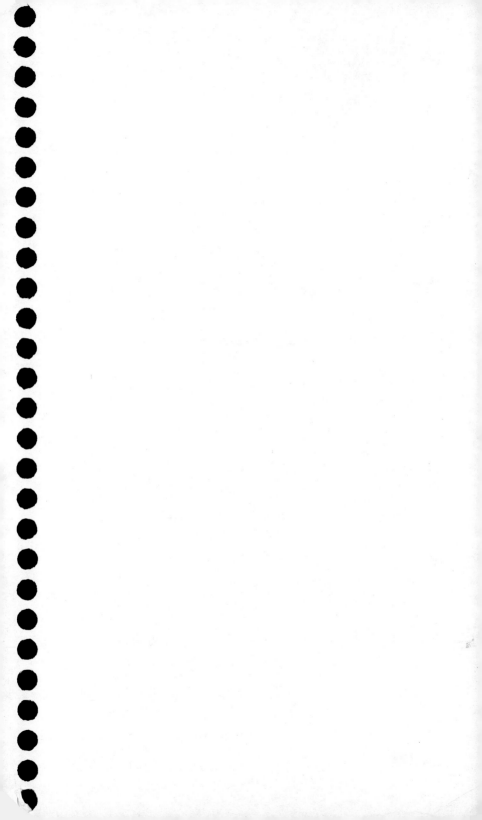